International Handbook of
Multigenerational Legacies of Trauma

The Plenum Series on Stress and Coping

Series Editor:
Donald Meichenbaum, *University of Waterloo, Waterloo, Ontario, Canada*

Editorial Board: Bruce P. Dohrenwend, *Columbia University* •Marianne Frankenhauser, *University of Stockholm* • Norman Garmezy, *University of Minnesota* • Mardi J. Horowitz, *University of California Medical School, San Francisco* • Richard S. Lazarus, *University of California, Berkeley* • Michael Rutter, *University of London*• Dennis C. Turk, *University of Pittsburgh* • John P. Wilson, *Cleveland State University* • Camille Wortman, *University of Michigan*

Current Volumes in the Series:

BEYOND TRAUMA
Cultural and Societal Dynamics
Edited by Rolf J. Kleber, Charles R. Figley, and Berthold P. R. Gersons

COMMUTING STRESS
Causes, Effects, and Methods of Coping
Meni Koslowsky, Avraham N. Kluger, and Mordechai Reich

COPING WITH CHRONIC STRESS
Edited by Benjamin H. Gottlieb

COPING WITH WAR-INDUCED STRESS
The Gulf War and the Israeli Response
Zahava Solomon

ETHNICITY, IMMIGRATION, AND PSYCHOPATHOLOGY
Edited by Ihsan Al-Issa and Michel Tousignant

HANDBOOK OF SOCIAL SUPPORT AND THE FAMILY
Edited by Gregory R. Pierce, Barbara R. Sarason, and Irwin G. Sarason

INTERNATIONAL HANDBOOK OF MULTIGENERATIONAL LEGACIES
OF TRAUMA
Edited by Yael Danieli

PSYCHOTRAUMATOLOGY
Key Papers and Core Concepts in Post-Traumatic Stress
Edited by George S. Everly, Jr. and Jeffrey M. Lating

STRESS AND MENTAL HEALTH
Contemporary Issues and Prospects for the Future
Edited by William R. Avison and Ian H. Gotlib

TRAUMATIC STRESS
From Theory to Practice
Edited by John R. Freedy and Stevan E. Hobfoll

A Continuation Order Plan is available for this series. A continuation order will bring delivery of each new volume immediately upon publication. Volumes are billed only upon actual shipment. For further information please contact the publisher.

International Handbook of Multigenerational Legacies of Trauma

Edited by

Yael Danieli

Group Project for Holocaust Survivors and Their Children
New York, New York

PLENUM PRESS • NEW YORK AND LONDON

Library of Congress Cataloging-in-Publication Data

On file

ISBN 0-306-45738-5

© 1998 Plenum Press, New York
A Division of Plenum Publishing Corporation
233 Spring Street, New York, N.Y. 10013

http://www.plenum.com

Printed in the United States of America

To the children yet unborn
with the hope that we leave them a better world in which to grow

Contributors

Petra G. H. Aarts, Aarts Psychotrauma Research, Consultancy and Training, Rozenstraat 55, 1016 NN Amsterdam, The Netherlands

Dan Aferiot, Mount Sinai Traumatic Stress Studies Program, Mount Sinai School of Medicine and Bronx Veterans Affairs Hospital, Bronx, New York 10468

Michelle R. Ancharoff, Department of Veterans Affairs Outpatient Clinic, National Center for Posttraumatic Stress Disorder, Boston, Massachusetts 02114

Nanette C. Auerhahn, Bellefaire Jewish Children's Bureau, Shaker Heights, Ohio 44118

Katharine G. Baker, 3 Chesterfield Road, Williamburg, Massachusetts 01096

Dan Bar-On, Department of Behavioral Sciences, Ben Gurion University of the Negev, Beer Sheva 84105 Israel

David Becker, Instituto Latinoamericano de Salud Mental y Derechos Humanos, Nunez de Arce 3055, Nunoa, Santiago, Chile

Murray M. Bernstein, Department of Social Work, Zablocki Veterans Administration Medical Center, Milwaukee, Wisconsin 53295

Karen Binder-Brynes, Mount Sinai Traumatic Stress Studies Program, Mount Sinai School of Medicine and Bronx Veterans Affairs Hospital, Bronx, New York 10468

Ann Buchanan, University of Oxford, Department of Applied Social Studies, Oxford OX1 2ER, United Kingdom

J. Boehnlein, Department of Psychiatry, Oregon Health Sciences University, Portland, Oregon 97201

Dennis S. Charney, Clinical Neurosciences Division, National Center for PTSD, VA Connecticut Healthcare System, West Haven Campus, West Haven, CT 06516

Cheryl Cottrol, Clinical Neurosciences Division, National Center for PTSD, VA Connecticut Healthcare System, West Haven Campus, West Haven, CT 06516

William E. Cross, Jr., School of Education, University of Massachusetts, Amherst, Massachusetts 01003–4160

Yael Danieli, Director, Group Project for Holocaust Survivors and Their Children; Private Practice, 345 East 80th Street, New York, New York 10021

Margarita Diaz, Instituto Latinoamericano de Salud Mental y Derechos Humanos, Nunez de Arce 3055, Nunoa, Santiago, Chile

Barbara H. Draimin, The Family Center, 66 Reade Street, New York, New York 10007

Aline Drapeau, Department of Psychiatry, Montreal Children's Hospital 4018, Montreal, Quebec, Canada

Bonnie Duran, First Nations, 4100 Silver SE Albuquerque, New Mexico 87108

Eduardo Duran, First Nations, 4100 Silver SE Albuquerque, New Mexico 87108

Lucila Edelman, Equipo Argentino de Trabajo e Investigacion Psicosocial, Rodriquez Peña 279 "A" (102o), Buenos Aires, Argentina

Abbie Elkin, Mount Sinai Traumatic Stress Studies Program, Mount Sinai School of Medicine and Bronx Veterans Affairs Hospital, Bronx, New York 10468

Ferenc Erős, Institute of Psychology, Hungarian Academy of Sciences, Teréz Krts. 13, H–1067 Budapest, Hungary

Irit Felsen, Jewish Family Service of Metrowest, Mountain Lakes, New Jersey 07046

Lisa M. Fisher, Department of Veterans Affairs Outpatient Clinic, National Center for Posttraumatic Stress Disorder, Boston, Massachusetts 02114

Alan Fontana, Department of Veterans Affairs, Northeast Program Evaluation Center, Veterans Affairs Medical Center, West Haven, Connecticut 06516

Dafna Fromer, Department of Behavioral Sciences, Ben Gurion University of the Negev, Beer Sheva 84105 Israel

Marie-Anik Gagné, Health Systems Research Unit, Clarke Institute of Psychiatry, 250 College Street, Toronto, Ontario, M5T 1R8 Canada

Abdu'l-Missagh Ghadirian, Faculty of Medicine, McGill University, Montreal, Quebec, Canada H3A 1A1

Julia B. Gippenreiter, Moscow State University, Psychology Faculty, Moscow, Russia 117463

Gertrud Hardtmann, Technical University, Berlin, Germany

Alisa Hoffman, Department of Psychiatry and Biobehavioral Sciences, Neuropsychiatric Institute, UCLA School of Medicine, Los Angeles, California 90024

Edna J. Hunter-King, Advisory Committee on Former Prisoners of War, Department of Veterans Affairs, Washington, DC 20420

Christine Johnson, Postdoctoral Fellow, Center for Family Research in Mental Health, Iowa State University, Ames, Iowa 50014

Anie Sanentz Kalayjian, Department of Psychology, Fordham University, 113 West 60th Street, New York, New York 10023-7412; Private Practice, 130 West 79th Street, New York, NY 10024

Alice Kassabian, School of Social Work, Virginia Commonwealth University, Arlington, Virginia 22201; Private Practice, 133 Maple Avenue East, Suite 306, Vienna, Virginia 22180

J. David Kinzie, Department of Psychiatry, Oregon Health Sciences University, Portland, Oregon 97201

Eduard Klain, Clinic for Psychological Medicine, Kišpatićeva 12, HR–10000, Zagreb, Croatia

Diana Kordon, Equipo Argentino de Trabajo e Investigacion Psicosocial, Rodriquez Peña 279 "A" (102o), Buenos Aires, Argentina

Éva Kovács, Institute for East European Studies, Budapest, Hungary

John H. Krystal, Clinical Neurosciences Division, National Center for PTSD, VA Connecticut Healthcare System, West Haven Campus, West Haven, CT 06516

Diane Kupelian, 1545 18th Street, N.W., Washington, D.C. 20036

Darío Lagos, Equipo Argentino de Trabajo e Investigacion Psicosocial, Rodriquez Peña 279 "A" (102o), Buenos Aires, Argentina

Dori Laub, Yale University School of Medicine, New Haven, Connecticut 06520

Carol Levine, Families and Health Care Project, United Hospital Fund, 350 Fifth Avenue, New York, New York 10018

Seymour Levine, Department of Psychology, University of Delaware, Newark, Delaware 19716

Martijn W. J. Lindt, Faculty of Educational Sciences, University of Amsterdam, 1091 GM Amsterdam, The Netherlands

Nada Martinek, Department of Psychiatry, The University of Queensland, Brisbane, Australia

Lockhart McKelvy, The Family Center, 66 Reade Street, New York, New York 10007

Andrew Morgan, Clinical Neurosciences Division, National Center for PTSD, VA Connecticut Healthcare System, West Haven Campus, West Haven, CT 06516

James F. Munroe, Department of Veterans Affairs Outpatient Clinic, National Center for Posttraumatic Stress Disorder, Boston, Massachusetts 02114

Kathleen Olympia Nader, Consultant on Trauma and Traumatic Grief, P.O. Box 2316, Austin, Texas, 78767

Donna K. Nagata, Department of Psychology, University of Michigan, Ann Arbor, Michigan 48109

Linda M. Nagy, Clinical Neurosciences Division, National Center for PTSD, VA Connecticut Healthcare System, West Haven Campus, West Haven, CT 06516

Abiola I. Odejide, Department of Communication and Language Arts, University of Ibadan, Ibadan, Nigeria

Adebayo Olabisis Odejide, Department of Psychiatry, College of Medicine, University College Hospital, Ibadan Nigeria

Tal Ostrovsky, Department of Behavioral Sciences, Ben Gurion University of the Negev, Beer Sheva 84105 Israel

Beverley Raphael, Director, Centre for Mental Health, NSW Health Department, North Sydney, NSW 2059 Australia

Ann Rasmusson, Clinical Neurosciences Division, National Center for PTSD, VA Connecticut Healthcare System, West Haven Campus, West Haven, CT 06516

Robert Rosenheck, Department of Veterans Affairs, Northeast Program Evaluation Center, Veterans Affairs Medical Center, West Haven, Connecticut 06516

Gabriele Rosenthal, University of Kassel, Faculty of Social Work 34109, Kassel, Germany

Cécile Rousseau, Department of Psychiatry, Montreal Children's Hospital 4018, Montreal, Quebec, Canada

William H. Sack, Department of Psychiatry, Oregon Health Sciences University, Portland, Oregon 97201

Akinade Olumuyiwa Sandra, Department of Public Administration, Obafemi Awolowo University, Ile-Ife, Nigeria

Jim Schmeidler, Mount Sinai Traumatic Stress Studies Program, Mount Sinai School of Medicine and Bronx Veterans Affairs Hospital, Bronx, New York 10468

Larry Siever, Mount Sinai Traumatic Stress Studies Program, Mount Sinai School of Medicine and Bronx Veterans Affairs Hospital, Bronx, New York 10468

Ronald L. Simons, Department of Sociology and Center for Family Research in Mental Health, Iowa State University, Ames, Iowa 50014

Michael A. Simpson, National Centre for Psychosocial and Traumatic Stress, P.O. Box 51, Pretoria 0001, South Africa

Zahava Solomon, The Bob Shapell School of Social Work, Tel Aviv University, Tel Aviv 69978 Israel

Stephen M. Southwick, Clinical Neurosciences Division, National Center for PTSD, VA Connecticut Healthcare System, West Haven Campus, West Haven, CT 06516

Stephen J. Suomi, Laboratory of Comparative Biology, National Institute of Child Health and Human Development, Bethesda, Maryland 20892

Patricia Swan, Aboriginal Health Resource Cooperative, Box 1565, Strawberry Hills 2012 NSW Australia

Mikihachiro Tatara, Department of Psychology, Hiroshima University, Hiroshima, Japan 739

Júlia Vajda, Institute of Sociology, ELTE University, Budapest, Hungary

Wybrand Op den Velde, Department of Psychiatry, Saint Lucas Andreas Hospital, P.O. Box 9243, 1006 AE Amsterdam, The Netherlands

Bettina Völter, University of Kassel, Faculty of Social Work, 34109, Kassel, Germany

Milton Wainberg, Mount Sinai Traumatic Stress Studies Program, Mount Sinai School of Medicine and Bronx Veterans Affairs Hospital, Bronx, New York 10468

David K. Wellisch, Department of Psychiatry and Biobehavioral Sciences, Neuropsychiatric Institute, UCLA School of Medicine, Los Angeles, California 90024

Skye Wilson, Mount Sinai Traumatic Stress Studies Program, Mount Sinai School of Medicine and Bronx Veterans Affairs Hospital, Bronx, New York 10468

Rachel Yehuda, Mount Sinai Traumatic Stress Studies Program, Mount Sinai School of Medicine and Bronx Veterans Affairs Hospital, Bronx, New York 10468

Maria Yellow Horse Brave Heart, Graduate School of Social Work, University of Denver, Denver, Colorado 80208

Susan Yellow Horse-Davis, Graduate School of Social Work, University of Denver, Denver, Colorado 80208

Foreword

Psychological professions have been slow to recognize the powerful psychic consequences of extreme suffering. They have been even slower to recognize the reverberations of that suffering in subsequent generations. While that professional neglect has hardly ceased, the contributors to this volume have done much to overcome it.

Working with survivors of Hiroshima and of Auschwitz, and also with American veterans of Vietnam, I could observe much that suggested that their overwhelming experiences could be transmitted in some way to the children of those interviewed. But I was unable to pursue that demanding question. I can appreciate, as will readers of this volume, the extraordinary achievement of pulling together such intergenerational studies from virtually every part of the world.

In doing so, Yael Danieli and the contributing authors have provided us with a record as valuable as it is disturbing of ongoing twentieth-century pain. There is a paradox here. By confronting the human consequences of genocidal projects that threaten the continuity of human life, we contribute precisely to that continuity. In that sense, the essays themselves are quiet expressions of protest against the inhumanity they describe.

All survivors undergo a struggle with what I call formulation—with giving form or meaning to an otherwise incomprehensible experience and, above all, to their survival. There is powerful evidence in this book that the offspring of survivors must do the same, except that in their case the meaning sought has to do with their own relationship to an event that took place before they were born. Their parents' experiences loom as both dreadful and mysterious, almost unknowable.

Recent studies emphasize the difficulties that even those directly exposed to extreme trauma have in taking in that experience and re-creating it in some form. How much greater is the problem of death-related knowledge for the next generation. But probing just that difficulty can teach us a great deal about the ways in which the mind explores or resists currents that are both powerful and amorphous. There can be no form of insight more precious to us—not just to those who study the mind but to everyone—in our struggles to navigate the very threatening world of the end of the second millennium.

ROBERT JAY LIFTON

Preface

This book is the culmination of a long journey, a complex and deeply rewarding one. It began for me over 25 years ago in the initial session with SL, a frail-looking, agitated young man who intermittently interrupted his seemingly uncontrollable, incoherent rambling with a refrain-like phrase, "My mother gave me gray milk," that quickly become a leitmotif of his therapy. Although I was not always aware of it, it also formed an indelible metaphor portending the development of my thinking and understanding in the following decades on the what and how of transmission of the effects of the Nazi Holocaust in particular and of trauma in general.

SL's father was "from Auschwitz," the sole survivor of a family that had included a wife and two sons who perished in the ovens. SL was named after his murdered half-brothers. His father met SL's 17-year-younger "beautiful" mother upon arriving in the United States. He is "very old." SL believed that, although American-born, his mother must have absorbed ashes from his father and passed them to him through her milk.

For many years, as I heard myriad survivors and their children share their legacies and attempt to break what I later studied as the "conspiracy of silence" (Danieli, 1982), I relived, with them, that alarming combined sense of acute pain, flooding helplessness, and outrage, particularly when conceiving their pain as "Hitler's posthumous victory."

Increasingly, clinicians and researchers have begun to examine the intergenerational consequences of exposure to a variety of traumata. Empirical research in this field is gathering momentum, and its social and public health significance is thus only now becoming more widely acknowledged. Given a lifetime posttraumatic stress disorder (PTSD) rate of 7.8% in the general population of the United States (Kessler *et al.*, 1995) it is a relatively common psychiatric disorder; even if only a minority is or will be involved in parenting, the number of children upon whom intergenerational effects will have an impact is enormous. In other groups and societies, where the rates of trauma exposure are much higher, an ever greater proportion of the population is affected, with consequent intergenerational implications.

Events such as the fall of the Berlin wall and the end of the Cold War symbolized by it, followed by the phenomenon of large groupings of people fragmented into smaller ones, usually on ethnic grounds, made imperative a worldwide dialogue, that is only in its beginning stages, about the issues raised in this book. More international networking among clinicians and researchers is leading to more exploration in this more open climate.

An earlier book, *International Responses to Traumatic Stress* (Danieli *et al.*, 1996), grew out of the appalling realization of the global scope of trauma and victimization and the necessity of international endeavors on behalf of the victims. The focus of that study was on the international agencies and programs and nongovernmental organizations working in this field.

That book was for the present—to "provide a home" for all those who from different viewpoints are interested in helping victims. The present book is intended to provide a home for the future. It establishes that effects of current actions may go beyond a lifetime, and that intervention and prevention measures thus have not only lifelong but also intergenerational means and consequences.

The authors of the chapters in this volume were recruited from around the world and from many different disciplines. They responded to the suggested guidelines rather differently, reflecting, in part, various stages of anguish in confronting their subjects, as well as different ways of knowing and means of access. Many belong to the populations they write about, which makes harder their struggle to create enough distance for writing, yet adds authenticity to the words they give voice to. Some are passionate, some poetic. Some used conclusions drawn from data as testimony for advocacy.

This is a profoundly disturbing book. It cannot be read from a cool, scientific or clinical distance because the topics covered challenge not only scientific neutrality but also the limits of our humanity. The extent of the suffering it chronicles cannot be denied. It pulls the reader toward advocacy, a role with which many clinicians and researchers feel uncomfortable, and from which they tend to shy away.

But the purpose of the book goes beyond documentation, description, and making available international scholarship. It is also intended to be used in practical ways to relieve and to prevent the suffering, and contribute to *informed advocacy*. It emphasizes to policymakers that the consequences of decisions that are frequently made with largely short-term considerations in mind cannot only be lifelong but also multigenerational.

The book confirms the universal existence of intergenerational transmission of trauma and its effects, and it validates the concern shared by many experts about the effects of the phenomenon. In the past, multigenerational transmission has been treated as a secondary phenomenon, perhaps because it is not as obviously dramatic as the horrific images of traumatized people. The mind recoils when viewing such images; and it does not take in that children not yet born could inherit a legacy and memories not of their own but that, nevertheless, will shape their lives. It is bad enough to see images of children victimized today; that the same images may shape the lives of generations to come, sometimes unconsciously, often by design, is even harder to comprehend, and accept.

I, and the readers of this book, owe a great debt of gratitude to the authors. Their scholarship and humanity offer hope for the future that justice will finally be done. A day of reckoning can help reassert order over chaos and anarchy and begin to give a sense of closure. Justice can restore a people's faith but not their innocence. Taking the painful risk of bearing witness does not mean that the world will listen, learn, change, and become a better place for our generation and generations to come.

It is fitting that this book is published in the year of the fiftieth anniversary of the Universal Declaration of Human Rights. The powerful accounts contained in the following pages should compel us to rededicate ourselves to converting the principles so clearly stated in that Declaration into living reality.

REFERENCES

Danieli, Y. (1982). Therapists' difficulties in treating survivors of the Nazi Holocaust and their children. (Doctoral dissertation, New York University, 1981). *University Microfilms International*, #949-904.

Danieli, Y., Rodley, N. S., & Weisaeth, L. (Eds.) (1996). *International Responses to Traumatic Stress; Humanitarian, Human Rights, Justice, Peace and Development Contributions, Collaborative Actions and Future Initiatives.* Published for and on behalf of the United Nations by Baywood Publishing Company, Inc., Amityville, New York.

Kessler, R. C., Sonnega, A., Bromet, E., Hughes, M., & Nelsen, C. B. (1996). Posttraumatic stress disorder in the National Comorbidity Survey. *Archives of General Psychiatry, 52,* 1048-1060.

Acknowledgments

First and foremost, I thank the contributors, who not only generously contributed their scholarship but also attended to this book with such care and dedication. They enriched my world and joined in making the book a labor of love. So did Robert Jay Lifton by contributing the Foreword, and Frederick Terna, a survivor of the Nazi Holocaust, by designing the figure for my Trauma and the Continuity of Self: A Multidimensional, Multidisciplinary Integrative (TMCI) Framework in the Introduction.

Joe Sills reviewed and commented on the entire book. His continued editorial assistance has been indispensable to its realization. Andrei Novac commented on all the chapters related to the Nazi Holocaust. Vladimir Kasnar, Donna Nagata, and Dinko Podrug reviewed specific chapters.

Roger Clark, Brian Engdahl, and William Schlenger gave invaluable editorial and collegial help with my Introduction and Conclusions and Future Directions and provided constant friendship, encouragement, and support. Discussions with Helen Duffy, John Krystal, Richard L. Libowitz, Andrei Novac, Elsa Stamatopoulou, and Frederick Terna helped elucidate specific issues raised in those two chapters. Kathleen Fraleigh and Irene Melup commented on, and Kathleen Hunt helped edit, the Conclusions and Future Directions.

John Wilson supported the idea of the book at its inception, and Matthew J. Friedman and Paula P. Schnurr included its summary in *The National Center for Post-Traumatic Stress Disorder PTSD Research Quarterly* (Danieli, 1997). This book has been blessed with the kind of generosity that helps transcend its sometimes heart-wrenching substance. I am thankful for that as well.

REFERENCE

Danieli, Y. (1997). International Handbook of Multigenerational Legacies of Trauma. *The National Center for Post-Traumatic Stress Disorder PTSD Research Quarterly, 8*(1), 1–6.

Contents

Introduction

History and Conceptual Foundations

YAEL DANIELI

This is the first book on traumatic stress that examines multigenerational effects of trauma across various victim/survivor populations around the world from multidimensional, multidisciplinary perspectives. It seeks to provide a comprehensive picture of the knowledge accumulated worldwide to date, including clinical, theoretical, research, and policy perspectives.

The few existing books in the literature that examine intergenerational transmission of trauma focus mostly on a single event (e.g., the Nazi Holocaust), utilizing a singular aspect or methodology (e.g., clinical or research) (Bar-On, 1989, 1994; Bergmen & Jucovy, 1982; Hass, 1990; Kogan, 1995; Nagata, 1993; Prince, 1985; Sigal & Weinfeld, 1989; Wardi, 1992). This book is the first endeavor to present and integrate multiple approaches with multiple populations around the world in an area that, although relatively new, is of great psychosocial importance. It contains chapters that explore for the first time in print, for some populations, issues of multigenerational effects of trauma.

The contributors to this volume were asked to describe and analyze traumatic events in a context that includes cultural, political, economic, and other appropriate dimensions using a longitudinal perspective on life before, during, and after the trauma. They were also requested to review relevant literature (including historical, literary, and journalistic sources), make explicit their theoretical/conceptual framework, and examine basic concepts such as "transmission," "legacies," intergenerational/multigenerational "effects," what is being transmitted, and "mechanisms of transmission." To enable evaluation of generalizability, they were requested to describe in detail their sample/case(s) and the assessment methodology utilized. They were also asked to address the heterogeneity of the phenomena and provide their explanation for the variability of findings in the field. Finally, they were asked to make clinical, research and policy recommendations, and draw relevant implications (e.g., legal, political, sociocultural, religious).

The edited format was chosen to preserve as much as possible both the richness and authenticity of the material, as well as its multidimensional and interdisciplinary perspective. This allowed for some repetition, including within the literature reviews, to enable the reader to comprehend fully the thinking of the authors. Many of the contributors, writing of populations that have been attended to only recently or for the first time, articulate a sense of alarm, outrage, and concern reminiscent of the early writers on the long-term and intergenerational effects of the Nazi Holocaust, who pioneered the field of multigenerational legacies of trauma.

YAEL DANIELI • Director, Group Project for Holocaust Survivors and Their Children; Private Practice, 345 East 80th Street, New York, New York 10021

International Handbook of Multigenerational Legacies of Trauma, edited by Yael Danieli. Plenum Press, New York, 1998.

Multigenerational transmission of trauma is an integral part of human history. Transmitted in word, writing, body language, and even in silence, it is as old as humankind. It has been thought of, alluded to, written about, and examined in both oral and written histories in all societies, cultures, and religions.

Nevertheless, only scant attention has been paid in religious and classical literary texts to the intergenerational transmission of *victimization*. To the extent that it discusses intergenerational transmission of trauma, the Bible's primary emphasis is on the multigenerational transmission of *perpetrators'* legacies. The Bible, moreover, reflects the complexity of these issues. In the earlier books of the Old Testament, God is portrayed as "visiting the iniquity of the fathers upon the children unto the third and fourth generation of those that displeased and reject [Him] but showing mercy unto generations of those that love [Him], and keep [His] commandments" (Exodus 20:5).

However, the later books reverse this position. In Jeremiah's well-known words, "They shall no longer say, the fathers have eaten a sour grape, and the children's teeth are blunted. But everyone shall die for his own sins; every man that eateth the sour grape, his teeth shall be blunted" (31:29–30). And Ezekiel wrote, "The son shall not bear the iniquity of the father" (18:20).

Numerous commentaries attempted to understand this reversal. One notes that the change followed the catastrophic destruction of the Temple and the dispersion into exile of the people of Israel. If the prophets had continued to hold that this terrible punishment would extend into future generations, there would have been no hope. The change reflects their attempt to forestall the earlier demoralizing projection of total hopelessness onto future generations.

These Biblical metaphors also suggest what could be currently framed as various modes of coping with traumatic memories. Important contemporary, differing points of view and even controversies among victim/survivor populations and among professionals working with them have their parallels in the Bible for (post)traumatic intergenerational responses, memories, their functions and purposes, and lessons drawn from them, for example, about prevention ("Never again").

Thus, the rescued wife of Lot was turned into a pillar of salt for *looking back* at the burning city of Sodom. In the wake of the destruction of their world, Lot's daughters believed their aging father to be the last man on earth. They got him drunk, had him impregnate them, and gave birth to his sons (Genesis 19).

Another relevant Biblical metaphor that illustrates the wish that the passing of generations would eradicate the effects of trauma is the banishment of the Israelites that were led by Moses out of slavery in Egypt to wander in the desert for 40 years and be forbidden entry to the promised land. The 40 years of wandering in the desert ensured that they died in exile, and that their children, "who had not known slavery," would be the ones to built the new land (Numbers 14).

Euripides reflects the complexity seen in the Bible. He writes both that "the gods Visit the sins of the fathers upon the children" (*Phrixus,* undated fragment 970) and that "when good men die their goodness does not perish. . . . As for the bad, All that was theirs dies and is buried with them" (*Temenidae,* undated fragment 734). Later authors, however, echo the early Biblical vision of cross-generational retribution. Horace (23 B.C.) says that the children, though guiltless, must suffer for the sins of the father; Shakespeare (1596/1597; see also 1599) wrote that the sins of the father are to be laid upon the children; and Hawthorne (1851) states as the author's moral—the truth that the wrongdoing of one generation lives into successive ones.

A great text of the twentieth century, the Charter of the United Nations, begins: "We the peoples of the United Nations, determined to save succeeding generations from the scourge of war, which twice in our lifetime has brought untold sorrows . . ."

INTERGENERATIONAL TRANSMISSION AND THE FIELD OF TRAUMATIC STRESS

Within the field of traumatic stress, intergenerational transmission of trauma is a relatively recent focus. It was first observed in 1966 by clinicians who were alarmed by and concerned about the number of children of survivors of the Nazi Holocaust seeking treatment in clinics in Canada (Rakoff, 1966; Rakoff, Sigal, & Epstein, 1966; Trossman, 1968). Subsequent pioneers, in the United States (Axelrod, Schnipper, & Rau, 1980; Barocas & Barocas, 1973, 1979; Danieli, 1980, 1981a; Fogelman & Savran, 1979; Kestenberg, 1972, 1989), and later in Israel (Davidson, 1980; Klein, 1971), further explored and enriched our knowledge and understanding of the "second generation." More recently, concern has also been voiced about the transmission of pathological intergenerational processes to the third and succeeding generations (Rosenthal & Rosenthal, 1980; Rubenstein, Cutter, & Templer, 1990).

Some comprehensive reviews of the psychiatric literature on the long-term effects of the massive traumata experienced by Holocaust survivors and of their treatment can be found in articles by Krystal (1968), Krystal and Niederland (1971), Chodoff (1975), Dasberg (1987), and Krystal and Danieli (1994), and on aging survivors in particular in Danieli (1994a, 1994b).

Reviews of the intergenerational transmission and treatment of the psychological effects of the Holocaust on survivors' offspring (children born after the war) can be found in Russell (1980), Danieli (1982a), Bergman and Jucovy (1982), Sigal and Weinfeld (1989), and Steinberg (1989). An updated, comprehensive multigenerational bibliography on the medical and psychological effects of concentration camps and related persecutions is provided by Krell and Sherman, 1997).

Not until 1980 did the evolving descriptions of the "survivor syndrome" in this literature find their way into the *Diagnostic and Statistical Manual of Mental Disorders* (DSM-III; American Psychiatric Association, Third Edition, 1980, pp. 236–238) as a separate, valid category: posttraumatic stress disorder (PTSD). The recognition of possible *intergenerational* transmission of victimization-related pathology still awaits inclusion in future editions. Although it is hard to conceive of PTSD (American Psychiatric Association, 1994) in isolation, its multigenerational aspects have been treated as an offshoot, off-center, as "secondary." Until it is included in the *Diagnostic and Statistical Manual of Mental Disorders,* the behavior of some children of survivors may be misdiagnosed, its etiology misunderstood, and its treatment, at best, incomplete (see also Krell, 1984).

As in other areas of traumatology, these initial clinical reports were followed by more systematic investigation. There are over 400 entries on children of survivors alone in the aforementioned bibliography (Krell & Sherman, 1997). Much of this vast and complex literature is reviewed throughout this volume, particularly in Chapters 1, 2, 3, 4, 16, 18, 19, and 37.

Rosenheck (1985, 1986) has described comparable processes of intergenerational transmission in sons of World War II veterans who are Vietnam veterans who exhibited "malignant PTSD" and in children of Vietnam veterans who demonstrated "secondary traumatization" (Rosenheck & Nathan, 1985; see also Jurich, 1983: "The Saigon of the Family's Mind"). Jordan *et al.* (1992) summarized a variety of problems that have been found to be associated with combat-related PTSD that can negatively affect the family of combat veterans.

Among *wives* of veterans with PTSD, Verbosky and Ryan (1988) found increased levels of stress and feelings of worthlessness as a result of attempts to cope adequately with the veteran's PTSD symptoms.

The multigenerational legacies of the growing number of "forgotten generations" that appear in this book have not previously received adequate exploration within the field of traumatic stress. These include the second generation of Hibakusha, the Japanese survivors of the atomic bomb; children of collaborators; offspring of both the Turkish genocide of the Armenians and the Khmer Rouge genocide in Cambodia; those revealed after the fall of communism, such as in the former Yugoslavia, unified Germany, and Hungary; indigenous peoples such as the Australian aborigines, Native Americans, and Africans; and those following repressive regimes including Stalin's purge, the dictatorships in Chile and Argentina, South Africa under apartheid, and the Baha'is in Iran.

The Conspiracy of Silence

It was in the context of studying the phenomenology of hope, in the late 1960s, that I first interviewed in depth, among others, survivors of the Nazi Holocaust. To my profound, yet retrospectively unsurprising, anguish and outrage, all of my interviewees without exception asserted that no one, including mental health professionals, listened to them or believed them when they attempted to share their Holocaust experiences and their related, continuing suffering. They, and later their children, concluded that nobody who had not gone through the same experiences could understand. Many thus bitterly opted for silence about the Holocaust and its aftermath.[1]

The reactions of society at large to survivors have a significant negative effect on their posttrauma adaptation and their ability to integrate their traumatic experiences. After liberation, as during the war, survivors of the Holocaust encountered a pervasive societal reaction consisting of indifference, avoidance, repression, and denial of their Holocaust experiences. Like other victims, survivors' war accounts were too horrifying for most people to listen to or believe. Their stories were therefore easy to ignore or deny. Even people who were consciously and compassionately interested played down their interest, partly rationalizing their avoidance with the belief that their questions would inflict further hurt. Similar to other victims who are blamed for their victimization ("You are stupid to live near the Bhopal plant"), survivors were faced with the pervasive myth that they had actively or passively participated in their own destiny by "going like sheep to the slaughter." Additionally, bystander's guilt for having knowingly neglected to do anything to prevent Nazi atrocities, or for having been spared their fate, led many to regard the survivors as pointing an accusing finger at them and projecting onto the survivors the suspicions that they had performed immoral acts in order to survive. Like other victims, they were also told to "let bygones be bygones" and get on with their lives.

As stated earlier, such reactions forced survivors to conclude that nobody cared to listen and that "nobody could really understand" unless they had gone through the same experiences. In their interactions with nonsurvivors, they became silent about the Holocaust. The resulting *conspiracy of silence* between Holocaust survivors and society (Danieli, 1981a, 1982a, 1988d), including mental health and other professionals (Danieli, 1982b, 1984), has proven detrimental to the survivors' familial and sociocultural reintegration by intensifying their already profound sense of isolation, loneliness, and mistrust of society. This has further impeded the possibility of their intrapsychic integration and healing, and made their task of mourning their massive losses impossible. The silence imposed by others proved particularly painful to those who had survived the war determined to bear witness.

---

[1]This led to the founding, formally in 1975 in the New York City area, of the Group Project for Holocaust Survivors and their Children that provides them with psychological help that had been missing for over 30 years, and trains professionals to work with this and other victim/survivor populations (Danieli, 1982c, 1989).

The only option left to survivors, other than sharing their Holocaust experiences with each other, was to withdraw completely into their newly established families. In some families, the children were used as a captive audience. Where both parents were survivors, the one who suffered the greater loss rarely did the talking. His or her account was either related by the other spouse or remained for the children an awesome mystery, fraught with myths and fantasies. Children of such families, although remembering their parents' and lost families' war histories "only in bits and pieces," attested to the constant psychological presence of the Holocaust at home, verbally and nonverbally, or in some cases, reported having absorbed the omnipresent experience of the Holocaust through "osmosis."

In contrast, other survivor parents welcomed the conspiracy of silence because of their fear that their memories would corrode their own lives and prevent their children from becoming healthy, normal members of society. But despite a family-stated tenet that "everything was alright," the children grew up in painful bewilderment; they understood neither the inexplicable torment within the family, nor their own sense of guilt. As Bettelheim (1984) observed, "What cannot be talked about can also not be put to rest; and if it is not, the wounds continue to fester from generation to generation" (p. 166).

Children of survivors seem to have consciously and unconsciously absorbed their parents' Holocaust experiences into their lives. Like their parents, many children of survivors manifest Holocaust-derived behaviors, particularly on the anniversaries of their parents' traumata. Moreover, some have internalized as parts of their identity the images of those who perished. Each survivor's family tree is steeped in murder, death, and losses, yet its offspring are expected to reroot that tree and reestablish the extended family, and start anew a healthy generational cycle.

Accepting psychological problems threatened the parents' need to deny the Holocaust's long-term emotional effects, which they also viewed as evidence of Hitler's posthumous victory. Worse, openly acknowledging their own psychological problems or those of their children diminished their self-image as perfect parents and their view of their offspring as "perfectly normal." Some experienced anything that may imply loss of control over, or mastery of, any situation as a total, retraumatizing threat. They also strongly resisted being stigmatized or labeled "crazy" (stemming from the Nazi practice of gassing the sick and mentally ill), particularly by doctors that they had learned not to trust.

The extrafamilial conspiracy of silence interacted with the intrafamilial one in yet another context. The phrase *conspiracy of silence* has also been used to describe the interaction of Holocaust survivors and their children with psychotherapists when Holocaust experiences were mentioned or recounted,[2] as it had been used to describe the pervasive interaction of survivors with society in general. Elsewhere (Danieli, 1988a) within the context of describing professionals' *bystander's guilt,* I summarized,

> Some therapists . . . were also afraid that survivors were fragile . . . overlooking the fact that these were people who had not only survived but also had rebuilt families and lives despite immense losses and traumatic experiences. [They] also tended to attribute fragility to survivors' offspring. . . . Some . . . feared that demonstrating the long-term negative effects of the Holocaust [on survivors and their offspring] was tantamount to giving Hitler a posthumous victory. In contrast, others feared that demonstrating these individual's strengths was

---

[2]For example, see Barocas and Barocas (1979), Krystal and Niederland (1968), and Tanay (1968). Elsewhere, I have reviewed in detail the literature on the conspiracy of silence (Danieli, 1982a, 1988d) and described its harmful long-term impact on the survivors (Danieli, 1981a, 1989), their families (Danieli, 1981a, 1985, 1988b), and their psychotherapies (Danieli, 1984, 1988c, 1992).

equivalent to saying that because people could adapt, "it couldn't have been such a terrible experience, and it is almost synonymous with forgiving the Nazis." (p. 226)

Although it is difficult to acknowledge the damage to the survivor parents, it is even more difficult to accept that it may continue in the offspring, who are the future.

The ubiquity of countertransference reactions in this and other populations has now moved to the forefront of our concern in the preparation and training of professionals who work with victims and trauma survivors.[3] Our work calls on us to confront, with our patients and within ourselves, extraordinary human experiences. This confrontation is profoundly humbling in that at all times, these experiences challenge our view of the world we live in and test the limits of our humanity.

The conspiracy of silence reverberates throughout this volume, in the experience of numerous victim/survivor populations. Hardtmann mentions in Chapter 4 of this book that it took 13 years for her first study on children of Nazis, which appeared in 1982 in English, to be translated into German. A later publication (Heimannsberg & Schmidt, 1993) is aptly entitled *The Collective Silence: German Identity and the Legacy of Shame.* The impact of the conspiracy of silence is chillingly evident in an interview with Ms. Robie Mortin, a survivor of the week-long rampage of a white mob in Florida, USA in 1923, during which the largely black town of Rosewood was burned to the ground, and many were killed and wounded, and others, especially children, were forced to flee and hide for days in the swamps. Ms. Mortin said that her life was ruined, and her birthright taken away, by that week. "My grandma told me not to say a word. My grandma said never to look back. We weren't supposed to talk about Rosewood." As Hannaham (1996) states, "What's left in posterity [is] what Parks (1995), in her drama *The America Play* (1992, 1994), calls 'the Great Hole of History'" (p. 24). Conversely, in O'Hara's (1996) play, *Insurrection: Holding History,* Ron feels that he is "holding history" when he wraps his arms around his great-great grandfather, who was a slave.

This book advances significantly a major goal in the field of traumatic stress—to dissipate the multidimensional silence, this time about multigenerational legacies of trauma.

TRAUMA AND THE CONTINUITY OF SELF: A MULTIDIMENSIONAL, MULTIDISCIPLINARY INTEGRATIVE (TCMI) FRAMEWORK

The attempt to delineate and encompass the nature and extent of the destruction of catastrophic massive trauma, having to account for the different contextual dimensions and levels of it, and the diversity in and in response to it, dictated the formulation of a multidimensional, multidisciplinary integrative framework. The TCMI framework will thus help guard against

---

[3]As early as 1980 (Danieli, 1980), when I published the preliminary thematic overview of my study of the difficulties of these psychotherapists, I stated, "While this cluster [of countertransference reactions] was reported by professionals working with Jewish Holocaust survivors and their offspring, I believe that other victim/survivors populations may be responded to similarly and may suffer . . . similar [consequences] (p. 366)." These insights and hypotheses about the ubiquity of countertransference reactions in other victim populations have now moved to the forefront of our concern in the preparation and training of professionals who work with victims and trauma survivors.

Indeed, the ensuing literature reflected a growing realization among professionals working with other victims/survivors of the need to describe, understand, and organize different elements and aspects of the conspiracy of silence among them (See Danieli, 1994c; Figley, 1995; Herman, 1992; Hudnall Stamm, 1995; Pearlman & Saakvitne, 1995; Wilson & Lindy, 1994), and the recognition that countertransference reactions (or equivalent phenomena) are ubiquitous, integral to, and expected in our work. In reality, countertransference reactions are the building blocks of the societal as well as professional conspiracy of silence.

the reductionistic impulse to find unidimensional explanations for such complex phenomena. The reader should recognize that underlying each of these dimensions there is a distinct philosophical view of the nature of humankind that informs what the professional *thinks* and *does*. The chapters in this book illustrate and elaborate on the elements that constitute the TCMI framework.[4]

An individual's identity involves a complex interplay of multiple spheres or systems. Among these are the biological and intrapsychic; the interpersonal—familial, social, and communal; the ethnic, cultural, ethical, religious, spiritual, and natural; the educational/professional/occupational; the material/economic, legal, environmental, political, national, and international. Each dimension may be a subject of one or more disciplines, which may overlap and interact, such as biology, psychology, sociology, economics, law, anthropology, religious studies, and philosophy. These systems dynamically coexist along the time dimension to create a continuous conception of life from past through present to the future. Ideally, the individual should simultaneously have free psychological access to, and movement within, all these identity dimensions. Figure 1 illustrates the TCMI network.

Exposure to trauma causes a *rupture,* a possible regression, and a state of being "stuck" in this free flow, which I have called *fixity.* The time, duration, extent, and meaning of the trauma for the individual, the survival mechanisms/strategies utilized to adapt to it (e.g., see Danieli, 1985), as well as postvictimization traumata variously described as the *conspiracy of silence* (Danieli, 1982b), the second wound (Symonds, 1980), the *third traumatic sequence* (Keilson, 1992), cutoff (Bowen, 1978), and *homecoming stress* (Johnson et al., 1997)[5] will determine the elements and degree of rupture, the disruption, disorganization, and disorientation, and the severity of the fixity. The fixity may render the individual vulnerable, particularly to further trauma/ruptures, throughout the life cycle. This TCMI framework allows evaluation of whether and how much of each system was ruptured or proved resilient, and may thus inform the choice of optimal systemic interventions. For example, the Nazi Holocaust not only ruptured continuity but also destroyed all the individual's existing supports. The ensuing, pervasive conspiracy of silence between survivors and society, including mental health professionals, deprived them and their children of potential supports (Danieli, 1985).

Integration of the trauma must take place in *all* of life's relevant dimensions or systems and cannot be accomplished by the individual alone. Routes to integration may include reestablishing, relieving, and repairing the ruptured systems of survivors and their community and nation, and their place in the international community. For example, in the context of examining the right to restitution, compensation, and rehabilitation for victims of gross violations of human rights and fundamental freedoms from the victims' point of view, for the United Nations Commission on Human Rights, I interviewed victim/survivors of the Nazi Holocaust, Japanese Americans, and victims from Argentina and Chile. Based on these interviews, I suggested the following goals and recommendations (Danieli, 1992):

> *Reestablishment of the victim's . . . value, power . . . and dignity, [through] . . . reparation* . . . accomplished by compensation, both real and symbolic; restitution; rehabilitation; and commemoration. *Relieving, the victim's stigmatization and separation from society . . .* is accomplished by commemoration; memorials to heroism; empowerment; and education. Lastly, . . . *repairing the nation's ability to provide and maintain equal value under law and the provisions of justice* [which] is accomplished by apology; securing public records;

---

[4]For an overview of how this framework relates to international responses to traumatic stress, see Danieli, Rodley, and Weisaeth (1996).
[5]A brief discussion comparing these concepts can be found in the concluding chapter of this volume.

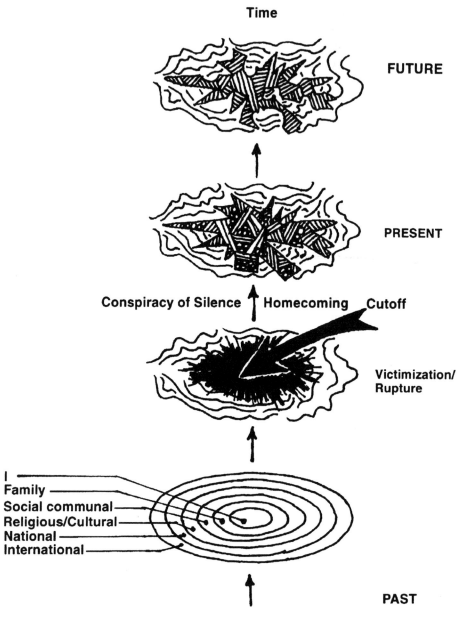

Figure 1. The TCMI framework.

prosecution; education; and creating mechanisms for monitoring, conflict resolution and preventive interventions. (E/AC57/1990/22, pp. 211–212)

In some respects this multidimensional, interdisciplinary integrative framework resembles formulations postulated by others (e.g., Archibald, Long, Miller, & Tuddenham, 1962; Elder & Clipp, 1989; Engel, 1977, 1996; Harvey, 1996). Wong (1993) similarly suggests that psychological resources and deficits are not opposite poles of the same continuum but coexist in a state of dynamic tension and balance.

To fulfill the reparative and preventive goals of psychological recovery from trauma, perspective and integration through awareness and containment must be established so that one's sense of continuity, belongingness, and rootedness are restored (see also Krystal, 1988; Lifton, 1979). To be healing and even potentially self-actualizing, the integration of traumatic experiences must be examined from the perspective of the *totality* of the trauma survivors' and family members' lives (Danieli, 1981b, 1985).

Systems can change and recover independently of other systems. For example, there may be progress in the social system but not in the political system. Although there can be isolated, independent recovery in various systems or dimensions, they may also be related and interdependent. For example, Matussek (1971/1975) found that survivors "in the USA and in Israel. . . have been more successful in coping with their concentration camp past than . . . in Germany, which, for them, is still the country of their persecutors" (p. 137; also see Kleinplantz, 1980, for comparisons between North American and Israeli children of survivors).

The Intergenerational Context

The intergenerational perspective reveals the impact of trauma, its contagion, and repeated patterns within the family. It may help explain certain behavior patterns, symptoms, roles, and values adopted by family members, family sources of vulnerability as well as resilience and strength, and job choices (following in the footsteps of a relative, a namesake) through the generations.

Viewed from a family systems perspective, what happened in one generation will affect what happens in the older or younger generation, though the actual behavior may take a variety of forms. Within an intergenerational context, the trauma and its impact may be passed down as the family legacy even to children born *after* the trauma. In response to some trends in the literature to pathologize, overgeneralize, and/or stigmatize survivors' and children of survivors' Holocaust-related phenomena, as well as differences emerging between the clinical and the research literature, I have emphasize the *heterogeneity* of adaptation among survivors' families (Danieli, 1981a; 1988b).

Studies by Rich (1982), Klein (1987) and Sigal and Winfeld (1989) have empirically validated my descriptions (Danieli, 1981a; 1988b) of at least four differing postwar "adaptational styles" of survivors' families: the *Victim* families, *Fighter* families, *Numb* families, and families of *"Those who made it."* This family typology illustrates lifelong and intergenerational transmission of Holocaust traumata, the conspiracy of silence, and their effects. Findings by others such as Klein-Parker (1988), Kahana, Harel, and Kahana (1989), Kaminer and Lavie (1991), and Helmreich (1992) confirm a *heterogeneity* of *adaptation* and *quality of adjustment* to the Holocaust and post-Holocaust life experiences.

The family is a carrier of conscious and unconscious values, myths, fantasies, and beliefs that may not be shared by the larger community or culture. Yet the role of the family as vehicle for intergenerational transmission of core issues of living and of adaptive and maladaptive ways of defining and coping with them may vary among cultures. The awareness of the possibility of pathogenic intergenerational processes and the understanding of the mechanisms of transmission should contribute to our finding effective means for preventing their transmission to succeeding generations (Danieli, 1985, 1993).

The identity dimensions contained in the framework also serve as pathways for intergenerational transmission. Different cultures capitalize on different pathways to acculturate their young. Thus, beyond the familial, from parents to offspring, entire bodies of human endeavor are vehicles of transmission: oral history, literature and drama, history and politics, religious ritual and writings, cultural traditions and the study thereof, such as anthropology, biology, and genetics. And the various disciplines examine, from their different perspectives, these identity dimensions.

Beyond their psychosocial implications, multigenerational effects of trauma may carry legal (e.g., issues of compensation and restitution, the current debate with regard to the need to form an international criminal court) and political (e.g., wars and cycles of violence, ethnic and racial strife) implications.

Vulnerability and/or Resilience?

The literature is in disagreement regarding the role of prior trauma in subsequent trauma response. Two contrasting perspectives exist. The vulnerability perspective holds that trauma leaves permanent psychic damage that renders survivors more vulnerable when subsequently faced with extreme stress. The resilience perspective (Harel, Kahana, & Kahana, 1993; Helmreich, 1992; Kaminer & Lavie, 1991; Leon et al., 1981; Shanan, 1989; Whiteman, 1993) postulates that coping well with initial trauma will strengthen resistance to the effects of future trauma. In other words, survivors of previous trauma will manifest more resilience when faced with adversity. In a sense, people who may succumb to a trauma's effects can be contrasted with those who do not. The latter may well be described as resilient, or more resistant to the negative effects of trauma. Both perspectives recognize individual differences in response to trauma, recognize that exposure to massive trauma may overwhelm predisposition and previous experience, and that posttrauma environmental factors play important roles in adaptation (see also Eberly, Harkness, & Engdahl, 1991; Engdahl, Harkness, Eberly, Page, & Bielinski, 1993; see also Ursano, 1990).

With survivors, it is especially hard to draw conclusions based on outward appearances. Survivors often display external markers of success (i.e., occupational achievement or establishing families) that in truth represent survival strategies. Clearly, these accomplishments may facilitate adaptation and produce feelings of fulfillment in many survivors. Thus, the external attainments represents significant adaptive achievement in their lives. However, there are also other facets of adaptation that are largely internal and intrapsychic (Engdahl, Dikel, Eberly, & Blank, 1997).

Similarly, although some of the literature on children of survivors reports good adjustment (e.g., Leon et al., 1981), Solomon, Kotler, and Milkulincer (1988) demonstrated in them a special vulnerability to traumatic stress. Despite optimistic views of adaptation, even survivors in the "those who made it" category still experience difficulties related to their traumatic past, suggesting that the overly optimistic views may describe defense rather than effective coping. In fact, it is within this category that we observe the highest rates of suicide among survivors as well as their children. It is important to note that the disagreement in the literature regarding the issue of vulnerability and/or resilience could be a result of professionals' countertransference reactions, as described earlier in this chapter.

The findings that survivors have areas of vulnerability and resilience is no longer paradoxical when viewed within a multidimensional (TCMI) framework for multiple levels of posttraumatic adaptation. And tracing a history of multiple traumata along the time dimension at different stages of development reveals that although for many people time heals ills, for *traumatized* people, time may not heal, but may magnify their response to further trauma (Yehuda et al., 1995) and may carry intergenerational implications.

AN INTERNATIONAL HANDBOOK ON MULTIGENERATIONAL LEGACIES OF TRAUMA

The structure of this book follows the developmental foci of the field of multigenerational legacies of trauma (rather than a chronology of the traumatic events themselves). It is thus divided into 11 sections that progress from the Nazi Holocaust, to World War II, to genocide, to the Vietnam War, to intergenerational effects revealed after the fall of Communism; in indigenous peoples; following repressive regimes, crime and urban violence, infectious and life-threatening diseases, and the emerging biology of intergenerational trauma, to a final synthesizing conclusion.

Part I consists of five chapters that explore the nature and prevalence of multigenerational effects of the Nazi Holocaust on its victims as well as its perpetrators, from theoretical, clinical, and empirical points of view. Auerhahn and Laub (Chapter 1), using case examples, delineate 10 forms of intergenerational knowing (remembering) trauma, modes of transmission, and implications for prevention and healing. Felsen (Chapter 2) provides a rich and complex review of nonclinical, controlled studies carried out in North America up to 1996, addresses the discrepancies between clinical and empirical reports, and proposes a unifying conceptual framework for the various findings. Solomon (Chapter 3) reviews and analyzes from several prisms all published empirical studies carried out on the well-being of the "second generation" in Israel up to 1995. Hardtmann (Chapter 4) focuses on (grand) children of Nazis and describes psychoanalytically their parents' use of denial, splitting, projection, and projective identifications to defend against, yet transmit to them, their past, and suggests treatment recommendation and further exploration. Bar-On, Ostrovsky, and Fromer (Chapter 5) describe seminars for German and Israeli youth struggling to work through personal and collective identity as they confront the Holocaust and each other.

Part II consists of six chapters that report on the family and intergenerational aspects of some of the significant groups affected by World War II. Two chapters describe groups in the United States: Bernstein (Chapter 6) touches upon some intergenerational implications of conflicts in adjustment in American prisoners of war, whereas Nagata (Chapter 7), based on a national survey and in-depth interviews, reports multiple effects of the Japanese American internment upon the third generation (Sansei) children of former internees. From Japan, focusing on Hibakusha Nisei (children of atomic-bomb survivors), Tatara (Chapter 8) illustrates the importance of the physiological, political, socioeconomic, cultural, and social dimensions to understanding the nature of their intergenerational trauma. Three chapters describe groups of "children of the war" in The Netherlands: Op den Velde (Chapter 9) reports on the diverse problems and specific family (psycho)dynamics of children of war sailors and civilian Resistance veterans, whereas Lindt (Chapter 10) describes the recently begun process of emergence toward integration from their (taboo) outcast societal status as children of collaborators (*quislings*). Aarts (Chapter 11) focuses on clinical and empirical findings of intergenerational effects in families of World War II survivors from the Dutch East Indies.

Part III consists of two chapters that describe the nature of effects on survivors, their cultures, and families of genocide and migration: Kupelian, Kalagjian, and Kassabian (Chapter 12) studied the impact of Turkish persecution and genocide of the Armenians on their ethnic identity, psychopathology, and its meaning in the second and third generations; Kinzie, Boehnlein, and Sack (Chapter 13) describe effects of the Cambodian genocide on its survivors, their families, parenting ability, and their children.

Part IV consists of three chapters addressing aspects of intergenerational transmission of the Vietnam War. Rosenheck and Fontana (Chapter 14) raise key sampling considerations, and empirically comparing Vietnam veterans whose fathers served in combat with those who did not, conclude that intergenerational effects of trauma emerge when the second generation itself has PTSD, and are more related to intergenerational processes during the homecoming period than to differences in premilitary vulnerability. Hunter-King's (Chapter 15) survey of children of service personnel missing in action indicates the mother's critical role in determining their coping and the preventive value of adequate support to the families. Ancharoff, Munroe, and Fisher (Chapter 16) examine several mechanisms of transmission, interventions, and clinical implications.

Part V consists of three chapters that examine intergenerational effects revealed after the fall of Communism, central to which are issues of submerged ethnic identity. Klain (Chapter 17) traces, from psychohistorical, psychoanalytic, and group analytic perspectives, current interethnic conflicts in the former Yugoslavia to historically remote, transgenerationally transmitted affects and memories of wartime events by families, communities, and nations, and makes therapeutic and preventive recommendations. Rosenthal and Völter (Chapter 18) compare sociologically how traumatic history is transmitted in (three generations) Jewish and non-Jewish German and Israeli family constellations (of victims, perpetrators, and Nazi followers), and in former East and West Germany after unification. Erős, Vajda, and Kovács (Chapter 19) describe processes of transformation of Jewish identity in Hungary as a function of intergenerational responses to the social and political changes.

Part VI consists of five chapters that address aspects of multigenerational transmission of trauma in indigenous peoples in their own lands and as slaves taken from their lands. Three chapters demonstrate the unsurprisingly similar continuing effects of colonialism. Raphael, Swan, and Martinek (Chapter 20) review and analyze the extensive and pervasive ongoing transgenerational effects of dispossession, deprivation, and discrimination, in particular the systematic removal and subsequent abuse of children ("stolen generations") of Australian aboriginal people. Duran, Duran, Brave Heart, and Yellow Horse-Davis (Chapter 21) propose "historical trauma" and postcolonial paradigms for understanding and healing the American Indian "soul wound," and Gagné (Chapter 22) outlines a sociological perspective to examine intergenerational effects of colonialism and dependency in (Canadian) First Nations Citizens. Examining theories of the sources of ethnic conflicts, Odejide, Sanda, and Odejide (Chapter 23) suggest that their recurrence (in Nigeria) reflects intergenerational effects of the civil war. Cross (Chapter 24) differentiates adjustment patterns linked to slavery from aspects of American black psychology that are the product of contemporary racism and economic neglect—the legacy of slavery for American whites.

Part VII consists of six chapters that describe the multigenerational effects of repressive regimes. Four chapters emphasize the significance of whether (societies and) families coped with the legacy of the repression through concealment or openness. Baker and Gippenreitner (Chapter 25) studied grandchildren of Stalin's purge victims utilizing Bowen Family Systems Theory; Becker and Diaz (Chapter 26) and Edelman, Kordan, and Lagos (Chapter 27), writing of the postdictatorship years in, respectively, Chile and Argentina, discuss the continuing trauma generated not only by uncertainty regarding the fate of loved ones and the resulting lack of closure, but also by the unfulfilled promise of postdictatorial regimes, which has given rise to impunity as a new traumatic factor. Based on data on the impact of family trauma on two groups of children from contrasting cultures (Southeast Asian and Central American), Rousseau and Drapeau (Chapter 28) discuss the influence of the child's culture of origin and stage of development on the transmission of trauma. Simpson (Chapter 29), drawing from work with South African apartheid-era victims and perpetrators, explores the continuing effects of unresolved conflicts on individuals, families, communities, and nations. Ghadirian (Chapter 30) reviews the roots of persecution of Baha'is, and reports strengthened beliefs and capacity for forgiveness in children of Iranian Baha'i martyrs.

Part VIII consists of three chapters that address intergenerational aspects of crime and domestic violence. Buchanan (Chapter 31) provides a systematic review of the multidisciplinary, worldwide literature on intergenerational child maltreatment ("cycle of abuse") and a corresponding body of recommendations, and Simons and Johnson (Chapter 32) examine competing explanations and related treatment implications for the intergenerational transmission of domestic violence. From two clinical studies, Nader (Chapter 33) concludes that children whose parent(s) were previously traumatized may be at increased risk both of traumatic exposure and of elevated symptom levels following a traumatic event.

Part IX consists of two chapters that address multigenerational effects of infectious and life-threatening diseases. Focusing on AIDS, Draimin, Levine, and McKelvy (Chapter 34) underline its uniqueness and disruptive and distorting effects on the normal sequence of generations. Wellisch and Hoffman (Chapter 35) describe the psychological and treatment implications for daughters of mothers with breast cancer of confronting their mother's (potentially terminal) illness and their own risk of contracting it.

Part X consists of three chapters that depict the emerging biology of intergenerational trauma. Suomi and Levine (Chapter 36) examine psychobiological processes involved in the transmission of behavioral and physiological sequelae based on data from prospective animal studies, including primates; Yehuda *et al.* (Chapter 37) demonstrate that offspring of Holocaust survivors are more vulnerable than controls to developing PTSD, and show similar neuroendocrine alterations to survivors with PTSD. Krystal *et al.* (Chapter 38) review the initial clinical evidence of genetic contributions to PTSD and recommend future research and related treatment directions.

Part XI, the editor's concluding chapter, notes striking similarities as well as enriching, instructive differences in the diversity of the contributions. It summarizes major findings and emerging themes, and maps them along the dimensions delineated in the proposed TCMI framework and includes recommendations for the future. Important foci are aspects of the time dimension, resilience, "mechanisms of the transmission" of trauma, role of the conspiracy of silence, the importance of culture as transmitter, buffer and healer, and justice.

REFERENCES

American Psychiatric Association. (1980). *Diagnostic and statistical manual of mental disorders* (3rd ed.). Washington, DC: Author.

American Psychiatric Association. (1994). *Diagnostic and statistical manual of mental disorders* (4th ed). Washington, DC: Author.

Archibald, H. C., Long, D. M., Miller, C., & Tuddenham, R. D. (1962). Gross stress reaction in combat—a 15-year follow-up. *American Journal of Psychiatry, 119,* 317–322.

Axelrod, S., Schnipper, O. L., & Rau, J. H. (1980). Hospitalized offspring of Holocaust survivors: Problems and dynamics. *Bulletin of the Menninger Clinic, 44,* 1–14.

Bar-On, D. (1989). *Legacy of silence: Encounters with children of the Third Reich.* Cambridge, MA: Harvard University Press.

Bar-On, D. (1994). *Fear and hope: Life-stories of five Israeli families of Holocaust survivors, three generations in a family.* Tel Aviv: Lochamei Hagetaot-Hakibbutz Hameuchad. (Hebrew)

Barocas, H. A., & Barocas, C. B. (1973). Manifestations of concentration camp effects on the second generation. *American Journal of Psychiatry, 130*(7), 820–821.

Barocas, H. A., & Barocas, C. B. (1979). Wounds of the fathers: The next generation of Holocaust victims. *International Review of Psycho-Analysis, 6,* 1–10.

Bergman, M. S., & Jucovy, M. E. (Eds.). (1982). *Generations of Holocaust.* New York: Basic Books.

Bettelheim, B. (1984). Afterword to C. Vegh, *I didn't say goodbye* (R. Schwartz, trans.). New York: Dutton.

Bowen, M. (1978). *Family therapy in clinical practice.* New York: Jason Aronson.

Braham, R. L. (Ed.). (1988). *The psychological perspectives of the Holocaust and of its aftermath.* New York: Columbia University Press.

Chodoff, P. (1975). Psychiatric aspects of the Nazi persecution. In S. Arieti (Ed.), *American handbook of psychiatry* (Vol. 6, 2nd ed., pp. 932–946). New York: Basic Books.

Danieli, Y. (1980). Countertransference in the treatment and study of Nazi Holocaust survivors and their children. *Victimology: An International Journal, 5*(2–4), 355–367.

Danieli, Y. (1981a). Differing adaptational styles in families of survivors of the Nazi Holocaust: Some implications for treatment. *Children Today, 10*(5), 6–10, 34–35.

Danieli, Y. (1981b, March 15–16). Exploring the factors in Jewish identity formation (in children of survivors). In *Consultation on the psycho-dynamics of Jewish identity: Summary of proceedings* (pp. 22–25). American Jewish Committee and the Central Conference of American Rabbis.

Danieli, Y. (1982a). Families of survivors of the Nazi Holocaust: Some short- and long-term effects. In C. D. Speilberger, I. G. Sarason, & N. Milgram (Eds.), *Stress and anxiety* (Vol. 8, pp. 405–421). New York: McGraw-Hill/Hemisphere.

Danieli, Y. (1982b). Therapists' difficulties in treating survivors of the Nazi Holocaust and their children (doctoral dissertation, New York University, 1981). *University Microfilms International,* #949-904.

Danieli, Y. (1982c). Group project for Holocaust survivors and their children. Prepared for National Institute of Mental Health, Mental Health Services Branch, Contract #092424762, Washington, DC.

Danieli, Y. (1984). Psychotherapists' participation in the conspiracy of silence about the Holocaust. *Psychoanalytic Psychology, 1*(1), 23–42.

Danieli, Y. (1985). The treatment and prevention of long-term effects and intergenerational transmission of victimization: A lesson from Holocaust survivors and their children. In C. R. Figley (Ed.), *Trauma and its wake* (pp. 295–313). New York: Brunner/Mazel.

Danieli, Y. (1988a). Confronting the unimaginable: Psychotherapists' reactions to victims of the Nazi Holocaust. In J. P. Wilson, Z. Harel, & B. Kahana (eds.), *Human adaptation to extreme stress* (pp. 219–238). New York: Plenum Press.

Danieli, Y. (1988b). The heterogeneity of postwar adaptation in families of Holocaust survivors. In R. L. Braham (Ed.), *The psychological perspectives of the Holocaust and of its aftermath* (pp. 109–128). New York: Columbia University Press.

Danieli, Y. (1988c). Treating survivors and children of survivors of the Nazi Holocaust. In F. M. Ochberg (Ed.), *Post-traumatic therapy and victims of violence* (pp. 278–294). New York: Brunner/Mazel.

Danieli, Y. (1988d). On not confronting the Holocaust: Psychological reactions to victim/survivors and their children. In *Remembering for the future, Theme II: The impact of the Holocaust on the contemporary world* (pp. 1257–1271). Oxford, UK: Pergamon Press.

Danieli, Y. (1989). Mourning in survivors and children of survivors of the Nazi Holocaust: The role of group and community modalities. In D. R. Dietrich, & P. C. Shabad (Eds.), *The problem of loss and mourning: Psychoanalytic perspectives* (pp. 427–460). Madison, CT: International Universities Press.

Danieli, Y. (1992). Preliminary reflections from a psychological perspective. In T. C. van Boven & C. Flinterman (Eds.), *Seminar on the Right to Restitution, Compensation and Rehabilitation for Victims of Gross Violations of Human Rights and Fundamental Freedoms.* Also in Neil Kritz (Ed.), *Readings on the Transitional Justice: How Emerging Democracies Reckon with Former Regimes.* Washington, DC: United States Institute of Peace.

Danieli, Y. (1993). The diagnostic and therapeutic use of the multigenerational family tree in working with survivors and children of survivors of the Nazi Holocaust. In J. P. Wilson & B. Raphael (Eds.), *The international handbook of traumatic stress syndromes* (pp. 889–898). New York: Plenum Press.

Danieli, Y. (1994a). As survivors age—Part I. *National Center for Post-Traumatic Stress Disorder Clinical Quarterly, 4*(1), 1–7.

Danieli, Y. (1994b). As survivors age—Part II. *National Center for Post-Traumatic Stress Disorder Clinical Quarterly, 4*(2), 20–24.

Danieli, Y. (1994c). Countertransference, trauma and training. In J. P. Wilson & J. Lindy (Eds.), *Countertransference in the treatment of post-traumatic stress disorder* (pp. 368–388). New York: Guilford.

Danieli, Y., & Krystal, J. H. (1989). *The initial report of the Presidential Task Force on Curriculum, Education and Training of the Society for Traumatic Stress Studies.* Chicago: Society for Traumatic Stress Studies.

Danieli, Y., Rodley, N. S., & Weisaeth, L. (Eds.). (1996). *International responses to traumatic stress: Humanitarian, human rights, justice, peace and development contributions, collaborative actions and future initiatives.* Published for and on behalf of the United Nations. Amityville, NY: Baywood.

Dasberg, H. (1987). Psychological distress of Holocaust survivors and offspring in Israel, forty years later: A review. *Israel Journal of Psychiatry and Related Sciences. 23*(4), 243–256.

Davidson, S. (1980). Transgeneration transmission in the families of Holocaust survivors. *International Journal of Family Psychiatry, 1*, pp. 95–112.

Dimsdale, J. E. (Ed.) (1980). *Survivors, victims and perpetrators: Essays on the Nazi Holocaust.* New York: Hemisphere.

Eberly, R. E., Harkness & Engdahl, B. E. (1991). An adaptational view of trauma response as illustrated by the prisoner of war experience. *Journal of Traumatic Stress (4)*, 363–380.

Elder, G. H., Jr. and Clipp, E. C. (1989). Combat experience and emotional health: impairment and resilience in later life. *Journal of personality, 57*(2), 311–341.

Engdahl, B. E., Dikel, T. N., Eberly, R., & Blank R. A. (1997). Posttraumatic Stress Disorder in a community sample of former prisoners of war: A normative response to severe trauma. *American Journal of Psychiatry 154*(11), 1576–1581.

Engdahl, B. E., Harkness, A. R., Eberly, R. E., Page, W. E., & Bielinski, J. (1993). Structural models of captivity trauma, resilience, and trauma response among former prisoners of war 20 to 40 years after release. *Social Psychiatry and Psychiatric Epidemiology, 28*, 109–115.

Engel, G. L. (1977). The need for a new medical model: A challenge for biomedicine. *Science, 196*, 129–136.

Engel, G. L. (1996). From biomedical to biopsychosocial: I. Being scientific in the human domain. *Families, Systems and Health: The Journal of Collaborative Family Health Care, 14*(4), 425–433.

Euripides. (Undated). *Phrixus,* fragment 970.

Euripides. (Undated). *Temenidae,* fragment 734.

Figley, C. R. (Ed.). (1995). *Compassion fatigue: Coping with secondary traumatic stress disorder in those who treat the traumatized.* New York: Brunner/Mazel.

Fogelman, E., & Savran, B. (1979). Therapeutic groups for children of Holocaust survivors. *International Journal of Group Psychotherapy, 29*(2), 211–235.

Hannaham, J. (1996). Holding history. *Public Access: The program of the Joseph Papp Public Theater/New York Shakespeare Festival, 3*(2), 22–26.

Harel, Z., Kahana, B., & Kahana, E. (1993). Social resources and the mental health of aging Nazi Holocaust survivors and immigrants. In J. P. Wilson & B. Raphael (Eds.), *International handbook of traumatic stress syndromes* (pp. 241–252). New York: Plenum Press.

Harvey, M. R. (1996). An ecological view of psychological trauma and trauma recovery. *Journal of Traumataic Stress, 9*(1), 3–23.

Hass, A. (1990). *In the shadow of the Holocaust: The second generation.* London: I. B. Tauris.

Hawthorne, N. (1851). Preface, *The House of the Seven Gables.*

Heimannsberg, B., & Schmidt, C. J. (Eds.). (1993). *The collective silence: German identity and the legacy of shame* (C. O. Harris & G. Wheeler, Trans.). San Francisco: Jossey-Bass.

Helmreich, W. B. (1992). *Against all odds: Holocaust survivors and the successful lives they made in America.* New York: Simon & Schuster.

Herman, J. L. (1992). *Trauma and recovery.* New York: Basic Books.

Horace, Q. H. F. (23 BC). *Odes* III, 6:1.

Hudnall Stamm, B. (Ed.). (1995). *Secondary traumatic stress: Self-care issues for clinicians, researchers, and educators.* Lutherville, MD: Sidran Press.

Johnson, D. R., Lubin, H., Rosenheck, R., Fontana, A., Southwick, S., & Charney, D. (1997). The impact of the homecoming reception on the development of posttraumatic stress disorder: The West Haven Homecoming Stress Scale (WHHSS). *Journal of Traumatic Stress, 10*(2), 259–277.

Jordan, B. K., Marmar, C. R., Fairbank, J. A., Schlenger, W. F., Kulka, R. A., Hough, R. L., & Weiss, D. S. (1992). Problems in families of male Vietnam veterans with posttraumatic stress disorder. *Journal of Consulting and Clinical Psychology, 60*(6), 916–926.

Jurich, A. P. (1983). The Saigon of the family's mind: Family therapy with families of Vietnam veterans. *Journal of Marital and Family Therapy, 9*(4), 355–363.

Kahana, B., Harel, Z., & Kahana, E. (1988). Predictors of psychological well-being among survivors of the Holocaust. In J. P. Wilson, Z. Harel, & B. Kahana (Eds.), *Human adaptation to extreme stress: From Holocaust to Vietnam* (pp. 171–192). New York: Plenum Press.

Kahana, B., Harel, Z., & Kahana, E. (1989). Clinical and gerontological issues facing survivors of the Nazi Holocaust. In P. Marcus, & A. Rosenberg (Eds.), *Healing their wounds: Psychotherapy with Holocaust survivors and their families* (pp. 197–211). New York: Praeger.

Kaminer, H., & Lavie, P. (1991). Sleep and dreaming in Holocaust survivors: Dramatic decrease in dream recall in well-adjusted survivors. *Journal of Nervous and Mental Disease, 179*(11), 664–669.

Keilson, H. (1992). *Sequential traumatization in children.* Jerusalem: Hebrew University, Magnes Press.

Kestenberg, J. (1972). Psychoanalytic contributions to the problem of children of survivors from Nazi persecution. *Israeli Annals of Psychiatry and Related Disciplines, 10,* 311–325.

Kestenberg, J. (1989). Transposition revisited: Clinical, therapeutic, and developmental considerations. In P. Marcus & A. Rosenberg (Eds.), *Healing their wounds: Psychotherapy with Holocaust survivors and their families* (pp. 67–82). New York: Praeger.

Klein, H. (1971). Families of Holocaust survivors in the Kibbutz: Psychological studies. In H. Krystal & W. C. Niederland (Eds.), *Psychic Tramatization aftereffects in Individual and Communities* (pp. 69–72). Boston: Little, Brown.

Klein, M. E. (1987). Transmission of trauma: The defensive styles of children of Holocaust survivors. Doctoral dissertation, California School of Professional Psychology. University Microfilms International, #8802441.

Klein-Parker, F. (1988). Dominant attitudes of adult children of Holocaust survivors toward their parents. In J. P. Wilson, Z. Harel, & B. Kahana (Eds.), *Human adaptation to extreme stress* (pp. 193–218). New York: Plenum Press.

Kleinplatz, M. M. (1980, August). *Contribution of support to the adaptation of survivors' children in two cultures.* Paper presented at the annual meeting of the American Psychological Association, Montreal, Canada.

Kogan, I. (1995). *The cry of mute children: A psychoanalytic perspective of the second generation of the Holocaust.* New York: Free Association Books.

Krell, R. (1984). Holocaust survivors and their children: Comments on psychiatric consequences and psychiatric terminology. *Comprehensive Psychiatry, 25*(5), 521–528.

Krell, R., & Sherman, M. (1997). *Medical and psychological effects of concentration camps on Holocaust survivors.* New Brunswick, NJ: Transaction Publishers.

Krystal, H. (1968). *Massive psychic trauma.* New York: International Universities Press.

Krystal, H. (1988). *Integration and self-healing.* Hillsdale, NJ: Analytic Press.

Krystal, H., & Danieli, Y. (1994). Holocaust survivor studies in the context of PTSD. *National Center for Post-Traumatic Stress Disorder PTSD Research Quarterly, 5*(4), 1–5.

Krystal, H., & Niederland, W. G. (1968). Clinical observations on the survivor syndrome. In H. Krystal (Ed.), *Massive psychic trauma* (pp. 327–348). New York: International Universities Press.

Krystal, H., & Niederland, W. G. (Eds.). (1971). *Psychic traumatization: Aftereffects in individuals and communities.* Boston: Little, Brown.

Lifton, R. J. (1979). *The broken connection.* New York: Simon & Schuster.

Matussek, P. (1975). *Internment in concentration camps and its consequences* (D. Jordan & I. Jordan, Trans.). New York: Springer-Verlag. (Original published 1971)

Nagata, D. K. (1993). *Legacy of injustice: Exploring the cross-generational impact of the Japanese American internment.* New York: Plenum Press.

Niederland, W. G. (1961). The problem of the survivor: Some remarks on the psychiatric evaluation of emotional disorders in survivors of the Nazi persecution. *Journal of the Hillside Hospital, 10*(3–4), 233–247.

Niederland, W. G. (1964). Psychiatric disorders among persecution victims: A contribution to the understanding of concentration camp pathology and its aftereffects. *Journal of Nervous and Mental Diseases, 139,* 458–474.

O'Hara, R. (1996). *Insurrection: Holding history.* Play directed by the author, produced by the Joseph Papp Public Theater/New York Shakespeare Festival, December 1996. Unpublished manuscript.

Parks, S.-L. (1995). The America Play (1992, 1994). In S.-L. Parks (Ed.), *The America Play and other works* (pp. 157–199). New York: Theatre Communications Group.

Pearlman, L. A., & Saakvitne, K. W. (1995). *Trauma and the therapist: Countertransference and vicarious traumatization and psychotherapy with incest survivors.* New York: W. W. Norton.

Prince, R. M. (1985). *The legacy of the Holocaust: Psychohistorical themes in the second generation.* Ann arbor, MI: UMI Research Press.

Rakoff, V. A. (1966). Long-term effects of the concentration camp experience. *Viewpoints: Labor Zionist Movement of Canada, 1,* 17–22.

Rakoff, V. A., Sigal, J. J., & Epstein, N. B. (1966). Children and families of concentration camp survivors. *Canada's Mental Health, 14,* 24–26.

Rich, M. S. (1982). *Children of Holocaust survivors: A concurrent validity study of a survivor family typology.* Unpublished doctoral dissertation, California School of Professional Psychology, Berkeley.

Rosenheck, R. (1985). Father–son relationships in malignant post Vietnam stress syndrome. *American Journal of Social Psychiatry, 5,* 19–23.

Rosenheck, R. (1986). Impact of posttraumatic stress disorder of World War II on the next generation. *Journal of Nervous and Mental Disease, 174*(6). 319–327.

Rosenheck, R., & Nathan, P. (1985). Secondary traumatization in children of Vietnam veterans. *Hospital and Community Psychiatry, 36*(5), 538–539.

Rosenthal, P. A., & Rosenthal, S. (1980). Holocaust effect in the third generation: Child of another time. *American Journal of Psychotherapy, 34*(4), 572–580.

Rubenstein, I., Cutter, R., & Templer, D. I. (1990). Multigenerational occurrence of survivors syndrome symptoms in families of Holocaust survivors. *Omega Journal of Death and Dying, 20*(3), 239–244.

Russell, A. (1980). Late effects-influence on children of concentration camp survivors. In J. E. Dimsdale (Ed.), *Survivors, victims, and perpetrators* (pp. 175–204). New York: Hemisphere.

Shakespeare, W. (1596/1597). *The Merchant of Venice,* Act III, i:1.

Shakespeare, W. (1599). *Julius Caesar,* Act III, ii:79.

Shanan, J. (1989). Surviving the survivors: Late personality development of Jewish Holocaust survivors. *International Journal of Mental Health, 17*(4), 42–71.

Sigal, J. J. (1971). Second-generation effects of massive psychic trauma. In H. Krystal & W. G. Niederland (Eds.), *Psychic traumatization: Aftereffects in individuals and communities* (pp. 67–92). Boston: Little, Brown.

Sigal, J. J., & Weinfeld, M. (1989). *Trauma and rebirth: Intergenerational effects of the Holocaust.* New York: Praeger.

Solomon, Z., Kotler, M., & Milkulincer, M. (1988). Combat-related post-traumatic stress disorders among second generation Holocaust survivors: Preliminary findings. *American Journal of Psychiatry, 145,* 865–868.

Steinberg, A. (1989). Holocaust survivors and their children: A review of the clinical literature. In P. Marcus & A. Rosenberg (Eds.), *Healing their wounds: Psychotherapy with Holocaust survivors and their families* (pp. 23–48). New York: Praeger.

Symonds, M. (1980). The "second injury" to victims [Special issue]. *Evaluation and Change,* 36–38.

Tanay, B. (1968). Initiation of psychotherapy with survivors of the Nazi persecution. In H. Krystal (Ed.), *Massive psychic trauma* (pp. 219–233). New York: International Universities Press.

Terry, J. (1984). The damaging effects of the "survivor syndrome." In S. A. Luel & P. Marcus (Eds.), *Psychoanalytic reflections on the Holocaust: Selected essays* (pp. 135–148). New York: Holocaust Awareness Institute Center for Judaic Studies, University of Denver and Ktav Publishing House.

Trossman, B. (1968). Adolescent children of concentration camp survivors. *Canadian Psychiatric Association Journal, 13,* 121–123.

Ursano, R. J. (1990). The prisoner of war. *Military Medicine, (155),* 176–180.

Verbosky, S. J., & Ryan, D. A. (1988). Female partners of Vietnam veterans: Stress by proximity. *Issues in Mental Health Nursing, 9,* 95–104.

Wardi, D. (1992). *Memorial candles: Children of the Holocaust.* London: Tavistock/Rutledge.

Whiteman, D. B. (1993). Holocaust survivors and escapees—their strengths. *Psychotherapy, 30*(3), 443–451.

Wilson, J. P., & Lindy, J. (1994). *Countertransference in the treatment of PTSD.* New York: Guilford.

Wilson, J. P., & Raphael, B. (Eds.). (1993). *International handbook of traumatic stress syndromes.* New York: Plenum Press.

Wong, P. T. P. (1993). Effective management of life stress: The resource-congruence model. *Stress Medicine, (9),* 51–60.

Yehuda, R., Kahana, B. Schmeidler, J., Southwick, S. M., Wilson, S., & Giller, E. L. (1995). Impact of cumulative lifetime trauma and recent stress on current posttraumatic stress disorder symptoms in Holocaust survivors. *American Journal of Psychiatry, 152*(12), 1815–1818.

I

The Nazi Holocaust

1

Intergenerational Memory
of the Holocaust

NANETTE C. AUERHAHN and DORI LAUB

The struggle of man against power is the struggle of memory against forgetting.
—MILAN KUNDERA, 1978/1982, p. 3

The literature on Holocaust survival and second-generation effects has been prone to controversy beyond criticisms of research methodology, sample selection, and generalizability of
findings (e.g., Solkoff, 1992). A critical backlash has also been evident (Roseman & Handleman, 1993; Whiteman, 1993), even from among the children themselves (Peskin, 1981),
against the penchant of the early Holocaust literature to formulate the transmission of deep
psychopathology from one generation to the next. Such an unbending formulation has understandably aroused readers' strong skepticism and ambivalence, in part because to expose the
magnitude of the Nazi destruction is to confirm Hitler's posthumous victory (Danieli, 1984,
1985). But seeking to correct this early bias wherein Holocaust suffering is equated with psychopathology has, often enough, also created an overcorrection that discourages understanding the Holocaust as a core existential and relational experience for both generations. This
stance also has made it difficult to integrate the Holocaust literature with the posttraumatic
stress disorder (PTSD) literature (that followed it), which appears thus far not to have been
similarly burdened with the accusation that to explore negative effects is to pathologize and de-
mean survivors. What the extensive clinical and research material on the Holocaust—its contradictions as much as its consistencies—has taught us is the diversity of meanings of
Holocaust suffering for both generations that can neither be accounted for by narrow psychopathological diagnoses (Bergmann & Jacovy, 1982) nor be contradicted by survivors' and
their children's undeniable resiliency and coping. In the growing polemic between those who
stress the negative effects of trauma (e.g., Krystal, 1968), and those who focus on survivors'
strengths and coping skills (e.g., Harel, Kahana, & Kahana, 1988), our body of work (e.g.,
Auerhahn & Laub, 1984, 1987, 1990; Auerhahn & Prelinger, 1983; Laub & Auerhahn, 1984,

NANETTE C. AUERHAHN • Bellefaire Jewish Children's Bureau, Shaker Heights, Ohio 44118.   DORI LAUB
• Yale University School of Medicine, New Haven, Connecticut 065200.

International Handbook of Multigenerational Legacies of Trauma, edited by Yael Danieli. Plenum Press, New York, 1998.

1985, 1989; Peskin, Auerhahn, & Laub, 1997) has rejected the polarization of researchers into those who claim that no (ill) effects of the Holocaust are to be found in survivors and their children versus those who claim that there are (negative) effects. Instead, we have shifted the focus away from value-laden judgments of psychological health to the issue of knowledge, and have come to view both generations as heterogeneous and therefore as consisting of individuals with different kinds and degrees of Holocaust knowledge. We find that it is the very individualized quality of knowing massive psychic trauma that compellingly informs as well as shapes one's subsequent life experiences, world view, fantasy world, relationships, decision making, and action. Therefore, both character and psychopathology indelibly bear the marks of knowing trauma, and it is through this lens that we attempt to examine the intergenerational effects of massive psychic trauma. Much of our work has sought to examine the question of what kind of knowledge of the Holocaust is possible, and to trace the threads of different forms of traumatic knowledge as they have woven through the conscious and unconscious of both generations. Indeed, we view the ongoing debate among researchers and scholars as to the extent of impact the Holocaust has had on individuals as part of the continuing struggle of all of us to fully grasp the nature of massive psychic trauma.

In this chapter, we summarize our current understanding of the many ways massive psychic trauma is known, for central to the response to trauma are the issues of knowing and forgetting. The chapter focuses on the attempt to know, the defenses against knowledge, the different levels of knowing that are possible, the inevitable limits of knowing, and implications for healing, and will progress from an initial focus on survivors to a later focus on the next generation. That is because in our clinical work with survivors and their children, as well as in our work collecting oral histories of Holocaust survivors at the Fortunoff Video Archive for Holocaust Testimonies at Yale University, we have found that knowledge of psychic trauma weaves through the memories of several generations, marking those who know of it as secret bearers (Micheels, 1985). Furthermore, we have found that massive trauma has an amorphous presence not defined by place or time and lacking a beginning, middle, or end, and that it shapes the internal representation of reality of several generations, becoming an unconscious organizing principle passed on by parents and internalized by their children (Laub & Auerhahn, 1984). Traumatic memory thus entails a process of evolution that requires several generations in which to play itself out. We initially understood this to be the result of conflicts arising from the paradoxical yoking of the compulsions to remember and to know trauma with the equally urgent needs to forget and not to know it (Auerhahn & Laub, 1990), but now see the situation as infinitely more complex. For along with any conscious or unconscious needs to know or not to know exist deficits in our abilities to grasp trauma, name it, recall it, and, paradoxically, forget it. We know trauma because it thrusts itself upon us unbeckoned. But we also fail to know it and frequently forget it because we are incapable of formulating and holding such knowledge in mind. Often, we cannot form an initial memory; at other times, the memory, once held, disappears. This process is exemplified by our psychiatric nosology, which has repeatedly omitted and reinstated the diagnosis of trauma, under various names, over decades (Solomon, 1995). On the political level, Dennis Klein (1991, p. 3) has noted an equivalent process in the tendency of some to deny or marginalize the Holocaust, coining the term *history's memory hole* to describe this phenomenon. It is no wonder, then, that survivors are unable to complete the process themselves, leaving their children to carry on the working through of trauma. These children become burdened by memories that are not their own (see Auerhahn & Prelinger, 1983; Fresco, 1984). As one child of survivors told us, "I am a prisoner of an empty space." The child echoes what exists in parents' inner worlds; the child's psychic reality thereby reveals the indelible marks left by trauma.

FORMS OF TRAUMATIC MEMORY

In an earlier work (Laub & Auerhahn, 1993), we briefly discussed eight forms of knowing massive psychic trauma. In this chapter, we expand on these forms as well as add two new forms to the list. As before, we have organized the different forms of knowing along a continuum according to psychological distance from the traumatic experience. The different forms of remembering trauma range from not knowing; to screen memories (which involve the substitution of true but less traumatizing memories for those that cannot be brought to mind); to fugue states (in which events are relived in an altered state of consciousness); to retention of the experience as compartmentalized, undigested fragments of perceptions that break into consciousness (with no conscious meaning or relation to oneself); to transference phenomena (wherein the traumatic legacy is lived out as one's inevitable fate); to its partial, hesitant expression as an overpowering narrative; to the experience of compelling, identity-defining, and pervasive life themes (both conscious and unconscious); to its organization as a witnessed narrative; to its use as a metaphor and vehicle for developmental conflict; and, finally, to action knowledge. These different forms of knowing also vary in degree of encapsulation versus integration of the experience and in degree of ownership of the memory—i.e., the degree to which an experiencing "I" is present as subject. Variations in distance dictate variations in the presence of imaginative elaboration and play.

While we consistently and deliberately use the term *forms of knowing,* each form also progressively represents a consciously deeper and more integrated *level of knowing.* For example, the transition from fugue states to fragments represents a cognitive and emotional breakthrough, whereby material that was previously not consciously known at all becomes known in partial, undigested fragments. Witnessed narrative, while representing fuller conscious knowledge, is still sufficiently chained to perception and the particular witnessing situation not to permit such knowledge to be used in the playful elaboration of metaphor. We prefer, however, to refer to these phenomena as forms rather than levels, so as not to imply that there are stages of remembering through which one must go sequentially. Additionally, these various forms of knowing are not mutually exclusive and may coexist in an individual at any point in time. Nevertheless, we believe that survivors know mostly through retention of fragments of unintegrated memories or by reliving such memories in transference phenomena; children of survivors tend to know through particular themes that prove central to their lives; and those not directly affected know of trauma through experiencing their own conflicts and predicaments in its language and imagery.

Not Knowing

Trauma happens, often with no experiencing "I." While being powerfully present and exerting an eclipsing influence on ego functions, its historical truth may never have been fully grasped by the victim or have attained the status of a psychic representation. That is because massive psychic trauma breaks through the stimulus barrier and defies the individual's ability to formulate experience. It registers in a moment of the breakdown of functional barriers of the ego and hence creates a fragmentation of the self. Erecting barriers against knowing is often the first response to trauma. An adult facing severe trauma often reexperiences infantile remnants of primary traumatization while attempting to ward them off by primitive mechanisms of defense (e.g., denial, splitting, amnesia, derealization, and depersonalization). These early defense mechanisms result in a nonreceptivity to the experience and, in varying degrees, the splitting off of reality. Additionally, severe trauma undermines and, at times, destroys the psychic representation of that internal other whose presence is a prerequisite for the dialogue with oneself that engenders knowing (Laub & Auerhahn, 1989). As a result of these factors, trauma may remain irretrievable to conscious memory even years later, when acknowledgment and the lack thereof can continue to exist simultaneously, without integration.

There are various levels of not knowing. The first involves the presence of an absence, that is, evidence of a painful state of concurrent awareness in the survivor of a depleted self and of an intense experience that is disconnected and forgotten but nevertheless affectively permeates and compromises life strategies of adaptation and defense.

In her analytic hours, Leah, a Holocaust survivor, repeatedly talked about disappointments with her son. The analyst asked her to let go of her son and tell him what came to mind. She spoke of her loneliness, despite having friends who were available every evening—was it perhaps because of her earlier losses that she had never mourned? Her daughter was going to have a child; Leah was scared. Indeed, she felt scared all the time when not preoccupied with something. The analyst inquired about her associations to the idea of a child being born. "Yes," she said, "it died in my arms." She had a baby in the ghetto, who had died one day without having been ill. The analyst commented that Leah had never told him about the child. She replied that she did not think about it any longer, that she thought she had overcome it, and now practically did not know if it.

Rachel Peltz (1994), a psychologist and child of survivors, recently recounted a conversation with her father, who had lost a wife and child or children at the hands of Nazis. Dr. Peltz had never known for certain how many children her father had had or what their names were. When, during a drive together, she finally was able to bring herself to ask him, he became pale and the car was filled with his silence. Then, in a terribly embarrassed tone, he said, "I cannot remember." Dr. Peltz remarks plainly, "My father was a very loving and highly related person, but he couldn't remember who his children were."

This type of erasure of children who were killed in the war is presented in the videotaped testimony of the Holocaust survivor Bessie K., from which Lawrence Langer quotes in his book of collected essays, *Admitting the Holocaust* (1995, p. 143). In her testimony, Bessie K. recalled how she attempted to hide her baby boy in her coat while German guards were separating men, women, and children before forcing them into cattle trains:

> But the baby was short of breath, started to choke, and it started to cry, so the German called me back. He said in German, "What do you have there?" Now, I didn't know what to do, because everything was so fast and everything happened so suddenly. I wasn't prepared for it.
>
> To look back, the experience was—I think I was numb, or something happened to me, I don't know. But I wasn't there. And he stretched out his arms I should hand him over the bundle; and I hand him over the bundle. And this is the last time I had the bundle . . .

Soon after, in the Stutthof concentration camp, she met the doctor who, in the ghetto, before her deportation, had operated on an infected breast. She continued:

> And when she [the doctor] saw me there she was so happy to see me, and right away she says, "What happened, where's the baby, what happened to the baby?" And right there I said, "What baby?" I said to the doctor, "What baby? I didn't have a baby. I don't know of any baby."

Yet another survivor, Helen Landsbury (reported on the ABC news show *20/20,* 1995), has no recollections of her Holocaust experiences, nor does she recall reunification after the war with her two surviving siblings, with whom she was persecuted during some of the war years. Instead, she fondly remembers the prewar years of her early childhood and her postwar marriage to a non-Jewish British soldier. She left her siblings in Europe to begin a new life in England, where she raised her children as non-Jews and talked to her new family only about the "before," never about the war itself. She had no idea that her siblings, who eventually emigrated to the United States, were still alive, and that that they continued to search for her for 50 years. By the time they finally located her through the American Red Cross, she was in her seventies and facing ovarian cancer. At that point, she was finally able to acknowledge regret and a sense of loss over having given up her ties to Judaism, and over the gap in her memories. Herein we have an example of a woman who forgot not only her war experiences but also her living siblings, in addition to having relinquished her religious identity. We believe that the siblings as well as her religion were forgotten precisely because of their linkages to those war experiences that could not be brought to mind.

We have encountered other survivors who, to this day, deny that they ever were in the camps, despite irrefutable evidence to the contrary. This state of not knowing leaves survivors in grief not only for dead loved ones who cannot be recaptured even in memory but also for those lost autobiographical memories that give us a sense of who we are. The lack of knowledge that prevents the revival of despair that would accompany memory leaves survivors alone and unknown even to themselves, and leaves their children with a sense of void and mourning for a past they do not know (Auerhahn & Prelinger, 1983; Fresco, 1984). In many cases, these children, born after the Holocaust, carry those dead children who have been forgotten by the parents. In Dr. Peltz's case, for example, she named her own child after her unknown sister (see Auerhahn & Laub, 1994, for a more extensive discussion of the effects of erasure of trauma on the second generation).

Of course, it is not just survivors who can live in a twilight state between knowing and not knowing. Albert Speer, the architect of the Third Reich, lived for years with both denial and knowledge of Nazi atrocities according to a new biography by Gitta Sereny (1995) entitled *Albert Speer: His Battle with Truth.* Speer had come to believe that often-stated phrase of many victimizers, "I didn't know." Grand (1995), working with perpetrators of incest who had themselves been sexually abused as children, has described several examples of dissociative, ahistorical states in these perpetrators that seemed to exist without speech and without memory, allowing these victims-turned-aggressors to disavow a sense of agency with regard to the evil they had committed and to genuinely experience themselves as innocent.

Screen Memories

The example of Helen Landsbury, the Holocaust survivor who gave up her familial, ethnic, and religious identities, illustrates the creation of an alternative, possibly false, self that screens over the absence of memory. Such a path can readily lead to mythmaking or the creation of false memories that constitute another form of knowing that goes beyond the first level's awareness of an absence to the creation of a fiction that covers over that absence. These fictions, which often contain half-truths, hint at traumatic knowledge even while screening against it. There are various degrees of awareness of this mythmaking and of conscious intention in the fictionalization process itself.

An extreme and pathological form of this kind of dissociation and fictionalization is found in a Vietnam veteran seen by one of the authors in treatment. Tom is a 47-year-old, unmarried biological male who presented to a gender identity program for the initial purpose of helping him clarify his gender identification. As therapy progressed, the patient denied any ambivalence and became more and more insistent on undergoing sex reassignment surgery. He reported that since the age of 9, he had cross-dressed in private, wishing that he was "the other side." At the age of 21, he had joined the Navy, working for 4 years, first in engineering and then in radio communications. He served four 6-month tours on a ship off the coast of Vietnam, where his ship was frequently bombarded by heavy guns and artillery. For 20 years after discharge, Tom suffered from headaches and from hearing the bombarding sound of guns pounding in his sleep. Finally, at the age of 45, he moved his cross-dressing out of the privacy of his home and into the public domain: He went out cross-dressed as a female for the first time. The headaches disappeared and the pounding of the guns stopped. Both briefly returned when the staff of the gender identity program temporarily rejected his request for permission to begin taking female hormones. When permission was finally granted and he began living full time as a female, his headaches and flashbacks disappeared once again.

Tom refused to engage in any psychological exploration, preferring instead to concretize and live out his wish to be "the other side." He soon broke off treatment. His is an example of a case wherein the trauma that is blocked out has no voice, having had its connection to what is consciously experienced severed. Individuals with more ego strengths are generally more consciously aware of the movement from trauma to fiction, at times deliberately using art as a way both to tell and not tell their traumatic stories. Indeed, fictionalization is an inherent part of any attempt to recall trauma, for the truth of trauma can never be fully recaptured. Instead, we have found most true trauma stories to be factually accurate in many ways and factually inaccurate in many ways, containing the facts as perceived (an arduous, incomplete, and interpretive process) and as defended against. In many works of art that attempt to give voice to, or master, trauma, there often is a "lie," a distortion, covering over the as yet unworked through and unknown aspect of trauma.

British writer J. G. Ballard provides an example of an individual attempting to work through his traumas in his art and, in the process, fictionalizing the facts in such a way as to conceal—and thereby reveal—the unworked-through and most difficult aspects of the traumas. Ballard's 1984 novel *Empire of the Sun* (upon which the movie by the same name was based) describes his real-life childhood experiences while interned, along with his father, in a Japanese prisoner-of-war camp near Shanghai during World War II. The novel (and film) painfully detail a young boy's separation from both parents and subsequent experiences alone in a brutalizing prison camp over a period of 3 years. Asked in a radio interview why he chose to have the boy in the novel, who depicted his life, be interned alone rather than with his father, which was Ballard's actual experience, Ballard responded that his own experiences had been so awful that it was as if he were alone. We wonder, however, whether the writer is evading a truth: The brutalization may have been felt even more keenly precisely because it occurred in Father's helpless presence, underscoring Father's inability to protect. Perhaps it was *this* abandonment and its corrosive impact on the father–son relationship that Ballard could not bring himself to depict.

Not only artists but also patients may substitute a fictionalized story that can be told for a truthful one that cannot. We have seen patients who, at first, presented stereotypical abuse stories, only later to reveal atypical, more personal, and hence more painful stories, ones which they had felt, initially, could not justify their pain. They had been unable to allow themselves to know their own stories intimately.

Even when the facts are completely known, survivors often regard them as fiction while, simultaneously, accepting their authenticity. Aharon Appelfeld (Roth, 1988, p. 28), a survivor and Israeli novelist, has admitted, "Everything was so unbelievable that one seemed oneself to be fictional." Appelfeld consciously admits to writing a story that is believable as a substitute for the true story that is not believable and appears to be the fiction, acknowledging (Roth, 1988, p. 29; italics in original), *"The things that are most true are easily falsified."* Not only do nonvictims, at times, not believe survivors, but also survivors often do not believe themselves. Deena Harris, M.D., a daughter of survivors, narrates in the 1994 BBC film *Children of the Third Reich,* how she located a catalogue containing artwork done by her mother and her mother's classmates in a school for Jewish children in Dusseldorf, Germany, during the war years. The catalogue included information about the fate of each of the individuals featured. Dr. Harris gave the catalogue to her mother as a gift, which represented the mother's only written record of the existence and fate of her schoolmates. As her mother read through the album and noted that after most of the names the words "killed in the Holocaust" were inscribed, she looked up at her daughter and, to the latter's astonishment, said in a hushed tone of voice, "You know, until this moment, I thought that I had made it all up." (We are reminded herein of Freud's observation that when a fact first emerges from the unconscious, it often has attached to it a "no." Perhaps the unconscionable facts of massive psychic trauma can likewise impress us only if accompanied first by a denial of their reality.)

Among perpetrators, the use of screen memories has been noted by Bar-On (1993) and von Schlippe (1993) in the form of the guilty remembrance of true but minor atrocities or single vignettes of minor sins that are shamefully acknowledged, paradoxically reassuring perpetrators of retaining a conscience, while screening out a deeper guilt from greater atrocities that are "forgotten."

Our last example comes from the analysis of a son of a perpetrator (a Nazi concentration camp physician), conducted by Dr. Werner Bohleber (1994), and illustrates an active, deliberate destruction of truth.

Rolf was a 32-year-old engineering student who presented for treatment with examination problems and work disturbance. He reported sitting in front of his drawing board for hours, doing nothing, as the day would seem to fly by. He had no feeling of personal wholeness or of continuity of identity and felt, instead, that he consisted only of fragments.

Rolf's parents lived together for many years without getting married, for his father never divorced his first wife. Only after the first wife's death, when Rolf was 24 years old, did they finally get properly married. This illegitimacy was a great source of shame and secrecy in the family. Only when Rolf was 16 years old did his parents inform him, for the first time, about their marital status. When his mother tearfully confessed this to Rolf, he recalls that it made no difference to him. He had stated, "What I don't know cannot bother me." His father noted approvingly that Rolf was reacting sensibly.

Treatment initially focused on Rolf's difficulties with time. The analyst connected the patient's forgetfulness with regard to the time of sessions with the parents' prohibition against his knowledge of the family situation. Rolf brought up some biographical information about his father, specifically about his father's gambling, but stated that there was no point in talking about the past. The analyst expressed his sense that there was a veil over the past, as if it had been cut off so as to not allow it to affect him emotionally. Rolf then recalled how, as a child, he used to ask his mother about her wedding, but that she would evade his questions. One time, he discovered a white dress in her cupboard and asked if that was her wedding dress, whereupon Mother started to cry. He never asked her about the wedding again, not wanting to know.

At some point in treatment, the analyst had a troubled feeling that something was wrong with Rolf's story. He suspected that his father had had an incriminating Nazi past and looked into the relevant literature, quickly obtaining confirmation of the father's documented participation in medical experiments, murder, and atrocities. At first, the analyst assumed that Rolf was unaware of the facts. As he slowly confronted Rolf with them, he discovered, instead, that Rolf knew many of the facts all along, even while denying and rationalizing them with half-truths and excuses. He could not admit that his father had been a party to criminal acts, at one point observing, "All this seems so unreal to me . . . I cannot bring it together in my own mind, that this is supposed to be my father and that he did such things earlier in his life. It's as if it were two different people." All this was said without emotion and, indeed, much of Rolf's life was discussed without his knowing what his feelings were, and with the sensation of standing next to himself. Rolf expressed the belief that his father's past had nothing to do with him and that "when you don't talk about it, it is all gone."

In his discussion of Rolf's case, Dr. Bohleber (1994) focused on the paradoxical fact that the therapy was marked by the father's Nazi past despite, and also precisely because of, the patient's tendency to deny it. Such a stance made it seem unreal both to patient and analyst, and the analyst had to deliberately call to mind the cruelty, criminality, and inhumanity of the things hinted at and kept secret in order to ensure that they retained their psychic presence.

For the purpose of this chapter and our understanding of not knowing and of screen memories, what is noteworthy is the story about the parent's wedding and the secrecy of the patient's illegitimacy. During his childhood, Rolf had sensed that there was something wrong with his family, and that there was a secret about his parents. But behind the tale of their wedding, something painful was hidden that he was not allowed to touch. The scene in which he had asked his mother whether the white dress was her wedding dress made him realize that if he were to touch on the past, it would sadden his mother. In order not to cause her any pain, he gave up his desire to know—his curiosity and thirst for knowledge were lastingly damaged. With his parents' approval, he had adopted the motto, "What I don't know cannot bother me." Thus, his loyalty toward his parents undermind the value of truth and exposed him to constant doubts about what was true, undermining not only his ability to acquire professional skills and knowledge but also his ability to know himself and to let himself be known by others. He could not establish intimate relationships, not even in the transference.

Rolf's parents, too, never owned their involvement in atrocities and never consciously expressed guilt, shame, or regret with regard to this involvement. Instead, all the secrecy and shame were consciously experienced as connected to the inconvenient, legalistic matter of the parents' marital status and the patient's illegitimacy, both of which screened out a darker secret.

Fugue States

Although the first two forms of traumatic memory discussed, those of not knowing and of screen memories, are characterized by the disappearance of traumatic content or of a connection to an experiencing "I," other forms are marked instead by the intrusive *appearance* of split off, fragmented behaviors, cognitions, and affect, which are pieces of the traumatic memory or experience. These fragments (of behavior, cognition, or affect) may be actual (undigested and not worked through) percepts, screen memories, or condensations of real events. With the emergence of this fragment in the individual's behavior or psychic life, varying degrees of knowing are possible. Individuals exhibit different degrees of awareness that they are remembering, with the most extreme form being repeating an experience without the experience being integrated into memory at all; that is, at its most extreme, fragments are "recalled" without the individual knowing that the "I," or subject who experienced the event, is different from the one who recalls it—there is a collapse of the two at the moment of "recall," with no reflective self present. The experience simply *happens*—without any subject whatsoever. The affect is so intense that there is no signal experience of it. The individual becomes the affect, or the affect is shut off. In either case, the memory is not integrated, and the experience cannot be recounted.

This third form of knowing trauma involves actually reliving (rather than remembering). Such reliving is usually discussed in terms of flashbacks wherein an *entire* experience is reenacted. The most classic example is the "battle fatigue syndrome" described in World War II soldiers (Grinker & Spiegel, 1945). This form of reliving often involves the experience of vivid imagery, usually (but not always) visual in nature.

This form of traumatic memory contrasts with the previous ones in that what is known in fugue states is kept separate from the conscious self in such a way as to preserve the latter intact. The ego's protective mechanisms, however pathological, are still operative. The integrity of the experience itself is likewise preserved—it may be repressed and recovered as a *whole*.

Interestingly, the reliving of a whole experience in a fugue state, which characterizes soldiers in an acute delirium, has not, to our knowledge, been reported in Holocaust survivors. (Rachel Yehuda (personal communication, November 1995) reports a relatively low level of dissociative phenomena and the absence of a significant correlation between trauma and dissociation in Holocaust survivors as compared with other traumatized populations.) We wonder whether recovery of the trauma as a whole necessitates certain pre- and posttraumatic conditions—in particular, whether repression of the whole occurs only when there is the possibility of experiencing a whole—when there is a certain normalcy and integrity both coming into and going out of the experience; that is, in order to repress and "remember" (relive) trauma as a whole, there must be an entrance into it from a state of normalcy, as well as a subsequent return to such a state. The world must still have its rules, and the scaffolding of reality must remain. Holocaust survivors entered concentration camps after the demolition of all their preexisting structures. Social and family networks had been destroyed, as had their sense of predictability regarding self and others. After the experience of atrocity, most survivors found neither community nor significant others to whom to return.

Fragments

A fourth form of remembering involves the retention of parts of a lived experience in such a way that they are decontextualized and no longer meaningful. The individual has an image, sensation, or isolated thought, but does not know with what it is connected, what it means, or what to do with it. The fragment may, at times, be restricted to only a single perceptual modality as yet another way of eluding knowledge. What the observer sees in these cases is not a memory but, rather, a derivative, a symptom that infuses the individual's life. The individual may know that the symptom is irrational yet be unable to discount it.

Hans, a man in his mid-40s, consulted a psychoanalyst with a very specific wish. He wanted to recapture an elusive memory that seemed to be haunting his life. He was aware of bewildering states of unusual intensity, for which he sought a link in a forgotten memory.

Hans felt that things had been going badly over the previous 15 years, since he had broken up with a woman with whom he had had a 10-year relationship. He had not established a stable relationship with a woman since. There were also psychosomatic complaints that bordered on the delusional—electricity running through his body, ringing in the ears, and a particular sensitivity to noise, especially sirens. If ever he found himself at the scene of an accident, he felt compelled to speak to the injured person, to apologize for not being able to save his or her life. He could not bring himself to touch a pistol, felt unable to concentrate or read, and was aware of a fear of knowing that jeopardized his professional successes.

Hans had been born in 1938 to a Protestant family in a little town in eastern Germany. When he was six, Hans was hospitalized for a mysterious disease, later diagnosed as typhoid or meningitis. The most important and enigmatic figure in his recollections of the hospital was a Jewish female doctor from the nearby concentration camp Buchenwald. Her help in the hospital may have been needed because of the shortage of medical personnel. The boy and this doctor formed a special relationship, and she would spend hours talking to him. The girl he had sporadically dated for over a decade, as well as several of the women who had touched him emotionally, were all dark-haired and attractive like the Jewish doctor.

Toward the end of the second month of therapy, Hans confided that he felt he was close to the secret: The Jewish doctor had been killed, executed, and he was somehow responsible for that. He saw her lying down, her face covered with blood; a shot had been fired. Could he have mistakenly fired a pistol that was lying there, or somehow have pushed the hand of a German officer so that a pistol was fired?

In sessions that followed, the memory emerged more fully, with an unusual intensity of affect. Hans recalled an air-raid, with everyone taking cover in the basement. After the air raid, most of the people returned upstairs. Only he and the doctor had remained. The doctor had turned to him, said she would come back shortly, and left, but did not return. He walked into the adjacent room where she had gone, only to find her hanging from the ceiling. In panic he grabbed her body, trying to pull her down, screaming, "Auntie doctor, auntie doctor, please come down!" Perhaps this had been the final blow to her life, because in pulling, he might have choked her even more. Other personnel came running. One of the SS officers pulled out his pistol and shot her—perhaps she had still been alive? The little boy screamed and cursed the SS man, and had to be restrained. The image of sirens returned to him, together with images of being in an ambulance and of electric shocks. The analyst hypothesized that the electric shocks might have been administered in order to help him forget.

At this point in Hans's life, something began to change. He took a job caring for an old man, spending nights in the hospital, and attempted to address the man's depression. Fearing that the man might commit suicide, Hans removed the man's pistol, the first time he had touched a pistol since childhood. This successful attempt at saving somebody's life represented a movement beyond the fragments of behavior in which he would apologize to those injured in accidents. Having recovered the memory he had lost, its intrusive fragments no longer blocked Hans from pursuing his life. Many of his somatic symptoms receded at the same time. He was also able to start a relationship with a nurse in the hospital and thereafter broke off treatment.

Transference Phenomena

When unintegrated fragments from the past are enacted on the level of object relations, the survivor's "knowledge" is in the form of transference experiences. This form of knowing involves the grafting of isolated fragments of the past on to current relationships and life situations that become colored by these "memories." The fragmentary quality of these transplants is responsible for the resulting absurdity, inappropriateness, and distortions in present experience. As with the previous form of knowledge, there are degrees of meshing past with present, as well as degrees of self-knowledge about doing so. Transference reactions vary in intensity from the psychotic delusional state to the minipsychotic episode, to more classical neurotic transferences that involve retention of the observing ego (the individual is cognizant of the present but nevertheless views the present in light of the past). Thus, even if the survivor recognizes the irrationality of traumatic grafts, such grafts can continue to exert their influence, distorting reality according to past scripts. For detailed examples of such transferences, see Auerhahn, Laub, and Peskin (1993) and Laub and Auerhahn (1993).

Survivors may, at times, lead their lives in resonance with such transferences and attempt to have their children do the same. For example, self-discipline was often an absolutely necessary (if not sufficient) condition for survival in the Nazi concentration camps, where a shoelace tied incorrectly could mean death. Accordingly, obligations in the present may at times continue to be experienced as life-and-death matters, with consequences for superego functioning. Real life and real relationships do not possess the power to attenuate these imprints from the past, which insidiously spill into and permeate the present. Thus, the survivor's strong sense of obligation often contaminates leisure time. His or her sense of being driven is directly traceable to the concentration camp experience wherein failure or relaxation meant death. Likewise, separations continue to be experienced as final. This is a continuation of the inmates' attempts to stay together as a means of survival and human support under conditions where neither was possible. Children of survivors often inherit these messages, for example, that life is hard, one cannot experience pleasure, and families must stay together, without necessarily being able to trace these messages back to their parents' Holocaust experiences.

Overpowering Narratives

A sixth form of "holding" a traumatic experience does not involve derivatives that are enacted, but rather memories for which there is a more conscious knowing. The memory can be described and the event narrated. There is an "I" present—a person who remembers and relates to the experience that happened. This "I," or internal witness, holds the experience together and synthesizes it into a narrative. The moment the fragment comes to mind, however, it breaks away from the narrator, obliterating or, at the very least, obscuring the rest of current reality. The individual loses perspective: He or she is in the experience once again; he or she is the same age again. The narration occurs without emotional or rational perspective, without the sense of "I have lived through that x number of years ago, when I was a particular age, with particular people, and had particular wishes." The memory is timeless, the image frozen. Instead of interacting with current life, as in the previous form of traumatic memory, an overpowering narrative obliterates or obscures it. In transference phenomena, a derivative (not even a memory) is reenacted, rather than remembered, and infuses the rest of the individual's life through symptoms. The present form does consist of a memory, one that, however, crowds current reality out and occupies a great deal of psychological and emotional space. The individual is stuck with images and affect with which he or she cannot cope. He or she may stop such images in their tracks when pursuing daily life, so that they do not interfere. At night, however, during sleep, they assume a life of their own, appearing in regularly recurring nightmares that are not only remembered in vivid detail but also affectively color the day that follows. For instance, many Holocaust survivors retain memories of their last moments with loved ones from whom they were separated and fantasize last moments before those others were killed. These memories and fantasies remain compelling and painfully ever present, obscuring or obliterating the present. Survivors will often shift to the present tense when narrating these memories, which are regarded by some researchers (e.g., Shoshan, 1989, p. 193) as standing at the center of survivors' trauma and as being the memories that are "the most preserved." The continuous mourning evoked by these unworked-through memories often is replaced, in survivors' children, by a longing and nostalgia that is similar to a depressive state (Shoshan, 1989). These memories of final separations, from which survivors cannot find comfort, are often reevoked at moments of separation from their own children, at times causing both generations to dread separations and regard them as potentially final.

Particularly gruesome events such as public executions or acts of cannibalism have such staying power that they obliterate the survivor's sense of living in the present. These unintegratable memories endure as a split-off part, a cleavage, in the ego. Ever greater amounts of energy are required to maintain ego functions, until real life becomes a fringe phenomenon around the nucleus of the trauma. Some survivors of massive psychic trauma show a great deal of achievement in their professional lives, amassing wealth, substantial personal acclaim, and social status. But they experience it all as insubstantial. If one talks to them, one finds that there is no sense of enjoyment, no full sense of living. They are absorbed in the nightmare that they find at the center of it all. Indelible memories create a kind of parallel life.

Life Themes

A seventh form of knowing is that of living out life themes. Just as fragments move into transference phenomena, overpowering narratives are enacted as life themes, wherein a more complex degree of personality organization and sublimatory processes form a nucleus for one's identity and striving. Memory in the form of an overpowering narrative is transformed to the level of life themes when a degree of distance from the traumatic event is established, and when there is less immersion in the concrete details of the trauma. As opposed to the multiplicity of different transferences that might occur from fragments, a life theme tends to be unitary, an organizing principle that becomes the center of an individual's personality. It takes the form of an organizing principle around which relationships and aspirations find their place. It is like a center of gravity for the direction or course the individual's life takes. The individual limits and shapes his or her internal and interpersonal life according to the life theme, which is often not only played out in relationships (as are transferences) but can also become a cognitive style. Thus, life themes involve a unique personality configuration, deriving from the particular way that the individual perceived and distilled his or her traumatic legacy. Transference repetitions, in contrast, involve bombardment of unintegrated percepts of the past without necessarily entailing a theme. Transference phenomena may be seen as roughly analogous to the role of plots in a novel, whereas a life theme is more analogous to the overall theme of a novel.

Life themes enacted in close relationships are often found in children of Holocaust survivors. An example of an adaptive life theme is the tendency in children of survivors to become mental health workers—they have an interest in secrets, and a need to decode them and help those who suffer from them. An example of a negative life theme is the sense of futility involving human relationships in general, and verbal communication in particular, that characterizes some second-generation individuals. For these people, the events of the Holocaust could never be fully articulated or shared and, therefore, there could be no hope for ever achieving real intimacy. The issue of communication (literally, knowing another and ultimately knowing oneself) thus becomes a focal theme for many children of survivors (Danieli, 1985; Peskin et al., 1997).

David was a 30-year-old college graduate who lived in his father's home and worked in the family butcher store, where he performed common labor. His father's life was a replica and continuation of the concentration camp he had helped to build as a foreman: It consisted of hard labor without any leisure, holiday, or pleasure of any kind, except for pride and security in the ability to outwit and manipulate "the system," and emphasis on material possessions, acquisitions, and worldly achievements. Defenses—particularly disavowal of feeling—were continued, as the father evidenced contempt for human contact and Jewish tradition, and attempted not to feel anything but, instead, to work only, mimicking a machine that obeyed orders to produce, as he had once done in the camp. Only on the High Holy Holidays did he come alive, as he might once have been, when he chanted the ancient religious prayers and allowed himself to feel affect within the only world that still seemed right—that of the *shtetl* (the vanished Jewish communities in Eastern Europe).

David begrudgingly submitted to his father's grip on him, affected through his father's threats of suicide and death, and had neither friends and interests, nor hobbies. Like his father, David could not permit himself to feel or experience anything. For David, coming alive—in Jewishness, in relationships—was dangerous, as it risked going crazy, the imagined consequence of the abandonment of constriction or of religiosity. Without control, David imagined that all regulation of affect might be lost. To permit a range of feelings might necessitate experiencing overwhelming murderous or suicidal feelings. To think, he feared, would necessarily lead to action, especially, to the committing of mass murder. Defenses against the loss of control were obsessive rituals (e.g., having to remember broadcasts and names), inhibitions, phobias, and somatizations, as well as physical limitations (e.g., difficulties focusing, and difficulties walking due to pains in his knee).

At one point during college, David attempted to abrogate his religiosity overnight: He removed his *yarmulka* (skull cap), took a non-Jewish girl out on a date to a non-kosher restaurant, kissed her passionately, and attended a church concert with her. He subsequently became extremely anxious, afraid that he would have uncontrollable feelings and lose his sanity. He proceeded to take LSD; during the trip he experienced a range of feelings that he could not put into words because of their exquisite beauty and intensity. He felt totally alone in facing his inner life. By abrogating religion, he felt that he had lost the only intimate friend he had had—his personal God to whom he could pray and who would always respond. He withdrew from his frightening "nervous breakdown" into the aforementioned constricted lifestyle. Becoming aware of and knowing his own feelings and experiences, separate from those prescribed by his father as part of a special bond between them, constituted a transgression David could not commit for fear of losing the only bond that existed for him to another human being.

Witnessed Narratives

An eighth form of traumatic memory involves witnessing, in which the observing ego remains present as a witness. On this level, knowing takes the form of true memory. When the individual narrates on this level, there is a distance, a perspective retained by the observing ego. The ego is present and understands itself to be continuous with the remembered subject but currently at a different stage. The memory is very vivid but not immediate. An "I" remains present—there is a person who remembers and relates not only to the experiences that are recalled but to the experience of remembering as well (e.g., see Auerhahn & Laub, 1984; Laub & Auerhahn, 1993).

Trauma as Metaphor and More

A ninth form of knowing trauma is the use of the imagery and language of massive psychic trauma as metaphor and vehicle for developmental conflict. This form of traumatic memory parallels the witnessed narrative to the extent that the distance between event and witness is preserved, yet goes beyond (but paradoxically never reaches) the previous level of knowing in that an element of play vis-à-vis the event enters, enabling the event's use as a metaphor that has some latitude. The imagery of trauma becomes more conscious, colorful, plastic, and variable than that found in the other levels of knowing. It readily appears in free associations and in dream associations, and does not have to be inferred or drawn out from ingrained silent modes of action. There is a disengagement from the event and its legacy as the individual chooses only those aspects of the event that reverberate with his or her internal conflict. The developmental conflict, rather than the event, is paramount and is the moving force behind the search for an appropriate vehicle for expression; that is, the motive for this form of traumatic memory comes more from a need to organize internal experience than, as with the previous forms, from a need to organize the external historical reality.

Nevertheless, traumatic imagery is not without its impact on how developmental conflict resolves as well as how psychic structure emerges. Once a particular developmental conflict is expressed in the imagery of atrocity, it is altered by dint of the particular metaphor used. Thus, inner reality both shapes the ultimate assimilation of such events and is, in turn, shaped by it. Major historical acts of genocide and atrocity leave their imprint on the quality and resolution of infantile conflict. The following case example is presented to illustrate not only the use of the Holocaust as metaphor, but also especially the manner in which such use may organize the intrapsychic life of an individual.

Gail, a 33-year-old married mother of two, entered analysis suffering from periods of depression, guilt, and phobic inhibition. The classical unfulfilled and unfulfillable love story dominated the clinical picture. She was the only daughter of a Jewish family that was affected, albeit indirectly, by the Holocaust. Most of the paternal grandparents' extended families (siblings, cousins, uncles) had perished in Europe during World War II. Her father, though professionally accomplished, yielded to her mother in everything, sacrificing his ties to Judaism and to his orthodox parents. The daughter felt both intensely part of and cruelly deprived of Judaism's genuine customs and traditions, and yearned for the Jewish heritage that she considered to be her secret prohibited tie with her father.

A "forbidden" romance occurred in late adolescence with a boyfriend who was Jewish. He was the son of an immigrant, nonassimilated family, studying the same profession as her father's and ideologically committed to Zionism, Jewish history, and, in particular, the study of the Holocaust. This cherished romance was ended after less than a year by the boyfriend's death, emphasizing for Gail the forbidden and fated nature of such a relationship, and indeed of all love relationships, and reinforcing her unconscious choice as well as sense of destiny to remain banned, outside, and unaccomplished in her family and career.

It is of interest to follow the vicissitudes of the transference neurosis in this patient. Castration themes made their appearance as early as the first week of analysis in Gail's response to the new analytic situation. These took the form of vividly imagined Holocaust atrocities. Gail was tied to the couch and the analyst was a Nazi surgeon who was going to perform an abortion on her—chop her body into pieces and flush it down the toilet. The air flowing from the air-conditioning system was the poison gas of a gas chamber. This theme found expression in an early screen memory of a tonsillectomy, an operation in which her father was present and slowly faded away in "a green mist." Much later on, Gail called this "my Auschwitz." She later used the same term for her grandfather's death. He was a beloved, benign, protective male figure for whom she was in a chronic state of mourning, thus holding onto him and avoiding heterosexual contact. This compromise solution practiced in fantasy and in life took the form of a transference resistance in her analysis. She quickly withdrew from her initial perception of the analyst as the Nazi surgeon and came to see him as the reincarnation of some of the previous men in her life—her loving, protective, benign grandfather or the romantic boyfriend, who died so early. Her grandfather, boyfriend, and, on a certain level, her father, too, were seen as afflicted, dying men—well-intentioned and caring, yet smitten by death, disease, or life circumstances.

The transference relationship quickly assumed the same tenor. The analyst was seen as a secluded, forlorn figure, isolated from the mainstream of successful, battling professionals. Expressions of mourning and guilt for not having cared enough for him or even for having harmed these damaged men in her life were prevalent in the first 2 years of the analysis. In the first year, Gail once arrived in tears with a newspaper clipping in which a panel was announced, at which Holocaust survivors were going to speak of their experiences. Her analyst was among the panelists. She "had known it all along"; indeed, her unspoken fantasies of him had always been that he was carrying the scars of having escaped the gas chambers and ovens. While compassionately wanting to protect her "analyst–victim," she was doing her best to extract equal protection from him and thus have a mutual bond sealed forever. It is this phenomenon that we recognize as her particular transference resistance. Her attempt to forge a mutually protective, nurturant relationship with a man in a world colored and besieged by savage Holocaust imagery metaphorically expressed, effectively silenced yet nevertheless gave a specific, original stamp to her own internal conflict that centered around her lifelong sense of herself having been injured and castrated, as well as her own feelings of envy and repudiated vengeful and castrating wishes. To meet men in a real world—"a leap into a sea full of sharks" in which she experienced herself as a shark also—was the more dreadful because it was imbued with imagery of real atrocities the patient had known about as a child. The model for identification in such a world was either the butchered, bloody victim or the victorious, sadistic Nazi, who left behind him a trail of blood, infirmity, and destruction—both equally repellent. Therefore, whenever confronted with men and her own feelings toward them, she always withdrew into the "caring for the victim" stance. It was irrelevant whether she was victim or caretaker herself.

In many ways, this account sounds like a young woman's Oedipal dilemma, couched in prevalent events of history that lent themselves to metaphorical use: a secret, mutual adoration between daughter and father assuming the content of a secret ethnic and religious bond. The conflict and prohibition against this internally forbidden, secret love tie were projectively experienced as a possessive, jealous, destructive witch–mother–camp guard and a seductive, yet, in the last resort, withholding father who perhaps offered and teased but ultimately kept his treasures to himself. The basic question is whether such themes went beyond providing appropriate content to the time-honored developmental conflicts—whether the metaphor acquired a life of its own, subtly changing the actual objects and processes it stood for and producing structural changes. Can external reality change the contemporary unconscious, even while that unconscious makes use of reality to deal with its own conflicts (Appy, 1988)?

Action Knowledge

The deepest level of traumatic knowledge is perhaps the level of action knowledge, in which knowing becomes consciously consequential and thus determines subsequent action. Knowing on this level entails knowing not only the facts but also what to do with those facts (Laub & Auerhahn, 1985). An example of such knowledge is to be found in a little-known demonstration in Berlin in March 1943, of Christian women whose husbands were Jewish. At that time, there were 10,000 Jews living legally in Berlin, 8,000 of whom were employed by the armament industry. Two thousand of these individuals were the husbands of Christian women. In order to give the Fuhrer a birthday present, it was decided to make Berlin *Judenrein*—to send all 10,000 Jews to Auschwitz. Hundreds of Christian wives of Jewish men and their children began to demonstrate in front of Rosengarten Platz, where the men had been gathered. When the Gestapo threatened to start shooting, they dispersed, only to return day after day, until every one of the 2,000 men was released, including 25 who had already been sent to Auschwitz. Herein we have an example not only of individuals who knew both the fate of the Jews and their own ability to act and to say "no," but also an example of an act of resistance that has been forgotten by historians, perhaps because it challenges bystanders' claims not to have known and not to have had choices.

A second example of action knowledge is told by Peter Steinbach, a historian of German resistance, about his own father, who had been a middle-class police officer in Germany when World War II started. This story stands in direct contrast to the earlier one, discussed as an example of the use of screen memories, about Rolf and his family. The elder Steinbach enlisted in the army and was transferred to the Eastern front, where he promptly landed in the hospital due to illness. In the bed next to him lay an SS officer who was seriously wounded, and who was hallucinating about his involvement in mass shootings. Steinbach became extremely agitated and distraught, and secured a transfer to Norway, where he spent the rest of the war. After the war, the father, unlike most other German fathers, told his son about his war experiences and stated, "These were my choices. I wasn't heroic and I wasn't a great guy, but at least I didn't shoot Jews on the Eastern front. Now we have to live with what I did and didn't do" (Sa'adah, 1995). Not only had father known, during the war, what the Nazis were doing and what his choices were, but also, after the war, he was able to recognize the ways in which he had and had not compromised himself. This knowledge allowed for a dialogue with his son (underscoring for us the connection between knowing and telling; see Laub & Auerhahn, 1985) and, we suggest, allowed his son to pursue historical knowledge both personally and professionally as a student of the German resistance; that is, in the second generation, the erection of defenses against knowing trauma can result in the development of deficits with regard to other forms of knowledge, as we saw in the case of Rolf (in the section on screen memories), whose failure to acknowledge his father's culpability served as an impediment in his pursuit of academic and personal knowledge, as well as the case of David (in the section on life themes) who, like Rolf, neither knew what he felt nor could tolerate another knowing him intimately.

IMPLICATIONS FOR HEALING

Our focus in this chapter has been on what kind of intergenerational knowledge of trauma is possible. We believe that there are many levels of remembering and preserving the horror of atrocity, all of which range along a continuum of differences in the degree of presence of an observing ego and its synthetic functions. When ego functions preserve their integrity, and when defensive operations, although stretched, are still effective, the knowledge of massive trauma can be screened out through total repression or through relegation to dissociative states. When ego functions break down in their defensive capacity, phenomena of depersonalization, derealization, and nonreceptivity to experience set in. Percepts penetrate the stimulus barrier nevertheless and regain access to consciousness in a variety of ways, according to the balance between the power of the experience and the ego's capacity to deal with it. When the balance is such that the ego cannot deal with the experience, fragmentation occurs. Hence, the registration of massive psychic trauma predisposes the ego to a nonintegration of fragments. The most tangible form of knowing trauma is, in its crudest, undigested, and unassimilated version, like a split-off foreign body, casting a perpetual shadow on life events and therapeutic trials. This is the form of knowing that tends to characterize the generation of victims.

Therefore, although none of the various forms of traumatic memory are mutually exclusive, and several may, to a greater or lesser degree, coexist in any particular individual at any given point in time, it is generally true that victims know mostly through retention of unintegrated memories or by reliving such memories in transference phenomena. Children of victims tend to know through particular themes that prove central to their identities and characters, and children of perpetrators tend to know through screen memories, whereas those not directly affected by massive psychic trauma know of it through experiencing their own conflicts and predicaments in its language and imagery. Any movement from level to level within one individual does not occur in a simple, progressively linear fashion. Instead of a distinct transfer from one form of knowing to the next, there is an opening up of the walls between forms. During the process of healing, the traffic between forms is increased, and the permeability of boundaries is enhanced. Fragments may shift toward overpowering narratives; overpowering narratives and transferences may be realized as witnessed narratives. Yet there are limits to such movement. For example, the use of traumatic schemes as metaphor cannot be found in victims to whom the trauma is too real to be used playfully, and too present and unresolved to lend itself to the function of defense.

It is precisely the limits of movement and healing within the generation of victims that at times propel the second generation to attempt to heal the first by completing the transformation from one form of knowing to another. We have encountered numerous children of survivors and of Nazis who have attempted to repair their parents' lives by eliciting testimonies or writing down the parents' histories. Many are journalists or therapists, engaged in professions that valorize the spoken word, knowing, and the telling of stories (i.e., the witnessed narrative) as ways to impact on others and/or heal [see *The Collective Silence: German Identity and the Legacy of Shame* (Bar-On, 1993) for examples of children of Nazis]. We have met other children of survivors and of Nazis who appear to belatedly be attempting to enact the actions compelled by Holocaust knowledge: They are activists in political and social movements, preventing a second Holocaust, as they see it, and retroactively responding to the first, impacting on the world by living out a kind of action knowledge. Yossi Klein Halevi, a child of a Holocaust survivor as well as a journalist and former member of the Jewish Defense League, depicts his once fanatical activism, in a recent (1995) memoir, as a direct response to his and his father's Holocaust knowledge. Such children would agree with Hallie's (1982) suggestion that perhaps it is only those who resist evil who truly know it. They have accepted as their life theme the belief that traumatic knowledge is not neutral; it compels reaction and impels to action.

MODES OF TRANSMISSION

We would like to briefly address the question of modes of transmission of memory from one generation to the next. No doubt the pathways are multiple, complex, and mediated by numerous variables. Using a population of women who were sexually abused as children, Armsworth, Mouton, De Witt, Cooley, and Hodwerks (1993) and Stronck and Armsworth (1994) have researched the indirect effects of parents' childhood trauma on the second generation, specifically the manner in which parents' own traumatic past induces insecure attachment to their own mothers and disconnected, intrusive, and flawed parenting styles that result in insecure attachments in their own children. We have focused in much of our work (see especially Auerhahn & Laub, 1994; Auerhahn & Prelinger, 1983; Laub & Auerhahn, 1984, 1993; and Peskin *et al.,* 1997) on a second pathway of intergenerational effects, that of direct effects, or what is sometimes called *vicarious traumatization*—the fact that children both pick up on the defensive structures of traumatized parents and intuit the repressed, dissociated, and warded off trauma that lurks behind the aggressive and traumatic overtones that are found in adults' parenting styles. It is an irony of the PTSD literature that it is widely accepted that therapists working with victims of trauma will suffer vicarious traumatization (see such recent publications as Pearlman, 1995), yet the fact that a young child who cannot readily differentiate his or her boundaries from those of the parent on whom his or her life depends should pick up on the parent's warded off, dissociated, and trauma-tized self and be seriously impacted by identification is still in dispute (see Solkoff, 1992). We maintain that children of survivors are witnesses to the Holocaust—to a reality in which aggression surpassed anything predictable or even imaginable—for they cannot but be profoundly affected by it despite their, at times, outward silence, for their innermost psychological structures are shaken by Holocaust knowledge. Children of survivors can become chained to parents' versions of reality, which may become the matrix within which normal developmental conflict takes place. These children are less immediately constrained from giving expression to their parents' conflicted themes; their distance from the experience itself, as well as the compelling quality of their heritage, can make them inevitable spokesmen for it.

Parents who are survivors often convey Holocaust themes in nonverbal ways. All parents wish very much to raise and nurture their children, even while they also wish to have the children out of their way. Thus love and aggression, hate and adoration, are part and parcel of the normal vicissitudes of parenting for all of us. This is difficult enough for most parents. But for traumatized parents who have experienced in their bodies the consequences of unrestrained brutality, the fantasy of aggression is not something that they can comfortably allow as an outlet for frustration. The possibility of action is too real and threatening. Likewise, their child's normal expressions of aggression and hate resonate in traumatized parents with their own overwhelming and repressed rage at the same time that the aggression conjures up the rage of the perpetrator whose victims they came to be. Furthermore, children of survivors, like all children, must organize their own instinctual lives. In addition, they must organize the stories of atrocities and massive trauma to which they have been exposed. Indeed, children of survivors, stimulated by images of atrocity and murder, experience instinctual danger. Their parents' stories of violence, which are threatening and traumatizing per se, can become fused with the children's own aggression, as well as become screens onto which this aggression is projected, at the same time that these stories shape and organize the children's fantasies and instinctual lives. Thus, infantile aggression and sexuality, stimulated by parental care, can become fused with Holocaust content if Holocaust affect and imagery are evoked in that relationship. Children of survivors may sense that their very activities or even their own developmental steps reactivate the trauma of the parents, who often react to the children's aggression as well as to their individuation and separation with Holocaust-related imagery and intensity, supporting the children's identification with victimizers by making them feel that their feelings and legitimate needs are murdering the parents (Danieli, 1985; Peskin *et al.,* 1997).

Furthermore, children's normative developmental needs and conflicts may reactivate parents' traumatic histories. A child's individuation and differentiation, as in the adolescent's normative departure from home, can be experienced by a parent as a devastating abandonment from which the parent cannot imagine recovering. We have encountered a number of survivors who could not cope when their children separated and became different from the dream of the reconstituted family the parents had lived for. Leah, the survivor mentioned in the section on not knowing, provides an example. Leah had lost parents, siblings, and a "forgotten" baby boy during the Nazi Holocaust. Upon rejoining her husband after liberation, she was unable to get pregnant and so adopted a baby boy, following which she did become pregnant and gave birth to a girl. The little boy became the center of her new life. She found in him an intimate companion and confidante. During adolescence, the boy became involved in drugs and petty crime. Leah felt devastated and betrayed. She wondered what she could have done wrong. When the son, as an adult, single-handedly engaged in a campaign against co-workers who made anti-Semitic remarks, he experienced this as directly linked to fighting his mother's battles (a form of action knowledge). He could not understand why she did not perceive him as continuing her legacy, especially later, when he became an orthodox Jew and had nine children, raising them to be Talmudic scholars in an attempted recreation of the old *shtetl* as he imagined it. Taking things to the extreme, as children of survivors sometimes do, he became so observant that, as proscribed by ultra-Orthodox Judaism, he could not allow himself to touch Leah, because she was a woman and not his biological mother. Neither would he let his children stay in her house, because she did not keep kosher properly. For the son, this was his attempt to rebuild his mother's lost world, but for Leah, who had become more worldly and modern than her son, it was the straw that broke the proverbial camel's back. She endlessly mourned the otherness and estrangement of her son, who was not the same as her original child and her fantasy of him. The son who was to have restituted her vanished family was lost. Although he tried to negotiate with her a new and different relationship, she wanted little to do with him, refusing to accept him on any terms other than those that *she* had envisaged as a way of rebuilding the life that had been destroyed. She was inconsolable regarding her "second Holocaust" (Peskin *et al.,* 1997) and could accept no compromise. For his part, the son's fanaticism and adherence to ritual and the letter of the law precluded warmth and human contact with his mother, despite his love for her. He, too, felt alone and estranged, and believed that he could turn for a sense of connection only to God. He eventually practiced no profession and put all his trust in God to provide for his children. This further increased the rift from his mother, because the God he trusted so much had utterly failed her by letting her entire family perish. Ultimately, it was only through their mutual concern and love for these children, the third generation, that a very tenuous and conflicted connection between mother and son was maintained.

Not coincidentally, Leah's daughter became a journalist and married an assimilated Jewish American man who could not understand his wife's inability to psychologically take leave of her mother. The daughter felt continually forced to choose between mother and husband and, despite Leah's advice to get on with her life and cleave to her husband, could not tolerate her mother's pain of being left behind.

Thus, in Leah's case, a baby was erased and then unconsciously compared against and searched for in a son (the second generation) who was found wanting in his ability to bring lost loved ones to life, while another child, a daughter, continually accepted the burden of filling her mother's void, even at the cost of her own individuation–differentiation. The anticipated birth of yet another (daughter's) baby (the third generation, as mentioned earlier in the section on not knowing) finally resurrected the forgotten memory of that first baby even while other children of the third generation (those of the adopted son) allowed for a partial reapproachment and reconciliation with the limits of substitution. Children and grandchildren can thus serve as reactivators of trauma even while they also serve (and offer themselves) as opportunities (and second chances) for healing (Danieli, 1994).

CONCLUSION

The child of traumatized parents who unknowingly labors against a received, devitalized life, often takes for granted that life's dimensions of time and space are shrunken and retracted from the start. As long as both generations do not discern that their life expectations are diminished by the trauma, they remain in the grip of that event. For, while survivors' double reality of horrific past and present life might contaminate and destroy the very essence of an average, expectable environment with the actuality of chronic foreboding, their children may all too unwittingly normalize the parents' agony by feeling life as expectably low keyed and attenuated. Generational continuity may be the most poignant and consequential casualty of this chronic inattention. We have sadly encountered numerous instances of children of traumatized parents who either consciously forsook their right to become parents, felt fated never to have families of their own, or gave up on the possibility of intimacy. In all these instances, they unconsciously accepted the victimizers' verdict of unfitness by relinquishing their birthright to join the natural order of generations (Danieli, 1985; Peskin *et al.*, 1997). It behooves those of us who are mental health professionals to prevent the perpetuation of trauma that deprives the next generation of its right to a life of its own because of the misfortunes that befell the first. We must combat the impact of trauma that, by the use of brutal force, has become reality for survivors and, by mechanisms of repetition and reenactment, has been carried into the memories of the next generation.

REFERENCES

Appy, G. (1988, May). *The meaning of "Auschwitz" today.* Paper presented at the 4th annual Conference of the Sigmund Freud Center of Hebrew University, Jerusalem.

Armsworth, M., Mouton, S., De Witt, J., Cooley, R., & Hodwerks, K. (1993, October). *Survivors as mothers: Intergenerational effects of incest on parenting abilities and attitudes.* Paper presented at the 9th annual meeting of the International Society for Traumatic Stress Studies, San Antonio, TX.

Auerhahn, N. C., & Laub, D. (1984). Annihilation and restoration: Post-traumatic memory as pathway and obstacle to recovery. *International Review of Psycho-Analysis, 11,* 327–344.

Auerhahn, N. C., & Laub, D. (1987). Play and playfulness in Holocaust survivors. *Psychoanalytic Study of the Child, 42,* 45–58.

Auerhahn, N. C., & Laub, D. (1990). Holocaust testimony. *Holocaust and Genocide Studies, 5,* 447–462.

Auerhahn, N. C., & Laub, D. (1994, November). *The primal scene of atrocity: Knowledge and fantasy of the Holocaust in children of survivors.* Paper presented at the 10th annual meeting of the International Society for Traumatic Stress Studies, Chicago, IL.

Auerhahn, N. C., Laub, D., & Peskin, H. (1993). Psychotherapy with Holocaust survivors. *Psychotherapy, 30,* 434–442.

Auerhahn, N. C., & Prelinger, E. (1983). Repetition in the concentration camp survivor and her child. *International Review of Psychoanalysis, 10,* 31–46.

Ballard, J. G. (1984). *Empire of the sun.* New York: Simon & Schuster.

Bar-On, D. (1993). Holocaust perpetrators and their children: A paradoxical morality. In B. Heinmannsberg & C. J. Schmidt (Eds.), *The collective silence: German identity and the legacy of shame* (pp. 195–208). San Francisco: Jossey-Bass.

Bergmann, M., & Jacovy, M. (1982). *Generations of the Holocaust.* New York: Basic Books.

Bohleber, W. (1994, December). *Fragments of an analysis of the son of a Nazi concentration camp physician.* Paper presented at the meeting of the American Psychoanalytic Association, New York.

British Broadcasting Company, producers. (1994). *Children of the Third Reich.*

Danieli, Y. (1984). Psychotherapists' participation in the conspiracy of silence about the Holocaust. *Psychoanalytic Psychology, 1*(1), 23–42.

Danieli, Y. (1985). The treatment and prevention of the long-term effects of intergenerational transmission of victimization: A lesson from Holocaust survivors and their children. In C. Figley (Ed.), *Trauma and Its Wake* (pp. 295–313). New York: Brunner-Mazel.

Danieli, Y. (1994). As survivors age: Part I. *National Center for PTSD Clinical Quarterly, 4*(1), 1–7.

Fresco, N. (1984). Remembering the unknown. *International Review of Psycho-Analysis, 11,* 417–427.

Grand, S. (1995, November). *Illusions of innocence: Dissociative states in perpetrators of incest.* Paper presented at the 11th annual meeting of the International Society for Traumatic Stress Studies, Boston, MA.

Grinker, R. R., & Spiegel, J. P. (1945). *Men under stress.* Philadelphia: Blakiston.

Hallie, P. (1979). *Lest innocent blood be shed: The story of the village of Le Chambon and how goodness happened there.* New York: Harper & Row.

Hallie, P. (1982, November). Remarks at the Yale Conference on the Holocaust, Yale University, New Haven, CT.

Harel, Z., Kahana, B., & Kahana, E. (1988). Psychological well-being among Holocaust survivors and immigrants in Israel. *Journal of Traumatic Stress, 1,* 413–429.

Klein, D. (1991). History's memory hole. *Dimensions: A Journal of Holocaust Studies, 6,* 3.

Klein Halevi, Y. (1995). *Memoirs of a Jewish extremist: An American story.* Boston: Little, Brown.

Krystal, H. (Ed.). (1968). *Massive psychic trauma.* New York: International Universities Press.

Kundera, M. (1982). *The book of laughter and forgetting.* New York: Penguin. (Originally published 1978)

Langer, L. L. (1995). *Admitting the Holocaust.* New York: Oxford University Press.

Laub, D., & Auerhahn, N. C. (1984). Reverberations of genocide: Its expression in the conscious and unconscious of post-Holocaust generations. In S. A. Luel & P. Marcus (Eds.), *Psychoanalytic reflections on the Holocaust: Selected essays* (pp. 151–167). Denver: Center for Judaic Studies of the University of Denver and New York: Ktav Publishing House.

Laub, D., & Auerhahn, N. C. (Eds.). (1985). Knowing and not knowing the Holocaust. *Psychoanalytic Inquiry, 5,* 1–8.

Laub, D., & Auerhahn, N. C. (1985). Prologue. *Psychoanalytic Inquiry, 5,* 1–8.

Laub, D., & Auerhahn, N. C. (1989). Failed empathy—a central theme in the survivor's Holocaust experience. *Psychoanalytic Psychology, 6*(4), 377–400.

Laub, D., & Auerhahn, N. C. (1993). Knowing and not knowing massive psychic trauma: Forms of traumatic memory. *International Journal of Psycho-Analysis, 74,* 287–302.

Micheels, L. J. (1985). Bearer of the secret. *Psychoanalytic Inquiry, 5,* 21–30.

Pearlman, L. A. (1995). *Trauma and the therapist: Countertransference and vicarious traumatization.* New York: W. W. Norton.

Peltz, R. (1994, April). In the shadow of the empty core: Survival through bearing witness. Opening remarks, panel presentation at 14th annual meeting of Division 39 of the American Psychological Association, Washington, DC.

Peskin, H. (1981). Observations on the First International Conference on Children of Survivors. *Family Process, 20,* 391–394.

Peskin, H., Auerhahn, N. C., & Laub, D. (1997). The second holocaust: Therapeutic rescue when life threatens. *Journal of Personal and Interpersonal Loss, 2,* 1–25.

Roseman, S., & Handleman, I. (1993). Modeling resiliency in a community devastated by man-made catastrophes. *American Imago, 49,* 185–226.

Roth, P. (1988, February 28). A talk with Aharon Appelfeld. *New York Times Book Review,* pp. 1, 28–31.

Sa'adah, A. (1995, July). Remarks at the Coming Home from Trauma Conference organized by the International Trauma Center at Yale University, Bailey Farms, NY.

Sereny, G. (1995). *Albert Speer: His battle with truth.* New York: Knopf.

Shoshan, T. (1989). Mourning and longing from generation to generation. *American Journal of Psychotherapy, 43*(2), 193–207.

Solkoff, N. (1992). Children of survivors of the Nazi Holocaust: A critical review of the literature. *American Journal of Orthopsychiatry, 62,* 342–357.

Solomon, Z. (1995). Oscillating between denial and recognition of PTSD: Why are lessons learned and forgotten? *Journal of Traumatic Stress, 8,* 271–282.

Stronck, K., & Armsworth, M. (1994, November). *Intergenerational transposition of disturbances to the self and quality of attachment relationships between mothers with a history of trauma and their adult children.* Paper presented at the 10th annual meeting of the International Society for Traumatic Stress Studies, Chicago, IL.

von Schlippe, G. (1993). "Guilty!" Thoughts in relation to my own past: Letters to my son. In B. Heinmannsberg & C. J. Schmidt (Eds.), *The Collective Silence: German Identity and the Legacy of Shame* (pp. 209–226). San Francisco: Jossey-Bass.

Whiteman, D. (1993). Holocaust survivors and escapees—their strength. *Psychotherapy, 30,* 443–451.

2

Transgenerational Transmission of Effects of the Holocaust
The North American Research Perspective

IRIT FELSEN

Over the past three decades, since the publication of the first article (Rakoff, Sigal, & Epstein, 1966) suggesting the transmission of effects of the Holocaust traumata to the second generation, several hundred articles and dozens of doctoral dissertations have been written on this topic. Clinical reports suggest special characteristics of children of survivors, and particular problems in the relationships between children and parents in survivor families, supporting the hypothesis of intergenerational transmission of Holocaust trauma. Empirical studies, on the other hand, have rendered a much less consistent view. Many of the early empirical works have been criticized (Solkoff, 1981) for biased samples, lack of control groups, reliance upon anec- dotal data, and presumption of psychopathology. Studies conducted during the past 15 years have remedied many of these methodological flaws. Most importantly, the number of controlled studies significantly increased after the 1970s, and the focus shifted onto nonclinical samples drawn from the generational population.

This chapter presents a review of the findings of empirical, controlled studies of North American, nonclinical samples of Holocaust offspring (HOF), including not only published articles but also an extensive list of over 30 unpublished doctoral dissertations. A conceptual framework is proposed, which organizes and unifies the diverse empirical observations regarding cognitive-affective, interpersonal, and defensive styles among HOF, and offers possible explanations for the discrepancies between clinical reports and empirical studies.

REVIEW OF THE EMPIRICAL RESULTS

Sigal (1973) summarized the paradigm of transgenerational transmission, which posits that parents, having experienced similar deprivation, subsequently developed similar distorted practices for human relations. These distorted capacities would be displayed, in the course of

---

IRIT FELSEN • Jewish Family Service of Metrowest, Mountain Lakes, New Jersey 07046

International Handbook of Multigenerational Legacies of Trauma, edited by Yael Danieli. Plenum Press, New York, 1998.

rearing their children, in the form of specific parent–child relationships, which would then result in specific and defined behavioral and experiential outcomes common to their children. Each of the three elements of this paradigm has been empirically investigated: the identification of the nature and specificity of the survivors' traumatization, the search for specific child-rearing practices associated with particular intrafamilial parent–child relationships in survivor families that could be postulated as the vehicle of intergenerational transmission, and the search for subsequent similarities in behavioral and experiential characteristics of HOF.

An important distinction has been made (Kendler, 1988; Schwartz, Dhorenwend, & Levav, 1994) between two different types of transmission of personality traits and psychiatric disorders. In "direct and specific" transmission, children learn to behave and think in disordered ways similar to those of their parents, resulting in higher rates among the children for the same disorders suffered by the parents. In "non-direct and general" transmission, the problems of the children are due to the parents' disorders, not through modeling and learning, but due to the disorder causing the parent to have difficulties in parenting. The parents' disorder thus causes a global deficit in the children that may underlie many types of psychiatric disorders, not necessarily the same ones with which the parents are affected.

The assessment of the degree of parental traumatization, and its effects among HOF, is presented first. This is followed by a review of empirical studies that explored direct transmission of symptoms of the Survivor Syndrome, and then those that investigated evidence of indirect transmission of effects related to the Holocaust.

Degree of Parental Traumatization

Considerable heterogeneity existed before the war among the survivors in aspects such as socioeconomic status, education, and occupational skills. There was also great heterogeneity in the traumatic experiences themselves and the interactions of specific Holocaust experiences with pre- and postwar conditions are further sources of variability among survivors (Klein, Zellermayer, & Shanan, 1963; Solkoff, 1981). Despite this heterogeneity, certain psychological features have been universally observed to characterize survivors, and have been demonstrated to be relatively independent of pre- and postwar personality characteristics. The clinical entity typical of this population, dubbed the "Survivor Syndrome," is characterized by the persistence, to varying degrees, of multiple symptoms, among which prevail chronic depressive and anxiety reactions, guilt, unresolved mourning, agitation, insomnia, nightmares, and far-reaching somatization (Eitinger, 1961; Niederland, 1968).

Operational quantification of the severity of the survivors' traumatization has been demonstrated to be extremely complex. Many studies use "categories" to quantify traumatization (the categories typically being concentration camp inmates, labor camp survivors, those who were n the ghetto, those who were in hiding, and those who were in the resistance). However, there is no universal agreement concerning the relative severity of traumatization for these categories. Some studies (Kanter, 1970; Klein *et al.,* 1963) found survivors who had been in hiding to have been most adversely affected. Sigal and Weinfeld (1989) found that the most severe consequences were observed for the concentration camp experience. On the other hand, Alexandrowicz (1973) found no differences between survivors of concentration camps and those who escaped to the U.S.S.R., consistent with the clinical observations of Winik (1968).

These contradictory observations suggest that these categories might not give an accurate measure of individuals' traumatic experience and its subsequent long-lasting effects on the survivors themselves. Perhaps it is not surprising, therefore, that, although there is some empirical support suggesting that the severity of adverse effects in HOF is indeed related to the degree of parental traumatization, there are inconsistent reports as to the relationship between specific categories of parental Holocaust experiences and effects in the children. Lichtman (1983) found that children of survivors who had been in hiding showed higher scores on paranoia, anxiety, and hypochondriasis than did other HOF, and Sigal and Weinfeld (1989) found that they were overrepresented in their subsample of HOF who sought psychotherapy. However, Magids (1994) found no differences in personality characteristics measured by the Sixteen Personality Factors Questionnaire (16-PF) between 50 children of hidden child survivors and 50 controls. Wanderman (1980) found essentially no differences between 70 children of concentration camp survivors, 29 other HOF, and 32 children of refugees with regard to difficulties in separation–individuation or the polarization in the perceptions of parents. Gross (1988) observed a "trend" (no statistical data were given) among 108 HOF for higher parental traumatization to be related to higher group dependence in sons, whereas low traumatization was related to higher self-sufficiency in daughters. However, no correlations were observed between the severity of traumatization and the children's perceptions of their parents' parenting styles. Similarly, Weiss (1988), using the Cornell Parent Behavior Inventory, observed no differences in perceived parental child-rearing practices between children of concentration camp or labor camp survivors, other HOF, and children of refugees. Likewise, Sigal and Weinfeld (1989) found no differences between children of two concentration camp survivors and controls.

Klein *et al.* (1963) suggested that a more sensitive measure of traumatization would be achieved using specific determinants of oppression, among which they enumerated the destruction of family, slavery and isolation, emotional and social deprivation, chronic frustration, humiliation, insecurity, fear of death, disregard of personality, hunger, sleep deprivation, physical traumatization, and infectious diseases. It has been suggested (Eissler, 1963) that the most extreme traumatizing factor was that of experiencing the murder of one's own children. Several authors have attempted to explore the relationship between effects in HOF and specific determinants. Hammerman (1980) found only little support for a relationship between the number of relatives lost and identity development in HOF. Blumenthal (1981) found no relation between the number of surviving members of the parent's family of origin and effects in the children. Similarly, Schulman (1987) found that the number of relatives lost, number of surviving siblings, and length of internment were not relevant indicators of depression in HOF. In contrast, Goodman (1978) found that the length of internment in a concentration camp was on average twice as long for the parents of HOF who sought therapy as for parents of non-help-seeking HOF.

The age at which traumatization was experienced is considered another potential determinant of the severity of traumatization, following expectations from the literature that those survivors who experienced traumatization during adolescence would be particularly damaged (Danto, 1968; Fink, 1968; Grubrich-Simitis, 1981; Segall, 1974). Contrary to such clinical observations, it was found (Budick, 1985) that the children of survivors who had been adolescents during the war did not show poorer interpersonal adjustment and coping, nor greater narcissim, than other HOF or controls. Baron, Reznikoff, and Glenwick (1993), with 241 HOF and 109 controls, and using the California Psychological Inventory, O'Brien Multiple Narcissim Inventory, and Kobasa Hardiness Scale, concluded that their findings failed to support their prediction that early loss and having been younger during traumatization would be related to a higher degree of pathology and narcissistic injury in the children of such survivors. Similarly, Walisever (1995) found that HOF whose mothers lost their own mothers in the Holocaust did not differ in their attachment style from other HOF. In contrast, despite the lack of differences when comparing the entire sample of HOF with controls, Gertler (1986) found that HOF whose parents lost a spouse or child in the Holocaust exhibited significantly greater problems in aggression, compliance, dependency, and intimacy.

Another approach to the assessment of parental traumatization uses the children's perceptions thereof. Blumenthal (1981) found evidence for a relation between the children's perceptions of parental traumatization and psychopathology in the children. Lichtman (1983) observed significant correlations between the types of communication most frequently employed by the parents who had undergone the most severe traumatization (as perceived by their children) and all variables measuring personality traits in their children. Guilt-inducing communication, experiential nonverbal communication, and indirect communication were related significantly to characteristics among HOF such as paranoia, hypochondriasis, anxiety, and low ego strength. Schleuderer (1990), using the Millon Clinical Multiaxial Inventory-II (MCMI-II) found statistically significant correlations between the children's rating of their mother's traumatization and their scores on the Histrionic, Narcissistic, and Debasement Scales. However, the ratings of mothers in the midrange of traumatization were most related to effects in the children, a finding that raises questions about the accuracy of assessment of parental traumatization as it is reflected in conscious perceptions of their children.

The assessment of the effects of parental traumatization on the children is further complicated by the fact that the degrees of traumatization of both parents are relevant. Karr (1973) found (using Minnesota Multiphasic Personality Inventory (MMPI), Nettler Alienation Scale, Srole Anomie Scale, and the Brenner Scale of Jewish Identification) more adverse effects among children of two concentration camp or labor camp survivors in comparison to HOF with one survivor parent and to children of refugees. This observation supports the view (Sigal, Silver, Rakoff, & Ellin, 1973) that having one survivor parent and one who is not might mitigate the effects on the children. In contrast, Antman (1986) found no differences between HOF with two survivor parents and controls on self-actualization and self-esteem, whereas HOF with one survivor parent fared less well than these two groups, and Gertler (1986) found no differences in the quality of interpersonal adjustment between 62 HOF with two survivor parents, 36 HOF with one survivor parent, 37 children of Jewish immigrants, and 49 children of American-born parents.

There is considerable indication in the empirical literature that effects of parental traumatization on the children are related to the gender of the traumatized parent (Karr, 1973; Keller, 1988; Lichtman, 1984; Schulman, 1987). Lichtman (1984), using MMPI scales, Welsh's Scale of Anxiety, Baron's Scale of Ego Strength, Mosher Forced Choice Scale of Guilt, and Hogan's Empathy Scale, as well as a Communication Questionnaire developed by the author (Lichtman, 1983), found that the gender of the survivor parent, as well as that of the child, were important factors in determining the effects of Holocaust-related communication. Frequent, willing, and factual maternal communication about the Holocaust was related to higher paranoia, lower ego strength, and lower empathy in HOF. Paternal communication, on the other hand, was related inversely to depression and hypochondriasis among the children. Daughters of mothers who used more guilt-inducing communication scored significantly higher on anxiety, paranoia, and hypochondriasis, and had lower ego strength, whereas, for sons, exposure to maternal guilt-inducing communication was related only to higher educational achievements. Indirect communication by either parent was related significantly to depression, anxiety, paranoia, hypochondriasis, and lower ego strength in daughters, but to *lower* depression scores and higher incomes among sons. It would appear that female HOF were generally more adversely affected than males by their parents' traumatization and reacted with symptoms of withdrawal, fear, somatic complaints, and low self esteem (consistent with Karr, 1973).

Chayes (1987), in one of the few studies that assessed directly both survivors and their children, found that, consistent with clinical formulations that focus on the mother's role vis-à-vis the infant and child, a moderate relationship was observed between the mothers' emotional unavailability and overcontrol, and levels of pathology in HOF, whereas no such relationship was seen for fathers. Also, psychopathology in HOF was inversely related to the mother's level of mourning, indicating that unacknowledged mourning is related to greater pathology in the children. No relationship was observed between HOF's pathology and the father's level of mourning. In contrast, Schleuderer (1990) found that having a survivor father, regardless of his level of traumatization, was related to higher scores on rage-related MCMI-II subscales as well as Histrionic, Narcissistic, and Paranoid Scales. The author concluded that an important route of intergenerational transmission is the father, consistent with clinical observations (Danieli, 1982; Kestenberg, 1982) that the traumatization of the Holocaust contains an added degradation for male survivors, due to their "failure" to protect loved ones.

It has been suggested that the effects of traumatization can be better understood in the context of differential coping and adaptation styles, rather than by focusing on parameters of the traumatic experiences themselves. Danieli (1981, 1982, 1985) delineated four adaptational styles observed in her clinical work with families of survivors, which she termed "Numb," "Victim," "Fighters," and "Those Who Made It." The Numb were described as emotionally depleted by their exposure to trauma, unable to relate warmly to themselves or to others, and isolated from the community, tending to avoid affiliation even with other survivors. Victims were described as depressed, fearful of a recurrence of the traumatic events, and quarrelsome and guilt-inducing with others. Fighters adopt a confrontational, defiant stance in their dealings with the world, show intolerance of any sign of weakness in themselves or others, push themselves and those close to them to achieve, and are determined that no one should ever again experience what happened to them. Those Who Made It are successful socioeconomically and distance themselves from the traumatic events of the past and those with whom they experienced them. Danieli's description of the four adaptational styles encompasses most of the diverse (and sometimes contradictory) features reported as typical of various survivors and their children.

Empirical validation for Danieli's typology has been demonstrated in several studies. Rich (1982) developed a questionnaire and structured interview that differentiated among types of HOF consistent with Danieli's taxonomy. It was further suggested that "types produce types," because each parental type provides environmental opportunities that enhance, among the children, its own predominant typological components. Klein (1987), with a sample of 54 children of concentration camp or labor camp survivors, and using instruments that included the Defense Mechanism Inventory and the Symptom Checklist-90-R (SCL-90-R), suggested that the four family types may be organized along two dimensions. Victim and Those Who Made It were viewed as opposite ends of a continuum ranging from insulated to assimilated, whereas Numb and Fighter were seen to range from passive internalization to active externalization. Using this conceptualization, the defensive styles demonstrated by HOF were consistent with predictions, the Victim exhibiting projection, the Numb exhibiting turning against the self, and Those Who Made It using primarily intellectualization. The prediction that the Fighter would use turning against the object was not confirmed, as Fighters also used intellectualization. Finally, those in the Victim and Numb groups showed a higher level of symptom distress than the other types, taken as indicating that they were less effective in distancing themselves from their parents' trauma. Sigal and Weinfeld (1989) asked their subjects to rate each of their parents using adjectives and statements from Danieli's descriptions of the four types. Principal component analyses yielded the same four factors for fathers and mothers separately. Factor I was labeled Schizoid Personality, and Factor II, Paranoid Personality, corresponding, respectively, to Danieli's Numb and Victim. Factor III, labeled Depressive/Masochistic Personality, corresponded roughly to Danieli's Victim/Numb, and Factor IV was Type A/Normal Aggressive Personality, corresponding to Danieli's Fighter/Those Who Made It.

In summary, there are inconsistencies in the operationalization of the degree of parental traumatization. The definition of "survivorhood" itself varies quite widely; some studies restrict their sample to concentration camp survivors; others include all those who survived the Holocaust in Nazi-occupied territory; and still others even include all those who survived the war in Europe including the U.S.S.R. (Hammerman, 1980). Some define HOF status as having two survivor parents, others require only one, and not all provide a breakdown of the effects according to the gender of the survivor parent. Studies of HOF based on either categories of parental experiences or specific determinants of parental traumatization rendered inconsistent findings, suggesting that important aspects of the traumatization were not properly assessed. Conceivably, phenomena in the children's generation are different than those in the survivors and are not as directly related to types of determinants of traumatization. For HOF, the transmission and mitigation of effects seem to be also influenced by the parents' style of adaptation to trauma.

Direct Transmission of Survivor Syndrome Symptoms

Initial clinical observations (Barocas & Barocas, 1973; Sigal *et al.,* 1973) suggested the possibility of transmission to HOF of symptoms resembling those of the Survivor Syndrome. Thus, empirical studies looked for evidence in HOF of personality traits such as depression, anxiety, somatization, guilt, and problems in regulation of aggression. Rubinstein, Cutter, and Templer (1990) examined both children and grandchildren of survivors, using the MMPI and Templer's Death Anxiety Scale for the children, and the Louisville Behavior Checklist (completed by parents) and School Behavior Checklist (completed by teachers) for the grandchildren. HOF demonstrated greater psychopathology on the MMPI than did controls. Ratings of the third generation by their parents also indicated more pathology, with higher ratings than controls on fear, neurotic behavior, aggression, social withdrawal, and inhibition, findings supported by their ratings by teachers.

Contrary to these findings, controlled research has not, on the whole, supported expectations for a greater pathology in HOF. Leon, Butcher, Kleinman, Goldberg, and Almagor (1981) are among the few authors that assessed both survivors and their offspring. Participants completed the MMPI and versions of the Current Life Functioning Form (constructed for the purpose of the study). Although survivors scored lower on mental health than controls, no differences were observed between HOF and controls. Sigal and Weinfeld (1989) randomly sampled the general Jewish community using a Jewish name-identification procedure applied to the voter registration list in Montreal. Theirs was an unusually large sample, with 242 HOF subjects, 76 children of other Jewish immigrants, and 209 children of Canadian-born Jewish parents. Their sample is noteworthy also for its relatively high response rate (76% for HOF, 63% for children of immigrants, and 46% for children of native Canadians), in comparison to most other studies, which are typically around 50%. They found no differences between HOF and controls on the total score or the individual scales of the Psychiatric Epidemiological Research Instrument (PERI), and no evidence for higher proportion of deviantly high scorers among HOF. In addition, no differences were found between the groups on questions of whether they had experienced anxiety or depression in the preceding 12 months, or had contemplated suicide during that time or at any time in the past. HOF were less phobic than controls, and no differences were observed regarding dealing with death. The authors concluded that, contrary to most clinical reports, their analyses did not yield much evidence that HOF have greater difficulties than controls with the control of aggression, anxiety, depression, phobias, low self-esteem, or psychosomatic complaints. Sigal and Weinfeld did find an indication of a higher suicide rate among siblings of HOF (although they had fewer siblings than did controls). In light of the lack of other differentiating findings, the psychological context leading to a higher suicide rate among HOF is not clear, suggesting that the questions asked did not assess some relevant aspects of the experiences of HOF.

Although there is almost unanimous agreement that no psychopathology has been observed in HOF, there is considerable evidence for differences between HOF and controls regarding some of the manifestations of the Survivor Syndrome, including depression, anxiety, regulation of aggression, and somatoform complaints. It has been suggested that this characteristic pattern reveals a "Child of Survivor Complex" (Budick, 1985) which, unlike a syndrome, does not imply a pathological level of functioning but rather a psychological profile typical of HOF.

Studies revealed that HOF scored higher than controls on depression (Wanderman, 1980), anxiety (Lichtman, 1984, using the MMPI), and expression of anger, paranoia, and overall pathology as measured by the SCL-90-R (Lowin, 1983). Schwarz (1986) observed that a sample of 70 HOF scored significantly higher in symptomatology in comparison with the SCL-90-R test norms. Karr (1973), using MMPI-derived scales, found that HOF of two survivor parents tended to indicate difficulties in impulse control, a tendency toward depression and anxiety, and feelings of alienation from society. Kleinplatz (1980), with a North American sample of HOF and controls, and a parallel Israeli sample (with 16 subjects in each of the four groups), found no differences on individuation (consistent with Wanderman, 1980), whereas differences in expression of aggression and feelings of depression, alienation, and apathy indicated that controls were functioning better than HOF. Budick (1985), using the Personal Attitudes Inventory and a structured interview, found HOF to be significantly more hostile and less trusting than controls, and male HOF to be more anxious than male controls, whereas no differences were observed regarding depression. HOF also scored significantly higher on hypochondriasis, in contrast to Sigal and Weinfeld (1989), who observed that HOF were not more problematic than controls with respect to psychosomatic complaints.

Differences in other cognitive-affective variables associated with depression have been reported in studies in which HOF did not differ from controls in total depression scores. Blumenthal (1981), using Baron's Ego Strength Scale, found HOF revealed frequent worries and fears, a reluctance to behave aggressively, and denial of aggressive impulses. HOF were also demonstrated to exhibit higher levels than controls of cognitive distortions associated with depression (Finer-Greenberg, 1987). Gertz (1986), with 47 HOF who belonged to an HOF support group, 64 other HOF, and 53 controls, saw evidence among HOF of guilt, fear, alienation, difficulty expressing emotions, Holocaust-related dreams, and a feeling that they are a replacement for a perished relative they never met, consistent with the phenomenon of "transposition" (Danieli, 1981; Kestenberg, 1982). Weiss, O'Connell, and Siiter (1986), using the Brief Mental Health Index, Nettler Alienation Scale, and Srole Anomie Scale, found that HOF scored higher than controls on guilt. Jurkowitz (1996), with 91 survivors, 91 HOF, and 91 grandchildren of survivors, concluded that there was evidence for transmission of depression, shame, and guilt across the three generations. Lovinger (1986), using projective and standardized instruments (including the thematic apperception test (TAT), Rosenzweig Projective Test, Defense Mechanism Inventory, Insolvable Puzzles, Multiple Affective Adjective List, and Moos Family Environment Scale) with 25 children of concentration camp survivors, showed that HOF projected more hostility than controls, were more likely to internalize aggression, reported feeling more depressed, were less expressive in communicating feelings, and less assertive and self-sufficient in making decisions.

In contrast, some studies failed to find evidence for transmission of salient symptoms of the Survivor Syndrome. Rustin (1971), comparing 77 children of concentration camp survivors and 77 controls using the Mosher Incomplete Sentence Test, Buss–Durkee Hostility–Guilt Inventory, and Brenner Scale of Jewish Identification, observed no transmission of guilt, hostility, or difficulties in the regulation of aggression. Similarly, Schleuderer (1900) found no differences between 100 HOF and 30 controls on MCMI-II scales measuring anxiety, somatoform, and dysthymic traits.

In summary, despite some inconsistencies, there does seem to be an accumulation of reports reflecting statistically significant differences between HOF and controls, albeit within the normative range of psychological functioning, demonstrating a common constellation of personality characteristics in HOF. The typical characteristics include a higher tendency to depressive experiences, mistrustfulness, elevated anxiety, difficulties in expressing emotions (especially hostile ones) accompanied by difficulties in the regulation of aggression, higher feelings of guilt and self-criticism, and a higher incidence of psychosomatic complaints.

Evidence for Effects of Indirect Transmission

Studies investigating transmission of indirect and nonspecific pathology examined the hypothesis that long-term effects of extreme traumatization lead to subsequent impairments in the survivors' capacity for parenting, which then exert cumulative traumatic effects (Khan, 1963) and lead to a variety of problems in the children. In addition to external difficulties following their liberation, many internal experiences of survivor parents, and especially mothers, could conceivably interfere with their capacity for cathecting and empathizing with their newborn babies. These factors could include excessive parental narcissim, massive pent-up impulses of hate and revenge seeking an outlet, as well as conscious and unconscious reservations against the cathexis of new objects, whether as a defense against repeated object loss or because, as a result of unresolved mourning, a great part of libidinal drives are not available (Grubrich-Simitis, 1981). A form of ego-regression in the survivors, referred to as "armoring of the ego," could be experienced by HOF as an inability to win their mother's interest in them, or as being of no value to her.

HOF have also been described as imbued with a variety of parental expectations that differ from the usual for parent–child relationships (Grubrich-Simitis; 1981; Levine, 1982; Rosenman, 1984; Sonnenberg, 1974), their identification with which leads to selective and premature ego development. A few of the "missions" described in clinical reports that HOF are expected to fulfill include serving as a bridge to life, replacing lost idealized love objects, acting out the parents' defensively warded-off hate, proving the failure of the persecutors' intentions to destroy a whole people, and being a solace to their parents. Communications of this kind from the parents are presumed to be organized in the mental life of HOF according to phase-specific drive wishes, ego needs, and anxieties, and to be particularly activated whenever conflicts involve separation–individuation, differentiation, rivalry, and working through of aggressive impulses, thus leading to impediments in separation–individuation and in identity formation in HOF.

The extreme emotional pain suffered by the survivors might also make it impossible for their children to fulfill "loyal obligations" to them (Boszormenyi-Nagy & Spark, 1973), since efforts to ease their pain might prove unsuccessful, and might be perceived by the children as reflecting their own failure rather than the parents' unresolved mourning and lingering depression. Although some Holocaust survivors might have had difficulty in meeting their children's emotional needs, others, who had lost their own parents in the Holocaust, might have focused all their attention on their children. The ensuing feeling in the children that their parents' total reason for being was for their (the children's) welfare might put great pressure on the children to meet unrealistic expectations. They might become overachievers, or they might just give up the quest to become something they cannot and be discouraged from pursuing academic as well as other achievements in life (Barocas & Barocas, 1979; Kestenberg, 1982).

From the perspective of structural family therapy (Minuchin, 1974), a useful parameter in evaluating family functioning is the clarity of boundaries within the family system. All families can be characterized according to their position on a continuum ranging from diffuse boundaries, typical of "enmeshed" families, to overly rigid boundaries, which typify "disengaged" families. Families of Holocaust survivors have been frequently characterized as enmeshed, due to features such as parental overvaluation of the children, overprotectiveness of the children toward their parents, and unclear boundaries between the spousal subsystem and the children. It was posited that the lack of differentiation discourages autonomous exploration and mastery of problems, thus inhibiting the development of cognitive-affective skills in the children. Overinvested parents might make it difficult for their children to grow emotionally and separate from them, as this would be perceived as disloyal in a family sensitive to loss. Hanover (1981) compared group means of 24 HOF and 20 controls on 18 dimensions of the Children's Report of Parental Behavior. Although no differences were observed between HOF and controls on the degree of autonomy or with regard to acceptance of individuation, HOF perceived both parents as exhibiting significantly greater possessiveness, as well as being more rejecting, intrusive, employing control through guilt, exercising hostile control, and practicing inconsistent discipline and withdrawal of relationship.

Several investigators who examined whether Holocaust families do indeed demonstrate higher degrees of enmeshment did not find evidence to support this notion. Zlotogorski (1983, 1985), using the Satisfaction with Well-Being Questionnaire and Washington University Sentence Completion Tests with 73 children of concentration camp or labor camp survivors and 68 controls, saw no significant differences between HOF and controls in levels of ego functioning in relation to perceptions of family cohesion and adaptability. The results indicated a great deal of variability in Holocaust families, who ranged from enmeshed to disengaged, as did controls, with the average survivor family characterized by structured separateness. Furshpan (1986), with 20 children of concentration camp survivors, 20 children whose parents had been in hiding, and controls, and using the Family Cohesion and Adaptability Scales and Family Structure Profile, did not find survivor families to exhibit greater enmeshment. In fact, children of concentration camp survivors, expected to be the most disturbed, perceived their families as "separated" or optimally functional. An unexpected result was that controls and children of concentration camp survivors scored similarly on perceived enmeshment, whereas the children of parents who had been in hiding scored higher than these groups. No differences were found between the HOF and controls on the level of family cohesion or the degree of satisfaction with it.

Weiss (1988) found no significant differences between survivor and control families in the degree of parental permissiveness. Sigal and Weinfeld (1989) asked their subjects to rate their parents as they saw them while they were growing up and at the current time, and how they would have preferred them to be. Male HOF reported their parents to be currently strict more often than did controls, and they also more often reported wishing their mothers would have been less strict in the past and less involved in their lives at present. Female HOF reported, more frequently than did controls, that their fathers had been too strict while they were growing up. The authors concluded that the observed differences suggest more difficulties with discipline in survivor families. Whereas the daughters and their fathers seem to have resolved these difficulties better, sons felt that their mothers were still currently too strict, suggesting that some issues related to the sons' autonomy had not yet been resolved. Overall, however, Sigal and Weinfeld concluded there was no support for the hypothesis that survivor families were more enmeshed than controls.

It had been pointed out (Schleuderer, 1990) that there is no evidence that differentially links the concepts of adaptability and cohesion (Olson, Sprenkle, & Russell, 1979) to separation and independence among offspring. Thus, although families of survivors were not generally observed to be more enmeshed, these observations do not preclude the possibility of difficulties in separation–individuation. Indeed, several studies that focused on the separation–individuation process and related variables found substantial evidence for differences between HOF and controls. Wanderman (1980) found that HOF reported significantly more difficulty in broaching with their parents the subject of moving out. Karr (1973) saw that HOF tended to live closer to their parents and demonstrated more unresolved ambivalence in their relationship with their parents. Whereas Schleuderer (1990) observed no differences between HOF and controls in the age at which they left home, and Shiryon (1988) found that leaving the parents' home for college was not reported to have been accompanied by difficulties, greater difficulties were reported by HOF at a later phase in their lives (mid- to late-20s) when conflicts around individuation peak with the need to make romantic, occupational, and other lifestyle choices. Similarly, Gertler (1986) observed that HOF tended to establish their own families later than did controls, supporting Shiryon's view that individuation might be accomplished later in the lives of HOF.

Wieder (1985), comparing 30 HOF with Jewish controls, observed support for the hypothesis that HOF would have the most difficulty with the differentiation process, followed by children of immigrants and then children of American-born parents. Rose and Garske (1987), comparing HOF with second-generation American Jews, non-Jewish children of Americans, and children of parents of non-Jewish Eastern European origin who survived the war as prisoners of war or in hiding, observed that HOF scored significantly lower than controls on feelings of independence and self-sufficiency on the Moos Family Environment Scale. Ofman (1981) saw that female HOF scored lower than all other subjects on autonomy and dominance, and higher on external locus of control and maternal overvaluation, but higher on boundary differentiation. For controls, the results were consistent with the prediction that parental overvaluation impedes differentiation in the children, whereas for HOF, overvaluation was positively and significantly correlated with boundary differentiation. Although the author concluded that this finding suggests a possible strengthening effect of parental Holocaust experiences on boundary differentiation, it would seem more consistent that it reflects in actuality an exaggerated and defensive emphasis on boundaries.

Felsen and Erlich (1990), comparing 32 HOF and 30 controls using the Tennessee Self-Concept Scale, observed less differentiation in the perceived identification of HOF with both parents on both the actual and the ideal, or ego and superego, levels. A higher degree of unresolved ambivalence in the identification of HOF with their parents was expressed in a relative rejection of identification with the mother (especially with her high self-criticism) and idealization of the father, which were not observed among noncontrols.

Karson (1989), using the Parental Relationship Inventory with 38 HOF and 40 controls, found HOF were significantly less well differentiated from their families of origin, perceived their parents as less able to respect boundaries between themselves and their children, and unable to focus on their own needs, investing their emotional energy in their children even after they leave home. HOF saw themselves as less able to maintain a sense of separateness from their parents and less autonomous, with concomitant difficulties in making their own decisions and placing their own needs before those of their parents. The mood surrounding the connection with parents was more angry and dysphoric for HOF, consistent with Karr's (1973) observations. The author concluded that the results offer evidence for perceived parental overinvolvement and for ambivalent dependency in HOF. Using the Bell Object Relations and Reality Testing Inventory, HOF demonstrated less developed object relations than controls and scored significantly higher on MCMI-II scales Borderline, Avoidant, Passive–Aggressive, and Self-Defeating Personality. Similarly, Lowin (1983), with 27 survivor families and 27 Jewish comparison families, found both survivors and HOF demonstrated significantly less mature overall levels of psychosocial development than controls and greater difficulties related to identity diffusion. Schleuderer (1990) found that HOF scored significantly higher than controls on MCMI-II scales measuring rage-related dynamics, mistrustfulness, suspiciousness, vigilance, and alertness to the possibility of betrayal. HOF also scored higher on Narcissism, interpreted as reflecting the incorporation of higher parental valuation into HOF's self-perceptions, and on the Histrionic scale, resulting from children's belief that parental love is contingent upon behaving in a certain way.

In summary, empirical studies provide substantial evidence that HOF experience greater difficulties than controls in the area of psychological separation–individuation. Although these difficulties have been unequivocally observed to be within the range of normal functioning and thus do not constitute a psychopathology, they bespeak a unique phenomenological experience with specific emotional and cognitive, as well as defensive and interpersonal, features.

Evidence for Patterns of Family Communication

Several studies examined the patterns of communication in survivor families, since depression in the survivors might be related to difficulties communicating about their wartime experiences, and effects in HOF might likewise hinder their capacity to acknowledge and communicate their own difficulties. Cahn (1987) examined the relationship between maternal communication and the children's symbolizing processes among 40 female HOF and 40 controls whose mothers were born in the United States. The instruments used included the Stroop Color Word Test, 5-minute monologues about a significant personal experience and about the mother's war experiences (or, for controls, a difficult experience in their mother's lives), a structured interview, and rating scales developed for the study to assess maternal communication. Some of the most salient findings showed that, although there were no differences between the groups in referential activity (RA) in the self-monologue, HOF scored significantly higher on RA in the parent monologue as compared to the self-monologue. In contrast, controls scored significantly lower in RA on the parent monologue. It was concluded that their mothers' difficulties were internalized and had a more significant role in the psychological world of HOF than for controls. Also, HOF's knowledge about their mother's experiences before and during the war (but not after) was related to their referential competence on the self-monologue, suggesting that impairments in symbolic activity are transmitted. The literature on symbol formation (see Cahn, 1987, for a review) suggests that the ability to symbolize and communicate one's experiences is an adaptive mechanism, while impairments therein might be related to vulnerability to depression. Lichtman (1983, 1984) found, as discussed earlier, that guilt-inducing, nonverbal and indirect styles of communication were more characteristic of severely traumatized parents and correlated with higher scores on anxiety, paranoia, depression, and low ego strength in HOF. Lichtman also observed that paternal communication seemed to be a positive influence whereas maternal communication had adverse effects on HOF. Keller (1988), using Family Adaptability and Cohesion Scales-III (FACES-III) and Lichtman's (1983) Communication Questionnaire, also found that paternal communication seemed to operate as a positive force, whereas maternal communication was related to negative effects in HOF's evaluations of the family's cohesion and adaptability, as well as their satisfaction with it. The finding that female HOF with frequent current communication with their parents described their fathers as providing frequent and willing communication about the Holocaust, and their mothers as seldom engaging in such communication, was explained as reflecting the daughters identifying with their mothers and then rejecting them if they are perceived as victims.

Schwarz (1986) administered a questionnaire to 70 HOF to measure the parents' style of communicating Holocaust experiences, the SCL-90-R, the Group Embedded Figure Test, and the Wechsler Adult Intelligence Scale-Revised (WAIS-R). Neither global level of symptomatology nor the level of psychological differentiation of HOF were related to the perceived level of parental communication. Higher levels of maternal Holocaust-related communication were related to higher levels of depression and greater personal hypersensitivity in HOF. The findings support the hypothesis of transmission of effects of the Holocaust with regards to symptomatology, but not in the realm of more neutral cognitive perceptual functioning. Sorscher (1991) found that HOF daughters had a higher awareness of parental nonverbal communication about the Holocaust and more Holocaust-related imagery than did sons. She suggested that the findings reflect different responses of the genders to trauma, whereby women demonstrate a higher vulnerability to trauma and a willingness to report symptoms, whereas men perhaps deny any such features as reflecting weakness.

The findings of Hammerman (1980) suggest that initiation by the child of Holocaust-related discussions, in addition to inclusion of both objective and subjective aspects of prewar as well as war experiences of the parents, is more important to identity development in the HOF than information itself. However, the findings, were seen only for male HOF and are limited by the sample size of only 11 male subjects.

Okner and Flaherty (1989) studied parental communication and psychological distress among 140 American and 54 Israeli HOF using the Buss and Durkee Hostility–Guilt Inventory, a demoralization scale from the PERI, and items from McNair's Profile of Mood Scale, the Center for Education of the Study of Depression Scale, Nettler's Measure of Alienation, and Rottler's Scale for Locus of Control. Israeli HOF reported more communication by their parents, but also a higher level of demoralization (which might be due to a higher level of demoralization in the general Israeli population). For all HOF, parental general communication correlated negatively with anxiety, depression, and demoralization, and positively with guilt. Parents' Holocaust-specific communication led to similar findings for American HOF, but only the negative correlation with demoralization was significant in the Israeli sample. It was concluded that parental communication about the Holocaust seems less important in Israel in determining the children's psychological outcome, reflecting the greater role played by Israeli society in shaping perceptions of the Holocaust, and highlighting possible limitations of generalizing findings interculturally.

In conclusion, empirical studies indicate that hindered intrafamilial communication about the parents' Holocaust experiences is associated with more adverse effects among HOF. The findings also suggest that gender plays an important role in determining the responses of HOF to parental communication, or lack thereof, and also demonstrate differences between Israeli and North American samples.

SOURCES OF INCONSISTENCIES IN THE EMPIRICAL FINDINGS

Some possible sources of inconsistencies among empirical studies of the intergenerational transmission of Holocaust traumata arise due to the many complex methodological problems they face, some aspects of which are outlined below.

"Clinical" and "Nonclinical" Subjects

The distinction between clinical and nonclinical samples has been discussed as an important source of possible bias (Solkoff, 1981, 1992). In some instances, subjects drawn from the general population were classified as "clinical" if they had, at some point in their lives, undergone psychotherapy. This criterion does not seem to be justified. A study (Goodman, 1978) that compared HOF who had been previously in therapy with those who had not found that, as a group, the former were more highly educated, held more advanced occupations, and earned a higher income, and saw very few significant differences between the two groups regarding levels of self-actualization and death anxiety. Also, although Gertler (1986) reported that 57% of his HOF subjects had therapy experience, he found no differences between HOF and controls in interpersonal adjustment. Schwarz (1986) found that HOF with therapy experience showed significantly higher levels of self-reported symptomatology, but were more psychologically differentiated than other HOF, who were relatively field dependent.

Based on their finding that HOF with two parents who had been in the resistance were more highly represented than other HOF among those who had sought therapy, Sigal and Weinfeld (1989) suggested that the past experiences of the parents of HOF who seek therapy are different from those of survivors whose children do not. Other explanations were that those who sought therapy had poorer relationships with their parents (although better than average relationships were seen for all HOF in this study), and also reported poorer relationships between their parents. The authors suggested that the discrepancy in the literature between empirical observations on nonclinical samples and clinical reports could be due to clinicians seeing only a subgroup of HOF who differ from the general HOF population. However, this possibility is diminished somewhat by the fact that a later analysis revealed no significant differences between HOF and controls who both sought therapy (Sigal, personal communication, August 1995).

Reliance on Volunteer Subjects

Most empirical studies recruit volunteer participants, often from various Jewish organizations. It could be hypothesized that volunteers for HOF-related studies are better adjusted than those who feel less secure and more defensive about the subject. On the other hand, one could claim that volunteers might be less well adjusted, and might seek a target population with which to identify in relation to their difficulties. Schleuderer (1990) pointed out that the higher scores obtained by HOF, as compared to controls, on Desirability (reflecting the wish to "look good") and on Debasement (reflecting the opposite tendency to present their emotional well-being in the worst possible light) suggest that, as a group, HOF have a conflictual attitude about how they perceive their emotional well-being and how they wish to present themselves.

Although some of these problems are encountered in many fields of psychological study, there are unique aspects of the study of the effects of the Holocaust that make it particularly emotionally charged. Subjects might have strong attitudes about their identity as children of Holocaust survivors, and might feel that not acknowledging problematic aspects of their own experience in relation to their parents' past might in some way belittle their parents' suffering. On the other hand, the recognition of long-lasting effects of the Holocaust, and especially of inter-generational effects, might be perceived as further victimization of the victims by "pathologiz-ing" them or their children, or might be experienced as granting the perpetrators success in damaging that which is most precious to the survivors, their children (see also Danieli, 1984). Furthermore, the assumption of intergenerational transmission might be perceived as assigning guilt and attributing the "victimizer" role to the survivor parents. Such affective and cognitive at-titudes might interfere with the motivations of subjects to participate in studies of HOF, as well as with what they choose to present on a conscious level, and need to be assessed carefully.

Conscious Perceptions

A large majority of the empirical studies rely upon self-reported perceptions of HOF, who describe themselves, their parents, and their perceived family interactions, leading to ob-vious potential biases inherent in the nature of the information gathered, which is direct, con-scious, and subjective. Such factors are particularly relevant when the issues assessed, such as separation–individuation, are laden with value judgments favoring certain outcomes, and when it is kept in mind that, in some studies, HOF obtained higher scores than controls in conformity (Schwartz et al., 1994) and social desirability (Schleuderer, 1990). Sigal and Weinfeld (1989), in discussing their finding that 65% of HOF reported that at least one of their parents suffered from specific psychological symptoms related to the war, but only 20% reported that they themselves suffered from similar symptoms, commented that it is possible that subjects are less willing to report negative characteristics about themselves than they are about their parents.

In-depth clinical interviews and projective measures might more successfully avoid these possible sources of bias. Wanderman (1980) showed that an in-depth analysis of one of her subjects (using interviews and projective testing) rendered very different results from those ob-tained with an impersonal, self-administered questionnaire. She mentioned that it was possi-ble that the contradiction between her results and those of Klein (1973), who did identify differences between children of concentration camp survivors and controls, could be due to Klein's inclusion of extensive clinical interviews and projective testing.

Instruments and Statistical Methods

Although many studies use questionnaires to tap specific issues related to the Holocaust, these are usually developed by the researcher and typically lack validation and normalization. Even when well-researched instruments are utilized, there are indications that some tools do not seem useful in this population. In some cases, specific questionnaires and structured interviews revealed significant differences between HOF and controls, whereas standard instruments did not (Gertz, 1986; Rich, 1982). Also, as discussed in more detail later, pencil-and-paper, mailed, impersonal instruments might be inadequate for the study of the effects of the Holocaust, due to the inherent nature of these effects.

Some of the discrepancies in the literature might be due to the statistical procedures em-ployed. Empirical findings show that although scores obtained by HOF often differ signifi-cantly from those of controls, they should not be expected to lie in the pathological range. Although analyses based on group means might be useful when it is assumed that grossly de-viant development has taken place, such an assumption does not seem adequate in the study of differences among groups that are essentially functioning adaptively. Indeed, in several studies

(Felsen & Erlich, 1990; Lichtman, 1984; Ofman, 1981) in which only few differences between HOF and controls emerged from analyses of group means, many significant differences were revealed using more sensitive correlational analyses.

Finally, there are several variables that have been observed to mediate the intergenerational transmission of Holocaust effects. Empirical studies that attempt to control for these variables are often faced with problems of insufficient statistical power, which can lead to sensitivity to only very dramatic effect and/or the observation of effects due to chance. Only a few authors report the relevant parameters required to assess the statistical limitations of their results, and many do not refer at all to such limitations.

DISCUSSION

Empirical studies of HOF have investigated a tremendously wide range of variables and have rendered a multitude of results. Perhaps the most prominent finding is that HOF are functioning within the normal range, and thus, as a group, do not demonstrate psychopathology, in contrast to what might have been expected based on clinical observations. However, many findings point to measurable differences between HOF and controls, suggesting a psychological profile typical of HOF that includes less differentiation from their parents, less feelings of autonomy and independence, elevated anxiety, guilt, and depressive experiences, and more difficulties in the regulation of aggression.

It has been suggested (Rose & Garske, 1987) that the differences observed are not unique to survivor families but typical of Jewish culture, which encourages independence and self-sufficiency to a lesser degree than American or Eastern European cultures. The whole sample of Jewish subjects, Holocaust-related or not, has been demonstrated to differ significantly from the general American population on some measures (Gerlter, 1986; Herskovic, 1989; Obermeyer, 1988; Rich, 1982; Rose & Garske, 1987; Schwarz, 1986; Weiss, 1988; Wieder, 1985), and thus comparisons between the scores of HOF and either control groups or the normalization data for psychological instruments must be done with particular caution concerning the possible influence of cultural factors. Comparison groups should therefore include children of Eastern European Jewish immigrants who were not directly related to the Holocaust. This was done by Leon et al. (1981), who observed that survivors and Jewish European immigrant parents exhibited common intrafamilial themes, indicating enhanced closeness between parents and children. They posited that these themes are cultural rather than specific to the influences of the Holocaust. The suggestion by Weiss et al. (1986) that their findings support attribution of effects in HOF to the parents' immigrant status is weakened by the fact that HOF scored higher on guilt than other children of immigrants, suggesting that a Holocaust background compounds the effects of immigration, and by the omission of a Jewish-immigrant non-Holocaust-related control group. It is possible that the characteristics observed as typical of Eastern European Jewish families provided the survivors with culturally available defenses and coping mechanisms that allowed them to make the leap of hope necessary to establish new families after the Holocaust. The culturally valued emphasis on the family might have functioned as a link to parental ideals, driving for the establishment of new families. Subsequently, the experience of parenthood itself served to reactivate further earlier identifications of the survivors with their own parents, in the pre-Holocaust world (Orenstein, 1981). The toll exerted by this adaptation, exhibited in elevated difficulties around separation–individuation observed in HOF, must be viewed along with its potentially highly adaptive role in the context of severe traumatization and loss.

A significant contribution to organizing many of the varied and, at times, conflicting empirical findings concerning HOF is offered by Danieli's typology (1981, 1985), which delineated four different types of survivors and their families who differ in their styles of adaptation, and which has been empirically validated (Rich, 1982; Klein, 1987; Sigal & Weinfeld, 1989). However, no integration has yet been accomplished between this descriptive typology of survivor families and a conceptual system or model of personality development that has an established validity outside the phenomena observed in HOF. Karson (1989), in an attempt to provide such a link, suggested that characteristics of HOF, such as less differentiation, sensitivity to loss, and subsequent avoidant behaviors, are consistent with theoretical formulations regarding the borderline personality (Masterson, 1981). However, this formulation does not seem merited. Extensive and varied psychodiagnostic assessments (including Karson's own findings) show that HOF function within the normative range and so do not exhibit the cognitive-affective deficits typical of borderline personality functioning. The kind of stormy affective and interpersonal style typical of the borderline personality was also not observed in studies of HOF, which revealed no differences in ego strengths (Zlotogorski, 1983; 1985), and found high occupational achievements and an overall positive adaptation (Sigal & Weinfeld, 1989). The characteristics mentioned by Karson seem to describe only a subsample of HOF, with other findings suggesting some HOF are characterized by a high degree of separateness and an overemphasis on self-definition and assertion (Wieder, 1985).

Based on this review of the empirical literature, it is proposed that, rather than focusing on whether the characteristics observed in HOF reflect a psychopathology, they can be better understood and conceptualized in the context of a theoretical model of normal personality development that is derived from an integration of psychoanalytic concepts of object relations, cognitive-developmental psychology, and attachment theory and research (for a detailed exposition, see Felsen, in preparation). It is proposed that these findings can be organized in an existing model (Blatt, 1991, 1995), which has been empirically demonstrated to be useful in a large variety of clinical and nonclinical populations unrelated to the Holocaust (Blatt, 1990; Blatt, D'Afflitti, & Quinlan, 1976), and which assumes that personality development occurs along two fundamental lines: a self-definition line and a relatedness line. In normal personality development, these two processes evolve in a mutually facilitating fashion, leading to the development of a consolidated, realistic, essentially positive, increasingly differentiated and integrated identity, and to the development of a consolidated, realistic, essentially positive, increasingly differentiated and integrated identity, and to the development of the capacity to establish increasingly mature, reciprocal, and satisfying interpersonal relations. Thus, normalcy can be defined as an integration of relatedness and self-definition. A relative emphasis on either interpersonal relatedness or self-definition defines two broad character styles, "anaclitic" or "introjective," respectively, which, in the extreme, also defines two broad categories of psychopathology. Introjective personalities share a basic focus on anger, aggression, self-definition, self-worth, living up to expectations imposed by internal standards, and accomplishments rather than feelings and relationships. Counteractive defenses are used (projection, reversal, reaction formation, intellectualization, introjection, identification with the aggressor, overcompensation), which all attempt to transform impulses and conflicts rather than to avoid or repress them. In the anaclitic configuration, individuals are more concerned about relatedness, at the expense of the development of the sense of self. The focus is on experiences of feelings and personal reactions and meanings, the cognitive style is more field dependent, and the primary instinctual mode is libidinal rather than aggressive, focusing on issues such as closeness and intimacy (with specific vulnerabilities to disruptions thereof, such as experiences of rejection, separation, and loss). Avoidant defenses, such as denial and repression, are utilized to deal with conflictual aspects within the self and in the environment.

It is proposed here that subsamples of HOF that have been empirically identified to be characterized by different, even contradictory, traits can be understood as placing an exaggerated emphasis on anaclitic or introjective development at the expense of the other. The relative emphasis demonstrated by a given individual will be determined by biological dispositions, cultural factors, gender, and family patterns (Blatt, 1990).

Empirical findings support the conclusion that Jewish Eastern European culture in general provided norms and values that put a relative emphasis on relatedness and interdependency within the family structure rather than on separateness and autonomy. The influences of the Holocaust in survivor families seem to compound this cultural emphasis on anaclitic traits even further, as evidenced by the particular family interactions reviewed previously.

Gender also seems to be an important determinant of the types of effects observed in HOF. Consistent with the literature about gender differences in general, the findings suggest that male HOF tend to respond to the same intrafamilial stressors with more introjective characteristics, whereas females display more anaclitic traits. It has been proposed (Vogel, 1994) that gender can be viewed as an organizing variable in personality development, and that personality development for girls can be described as a growing capacity for connectedness, rather than as a process of increasing individuation (Chodoroff, 1972; Gilligan, 1983; Miller, 1986), leading to an enhanced capacity of empathy in females, as well as to more permeable ego boundaries.

This model would suggest that daughters of survivors might be more vulnerable to the intergenerational transmission of parental trauma, a suggestion supported by empirical findings. Lichtman (1984) found that indirect communication by both parents was related significantly to depression, anxiety, paranoia, hypochondriasis, and low ego strength for female HOF, but to lower depression and higher income for male HOF. Schulman (1987) saw that female HOF scored lower than males on efficacy, were significantly more prone to anaclitic depressive experiences, and exhibited different affective reactions to hearing their parents talk about the Holocaust; they were more upset and curious than males. Karr (1973) found that male HOF tended to act our aggressive impulses, whereas female HOF tended to use reaction formation. Also, the fact that many studies reported difficulties in obtaining male HOF in equal numbers as females was interpreted by Rich (1982) as reflecting that men might be more comfortable with being noncompliant, or that women deal more easily with emotion-laden issues, whereas men need to defend against (and deny) any aspect of their upbringing that might connote defeat or powerlessness. Due to these differences, attempts to generalize and compare the findings of individual studies must take into consideration the gender composition of the samples used.

Additional factors that might lead to an overemphasis among HOF of either anaclitic or introjective traits are associated with particular features of the dynamics in survivor families. Erlich and Blatt (1985) proposed that the phenomenological experience of the self and the object evolves along two fundamental dimensions: the experiential modes of being and doing, the relative emphasis on which leads to the formation of different character styles. In the realm of doing, the object is perceived as involved in activities related to stimulation and satisfaction of drives and drive-derivatives, tending to or protecting the child. Experiences in the mode of being are related to feeling a sense of oneness, fusion, and omnipotence with the object as confirmation of adoration, reflected beauty, importance, or centrality of the child to the caring parent.

Shoshan (1989) commented that, to varying degrees, "survivors managed to overcome the deep depression resulting from the ongoing states of mourning by tireless 'doing,' while the state of primal 'being' was an unknown experience to them, as well as to their family members" (p. 198). The defensive overemphasis of survivors on doing at the expense of being could lead to a similar imbalance in their children, with relative deficits in the experiences of HOF in the realm of being. HOF born soon after the war, before some psychological rehabilitation could be achieved by the survivors, might have experienced a greater disruption, and might have been endowed with special roles and expectations (Grubrich-Simitis, 1981; Rosenman, 1984; Sonnenberg, 1974) that would predispose them toward the anaclitic developmental line. Although firstborn HOF have been reported to have been more adversely affected by their parents' Holocaust past (Klein, 1973), the differential effects of age reported in the literature are more consistent than those related to birth order. Gertler (1986) found that the oldest HOF in his sample (ages 36–41) were more compliant and found it harder to be sociable than subjects of ages 25–35. Tauber (1980) observed that, upon dividing her HOF sample according to age, the middle group (ages 26–30; $n = 33$) scored higher than both the younger (ages 18–25; $n = 28$) and older (ages 31–35; $n = 20$) groups on the subscales Personal, Self, and Behavior of the Tennessee Self-Concept Scale (reflecting more positive self-perceptions). Keller (1988) reported that the older the HOF, the more likely they were to describe their families as less adaptive, and their parents as engaging in indirect communication about the Holocaust. However, there seem to be reparative processes later in the lives of HOF, due to which they perceive themselves as less depressed and less anxious than they were when younger (Schwartz *et al.*, 1994).

Erlich and Blatt (1985) postulated that deficits in being would lead to a diminished sense of self. Indeed, HOF have been reported to score lower on autonomy and self-sufficiency (Karson, 1989; Ofman, 1981; Rose & Garske, 1987), and higher on external locus of control (Ofman, 1981), field dependence (Gross, 1988), and self-criticism (Wanderman, 1980; Felsen & Erlich, 1990). HOF also demonstrate difficulties in emotional expression (Gertz, 1986), especially of hostile feelings (Blumenthal, 1981; Kleinplatz, 1980; Lowin, 1983) and a tendency to internalize aggression (Lovinger, 1986). Other findings indicated higher levels among HOF of depressive experiences (Karr, 1973; Kleinplatz, 1980; Lovinger, 1986) and anxiety (Budick, 1985; Karr, 1973; Lichtman, 1984), more frequent worries and fears (Blumenthal, 1981; Gertz, 1986), higher vigilance and mistrustfulness (Budick, 1985; Lowin, 1983; Schleuderer, 1990), and higher overall level of symptomatology (Schwarz, 1986).

Since it requires successful integration of both experiential modes, one would expect HOF to exhibit difficulties related to the process of separation–individuation during adolescence and early adulthood. Later transitions in life, such as becoming a parent (Stern, 1995) or coping with the aging of survivor parents, might reactivate these difficulties. Various empirical studies did indicate that HOF have difficulties related to physical separation from their parents; they find it harder to breach the subject of moving out of their parents' homes (Wanderman, 1980), tend to live closer to their parents after moving out (Karr, 1973), and tend to establish their own families later than do controls (Gertler, 1986). Other studies showed evidence for problems in the process of separation–individuation among HOF (Karson, 1989; Shiryon, 1988; Wieder, 1985), as well as difficulties in the resolution of the stage of identity versus role diffusion (Lowin, 1983).

On the other hand, a deficit in being could also lead to a strengthening of the ego in many practical spheres, because the deficient sense of being can find compensatory outlets in an increased and expanded emphasis on doing (Erlich & Blatt, 1985), and such compensatory developments can be highly adaptive, driving toward higher achievements and efficacy. The underlying deficient sense of self can often go unnoticed in the shadow of the more apparent and real strengthening effects observed in highly adaptive achievements. This formulation is consistent with recent suggestions that experiencing stressful situations, including those of the Holocaust, may lead to certain resiliencies (Garmezy, 1987; Rieck, 1994; Rieck, Carmil, & Breznitz, 1994). Luthar and Zigler (1991) stated that a significant relationship between stress and adjustment does exist. Similarly, Meichenbaum and Novac (1978) emphasized the potential benefits to later coping of experiencing stressful situations. This type of poststress mode of adaptation is consistent with the survivors' own successes at attaining relatively high achievements (Helmreich, 1992) despite the objective external difficulties they had to face and their internal distress.

Indeed, several clinical reports revealed that HOF demonstrate remarkable ego strengths alongside some ego weaknesses (Kestenberg, 1980; Rosenman, 1984; Rosenman & Handelsman, 1992). These strengths seem to evolve from a precocious maturity, induced through a reversal of the usual parent–child roles in survivor families and accompanied with early practice of mediating issues between the parents. Empirical evidence supports this view. Podietz *et al.* (1984), with 53 HOF and 138 controls, concluded that there is a greater degree of engagement in survivor families, but emphasized the adaptive, functional, and positive aspects of the style of interactions of Holocaust families. Moskowitz (1992), comparing three generations of both survivor and control families, found that the survivor families scored significantly higher on self-efficacy. Studies have found that HOF, and especially males, scored higher than controls on motivation for success and academic achievements (Lichtman, 1984; Russell, Plotkin, & Heapy, 1985), consistent with similar findings from Israel (Last & Klein, 1984). Sigal and Weinfeld (1989) reported that 62% of HOF had at least a bachelor's degree, compared to 47.4% and 55.5% in their comparison groups. Similarly, Hanover (1981) reported that 75% of HOF were either employed as professionals or completing professional schools, compared with 55% of controls.

Simon (1995) examined the relationship between guilt and achievement motivation among 105 HOF and compared them to the test norms for the Kugler and Jones Guilt Inventory, Mehrabian Achieving Tendency Scale, and Cassidy–Lynn Achievement Motivation Questionnaire. HOF exhibited significantly higher levels of both state and trait guilt, and higher levels of actual achievements when compared with the general population. However, self-ratings of achievement motivation were significantly higher on only one subscale of the Cassidy–Lynn questionnaire. It is possible that self-perceptions of achievement motivation among HOF do not reveal elevated scores due to their higher self-criticism, which was observed elsewhere (Felsen & Erlich, 1990). Other findings suggest that these achievements are accompanied by vulnerabilities seen in elevated psychosomatic complaints (Leventhal & Ontell, 1989), as well as difficulties in personal contentment and emotional expression (Russell, 1980).

One reason for the discrepancy between clinical and empirical observations is that whereas any interaction contains both dimensions, there is a difference in visibility between the modes of being and doing. The experience of being is more private and less amenable to verbal elaboration. Being phenomena are not only specific contents of the mental apparatus but also an experiential mode in which the self and the object are perceived. In a "being-oriented" encounter, such as in the context of therapy, support groups, and in-depth, face-to-face interviews, aspects related to being might be more likely to emerge and find expression than in the empirical setting, with its emphasis on the subjects (as well as the researchers) engaging in a task-oriented interaction in a time-limited fashion, and in the context of a less personal relationship between them. (This is even more accentuated when impersonal data-acquisition procedures are utilized, such as mailing self-administered questionnaires.) As a result, one might expect clinical and empirical settings to render different perspectives on the experiences of HOF.

Indeed, there is a recurring theme in the literature that some aspects of the experiences of HOF are not well grasped in empirical studies and seem to defy measurement by standard psychological scales. Blumenthal (1981) reported that some HOF who scored within the normal range on Baron's Ego Strength Scale claimed, once the investigation was revealed, that they did experience emotional difficulties that they perceived as related to their HOF status, but the questionnaire was irrelevant to their specific problems. Wanderman (1980) found that an in-depth analysis of one of her subjects (using an interview and projective testing) rendered results that appeared very different from those obtained with an impersonal, self-administered questionnaire. In an Israeli study (Solomon, Kother, & Mikulincer, 1988), HOF who were screened prior to military service and found to be as qualified as recruits from control groups exhibited a greater psychological vulnerability, as evidenced by more prolonged symptomatology related to PTSD. However, this covert vulnerability was manifested only after exposure to severe stress situations.

Some reports based on clinical work and in-depth interviews do seem to offer glimpses into the relatively less visible realm of phenomena of "being." Kestenberg (1982) referred to a "transposition" into the world of the past, whereby the survivor's children tend, on one level of their existence, to enter a "time tunnel" during which scenes from the Holocaust are enacted. HOF have reported living in such a double reality, motivated by the wish to defend parents against facing the loss of significant others since they continue to live within the child (Rosenman, 1984). These experiences seem to evade typical empirical investigations. For example, although Gertz (1986) observed that the phenomenon of "transposition" was reported by almost one-fifth of HOF, it was not observable with the standardized instrument used in this study.

In summary, the empirical literature supports the conclusion that exposure to the trauma of the Holocaust had long-term effects on the offspring of survivors due to the parents' relative deficit in the experiential mode of being, leading to similar deficits in their children's experience, which are evidenced, among various subsamples of HOF, by an overemphasis of either anaclitic or introjective personality traits. Such an overemphasis represents potential psychological vulnerabilities that might be exacerbated, in some individuals, by additional characteristics that will determine the severity of pathology that will develop, as well as by exposure later in life to severe stress (Novac, 1994). This conceptualization seems useful in integrating clinical and empirical findings on HOF and opens new avenues for future research.

CONCLUSIONS AND IMPLICATIONS FOR RESEARCH AND CLINICAL WORK

There exists a rich body of empirical literature dealing with possible transmission of Holocaust traumata to the children of survivors. A wide range of individual and family characteristics has been studied, including psychopathological symptoms, personality traits, cognitive and defensive styles, and family interactions and communication patterns. On the whole, no evidence was obtained for psychopathology. However, despite some inconsistencies among various studies, a pattern emerges in which HOF demonstrate greater difficulties around the process and outcomes of separation–individuation, a greater proneness to anxiety, depressive experiences, and psychosomatic complaints, and difficulties in the expression of aggressive impulses and assertive behavior. Along with these vulnerabilities, there is evidence for significant ego strengths, as evidenced by both high achievement motivation and increased empathic capacities (Vogel, 1994). Kohut (1966) pointed out that the capacity to utilize relatively permeable ego boundaries toward highly adaptive accomplishments should be viewed not as a reflection of an ego weakness (i.e., as a relatively poor differentiation between self and other), but might in fact represent another form of highly adaptive achievements of psychologically mature personalities, as demonstrated, for example, by good therapists, good leaders, and others in the helping professions. Although findings indicate that HOF feel less differentiated from their parents, this is not necessarily maladaptive. Rosenman (1984) stressed that HOF often do not just conform to parental expectations but come to want the role and to feel self-actualized by being "rescuers." Empirical evidence supports this view, with 20% of HOF subjects in one study working in mental health professions in comparison to 12% of controls (Russell *et al.*, 1985).

The findings also point out the need to reconceptualize the roles of guilt, denial, and mourning in the context of massive, man-made trauma. As has been pointed out (Krell, 1984; Klein, 1973) and demonstrated empirically (Chayes, 1987), the dynamics in survivors are different than what has been traditionally conceptualized as adaptive or maladaptive in more normal mourning. Some denial of the damage (Danieli, 1981), of the extent of mourning (Chayes, 1987), and some adaptive meanings associated with guilt (Klein, 1973) must be considered as potentially beneficial in the context of severe trauma. Similarly, a reexamination of the concept of identification with the aggressor must be undertaken in these populations, especially since most findings point to difficulties in expression of aggression rather than to elevated aggression, and adaptive avenues of incorporating normal, healthy aggression should be explored both clinically and empirically.

The conceptualization offered here seems to help integrate the diverse empirical and clinical observations. Special personality characteristics, as evidence by particular cognitive-affective traits and psychological disorders, are viewed along a continuum (either anaclitic or introjective) that ranges from normal to pathological development and from less to more severe disturbances. It has been empirically demonstrated with many other populations that the distinction between anaclitic and introjective configurations is valid and useful in the study of different types of depression (Blatt, 1990; Blatt *et al.*, 1976), and in determining the differential responses of individual patients to different therapeutic interventions (Blatt & Felsen, 1993). The distinction, which can be relatively easily inferred from the patient's past history and style of personality, as well as by using specific psychodiagnostic procedures, can be useful in both empirical and clinical settings.

Topics for future empirical research include identifying anaclitic and introjective subgroups among clinical and nonclinical HOF and controls, investigating the composition of these subgroups in terms of key variables (gender, age, birth order, etc.), and examining whether, despite differences among HOF in cognitive-affective styles due to their different personality configurations, both anaclitic and introjective HOF show greater deficits in the realm of being. Such studies would currently be hampered by the fact that experiences in the realm of being, due to their very nature, are less well assessed by standard instruments. There is a need for new tools to overcome this problem, the development of which would need to rely (at least in the initial phase until less time-consuming forms could be developed and validated) on the use of intensive clinical interviews and projective testing. Such tools could be useful not only for future research on the effects of the Holocaust, but also possibly for developing research tools for other severely traumatized populations. For this purpose, it would be important for studies of HOF to adhere to standard psychiatric nomenclature and to incorporate more traditional psychoanalytic terminology with more recent research and theory related to PTSD in general. Further information might be gleaned by comparing, for example, in the Israeli army (Solomon *et al.*, 1988), HOF who developed PTSD under stress to those who did not, in order to investigate the variables contributing to the relative resiliency of some HOF.

Implications for clinical work with individuals who have been exposed to trauma include the need to recognize the importance of the style of adaptation to trauma in determining the response to the trauma itself and point to the potential usefulness of cognitive therapy in enhancing the individual's resiliencies and in emphasizing self-empowering, in contrast to self-blaming or victimizing, self-statements. The distinction between anaclitic and introjective might help in identifying, for those HOF who develop disorders, the particular aspects of their experience that were most salient in triggering the disturbance, were the most distressing to them, and should become the focus of therapy, as well as what kind of therapy would be most helpful. The relatively lower visibility of deficits in the experiential mode of being, which seems to characterize many HOF, highlights the need for clinicians to be aware of their patient's Holocaust-related background and its possible implications, even when the patient does not present this as relevant. Also, studies that examined styles of communication about the Holocaust suggest that exposure to severe trauma and loss, in the survivors themselves and in their offspring, leads to impeded communication, and that this in turn leads to more adverse effects in the children. Thus, it would seem that therapy that includes the family could be particularly useful in establishing more open communication, thereby alleviating some of the damaging effects of the "conspiracy of silence" for the primary victims as well as their children. Since it may be impractical with the aging survivor population, it seems important with HOF patients to reinforce a reopening of a dialogue, if not with the parents, then internally in therapy, about the individual's perceptions of the parents' war-related past and its role in the relationships in the family.

REFERENCES

Alexandrowicz, D. R. (1973). Children of concentration camp survivors. In E. S. Anthony & C. Koupernik (Eds.), *The child in his family: Vol. 2. The impact of disease and death* (pp. 385–392). New York: Wiley.

Antman, S. R. (1986). *Offspring of Holocaust survivors and the process of self-actualization and related variables* (Doctoral dissertation, California School of Professional Psychology, Fresno, 1986). *Dissertation Abstracts International, 46*, 2794.

Barocas, H. A., & Barocas, C. B. (1973). Manifestations of concentration camp effects on the second generation. *American Journal of Psychiatry, 130*, 820–821.

Barocas, H. A., & Barocas, C. B. (1979). Wounds of the fathers: The next generation of Holocaust victims. *International Review of Psycho-Analysis, 6*, 331–340.

Baron, L., Reznikoff, M., & Glenwick, D. S. (1993). Narcissism, interpersonal adjustment, and coping in children of Holocaust survivors. *Journal of Psychology, 127*, 257–269.

Blatt, S. J. (1990). Interpersonal relatedness and self-definition: Two personality configurations and their implications for psychopathology and psychotherapy. In J. L. Singer (Ed.), *Repression and dissociation: Implications for personality theory, psychopathology and health* (pp. 299–335). Chicago: University of Chicago Press.

Blatt, S. J. (1991). A cognitive morphology of psychopathology. *Journal of Nervous and Mental Disease, 179*, 449–458.

Blatt, S. J. (1995). The destructiveness of perfectionism: Implications for the treatment of depression. *American Psychologist, 50*, 1003–1020.

Blatt, S. J., D'Afflitti, J. P., & Quinlan, D. M. (1976). Experiences of depression in normal young adults. *Journal of Abnormal Psychology, 85*, 383–389.

Blatt, S. J., & Felsen, I. (1993). Different kinds of folks may need different kinds of strokes: The effect of patients' characteristics on therapeutic process and outcome. *Psychotherapy Research, 3*, 245–259.

Blumenthal, N. N. (1981). Factors contributing to varying levels of adjustment among children of Holocaust survivors (Doctoral dissertation, Adelphi University, 1918). *Dissertation Abstracts International, 42,* 1596.

Boszormenyi-Nagy, I., & Spark, G. M. (1973). *Invisible loyalties: Reciprocity in intergenerational family therapy.* Hagerstown, MD: Harper & Row.

Budick, C. (1985). An investigation of the effect of Holocaust survivor parents on their children (Doctoral dissertation, University of Rhode Island, 1985). *Dissertation Abstracts International, 46,* 4005.

Cahn, A. (1987). The capacity to acknowledge experience in Holocaust survivors and their children (Doctoral dissertation, Adelphi University, 1987). *Dissertation Abstracts International, 49,* 1381.

Chayes, M. (1987). Holocaust survivors and their children: An intergenerational study of mourning, parenting and psychological adjustment (Doctoral dissertation, Adelphi University, 1987). *Dissertation Abstracts International, 48,* 3675.

Chodoroff, P. (1972). The depressive personality: A critical review. *Archives of General Psychiatry, 27,* 666–673.

Danieli, Y. (1981). Differing adaptational styles in families of survivors of the Nazi Holocaust: Some implications for treatment. *Children Today, 10,* 6–10.

Danieli, Y. (1982). Families of survivors of the Nazi Holocaust: Some short- and long-term effects. In C. D. Spielberger, I. G. Sarason, & N. Milgram (Eds.), *Stress and Anxiety* (Vol. 8, pp. 405–421). New York: McGraw-Hill/Hemisphere.

Danieli, Y. (1984). Psychotherapist' participation in the conspiracy of silence about the Holocaust. *Psychoanalytic Psychology, 1*(1), 23–42.

Danieli, Y. (1985). The treatment and prevention of long-term effects and intergenerational transmission of victimization: A lesson from Holocaust survivors and their children. In C. R. Figley (Ed.), *Trauma and its wake: Vol. 1. The study and treatment of post-traumatic stress disorder* (pp. 295–313). New York: Brunner/Mazel.

Danto, B. L. (1968). The role of "missed adolescence" in the etiology of the concentration-camp survivor syndrome. In H. Krystal (Ed.), *Massive psychic trauma* (pp. 248–259). New York: International Universities Press.

Eissler, K. R. (1963). Die Ermordung von wievielen seiner Kinder muss ein Mensch symptomfire ertragen koennen, um eine normale Konstitution zu haaben? *Psyche, 17,* 241–291.

Eitinger, L. (1961). Psychiatric post conditions in former concentration camp inmates. In *Later Effects of Imprisonment and Deportation.* The Hague: World Veterans' Federation.

Erlich, H. S., & Blatt, S. J. (1985). Narcissim and object love: The metapsychology of experience. *Psychoanalytic Study of the Child, 40,* 57–79.

Felsen, I. V., & Erlich, H. S. (199). Identification patterns of offspring of Holocaust survivors with their parents. *American Journal of Orthopsychiatry, 60,* 506–520.

Finer-Greenberg, R. (1987). Factors contributing to the degree of psychopathology in first- and second-generation Holocaust survivors (Doctoral dissertation, California School of Professional Psychology, Los Angeles, 1987). *Dissertation Abstracts International, 49,* 1939.

Fink, H. F. (1968). Development arrest as a result of Nazi persecution during adolescence. *International Journal of Psychoanalysis, 49,* 327–329.

Furshpan, M. (1986). Family dynamics as perceived by the second generation of Holocaust survivors (Doctoral dissertation, State University of New York, Buffalo, 1986). *Dissertation Abstracts International, 47,* 271.

Garmezy, N. (1987). Stress, competence and development: Continuities in the study of schizophrenic adults, children vulnerable to psychopathology, and the search for stress-resistant children. *American Journal of Orthopsychiatry, 57,* 159–174.

Gertler, R. J. (1986). A study of interpersonal adjustment in children of Holocaust survivors (Doctoral dissertation, Pacific Graduate School of Psychology, 1986). *Dissertation Abstracts International, 47,* 4298.

Gertz, K. R. (1986). Psychosocial characteristics of children whose parent(s) survived the Nazi Holocaust and children whose parents were not in the Nazi Holocaust and implications for counseling children of survivors (Doctoral dissertation, University of California, Los Angeles, 1986). *Dissertation Abstracts International, 47,* 3312.

Gilligan, C. (1983). Do the social sciences have an adequate theory of moral development? In N. Haan, P. Bellak, M. Robins, & P. Sullivan (Eds.), *Social sciences: Moral inquiry.* Berkeley: University of California Press.

Goodman, J. S. (1978). The transmission of parental trauma: Second generation effects of Nazi concentration camp survival (Doctoral dissertation, California School of Professional Psychology, Fresno, 1978). *Dissertation Abstracts International, 39,* 4031.

Gross, S. (1988). The relationship of severity of the Holocaust condition to survivors' child-rearing abilities and their offsprings' mental health. *Family Therapy, 15,* 211–222.

Grubrich-Simitis, I. (1981). Extreme traumatization as cumulative trauma: Psychoanalytic investigations of the effects of concentration camp experiences on survivors and their children. *Psychoanalytic Study of the Child, 36,* 415–450.

Hanover, L. A. (1981). Parent–child relationships in children of survivors of the Nazi Holocaust (Doctoral dissertation, United States International University, 1981). *Dissertation Abstracts International, 42,* 770.

Helmreich, W. B. (1992). *Against all odds: Holocaust survivors and the successful lives they made in America.* New York: Simon & Schuster.

Herskovic, S. A. (1989). A comparative study of stress and coping strategies of adult children of Holocaust survivors and adult children of non-Holocaust survivors (Doctoral dissertation, United States International University, 1989). *Dissertation Abstracts International, 51,* 1029.

Jurkowitz, S. W. (1996). Transgenerational transmission of depression, shame and guilt in Holocaust families: An examination of three generations (Doctoral dissertation, California School of Professional Psychology, Los Angeles, 1996). *Dissertation Abstracts International, 57,* 2946.

Kanter, I. (1970). Extermination camp syndrome: The delayed type of double-bind (a transcultural study). *International Journal of Social Psychiatry, 16,* 275–282.

Karr, S. D. (1973). Second-generation effects of the Nazi Holocaust (Doctoral dissertation, California School of Professional Psychology, San Francisco, 1973). *Dissertation Abstracts International, 3,* 2935.

Karson, E. (1989). Borderline phenomena in children of Holocaust survivors (Doctoral dissertation, California School of Professional Psychology, Los Angeles, 1989). *Dissertation Abstracts International, 51,* 3135.

Keller, R. (1988). Children of Jewish Holocaust survivors: Relationship of family communication to family cohesion, adaptability and satisfaction. *Family Therapy, 15,* 223–237.

Kendler, K. (1988). Indirect vertical cultural transmission: A model for nongenetic parental influences on liability to psychiatric illness. *American Journal of Psychiatry, 145,* 657–665.

Kestenberg, J. S. (1980). Psychoanalyses of children of survivors from the Holocaust: Case presentations and assessment. *Journal of the American Psychoanalytic Association, 28,* 775–804.

Kestenberg, J. S. (1982). Survivors' parents and their children. In M. S. Bergmann & M. E. Jucovy (Eds.), *Generations of the Holocaust* (pp. 83–102). New York: Basic Books.

Khan, M. M. R. (1963). The concept of cumulative trauma. In M. M. R. Khan (Ed.), *The privacy of the self* (pp. 42–58). New York: International Universities Press.

Klein, H. (1973). Children of the Holocaust: Mourning and bereavement. In E. S. Anthony & C. Koupernik (Eds.), *The child in the family: Vol. 2. The impact of disease and death* (pp. 393–410). New York: Wiley.

Klein, H., Zellermayer, J., & Shanan, J. (1963). Former concentration camp inmates on a psychiatric ward. *Archives of General Psychiatry, 8,* 334–342.

Klein, M. E. (1987). Transmission of trauma: The defensive styles of children of Holocaust survivors (Doctoral dissertation, California School of Professional Psychology, Berkeley, 1987). *Dissertation Abstracts International, 48,* 3682.

Kleinplatz, M. (1980). The effects of cultural and individual supports on personality variables among children of Holocaust survivors in Israel and North America (Doctoral dissertation, University of Windsor, 1980). *Dissertation Abstracts International, 41,* 1114.

Kohut, H. (1966). Forms and transformations of narcissim. *Journal of the American Psychoanalytic Association, 14,* 243–272.

Krell, R. (1984). Holocaust survivors and their children: Comments on psychiatric consequences and psychiatric terminology. *Comprehensive Psychiatry, 25,* 521–528.

Last, U., & Klein, H. (1984). Impact of parental Holocaust traumatization on offsprings' reports of parental child-rearing practices. *Journal of Youth and Adolescence, 13,* 267–283.

Leon, G. et al. (1981). Survivors of the Holocaust and their children: Current status and adjustment. *Journal of Personality and Social Psychology, 41,* 503–516.

Leventhal, G., & Ontell, M. K. (1989). A descriptive demographic and personality study of second-generation Jewish Holocaust survivors. *Psychological Reports, 64,* 1067–1073.

Levine, H. B. (1982). Toward a psychoanalytic understanding of survivors of the Holocaust. *Psychoanalytic Quarterly, 51,* 70–92.

Lichtman, H. (1983). Children of survivors of the Nazi Holocaust: A personality study (Doctoral dissertation, Yeshiva University, 1983). *Dissertation Abstracts International, 44,* 3532.

Lichtman, H. (1984). Parental communication of Holocaust experiences and personality characteristics among second-generation survivors. *Journal of Clinical Psychology, 40,* 914–924.

Lovinger, M. (1986). Expression of hostility in children of Holocaust survivors (Doctoral dissertation, Case Western Reserve University, 1986). *Dissertation Abstracts International, 47,* 3530.

Lowin, R. G. (1983). Cross-generational transmission of pathology in Jewish families of Holocaust survivors (Doctoral dissertation, California School of Professional Psychology, San Diego, 1983). *Dissertation Abstracts International, 44,* 3533.

Luthar, S. S., & Zigler, E. (1991). Vulnerability and competence: A review of research on resilience in childhood. *American Journal of Orthopsychiatry, 61,* 6–22.

Magids, D. M. (1994). Personality comparison between offspring of hidden survivors of the Holocaust and offspring of American Jewish parents (Doctoral dissertation, Fordham University, 1994). *Dissertation Abstracts International, 55,* 5077.

Masterson, J. F. (1981). *The narcissistic and borderline disorders: An integrated developmental approach.* New York: Brunner/Mazel.

Meichenbaum, D., & Novac, R. (1978). Stress inoculation: A preventive approach. In C. Spielberger & I. Sarason (Eds.), *Stress and anxiety* (Vol. 5, Washington, DC: Hemisphere.

Miller, J. B. (1986). *Toward a new psychology of women* (2nd ed.). Boston: Beacon.

Minuchin, S. (1974). *Families and family therapy.* Cambridge, MA: Harvard University Press.

Moskowitz, T. B. (1992). The intergenerational transmission of self-efficacy among families of Jewish survivors of the Holocaust (Doctoral dissertation, Miami Institute of Psychology of the Caribbean Center for Advanced Studies, 1992). *Dissertation Abstracts International, 53,* 2071.

Niederland, W. G. (1968). Clinical observations on the "Survivor Syndrome." *International Journal of Psycho-Analysis, 49,* 313–315.

Novac, A. (1994, May). Clinical heterogeneity in children of Holocaust survivors. *Newsletter of the World Psychiatric Association,* pp. 24–26.

Obermeyer, V. R. (1988). Outmarriage and cohesion in Jewish Holocaust survivor families. *Family Therapy, 15,* 255–269.

Ofman, J. (1981). Separation–individuation in children of Nazi Holocaust survivors and its relationship to perceived parental overvaluation (Doctoral dissertation, California School of Professional Psychology, Berkeley, 1981). *Dissertation Abstracts International, 42,* 3434.

Okner, D. R., & Flaherty, J. F. (1989). Parental communication and psychological distress in children of Holocaust survivors: A comparison between the U.S. and Israel. *International Journal of Social Psychiatry, 35,* 265–273.

Olson, D. H., Sprenkle, D. H., & Russell, C. S. (1979). Circumplex model of marital and family systems: I. Cohesion and adaptability dimensions, family types, and clinical applications. *Family Process, 18,* 3–28.

Orenstein, A. (1981). The aging survivor of the Holocaust. The effects of the Holocaust on life-cycle experiences: The creation and recreation of families. *Journal of Geriatric Psychiatry, 14,* 135–154.

Podietz, L., Zwerling, I., Ficher, I., Belmont, H., Eisenstein, I., Shapiro, M., & Levick, M. (1984). Engagement in families of Holocaust survivors. *Journal of Marital and Family Therapy, 10,* 43–51.

Rakoff, V., Sigal, J. J., & Epstein, N. (1966). Children and families of concentration camp survivors. *Canada's Mental Health, 14,* 24–26.

Rich, M. S. (1982). Children of Holocaust survivors: A concurrent validity study of a survivor family typology (Doctoral dissertation, California School of Professional Psychology, Berkeley, 1982). *Dissertation Abstracts International, 43,* 1626.

Rieck, M. (1994). The psychological state of Holocaust survivors' offspring: An epidemiological and psychodiagnostic study. *International Journal of Behavioral Development, 17,* 649–667.

Rieck, M., Carmil, D., & Breznitz, S. (1993). The effects of war on civilians: The mixed albeit biased effects of stress. In L. Weisaeth (Ed.), *The individual meeting with trauma.* Oslo: Oslo University Press.

Rose, S. L., & Garske, J. (1987). Family environment, adjustment, and coping among children of Holocaust survivors: A comparative investigation. *American Journal of Orthopsychiatry, 57,* 332–344.

Rosenman, S. (1984). Out of the Holocaust: Children as scarred souls and tempered redeemers. *Journal of Psychohistory, 18,* 35–69.

Rosenman, S., & Handelsman, I. (1992). Rising from the ashes: Modeling resiliency in a community devastated by man-made catastrophe. *American Imago, 49,* 185–226.

Rubenstein, I., Cutter, F., & Templer, D. I. (1990). Multigenerational occurrence of survivor syndrome symptoms in families of Holocaust survivors. *Journal of Death and Dying, 20,* 239–244.

Russell, A. (1980). Late effects—influence on children of concentration camp survivors. In J. E. Dimsdale (Ed.), *Survivors, victims, and perpetrators* (pp. 175–204). New York: Hemisphere.

Russell, A., Plotkin, D., & Heapy, N. (1985). Adaptive abilities in nonclinical second-generation Holocaust survivors and controls: A comparison. *American Journal of Psychotherapy, 39,* 564–579.

Rustin, S. (1971). Guilt, hostility and Jewish identification among a self-selected sample of late adolescent children of Jewish concentration camp survivors: A descriptive study (Doctoral dissertation, New York University, 1971). *Dissertation Abstracts International, 32,* 1859.

Schleuderer, C. G. (1990). Issues of the phoenix: Personality characteristics of children of Holocaust survivors (Doctoral dissertation, University of Georgia, 1990). *Dissertation Abstracts International, 51,* 4066.

Schulman, M. D. (1987). Factors related to experiences of depression among children of Holocaust survivors (Doctoral dissertation, City University of New York, 1987). *Dissertation Abstracts International, 48,* 1820.

Schwartz, S., Dohrenwend, B. P., & Levav, I. (1994). Nongenetic familial transmission of psychiatric disorders? Evidence from children of Holocaust survivors. *Journal of Health and Social Behavior, 35,* 385–402.

Schwarz, R. P. (1986). The effect of parental trauma on offspring of Holocaust survivors (Doctoral dissertation, Columbia University, 1986). *Dissertation Abstracts International, 47,* 4314.

Segall, A. (1974). Spaetreaktion auf Konzentrationslagererlebnisse [Delayed reactions to concentration camp experiences]. *Psyche, 28,* 221–230.

Shiryon, S. (1988). The second generation leaves home: The function of the sibling subgroup in the separation–individuation process of the survivor family. *Family Therapy, 15,* 239–253.

Shoshan, T. (1989). Mourning and longing from generation to generation. *American Journal of Psychotherapy, 43,* 193–207.

Sigal, J. J. (1973). Hypotheses and methodology in the study of families of Holocaust survivors. In E. S. Anthony & C. Koupernik (Eds.), *The child in his family: Vol. 2. The impact of disease and death* (pp. 411–415). New York: Wiley.

Sigal, J. J., Silver, D., Rakoff, V., & Ellin, B. (1973). Some second-generation effects of survival of the Nazi persecution. *American Journal of Orthopsychiatry, 43,* 320–327.

Sigal, J. J. & Weinfeld, M. (1989). *Trauma and rebirth: Intergenerational effects of the Holocaust.* New York: Praeger.

Simon, D. A. (1995). Guilt and achievement motivation among children of Holocaust survivors: An exploratory study (Doctoral dissertation, California School of Professional Psychology, Los Angeles, 1995). *Dissertation Abstracts International, 57,* 1454.

Solkoff, N. (1981). Children of survivors of the Nazi Holocaust: A critical review of the literature. *American Journal of Orthopsychiatry, 51,* 29–42.

Solkoff, N. (1992). Children of survivors of the Nazi Holocaust: A critical review of the literature. *American Journal of Orthopsychiatry, 62,* 342–358.

Solomon, Z., Kother, M., & Mikulincer, M. (1988). Combat-related post-traumatic stress disorders among second generation Holocaust survivors: Preliminary findings. *American Journal of Psychiatry, 145,* 865–868.

Sonnenberg, S. M. (1974). Children of survivors. Workshop report. *Journal of the American Psychoanalytic Association, 22,* 200–204.

Sorscher, N. L. (1991). The effects of parental communication of wartime experiences on children of survivors of the Holocaust (Doctoral dissertation, Adelphi University, 1991). *Dissertation Abstracts International, 52,* 4482.

Stern, Z. Y. (1995). The experience of parenthood among children of Holocaust survivors: Reworking a traumatic legacy (Doctoral dissertation, Massachusetts School of Professional Psychology, 1995). *Dissertation Abstracts International, 56,* 3465.

Tauber, I. D. (1980). Second-generation effects of the Nazi Holocaust: A psychological study of a nonclinical sample in North America (Doctoral dissertation, California School of Professional Psychology, Berkeley, 1980). *Dissertation Abstracts International, 41,* 4692.

Vogel, M. L. (1994). Gender as a factor in the transgenerational transmission of trauma. *Women and Therapy, 15,* 35–47.

Walisever, H. B. (1995). The effect of traumatic loss on attachment and emotional organization: An intergenerational study (Doctoral dissertation, Long Island University, 1995). *Dissertation Abstracts International, 56,* 2345.

Wanderman, E. (1980). Separation problems, depressive experiences, and conception of parents in children of concentration camp survivors (Doctoral dissertation, New York University, 1980). *Dissertation Abstracts International, 41,* 704.

Weiss, E., O'Connell, A. N., & Siiter, R. (1986). Comparisons of second-generation Holocaust survivors, immigrants, and nonimmigrants on measures of mental health. *Journal of Personality and Social Psychology, 50,* 828–831.

Weiss, M. D. (1988). Parental uses of authority and discipline by Holocaust survivors. *Family Therapy, 15,* 199–209.

Wieder, J. A. (1985). Children of Holocaust survivors: Differentiation from family of origin and its relationship to family dynamics (Doctoral dissertation, California School of Professional Psychology, Los Angeles, 1985). *Dissertation Abstracts International, 46,* 4039.

Winik, M. F. (1968). Generation to generation: A discussion with children of Jewish Holocaust survivors. *Family Therapy, 15,* 271–284.

Zlotogorski, Z. (1983). Offspring of concentration camp survivors: The relationship of perceptions of family cohesion and adaptability to levels of ego functioning. *Comprehensive Psychiatry, 24,* 345–354.

Zlotogorski, Z. (1985). Offspring of concentration camp survivors: A study of levels of ego functioning. *Israel Journal of Psychiatry and Related Sciences, 22,* 201–209.

3

Transgenerational Effects of the Holocaust
The Israeli Research Perspective

ZAHAVA SOLOMON

"Second generation" has now become an accepted term in Israel to refer to adult children of Holocaust survivors. The term has been current in Israeli professional literature since at least the early 1980s and has made its way into music, film, literature, and other arts, as well as into common parlance. In Israel, as elsewhere, children of survivors themselves have banded together to form commemorative organizations and self-help groups, thereby defining themselves as a group of people with a good deal in common. Their assumption, and the assumption of all who use the term *second generation,* is that it is more than merely a biological marker and that somehow or other the trauma of the Holocaust has been transmitted from the survivors to their children. The current chapter investigates the content of this term in Israel.

THE SURVIVAL FAMILY

There is a great deal of literature, primarily but not solely clinical, on difficulties in survivor families (e.g., Danieli, 1981; Engel, 1962; Freyberg, 1980; Koening, 1964). This literature, which deals with survivors in many countries, recognizes that it could not have been easy for persons who underwent the earth-shattering experiences that the survivors did to rebuild their lives. The literature describes a generation of destitute and desperate refugees who hurried into hasty marriages out of the wish to recreate their lost families and to ease the piercing pain of loneliness (Danieli, 1981). Many of the marriages were made in disregard of the usual considerations, including compatibility, lifestyle and socioeconomic status, that generally affect the selection of partners (Danieli, 1981). Many of the marriages, it is asserted, were loveless unions of despair between persons whose Holocaust experience left them in a narcissistic state (Chodoff, 1975), unable to love, and too emotionally depleted to develop intimacy (Koening, 1964).

ZAHAVA SOLOMON • The Bob Shapell School of Social Work, Tel Aviv University, Tel Aviv 69978 Israel.

International Handbook of Multigenerational Legacies of Trauma, edited by Yael Danieli. Plenum Press, New York, 1998.

The children born into Holocaust families have been described, and have described them-selves, as individuals who were brought into the world with the mission of compensating their parents for the terrible losses they had suffered and for their discontent in their marital lives (e.g., Bar-On, 1994; Wardi, 1990). They were given the responsibility of mediating between their parents and keeping the family intact. In many cases, they were perceived as extensions of their parents, who interpreted any attempt on their part to achieve individuation and auton-omy as a threat.

The upheavals noted in the survivor generation and the special burdens these have im-posed on their children have generally been acknowledged. Much less clear, however, are the nature and extent of the psychological residuals that the parents' Holocaust trauma has left in the second generation. In recent years, there has been a certain amount of empirical study, but the professional literature is divided. Some investigators claim that the Holocaust has had a long-term detrimental impact on the survivors and their children (e.g., Barocas & Barocas, 1979; Danieli, 1981; Epstein, 1979; Kestenberg, 1972). Others maintain that the majority of the second generation do not manifest substantial psychological disturbance (e.g., Leon, Butcher, & Kleinman, 1981; Sigal & Weinfeld, 1989).

SURVIVORS IN ISRAEL

The question is further complicated by the fact that after the Holocaust, the survivors im-migrated to various parts of the world. The massive destruction and the collapse of social and cultural structures drove most of them from the blood-soaked lands where they had been born and raised to rebuild their lives in other countries. Their experiences in their adopted countries doubtless varied, but little is known either of the experiences themselves or of their differential impact on their adjustment and, presumably, the consequential mental health of their children.

The survivors who immigrated to Israel encountered a reality quite different from that of other survivors. Israel was a newly declared state that offered the survivors a Jewish national home, where they were among their own and, moreover, where they were called upon to partic-ipate actively in the monumental enterprise of nation building that was then in process. Their drive to "rebuild" themselves and to create new families and a new community after the de-struction of the Holocaust coincided with the national enterprise of building the Jewish state. Moreover, many of the survivors perceived the establishment of the State of Israel as evidence of the failure of the Nazis to destroy the Jewish people. This perception could have given spe-cial meaning to their survival and helped restore some of their massively injured self-esteem. In addition, the participation in the Arab–Israeli conflict presented many of the survivors with the opportunity to channel their pent-up aggressions toward the Arabs, and helped to replace their image as victims with a new self-concept of warriors fighting in a war of independence. This image was supported by the establishment of bereavement memorials, memorial museums, and a national anniversary, which deliberately emphasized the heroic nature of the survival.

Their adjustment may also have been facilitate by the fact that they were a large group of people who shared similar traumatic experiences. Indeed, not only the Holocaust survivors, but also most of the citizens of the new state, had been uprooted from their former homes and had to contend with the trials of adjusting to a new society.

On the other hand, the very same circumstances may have made the survivors' adjustment more difficult. They reached a country with minimal, scarce resources, most channeled to its survival and building, in the midst of or shortly after a bloody war of independence. It could thus not provide them a "cushioned" absorption, and they were generally left alone in their struggle. Moreover, manifestations of weakness and dependency were regarded as detrimental to the national effort of building a new state. As a result, expressions of grief, sadness, and bereavement were discouraged. In addition, the fact that many veteran Israelis had themselves lost loved ones in the Holocaust left them with intense feelings of guilt, which led them to reject and even blame the Holocaust survivors (for an extensive review, see Danieli, 1982; Segev, 1991; Solomon, 1995a, 1995b).

Whether immigration to Israel facilitated or impeded the survivors' "recovery" from the Holocaust trauma, one cannot rule out the possibility that the experience of the years immediately after the Holocaust may have had its own impact on the survivors and their children. The findings of transgenerational transmission of the Holocaust trauma might thus be different in Israel than in other parts of the world.

This chapter surveys the literature on the transgenerational transmission of the Holocaust experiences between survivors and their children in Israel. It examines the second generation's knowledge and attitudes, worldviews, intrapsychic characteristics, family relationships, and interpersonal and social functioning. A summary of the empirical studies is presented in Table 1.

KNOWLEDGE AND COMMUNICATION:
THE CONSPIRACY OF SILENCE

The literature on Holocaust survivors reveals two opposite trends in how the survivors communicated their traumatic experiences. Many survivors kept silent, unable to speak about the events, or denying their emotional impact. On the other hand, many survivors felt a strong need to tell: to recount their experiences over and over again. Psychologically, telling serves trauma survivors as a means of working through their emotional trauma, mourning their losses, perpetuating the memory of the martyred dead, and relieving their guilt feelings. Existentially, it is the fulfillment of the urgent moral obligation expressed by many survivors (e.g., Wiesel, 1972) to "bear witness," to testify to the truth of the Holocaust lest it be forgotten. For the survivors as a whole, sharing Holocaust experiences was the only way of bridging the chasm between the gruesome, nightmarish world they had inhabited under the Nazis and the human and humane world they wished to rejoin.

This urge to tell, however, confronted a conspiracy of silence. According to Danieli (1982), people were not only unwilling to listen to survivors' experiences, but they also refused to believe that the horrors had actually occurred. The prevailing social avoidance, repression, and denial often ensured that survivors, feeling betrayed and alienated, kept silent. Only in recent years, following profound changes in Israeli society, has the conspiracy of silence been broken (Segev, 1991). Today, there is a growing sensitivity and readiness to listen to the survivors' Holocaust' experiences (Solomon, 1995a).

Three Israeli studies examined how these two trends might affect the children of the survivors on the cognitive level. They looked at the second generation's information seeking (both of historical and personal Holocaust-related facts) and attitudes toward both the survivors and their persecutors.

Klein and Last (1974) found that in Israel, the second generation's historical knowledge of the Holocaust did not differ from that of children of non-Holocaust survivors. This finding contrasts with findings on the comparative knowledge of the second generation in other countries. In the same study, Klein and Last found that American children of Holocaust survivors knew more historical facts about the Holocaust than other American Jewish youth. The same pattern was revealed in the Canadian population, where offspring of concentration camp survivors were more knowledgeable about World War II than other Jews of their generation (Sigal & Wein-field, 1989).

Another study examined the intergenerational communication of Holocaust experiences in terms of the kinds of experiences the parents had (Kav Venaki, Nadler, & Gershoni, 1985). This study found that partisans generally shared their war experiences with their children more than concentration camp survivors, and that children of partisans knew more about their parents' Holocaust experiences than those of camp survivors. Children of partisans reported more verbal and nonverbal communication about the Holocaust in their homes than children of concentration camp survivors, and indicated that talking about the subject was more acceptable in their homes. On the other hand, the two second-generation groups gave similar reasons for both initiating and avoiding discussion of the Holocaust with their parents. Both stated that they asked about the Holocaust mainly because they wanted to learn about the family members who were killed, as well as their parents' past. Both said that the main reason they avoided asking their parents about the Holocaust was that their parents themselves tended to initiate such conversations (Gershoni, 1980). This study also found that children of partisans expressed more favorable attitudes toward Holocaust survivors than those whose parents had been in concentration camps (Kav Venaki *et al.,* 1985).

On the whole, the attitudes of the Israeli second-generation adolescents did not differ from other Israeli youths (Klein & Last, 1974, 1978). Both second-generation and other Israeli youths expressed empathy toward the survivors (Klein & Last, 1974) and hostility toward the Germans (Klein & Last, 1978). In contrast, American children of Holocaust survivors expressed more empathy with, and less anger at, the survivors (Klein & Last, 1974) and more hostility toward the Germans than other American Jewish youths (Klein & Last, 1978). The difference in the two countries seems to have been not so much in the attitudes of the second generation as in the attitudes of the Jewish population at large. Israeli adolescents expressed more hostility toward the Germans and less denial than their American peers.

Taken together, the studies presented in this section indicate that although in North America the children of survivors are those who bear the legacy of the Holocaust, in Israel the legacy is shared by the entire society and not by the second generation alone. The similarity of knowledge and attitudes in Israel across both second-generation and non-second-generation youth would seem to be the natural outcome of the teaching of the Holocaust in Israeli schools, the annual public commemorations, and the intense media coverage of the Holocaust around those commemorations.

WORLDVIEWS

Worldviews consist of beliefs that help their holders grasp and interpret their inner and outer worlds and their interrelationships (Fiske, & Taylor, 1991). Most people hold a positive worldview, for example, believing that the world is benevolent, just, and meaningful (Epstein, 1991; Janoff-Bulman, 1985; Lerner, 1980), derived from the warmth and nurturing they received in infancy (Bowlby, 1985). They also strive to maintain that view (Taylor & Brown, 1988) by assimilating new data, even where they confute their assumptions, into their existing schemes (Lerner, 1980). Exposure to trauma may make it difficult to merge this new information with the old schemes and thus force people to alter their worldviews (Epstein, 1991; Janoff-Bulman & Frieze, 1984; Thompson & Janigan, 1988).

During the Holocaust, its victims lived on a "different planet," governed by rules alien to the ones they had known before and inconsistent with the worldview they had previously held.

To survive, they had to adopt very different patterns of thought and behavior. They had to alter their worldviews, which no longer fit the reality with which they had to contend. Many survivors retained their altered schemata long after the Holocaust ended. In a study assessing the cognitive schema of Israeli Holocaust survivors 45 years after the event, we found that they perceived the world and the people in it as both less benevolent and more meaningful than the nonsurvivor controls (Prager & Solomon, 1995). Another study found that Holocaust survivors reported more optimistic beliefs about the future than did matching controls (Carmil & Breznitz, 1991). The question that arises is whether this trauma-generated worldview is transmitted to the next generation.

As can be seen in Table 1, the studies that assessed the worldviews of the second generation in Israel yielded mixed results. Two studies found that the second generation did not differ from controls in their moral perceptions, trust, and views of human nature, in their locus of control, degree of ethnocentricity, or tendency to a siege mentality (Antebi, 1989; Eisenberg, 1982). One study found that the second generation was more optimistic, more religious, and more moderate in its political views than the control group (Carmil & Breznitz, 1991). Yet another study found that children of partisans were more inclined to believe that another Holocaust was possible than were children of concentration camp survivors (Kav Venaki et al., 1985).

Taken together, these studies suggest that some of the survivors' worldviews were transmitted to their children. Surprisingly, though, what seems to have been transmitted were not the negative or pessimistic views that one might expect from the trauma, but a certain optimism.

INTRAPSYCHIC CHARACTERISTICS

The literature on the mental health of Holocaust survivors suggests that this is a high-risk population with special intrapsychic characteristics. The features noted by various clinicians and researchers include anxiety, depression, guilt, anhedonia, emptiness, despair, somatization, and obsessive preoccupation with traumatic memories of the Holocaust (e.g., Danieli, 1981; Eitinger, 1961; Niederland, 1968). The question of whether these problems are passed on to the second generation arises.

Studies of the mental health of the second generation again show mixed findings. Two studies compared the mental health of clinical populations with and without a Holocaust background. Aleksandrowicz's (1973) study of children with psychiatric problems found no difference in the diagnostic categories of those whose parents were Holocaust survivors and those whose parents were not. De Graaf's (1975) study of Israeli soldiers treated in army mental health facilities found that the second-generation Holocaust survivors showed more personality disorders and delinquent tendencies than other patients, though they did not differ in neurotic or depressive symptoms, or in adjustment difficulties.

A larger number of studies compared nonclinical populations. These found no difference between the second generation and comparable controls in anxiety (Keinan, Mikulincer, & Rybnicki, 1988), depression (Keinan et al., 1988), neuroticism (Goder, 1981), or most aspects of self-perception (Felsen & Erlich, 1990; Keinan et al., 1988). They did, however, find evidence of weaker superegos (Goder, 1986) and depleted ego strength (Schellekes, 1986), as well as greater self-criticism (Felsen & Erlich, 1990), higher levels of guilt feelings (Nadler, Kav Venaki, & Gleitman, 1985), and more difficulty in anger resolution, often manifested in the form of angry outbursts, acting out, and demanding behavior toward spouses and other close persons (Erel, 1989; Nadler et al., 1985). Schwartz, Dohrenwend, and Levev (1994), who studied a large sample of Israeli adults, found that although the second generation was not

Table 1. Studies of Israeli Holocaust Survivors' Offspring

	N	Sampling	Measures	Findings
Knowledge and communication				
Kav-Venaki, Nadler, & Gershoni (1985)	15 families in which both parents were expartisans; 15 families in which both parents were exprisoners in concentration camps	Nonclinical population	Individual interviews regarding communication behaviors	Greater legitimacy and openness in discussing Holocaust-related issues in the homes of expartisans than in the homes of exprisoners in concentration camps. Offspring of the former group have better knowledge of the Holocaust and hold more favorable attitudes than offspring of the second group.
Klein & Last (1974)	211 Israeli adolescents (13–14 yrs), 97 American Jewish adolescents (13–14 yrs)	Nonclinical population	Closed questionnaires: knowledge about the Holocaust; attitudes toward Holocaust victims	Knowledge about the Holocaust among the Israeli OHS was high and similar to this of their peers (nOHS). Attitudes toward Holocaust victims were also uniform among the Israeli adolescents: 73% of the sample report with realistic attitude (e.g., "They had no choice but to act as they did."). Most of adolescents expressed empathy (94%). Anger and contempt were almost completely absent.

Study	Sample	Population	Method	Results
Eisenberg (1982)	20 OHS; 20 controls	Nonclinical population	Standardized questionnaires: Locus of Control Scale, Philosophies of Human Nature Scale, Interpersonal Trust Scale, Mash Scale (Machiavellism and moral behavior)	There were no group differences.
Intrapsychic characteristics				
Aleksandrowicz (1973)	10 children, both parents Holocaust (HS) survivors; 15 children, one parent HS; 9 children, nOHS	Clinical population	Individual interviews, family interviews, psychological tests	The groups did not differ in the diagnostic categories.
De Graff (1975)	27 soldiers, OHS; 36 soldiers, nOHS	Clinical population	Individual interviews	OHS did not differ from the controls in neurotic traits, depressive syndrome, and maladjustment. OHS had higher levels of personality disturbances and delinquent traits.
Klein & Last (1978)	211 Israeli adolescents (13–14 yrs), 97 American Jewish adolescents (13–14 yrs)	Nonclinical population	Attitudes toward Germans and German children (questionnaires)	Attitudes of Israeli OHS were similar to those of their peers: more than two-third of the adolescents expressed hostility toward Germans. More than 40% of the adolescents would respond with negative affect toward the hypothetical German child, a third of them would avoid him.
Worldview				
Antebi (1989)	376 students, 20% OHS	Nonclinical population	Questionnaires regarding siege mentality, ethnocentric beliefs, and suspicion	There were no group differences.

(continued)

Table 1. *(Continued)*

Carmil & Breznitz (1991)	189 OHS; 191 controls	Nonclinical population	Questionnaires: demographic background, political attitudes, religious identity, future orientation	There were no group differences with regard to political preferences of right versus left parties. However, OHS hold more moderate political position than controls. More OHS identified themselves as religious than controls. OHS were more optimistic than controls.
Erel (1989)	5 couples in which one is OHS	Couples that applied to marital treatment	Individual interviews	OHS exhibited problems in expression of aggression.
Goder (1981)	20 OHS; 20 controls	Nonclinical population	Standardized questionnaire regarding personality characteristics	There were no group differences in nuroticism. Female OHS tend to be more depressed and to react according to their mood more than female controls. In addition, they have less clear and stable ideal-ego. Male OHS tend to be more extroverted, assertive, and dominant, than male controls. All OHS tend to have weaker superego than controls.
Keinan, Mikulincer, & Rypnicki (1988)	47 OHS; 46 controls	Nonclinical population	Standardized questionnaires: State-Trait Anxiety Inventory; Depressive Adjective Checklist; Semantic Differential Scale	The groups did not differ in level of anxiety and depression, or in self-perception.
Nadler, Kav-Venaki, & Gleitman (1985)	19 OHS; 19 controls	Nonclinical population	Rosenzweig Projective Test of Reactions to Frustration; structured interviews	OHS express more guilt and less external aggression than their counterparts.

Sachs (1988)	40 families of HS and their offspring	Nonclinical population	Standardized questionnaires: Family Adaptability and Cohesion Scale; Trait Anxiety Inventory; Depressive Adjective Checklist	In families whose family cohesion and adaptability scores were extreme (high or low), OHS manifested higher levels of anxiety and depression than those of families whose family functioning pattern moved in the moderate ranges.
Schellekes (1986)	20 couples in which one is OHS; 20 matched couples	Nonclinical population	Standardized questionnaire: Baron's Ego Strength Scale	OHS had lower ego strength than nOHS.
Schwartz, Dohrenwend, & Levav (1994)	291 OHS and 957 controls in the first stage; 147 and 476 (respectively) in the second	Nonclinical population	Standardized questionnaires: Psychiatric Epidemiology Research Interview, IES, PTSD Inventory	The two groups did not differ in level of psychopathology. OHS, however, manifested higher rates of past disorders.
Shafat, 1994	40 OHS; 43 controls	Nonclinical population	Standardized questionnaires: Children's Commitment toward Parents Questionnaire, Mental Health Inventory, Rosenberg Self-Esteem	OHS reported more commitment to undertake and perform unsolvable tasks in their relationships with their parents. This influences their emotional status: The more the OHS try to benefit their parents, the greater is their mental distress and the lower their mental well-being.
Family relationships				
Erel, 1989	5 couples in which one is OHS	Couples that applied to marital treatment	Individual interviews	OHS exhibited problems in separation–individuation and express high significance to their relations with their parents. There were no problems in parental functioning.

distinguished from controls in anxiety and depression at the time of the study, it differed in levels of *lifetime* psychopathology, since it reported higher rates of past anxiety and depression.

There are also indications that some of the second generation suffer more from their parents' traumatization than others. A gender-focused study found that second-generation women tended to be more depressive, moody, and emotionally labile than comparable controls, whereas second-generation men tended to be more extroverted, assertive, and dominant than controls (Goder, 1981). Another study found that offspring of Holocaust families with either very high or very low cohesion suffered from higher levels of anxiety and depression than those from families with more balanced cohesion and adjustment (Sachs, 1988). Yet another study found that members of the second generation who were expected to perform many unresolvable tasks in their relationships with their parents reported that the harder they tried, the greater their mental distress and the less their sense of their well-being (Shafat, 1994).

FAMILY RELATIONSHIPS

Creating a family was one of the most important aims of the survivors' lives. Children represented the survivors' endurance and continuity, served as the repository of what they had suffered and lost, guarded the family against the hostility of the outer world, and fulfilled myriad other possible and impossible functions that children ordinarily need to fulfill. The parent–child relationships in survivors families were usually highly intense.

Offspring of survivors have been found to be highly committed to their parents' welfare (Shafat, 1994) and to feel that they must fulfill their parents' expectations (Shafat, 1994). They have also been found to be dependent on their parents (Tal, 1992) and to have difficulties with separation–individuation (Erel, 1989; Tal, 1992) and intimacy (Tal, 1992). Some describe their families as enmeshed and their parents as overly involved in their lives (Nadler *et al.*, 1985). Others describe parental disengagement (Stepak, 1989), emotional inaccessibility (Tal, 1992), and lack of supportiveness (Tal, 1992).

Two studies investigated members of the second generation's identification with their parents. Here, results were contradictory. One study found lower correlations between the second-generations members' perceptions of themselves and their perceptions of their parents (Keinan *et al.*, 1988) than among controls. Another, however, found that survivors' children's perceptions of both their actual selves and their ideal selves were closer to their perceptions of their parents actual and ideal selves than those of a control group (Felsen & Erlich, 1990).

The importance of family and children has apparently extended to the families that the second generation itself created. Like their parents, the second generation assigns great importance to parenthood. One study found that members of the second generation who were in marital therapy placed the better part of their effort and energy into issues of child rearing (Erel, 1989). A study that assessed perceptions of parenthood among daughters of survivors found these women to manifest greater maternal anxiety and maternal distress, along with less maternal satisfaction and flexibility, than comparable controls (Marcus, 1988).

ADJUSTMENT AND VULNERABILITY

Studies that examined the functioning of the second generation in different areas have also yielded mixed outcomes. An analysis of demographic statistics by two Israeli sociologists, Yuchtman-Yaar and Menachem (1992), suggests a good level of social adjustment. This study found that whereas Holocaust survivors were economically less successful than comparable non-Holocaust immigrants to Israel, the second generation attained greater socioeconomic success than their peers. The researchers conclude that the parents' Holocaust experience led to high motivation and achievement needs in their offspring.

But findings on the second generation's coping with stress were less clear-cut. The coping styles of the second generation were found to be remarkably similar to those of their parents, especially their mothers (Rim, 1992). Among the typical mechanisms were minimization, replacement, and mapping. Nathan (1988) found that second-generation youths did not differ from their non-second-generation peers in social functioning, somatic and psychiatric health, and academic achievements, and, moreover, that they adjusted better than their peers without a Holocaust background to stressful life events (such as death or severe illness in the family). This finding led her to conclude that second-generation Holocaust survivors were more resilient than others and better equipped to deal with stress.

Similarly, our study of soldiers in the Israel Defense Forces during the 1982 Lebanon War (Solomon, Kotler, & Mikulincer, 1988) found no difference in the rates of "combat stress disorder" (mental breakdown during or shortly after battle action) among second-generation and non-second-generation combatants.

On the other hand, the same study (Solomon *et al.,* 1988) found that second-generation soldiers who did sustain a combat stress reaction showed greater vulnerability than their non-second-generation peers. Examination of recovery rates 2 and 3 years after the war showed that the casualties with a Holocaust survivor parent suffered more intense and enduring posttraumatic residues than those without Holocaust background. The comparative durability of the distress may be related to the nature of the combat breakdown. Soldiers who break down in combat generally suffer from feelings of shame and guilt at having let down their country and their buddies. Among members of the second generation, who were raised to undo the damage the Nazis inflicted on their parents' lives, these feelings cut deeper as the magnitude of the expectations intensified the failure implicit in the breakdown. Alternatively, the severity of the second-generation members' PTSD may be explained by the possibility that it is, in fact, a reactivation of a latent trauma that they suffered as a result of their parents' experiences.

However the findings are explained, the two studies suggest that members of the second generation cope well with stress, and perhaps even better than their non-second-generation peers, though those who fail to cope suffer deeper and more intense distress.

SUMMARY

On the whole, the various studies discussed show members of the second generation in Israel to be an essentially healthy and functioning population despite certain difficulties that apparently derive from their parents' Holocaust experience. The studies show that the second generation in Israel is no more prone to psychopathology than the rest of the population, but that it does suffer from distinct intrapsychic difficulties. Consistent with this, the studies indicate a family pattern of strong relationships, marked, on the one hand, by commitment and dedication to both the family of origin and the family of making, and, on the other, by a good deal of tension and difficulty. Along similar lines, the studies of the second generation's functioning suggest a high level of day-to-day coping as well as the ability to deal with stressful life events, but also indicate that there might be special difficulties under certain circumstances, as seen in the robustness of their posttraumatic stress disorder (PTSD) following combat breakdown. On the cognitive level, the survivors' experience has evidently not produced a suspicious or pessimistic worldview of their children. If anything, children of survivors showed greater optimism and more moderate political views than other Israelis of their generation.

The overall picture of a healthy, functioning population, able to build warm families and to cope with its problems, emerges from a literature that contains very different expectations. Most of the studies of both survivors and their offspring are conducted from a pathogenic perspective. For almost three decades, if not more, the bulk of the studies consisted of clinical impressions of clinical populations, either hospitalized or in some form of psychotherapy (e.g., Chodoff, 1963; Davidson, 1980; Eitinger, 1961; Gampel, 1992; Kogan, 1988), from which the researchers generalized to the survivors and the second generation as a whole. This literature naturally revealed pathology and led to the adaptation of a pathogenic perspective in subsequent studies. The assumption of pathology affected the selection and definition of the research questions, and the choice of instruments and procedures, and colored interpretation of the findings. Although most of the empirical studies reviewed here focused on nonclinical populations, the influence of the pathogenic approach is noticeable. Most of the outcome measures assess psychopathology (e.g., anxiety, depression) and maladjustment rather than, for example, emotional maturity and strengths.

Beyond its specific sources, the pathogenic bias in the studies of Holocaust survivors and their children is much the same as that which informs most of the traumatology literature (Antonovsky & Bernstein, 1986). It is consistent with the bias inherent in modern psychology, commencing with Freud, which has been constructed largely by generalizing from patients in psychoanalysis. It is fostered by the orientation of the mental health profession, whose work is to treat and study people in need of emotional help, and who thus naturally focus more on mental illness than on mental health. The pathogenic approach may also be fostered by the countertransference of those who treat or study the victims of man-made traumas (Danieli, 1982; Haley, 1974; McCann & Pearlman, 1980; Ofri, Solomon, & Dasberg, 1995). The intensity of such traumas, even when experienced by proxy, arouses strong emotions, including guilt, anger, and overidentification with the victim (Bergmann & Jucovy, 1982; Chodoff, 1980; Danieli, 1984; Prince, 1984). These feelings may make it difficult for therapists and researchers to maintain the professional neutrality that would be required to conceive of and explore the possibility of positive effects arising from trauma.

Much like that of traumatology in general, the literature on the long-term effects of the Holocaust tends to ignore possible salutogenic effects that, according to Antonovsky and Bernstein (1986), can also issue from stressful experiences. In recent years, there has been some correction in this bias, but more remains to be done.

Another line of reasoning is presented by Steinberg (1995) as a duality between the inner experience of the second generation and its overt level of functioning. She asserts that although there are similar levels of functioning between members of the second generation and controls, the former perceive themselves as more vulnerable and less adjusted. The author maintains that the empirical studies fail to reflect the true picture of the subjective experience of the offspring of survivors, due to the use of assessment tools that are not sufficiently sensitive in tapping subtle subjective effects.

An important finding of the studies was that second-generation Israelis' knowledge of the Holocaust and the attitudes toward the survivors and the perpetrators were similar to those of other Israelis of the same age (Klein & Last, 1974, 1978). This contrasts strikingly with the disparity in knowledge and attitudes of the second generation and the rest of the Jewish population in North America (Klein & Last, 1974, 1978; Sigal & Weinfeld, 1989).

The difference reflects the central role of the Holocaust in the Israeli experience. Though Israel was established after more than half a century of nation building on the part of successive waves of Jewish pioneers, its acquisition of statehood was seen as a direct response to the genocide in Europe. From its earliest days, and despite the conspiracy of silence, there was a strong public commitment to remember the Holocaust and to remind the citizens of Israel and the world of its ignominy. This remembering and reminding was more than a formal declaration. It was manifested in innumerable public and private acts that were part and parcel of life in Israel. Whereas in most parts of the world the Holocaust has been treated as a tragic historical occurrence, in Israel it has been experienced as a formative event with a profound, ongoing impact on the country's identity and on its political, social, and emotional life. Throughout most of the world, the Holocaust is the legacy of the survivors and their offspring. In Israel, it is the legacy of all.

Need for Further Study

Overall, there are relatively few studies of the second generation in Israel, and most of those are flawed. The majority of the studies discussed here are based on nonclinical populations and utilize objective standardized measures; most have very small samples (e.g., Kav Venaki *et al.,* 1985; Schellekes, 1986), and relied on "snowballing" to obtain their subjects (e.g., Shafat, 1994; Tal, 1992). These limitations cast doubt on the representativeness of the samples and limit the generalizability of the studies' findings. The choice of self-report measures has also been criticized as not adequately sensitive in tapping the internal experiences of children of Holocaust survivors, or as being too sensitive to social desirability (Steinberg, 1995).

Also problematic is the question of who is and is not included in the "second generation." The experiences of the Holocaust generation were highly varied. Although most survived in hiding or in camps, others immigrated or escaped from Nazi Europe without direct experience of these particular horrors. Some escaped shortly after Hitler came to power, others only after suffering considerable abuse. Most were uprooted, most lost loved ones, and some were imprisoned, such as in Siberia. Which of them are "Holocaust survivors," and which of their children fit into the category of the "second generation"? The difficulties of setting boundaries and defining second generation clearly compromise the research findings.

Many questions remain unanswered. How exactly is the Holocaust, or any trauma, transmitted from generation to generation? What possible positive impact can the parents' Holocaust experience have on their children? What determines whether the legacy is pathogenic or salutogenic? The centrality of the Holocaust in Israeli society emphasizes the need for crosscultural studies to examine the impact of sociocultural characteristics on the transgenerational transmission of Holocaust experiences.

REFERENCES

Aleksandrowicz, D. R. (1973). Children of concentration camp survivors. In E. J. Anthony, & C. Koupernick (Eds.), *The child and his family* (pp. 385–392). New York: Wiley.

Antebi, D. (1989). *Siege mentality in Israel.* Unpublished master's thesis, Tel Aviv University, Department of Psychology [Hebrew], Tel Aviv, Israel.

Antonovsky, A., & Bernstein, J. (1986). Pathogenesis and salutogenesis in war and other crises: Who studies the successful coper? In N. Milgram (Ed.), *Stress and coping in time of war: Generalizations from the Israeli experience* (pp. 52–65). New York: Brunner/Mazel.

Bar-On, D. (1994). *Fear and hope.* Tel Aviv, Israel: Ghetto Fighters' House [Hebrew].

Barocas, H., & Barocas, C. (1979). Wounds of the fathers: The next generation of Holocaust victims. *International Review of Psychoanalysis, 5,* 331–341.

Bergmann, M. S., & Jucovy, M. E. (1982). *Generations of the Holocaust.* New York: Basic Books.

Bowlby, J. (1985). *Attachment and loss: Separation*. New York: Penguin Books.

Carmil, D., & Breznitz, S. (1991). Personal trauma and world-view: Are extremely stressful experiences related to political attitudes, religious beliefs, and future orientation? *Journal of Traumatic Stress, 4*(3), 393–405.

Chodoff, P. (1963). Late effects of the concentration camp syndrome. *Archives of General Psychiatry, 6*, 323–333.

Chodoff, P. (1975). Psychiatric aspects of Nazi persecution. In Arieti (Ed.), *American handbook of psychiatry*, vol. VI, p. 933. Washington, DC: American Psychiatric Association.

Chodoff, P. (1980). Psychotherapy of the survivor. In J. E. Dimsdale (Ed.), *Survivors, victims, and perpetrators: Essays on the Nazi Holocaust* (pp. 205–217). New York: Hemisphere.

Danieli, Y. (1981). Families of survivors of the Nazi Holocaust: Some long- and some short-term effects. In N. Milgram (Ed.), *Psychological stress and adjustment in time of war and peace* (pp. 000–000). Washington, DC: Hemisphere.

Danieli, Y. (1982). *Therapists' difficulties in treating survivors of the Nazi Holocaust and their children*. Ph.D. dissertation, New York University, New York.

Danieli, Y. (1984). Psychotherapists' participation in the conspiracy of silence about the Holocaust. *Psychoanalytic Psychology, 1*, 23–42.

Davidson, S. (1980). The clinical effects of massive psychic trauma in families of Holocaust survivors. *Journal of Marital and Family Therapy, 6*, 11–21.

de Graaf, T. (1975). Pathological patterns of identification in families of survivors of the Holocaust. *Israel Annals of Psychiatry, 13*, 335–363.

Eisenberg, K. (1982). *The social world of the second generation of Holocaust survivors values and beliefs about interpersonal relations*. Unpublished master's thesis, Tel Aviv University, Department of Psychology [Hebrew], Tel Aviv, Israel.

Eitinger, L. (1961). Pathology of the concentration camp syndrome. *Archives of General Psychiatry, 5*, 371–379.

Engel, W. H. (1962). Reflections of the psychiatric consequences of persecution. *American Journal of Psychotherapy, 16*, 191–203.

Epstein, H. (1979). *Children of Holocaust: Conversations with sons and daughters of survivors*. New York: Putnam.

Epstein, S. (1991). Cognitive-experimental self-theory: An integrative theory of personality. In R. C. Curtis (Ed.), *The relational self* (pp. 111–137). New York: Guilford.

Erel, D. (1989). *Marital interaction of children of Holocaust survivors: The intergenerational transmission of posttraumatic impacts on marital functioning (An exploratory study of five couples in marital therapy)*. Unpublished master's thesis, Tel Aviv University, School of Social Work [Hebrew], Tel Aviv, Israel.

Felsen, I., & Erlich, S. (1990). Identification patterns of offspring of Holocaust survivors with their parents. *American Journal of Orthopsychiatry, 60*, 506–520.

Fiske, S. T., & Taylor, S. E. (1991). *Social cognition*. New York: McGraw-Hill.

Freyberg, J. T. (1980). Difficulties in separation–individuation as experienced by offspring of Nazi Holocaust survivors. *American Journal of Orthopsychiatry, 50*, 87–95.

Gampel, Y. (1992). Psychoanalysis, ethics, and actuality. *Psychoanalytic Inquiry, 12*, 526–550.

Gershoni, H. (1980). *Communication, knowledge and attitudes concerning the Holocaust among families of survivors*. Unpublished master's thesis, Tel Aviv University, Department of Psychology [Hebrew], Tel Aviv, Israel.

Goder, L. (1981). *Personality characteristics of the offspring of Nazi Holocaust survivors in Israel*. Unpublished master's thesis, Tel Aviv University, Department of Psychology [Hebrew], Tel Aviv, Israel.

Haley, S. A. (1974). When the patient reports atrocities. *Archives of General Psychiatry, 30*, 191–196.

Janoff-Bulman, R. (1985). The aftermath of victimization: Rebuilding shattered assumptions. In C. R. Figley (Ed.), *Trauma and its wake* (pp. 15–35). New York: Brunner/Mazel.

Janoff-Bulman, R., & Frieze, I. H. (1983). A theoretical perspective for understanding reactions to victimization. *Journal of Social Issues, 39*, 1–17.

Kav Venaki, S., Nadler, A., & Gershoni, H. (1985). Sharing the Holocaust experience: Communication behaviors and their consequences in families of ex-partisans and ex-prisoners of concentration camps. *Family Process, 24*, 273–280.

Keinan, G., Mikulincer, M., & Rybnicki, A. (1988). Perception of self and parents by second-generation Holocaust survivors. *Behavioral Medicine, 14*, 6–12.

Kestenberg, J. (1972). Psychoanalytic contributions to the problem of children of survivors from Nazi persecution. *Israel Annals of Psychiatry and Related Disciplines, 10*, 311–325.

Klein, H., & Last, U. (1974). Cognitive and emotional aspects of the attitudes of American and Israeli Jewish youth toward the victims of the Holocaust. *Israel Annals of Psychiatry and Related Disciplines, 12*, 111–131.

Klein, H., & Last, U. (1978). Attitudes toward persecutor representations in children of traumatized and nontraumatized parents: Cross-cultural comparison. *Adolescent Psychiatry, 6*, 224–238.

Koening, W. (1964). Chronic or persisting identity diffusion. *American Journal of Psychiatry, 120*, 1081–1083.

Kogan, I. (1988). The second skin. *International Review of Psycho-Analysis, 15*, 251–260.

Leon, G. R., Butcher, J. N., Kleinman, M., Goldberg, A., & Almagor, M. (1981). Survivors of the Holocaust and their children: Current status and adjustment. *Journal of Personality and Social Psychology, 41,* 503–516.

Lerner, M. J. (1980). *The belief in a just world.* New York: Plenum Press.

Marcus, D. (1988). *Emotional features in the experience of motherhood among daughters of Holocaust survivors.* Unpublished master's thesis, Haifa University, Department of Psychology [Hebrew], Haifa, Israel.

McCann, L., & Pearlman, L. A. (1990). Vicarious traumatization: A framework for understanding the psychological effects of working with victims. *Journal of Traumatic Stress, 3*(1):131–149.

Nadler, A., Kav-Venaki, S., & Gleitman, B. (1985). Transgenerational effects of the Holocaust: Aggression in second generation of Holocaust survivors. *Journal of Consulting and Clinical Psychology, 53,* 365–369.

Nathan, T. S. (1988). Shoa survivors' second generation adjustment in adolescence. *Studies on the Holocaust Period, 2,* 13–26 [Hebrew].

Niderland, W. G. (1968). The problem of the survivor. In H. Krystal (Ed.), *Massive psychic trauma* (pp. 8–22). New York: International Universities Press.

Ofri, I., Solomon, Z., & Dasberg, H. (1995). Attitudes of therapists toward Holocaust survivors. *Journal of Traumatic Stress, 8,* 229–242.

Ohel, N. (1994). *Perception of the family of origin, attachment styles, and the quality of marriage in the second generation of Holocaust survivors.* Unpublished master's thesis, Haifa University, School of Social Work [Hebrew], Haifa, Israel.

Prager, E., & Solomon, Z. (1995). Perceptions of world benevolence, meaningfulness, and self-worth among elderly Israeli Holocaust survivors and non-survivors. *Anxiety, Stress and Coping, 8,* 165–277.

Prince, R. M. (1984). *The legacy of the Holocaust: Psychohistorical themes in the second generation.* ?????, MI: V. M. F. Research Press.

Rim, Y. (1991). Coping styles of (first- and second-generation) Holocaust survivors. *Personality and Individual Differences, 12,* 1315–1317.

Sachs, H. (1988). *The relationship between family adaptability and cohesion levels, and anxiety and depression levels in Holocaust survivors offspring.* Unpublished master's thesis, Tel Aviv University, Department of Psychology [Hebrew], Tel Aviv, Israel.

Schellekes, S. (1986). *The implications of concentration camp interment for second generation survivors' marriages and interpersonal characteristics.* Unpublished master's thesis, Bar Ilan University, Department of Psychology [Hebrew], Bar Ilan, Israel.

Schwartz, S., Dohrenwend, B. P., & Levav, I. (1994). Nongenetic familial transmission of psychiatric disorders? Evidence from children of Holocaust survivors. *Journal of Health and Social Behavior, 35,* 385–402.

Segev, T. (1991). *The seventh million: The Israelis and the Holocaust.* Jerusalem, Israel: Maxwell-Macmillan-Keter Publishing [Hebrew].

Shafat, R. (1994). Commitment to parents as unresolvable problem in children of Holocaust survivors, *Sihot, 8,* 23–27 [Hebrew].

Sigal, J. J., & Weinfeld, M. (1989). *Trauma and rebirth.* New York: Praeger.

Solomon, Z. (1995a). From denial to recognition: Attitudes toward Holocaust survivors from World War II to the present. *Journal of Traumatic Stress, 8,* 215–228.

Solomon, Z. (1995b). Oscillating between denial and recognition of PTSD: Why are lessons learned and forgotten. *Journal of Traumatic Stress, 8,* 271–282.

Solomon, Z., Kotler, M., & Mikulincer, M. (1988). Combat-related posttraumatic stress disorder among second-generation Holocaust survivors: Preliminary findings. *American Journal of Psychiatry, 145,* 865–868.

Steinberg, A. (1995, July). *Coming home from trauma: Clinical directions in research with Holocaust survivors' children.* Paper presented at Coming Home from Trauma: The next Generation, Muteness and the search for a Voice, Yale Trauma Center, New Haven, CT.

Stepak, S. (1989). *Perception of family-system and personality characteristics among offspring of Holocaust survivors.* Unpublished master's thesis, Tel Aviv University, Department of Psychology [Hebrew], Tel Aviv, Israel.

Tal, I. 1992. *Separation–individuation and capacity for intimacy in children of Holocaust survivors.* Unpublished master's thesis, Tel Aviv University, Department of Psychology [Hebrew], Tel Aviv, Israel.

Taylor, S. E., & Brown, J. D. (1988). Illusion and well being: A social psychological perspective on mental health. *Psychological Bulletin, 103,* 193–210.

Thompson, S. C., & Janigian, A. S. (1988). Life schemas: A framework for understanding the search for meaning. *Journal of Social and Clinical Psychology, 7*(2/3), 260–280.

Wardi, D. (1990). *Memorial candels.* Jerusalem: Keer Publishing House [Hebrew].

Wiesel, E. (1972). *One generation after.* New York: Avon Books.

Yuchtman-Yaar, E., & Menahem, G. (1992). Socioeconomic achievements of Holocaust survivors in Israel: The first and second generation. *Contemporary Jewry, 13,* 95–123.

4

Children of Nazis

A Psychodynamic Perspective

GERTRUD HARDTMANN

The Nazi disaster—the most devastating period in German history for the lives, the culture, and the souls it ruined—is still only a marginal subject in German psychological research. In fact, up to the early 1980s, there were hardly any scientific publications. There are probably three reasons for the lack of research about this topic in Germany: (1) the long time of latency between the end of the Nazi area in 1945 and the beginning of the investigations in the 1980s; (2) the absence of theory to conceptualize the research data; and (3) the fact that *all* the investigators in Germany are part of the problem they are investigating.

Only after a long period of latency, starting in the early 1980s, have there been German investigations about "Children of Nazis." In 1982, for the first time, German scientists wrote on this topic in the American publication *Generations of the Holocaust* (Bergmann & Jucovy, 1982; Eckstaedt, 1982; Hardtmann, 1982; Rosenkötter, 1982). It took another 13 years until a German publisher took the risk to translate and republish in Germany extracts from this important book. Peter Sichrovski published his moving interviews with children of Nazis in 1987. And strong media interest was roused in Germany when Niklas Frank displayed in public the conflict with his father, who had been the chief of *Generalgouvernemt* Poland from 1939 until 1945, and had been sentenced to death in 1946 (Frank, 1987).

Dörte von Westernhagen (1987), a German journalist, conducted considerable research over several years in order to reconstruct the biography of her father, who had been a member of the *Leibstandarte Adolf Hitler* and had died as a soldier toward the end of the war. In a very vivid and sensitive way, the reader received an example of how the second generation labored to save what could be saved from the ruins of the Third Reich. The desire to comprehend her father, to get access to the inconceivable, to do justice to him and to her own wishes and disappointed longings, were laid open.

For years, Bar-On interviewed children of leading Nazis. He listened to them, individually and in groups, starting out with entirely German groups, later counseling mixed groups of the second and third generation of German children of persecutors and Jewish children of survivors from the United States and Israel. He described in detail the everyday experiences of the

GERTRUD HARDTMANN • Technical University, Berlin, Germany

International Handbook of Multigenerational Legacies of Trauma, edited by Yael Danieli. Plenum Press, New York, 1998.

Nazi children with their fathers and mothers, their unfulfilled hopes, their yearnings and disappointments, and their attempts, over and over again, to understand what was going on inside the psyche of their parents, their fathers' especially (Bar-On, 1989).

Naturally, all these investigators were initially concerned with saving the historical facts by exploring the specific experiences and events and preparing documentary material. Ready-made theoretical concepts to process and sort out the observations were not at hand. In the human science perspective, Bar-On tried to use the concepts of "partial relevance" by Rokeatch (1968) and Tetlock (1979), and the psychoanalytic concept of "working through" (Freud, 1914), and tried to draw theoretical conclusions from the "Milgram experiment" (Milgram, 1963). Recent field studies in France on right-wing youngsters and their ethnic conflicts utilize concepts of marginalization and concepts describing the process of acculturation or deculturation of French or Algerian adolescents in today's France. Certain social, not individual, factors are emphasized, above all employment, self-sufficiency, and the social appreciation connected thereto, that even out ethnic differences. The ethnic factors gained important—in a process of "ethnification"—the more the social conditions deteriorated (Dubet & Lapeyronnie, 1992).

A great problem in Holocaust research seems to be that different sciences (psychology, sociology, history, educational and political science) are investigating and explaining different parts of the phenomenon. But the whole phenomenon is not susceptible to a reliable interpretation. This need to cover the whole phenomenon is seemingly compensated on occasion by professional narcissism. The investigators try to sell a fraction as the whole and draw conclusions that are trespassing the boundaries of their special discipline. The uniqueness of the Holocaust seems to be unconsciously viewed as a provocation, urging a need to counter the incomprehensible with an—if late and ex-post but comprehensive—understanding. There is, and remains, some discomfort and frustration, however, that the different observations and conclusions cannot be joined in an integrated concept. A large number of details do not necessarily create a complete, whole picture.

Such efforts can be observed also with some psychotherapists who attempted to draw a complete portrait of the Führer's psychic structure using only fractional accounts (Miller, 1980; Stierlin, 1975). Focused only on the individual, they neglected the fact that National Socialism and the splitting of German society into Aryans and non-Aryans and projective identification, starting as early as 1933, was a collective effort Hitler could not have performed alone, even had he wished to. Working alliances between different disciplines could be helpful to avoid such misunderstandings.

Early on in my investigations, I gained much insight from studying the perspective of the victims observing the perpetrators. Ruth Klüger's description (1992) of a baker's daughter in Vienna maliciously frightening a Jewish child illegally visiting the cinema demonstrates that during the Nazi period, every "Aryan" person—even the children—had the power to persecute "non-Aryan" people. Any kind of mischievous, even playful, attitude against minorities was legalized and promoted by the authorities. Many people used this empowerment in their everyday lives (Goldhagen, 1996).

Primo Levi (1988) described how, in the concentration camp during mutual working hours, he was seemingly treated normally as a chemist by his German colleague, but later—abruptly—like a cheap object, dead and worthless. The relationship on the part of the persecutor was not determined by personal feelings, affection, or dislike, or even neutrality, but rather by impersonal conditions that he accepted completely: As a colleague, Primo Levi deserved to be treated as a colleague; as a prisoner, he did not deserve any respect. Like a chameleon, the colleague adapted his personal conduct completely to the social structure. But the social environment only proposed certain behavioral regulations, yet never compelled or forced people to abide by them.

A German court, in the case of a Jewish survivor seeking reparations, ruled that children who spent the first 3 years of their lives in a concentration camp could not have suffered any lasting traumatization or psychic damage, because they did not have conscious memory of that time. This conclusion has been proven wrong by Judith Kestenberg (1982) through numerous interviews. These children especially showed severe and quasipsychotic disturbances. This court's statement reveals more about the perpetrators than the victims. Following the logic of this court, children up to 3 years of age could be subjected to any psychic torture and injury without lasting effects.

The differentiating reports of the victims show that there was some freedom of choice during the Nazi period, even in the concentration camps. In their reports, the victims distinguish between guards who used their instructions to torture the prisoners, and others who preserved for themselves a small degree of humanity (Müller-Münch, 1982).

NAZI CHILDREN'S TRAUMA

My investigations are based solely on German children of the second and third generation. Their parents shared the National Socialist ideology and actively supported the persecution as far as their personal power and influence permitted. They had collaborated by denouncing Jews to the police, boycotting their businesses, expelling and banishing Jewish colleagues, and using concealed or open force as white-collar perpetrators in the administration, in the Gestapo, in concentration camps, or as members of an *Einsatzkommando* (special *Wehrmacht* execution units). Some of them were sentenced to death after 1945 and were executed; others lived in Germany incognito, often under false names, well into the 1950s and 1960s. Some even revealed themselves involuntarily through their own publications, as if they no longer had seriously considered personal criminal prosecution. After the war, most of them had merged inconspicuously into the German society from which they had initially emerged. None of the mothers and fathers had been guilty of criminal acts after 1945. This means that we are dealing with a phenomenon in which people who behaved lawfully under normal political conditions, used and abused their power under National Socialist rule to single out, humiliate, torture, and kill innocent citizens of their own country who had done them no harm.

The murder of the Jews began by giving them a bad name, "murdering their reputation"[1] through the propaganda of the Nazis that split the German people into Jews and Aryans, disparaging one and idealizing the other. Only a few Germans resisted this effort. It left traces as early as 1933 in everyday life. What started in the neighborhood, in the housing area, in the village, and in the city ended in Auschwitz. This knowledge was not passed on openly in the family narration; it nevertheless exists. To the question of what in the everyday life of their parents and grandparents could have been useful for Hitler in executing his plans for extermination, students of the third generation, interviewed in 1989, answered, "That's a mean question." It was "mean" because it aimed at the nucleus of the problem: the collaboration of many, indeed almost all, of the people in Germany. It was acknowledged only upon direct and specific questioning; otherwise, a veil of silence covered up the crimes.

Even if National Socialism was described in the families, the Holocaust was not mentioned. Instead, stories of everyday life during the war were told. German children relying only

---

[1] *Rufmord* in German.

on family narration for their knowledge of National Socialism would have had a fragmentary and deceiving, and thus false, picture. Even the complete defeat of 1945 was sometimes turned into a victory in family narration. It was called a "honorable defeat against a world full of enemies." Thanks to the intense historical research of scientists, passed over to the children by teachers and journalists, there is now, however, a knowledge of facts in the second and third generation.

My investigations are based on the following:

- Observations of the second and third generation in psychoanalytic treatment since 1976 (Hardtmann, 1982).
- Counseling a self-help group of children of Nazi functionaries in 1988 and 1989.
- Interviews with students of the third generation in East and West Berlin in 1988 and 1989.
- Social training courses with right-wing, radical delinquent youngsters in Berlin since 1991.

The material therefore derives from different sources. These observations can be compared to different microscopic adjustments and enlargements: The pictures perceived therein are connected but not congruent. The most superficial material is from the interviews, because the contact was very brief. The material that goes deeper is that from the self-help groups, because all members were tied together by a mutual experience—suffering from the Nazi fathers and mothers, as well as that based on observations in social training courses with the right-wing radical delinquent youth. However, I owe the deepest and farthest reaching revelations to my patients in psychoanalytic treatment, who suffered extremely from their parents' and their childhood experiences because they could not deal with them. They brought these experiences unprocessed into the treatment sessions and suffered deep affective disturbances and psychosomatic disorders. They felt insecure in the realistic perception of the self, because, in their childhood, they had been, again and again, exposed to parental projection and projective identification.

FAMILY DYNAMICS

I begin by describing the childhood experience of a patient. As a five-year-old child of a former SS leader, born after the war, one morning he went to get breakfast rolls from the bakery with the dog and let the dog carry the bag of rolls in his mouth. The father watched them through the window and saw that the bag was dragging in the dirt. With the words "I shall teach you to drag the one who gives you bread[2] through the dirt," he hit the child so hard that he had to be hospitalized with a broken arm.

I met this child as a grown-up in my office after he failed a university exam. He was pale and frightened, depressive, and lacking any self-confidence. Only after long treatment did the patient manage to get a grip on life. After the anxieties toward the father and the projection of these anxieties onto the examiners had been worked through, the patient finished his studies with an excellent exam.

This simple example shows typical characteristics of the *structure of relationship* between the first and second generation. The first generation—defeated, debased, returning from

---

[2]Bread in German being the synonym for subsistence, hence the one giving bread, *der Brötchengeber* as characteristic of the father.

the World War II laden with guilt and shame—suffered from chronically deficient self-esteem. Normally, these feelings were warded off with denial and reaction formation, for instance, with arrogance. In certain moments, beyond apprehension for children, the defense collapsed, and the fathers, suddenly overwhelmed with feelings, projected them onto the children, who felt like blind people slapped in the face. They found themselves abruptly and unpreparedly in a *quasipsychotic world* and were exposed to destructive action with which the fathers fought off their presumed "persecutors"—in this example, the (presumed) "despiser." In some cases, these children indeed later on turned into "persecutors"; the vast majority, however, had identified with the projections and had, in place of their parents, developed feelings of guilt and shame themselves. *Projections* and *projective identifications* determined the object relationships in their families. When the children became subject to negative projections, they saw themselves as the *Jews* of their parents.

Occasionally, the whole family would symbiotically join together (*folie à famille*) and project their own denied parts outward onto a third person. In this case, tight family ties between the generations were formed, which impeded the separation and individuation of the children, so important in adolescence. The mutual defenses—denial, splitting, and projection—tied the members of the family together like a sect because of the danger of being radically questioned outside the family. I observed similar phenomena with right-wing radical delinquents. The *Weltanschauung,* splitting, idealization of the self, disparagement of foreigners, and unquestioned anti-Semitism—almost word for word and entirely uncritically—had been taken over by them according to their own statements from their grandparents.[3]

Another characteristic was the *concrete* or *literal thinking* in the sense of *symbolic equations* (Segal, 1979), which occurred *along* with the symbolic thinking. This is important because the thinking apparatus as such was not disturbed but very much intact. Apparently, as Kestenberg has also noted with the children of the victims, the psychosis-like thinking structures differ from those of actual psychotic patients. Under the influence of strong, suppressed feelings that suddenly became relevant—an overflooding with affects—a *regression of thinking* took place. The breakfast rolls no longer symbolized the provider (*Brötchengeber*); they were literally equated with the provider, the father. The five-year-old was accused of having dragged the father in the dirt. This regression in the thinking of grown-ups is extremely frightening for children, because it translates into a language of concrete thought and action what really is a metaphorical language. Due to the strong emotion paralyzing the critical ability and the associated repelling, unpleasant self-perception, the actions were mostly of a destructive nature. The threat of such unforeseeable impulsive action lay like a shadow over the childhood of members of the second generation and paralyzed their healthy self-maintenance and their own aggression. The latter generally turned against the self in the sense of an identification with the aggressor (Freud, 1965). Because the children could not comprehend the biographical and historical context in which their parents' sudden emotional, erratic, and chaotic outbursts could be explained, they lived in an imperceivable world where the connection between certain feelings and specific incidents remained hidden. Some of them generally perceived emotions and affects as irrational, something that one can only fight, suppress, and control, but cannot use in a sensible way to understand more about oneself.

The *suppression of the feelings* led to an inner paralysis, a loss of liveliness, and a diffuse incapability in situations when difficult decisions in life had to be made. The children remained foreign to themselves, felt "alien in their own house," in their body, and in their soul, in some cases developing psychosis-like symptoms and symptoms of a split personality or a false self.

---

[3]Statements like these were very often heard: "My grandfather/grandmother or my father/mother told me . . ."

One patient, whose father had served in an *Einsatzkommando,* as an adult visited those places where her father had participated in shootings. At these places, she did not feel any emotion, whereas films—fiction!—often drew her tears. She suffered much from that and developed severe psychic and somatic defects, because she could not separate true and false, real and unreal, emotions. She could not acknowledge to herself or to others what was play/fantasy and what was earnest/reality. Sometimes she behaved like the mad farmer who calls the firefighters when there is a fire on the theater stage, but who is sound asleep as his own roof is ablaze.

One interviewee reported that in her family, a macabre "play" was even today enacted over and over again: The father, who hadn't been a Hitler-boy due to his young age, made grand Führer-speeches to the family, asserting that Germany was still "number one" in the world. The family had to listen silently without talking back. Whoever protested against this ritual, as did the only son, was kicked out. The speeches contained three recurring ideas:

- He saw himself surrounded by a world of enemies (paranoia).
- He felt himself superior to everybody else (omnipotence).
- He could not find peace until all "enemies" (the Jews) were eliminated (destructive fantasy).

He was incapable of turning his eyes inward and asking himself what enemies were threatening him from the inside and against what enemies did he have to prove constantly his superiority. He had to ward off feelings of weakness permanently, because he fought a hopeless battle on the wrong front—against the enemies on the outside, not on the inside—that robbed him of his peace until the end of his life. Self-observation and self-criticism were completely alien to him. This ego weakness did not prevent him from being extraordinarily successful on the job; it was thus only partial.

In the self-help group, the children of the second generation discussed their experiences with their Nazi fathers and mothers. Therein, they often described splitting:

- A father who had grown up in a parsonage was able to sing "The Daughter Zion"[4] with the child and simultaneously to be actively involved in the persecution of the Jews.
- A father and Nazi officer, deeply concerned with the scholastic career of his son, also made him spy on his teachers and at the end of the war ordered him (and the whole family) to be killed, an order luckily never executed.
- A mother had her children set the Christmas table for years after 1945 for "father returning from captivity," even though she knew he had been executed in 1946.
- A "loving father" was revealed in a war-crime trial to be a mass murderer.

None of the fathers and mothers had the courage, in view of the children, to face openly their own deeds. Silence, hiding, deceit, and lies were thereby inevitable, and undermined—often recognized only in retrospect—not only the trust in the parents but also trust in human relationships altogether. Who was to be trusted if one had been deceived and betrayed by one's closest relatives? Furthermore, fathers only known through fractional family narration had their identity completed by their children's wishful imagination and thereby turned into *phantom fathers,* with whom the children satisfied their yearning for a father to be respected and loved, at least in their imagination.

---

[4]Lyrics by Heinrich Ranke (1798–1876), set up to music by Georg Friedrich Händel, 1747:

> Tochter Zion, freue dich, jauchze laut Jerusalem!
> Sieh, dein König kommt zu dir, ja, er kommt der Friedefürst!
> Hosianna, Davids Sohn! Sei gegrüßet, König mild.

THEORETICAL REFLECTIONS

From the psychoanalytic standpoint, the most helpful to me were the concepts of projective identification by Klein (1952), Bion (1967) and Segal (1979). The denial and splitting preceding projection are, by my account, not yet symptoms of illness in the social and political context, as long as the subject remains open to the self-reliance and independence of the object, and as long as the object can actively resist the projection. In this context, Bion talks about *normal projection,* which happens every day and can be corrected at any time, and usually is corrected. Projections become pathological and politically dangerous only when the subject compulsorily identifies the object with projection, depriving it of independence. Such a distorted and, in the sense of the projection perceived, *bizarre object* (Bion, 1967) is *compulsorily identified* with the projection and treated accordingly. It is either disparaged or idealized, perceived and treated as the devil and the ultimate evil or as the incarnation of divinity and goodness. The subject thereby saves itself from a critical argument with the evil (or the good) within itself or the other. It pays for this *loss of self* with a false, usually idealized, self-image and an unrealistic and overweening self-assumption.

Such splitting becomes necessary if the subject cannot accept itself the way it is. The reasons are

- False because of too high and exaggerated expectations toward itself, in the sense of illusions of megalomania, and lowered self-esteem (with depressive personalities).
- An exceedingly unloving, punishing, and depreciating, unloving superego authority, which is surrendered—like formerly the heathenish gods—to devour a foreign object in place of the own self. To save one own's skin from the inner persecutor, the other is sacrificed, thereby serving as a scapegoat.

In both cases, a healthy and "sufficiently good" (Winnicott, 1958) self-love is missing. This self-esteem was not acquired in the family socialization and, even in the second and third generation, its absence leads to an alternation between over- and underestimating the self. The person does not manage to deal with faults, weaknesses, and good qualities, and to develop a realistic and healthy self-perception. Through *projective identification,* the projections are materialized and specified. They thereby leave the sphere of mere fantasy, become relevant to action, and produce effects with which, rather than with thoughts and mere imaginations, the subject must come to terms. Fantasies generally, if they are not relevant for action, do not leave traces in the outside world. They can therefore, even if they are important for the self and trigger feelings of shame and guilt, be put off easily. We all know the feeling experienced when waking from a nightmare, relieved that we have *just* dreamt. Actions can neither be revoked nor erased by a mere act of the imagination. They are withdrawn from the sole power of the subject by the fact that they cannot be renounced and develop a life of their own. The effects of a violent act, for instance, are visible and tangible. One can erase the traces, as the Nazis tried to do, and smear the references, but one cannot make it undone. Hannah Arendt (1967, 1971) has pointed out that historic facts, as opposed to those in natural science, can be lied away successfully to the extent that no trace is left in the memory of the people. In the helpless attempt to escape the effects of action, the only way left for the subject is to blot out the traces from his or her memory. Such thought could have been contained in the *Endlösung* (the "final solution," the Nazis' 1942 resolution for the extermination of the Jews). Surely today, we would know much less about the crimes committed in the concentration camps had some prisoners not survived to give evidence. Surely also, many Nazi crimes have long fallen into oblivion.

The subject, however, would try to obtain liberation through oblivion from something that actually happened, looses a part of its history, and therefore a part of its identity. In this way, the subject walks around *without a shadow* and becomes "face- and history-less" (Speier, 1987) and is yet permanently in restlessness and fear of being caught by its own shadow and its true face. It thereby enters a paranoid situation in which what is fantasized had a real cause, but in the past. The subject falls back on mechanisms that have proven effective with dreams, treating reality as if it were only a bad dream. Victims then appear like in a "movie"; they are thereby again erased by *derealization.* In this way, some fathers were even able to talk to their children about their crimes.

The self, mutilated and amputated by projection, is permanently threatened from the inside by the reappearance of the suppressed parts, and from the outside by the fact that the object normally resists the projective identification. It thus lives in a two-front war, threatened from both the inside and the outside, cleft and torn from itself. Cure would only be possible if an inner reconciliation and a destruction of the false self-image took place.

The bloated, omnipotent self resists this for different reasons:

- It feels flatteringly uprated with this false self-image and experiences the devaluation as a devastating defeat, because it does not have any loving parts that could alleviate and stop the fall. It thus suffers from fears of annihilation.
- The false self feels at home only in itself; its loss is not only experienced as a threat and collapse, but also as homelessness.

It thus attempts for all to maintain the projections and forces others to confirm them. Thereby, the projections appear like an outer reality.

For the children, the second generation in Germany, this means that they grew up with partially "face- and history-less parents." Insofar as they have identified with them, as, for instance, the right-wing radical youth, their own identity depends on an illussionary and brittle foundation. It is difficult for them to develop a defined identity of their own, to live a different history, and show a different face. To the extent that they develop this identity, they have to question the parental models and thus the yearning and loving feelings attached to them. They are orphans inside, reliant on surrogate mothers and fathers. The story of these surrogate mothers and fathers has not yet been written. From the psychoanalyst's perspective, it is not rare for the psychoanalyst to take over that function.

The process necessary for reparation of the self could also be described in terms of Edith Jacobson's theory on psychotic identifications (1954) and Margaret Mahler's considerations about the restitutive aspects of individuation (Mahler & Furrer, 1968). The different theoretical concepts concerning the interchange between internal world and external reality are well described by Kernberg (1980).

SOME CONSIDERATIONS ABOUT THERAPY

First, there must be special concern with projective mechanisms in therapy, be it by projection of parts of the self, or be it by projective transference by the patient identifying the therapist with a real object of the past. A *stable sense of reality* on the side of the therapist and *permanently open communications* about the projective character of affects, thoughts, and fantasies are much more important than to give early interpretations, in order to establish *stable self- and object-boundaries.* Second, the therapist must not fear *psychotic-like communications* by the patient, because they are not expression of a severely disturbed thinking apparatus but an expression of severely disturbed separation and individuation processes of the patient as a child; in other words, they are the result of the traumatic childhood experience of the patient. The origins therefore can be drawn back into the past by psychoanalytic exploration.

Third, the *setting depends very much on the patient,* because it is he or she who just must come in contact with his or her traumatization. Therefore it is better to give the patient time to develop a feeling of how many sessions are needed and over how long a period of time. It is my experience that every patient has not only his individual fate but also his *individual way of getting out.*

Fourth, but in special moments when the patient endures severe psychic pain, anger, and fear of loss because of the inevitably necessary but extremely harmful separation process (Mahler & Furrer, 1968) it is important to *encourage him or her no longer to deny but to confront the traumatizing experience* and work it through in the therapeutic alliance.

CONCLUSIONS

National Socialism left traces in the children of the victims and the perpetrators. Denial, splitting, projection, and projective identification are not only characteristics of the perpetrators during the Nazi period. These defense mechanisms were also maintained after 1945. Through denial and splitting, the majority of the German people entered an alliance with the Nazis against the Jewish minority in 1933. Thereby, they spared themselves from a critical argument with themselves and their own failures.

The children of the second generation have become objects of their parents' splitting and projective identification. They then lived either as projectively distorted, bizarre objects in a quasipsychotic world, or they shared these projections and thus became incapable of finding an independent identity of their own. Traces of the former identification are found in numerous physical and psychic symptoms; traces of the latter are found in uncritical symbiotic family ties (*folie à famille*). For cure, both groups depend on searching for objects of positive identification outside the family, because their parents never worked through their own shame and guilt.

On the subject's side, not only did splitting and projection take place during the national socialist period, but, above all, projective identifications. These became relevant for everyday action and led to an active implementation of the Nazi ideology into concrete destructive actions. In the families, the responsibility for what happened was retroactively denied, and thus a paranoid structure in the postwar years—now perpetuated—was established after the outer pressure for conformity had ceased. The suppressed parts, feelings of guilt and shame, were projected either onto the second generation or onto third-party outsiders (anti-Semitism *due to* Auschwitz).

Owing to the aftereffects of the National Socialist crime, the psychotic-like behavior in large groups (*folie nationale*) should be further explored. Temporary, literal identification of metaphors, for example, of the nation with the "father" and the "mother," splitting, and desire for blending correspond with quasipsychotic transferences, yet earlier than individuation and separation. It can be used for *inner politics* also, such transferring the responsibility for one's destructiveness onto the "Führer." Political power can be drawn from misuse of this longing, something that demagogues such as Hitler and Goebbels knew very well. They could support their power not only over all those who thought and felt in an anti-Semitic way and thereby share their projective identifications, but also over those who by no means thought in an anti-Semetic way but had not grown adult enough to take responsibility for themselves. Bot the anti-Semitic agitation speeches and the adjuration of the spiritual unity of the German people by the Nazis had to find an inner resonance within the listeners in order to take effect.

There were cases in which this resonance did not come forth and people had proven re-sistant to Nazi propaganda and resisted splitting. The resistance sprang from three sources:

1. From love of the other who was made a compulsory object of the projection by the Nazis; that was the case with many "Aryan" women who were married to Jewish men.
2. From love of oneself, one's self-reliance and independence, which revolted against a splitting between the inner beliefs in norms and values, and the outer conduct.
3. From a sober relationship with the nation: distanced, critical, self-conscious, indepen-dent, like children who have ultimately separated themselves from their parents, and have grown into adults.

REFERENCES

Arendt, H. (1967, February 25). *Truth and politics. The New Yorker,* pp. 49–88.
Arendt, H. (1971, November 18). *Lying and politics. The New York Review of Books,* pp. 30–39.
Bar-On, D. (1989). *The legacy of silence: Encounters with children of the Third Reich.* Cambridge, MA and London: Harvard University Press.
Bergmann, M. S., & Jucovy, M. E. (Eds.). (1982). *Generations of the Holocaust.* New York: Columbia University Press.
Bion, W. R. (1967). *Second thoughts.* New York: Basic Books.
Dubet, F., & Lapeyronnie, D. (1992). *Les quartiers d'Exil.* Paris: Seuil.
Eckstaedt, A. (1982). *A victim of the other side.* In M. S. Bergmann & M. E. Jucovy (Eds.), *Generations of the Holo-caust* (pp. 197–227). New York: Columbia University Press.
Frank, N. (1987). *Der Vater. Eine Abrechnung.* München: Bertelsmann.
Freud A. (1965). *Normality and pathology in childhood.* New York: International Universities Press.
Freud, S. (1914). *Erinnern, Wiederholen, Durcharbeiten.* Gesammelte Werkie X: 126–136; Standard Edition XII: 155ff.
Goldenhagen, D. J. (1996). *Hitler's willing executioners: Ordinary Germans and the Holocaust.* New York: Knopf. Also published in Germany *Hitlers bereitwillige Vollstrecker. Ganz gewöhnliche Deutsasche und der Holocaust.* Berlin: Siedler.
Hardtmann, G. (1982). *The shadows of the past.* In M. S. Bergmann & M. E. Jucovy (Eds.), *Generations of the Holo-caust* (pp. 228–244). New York: Columbia University Press.
Jacobson, E. (1954). *On psychotic identifications.* International Journal of Psycho-Analysis, *35,* 102–108.
Kernberg, O. (1980). *Internal world and external reality: Object relation theory applied.* Colchester, UK: Mark Patterson.
Kestenberg, J. and M. (1982). *The experience of survivor-parents.* In M. S. Bergmann & M. E. Jucovy (Eds.), *Gener-ations of the Holocaust* (pp. 46–61). New York: Columbia University Press.
Klein, M. (1952). *Notes on some schizoid mechanisms.* In J. Riviere (Ed.), *Developments in Psychoanalysis.* London: Hogarth Press. (Originally published 1946)
Klüger, R. (1992). *Weiter leben.* Göttingen: Wallstein.
Levi, P. (1988). *Ist das ein Mensch? Die Atempause.* München/Wien: Hanser. (Originally published 1947)
Mahler, M., & Furrer, M. (1968). *On human symbiosis and the vicissitudes of individuation.* New York: International Universities Press.
Mahler, M., Pine, F., & Bergmann, A. (1975). *The psychological birth of the human infant.* New York: Basic Books.
Milgram, S. T. (1963). Behavioral study of obedience. *Journal of Abnormal and Social Psychology, 67,* 371–378.
Miller, A. (1980). *Die Kindheit Adolf Hitlers.* In A. Miller, *Am Anfang war Erziehung* (pp. 169–231). Frankfurt/M.: Suhrkamp.
Müller-Münch, I. (1982). *Die Frauen von Maydanek: Vom zerstörten Leben der Opfer und der Mörderinnen.* Reinbek: Rowohlt.
Rokeatch, M. (1968). *Beliefs, attitudes and values.* San Francisco: Jossey-Bass.
Rosenkötter, L. (1982). *Child of persecutors.* In M. S. Bergmann & M. E. Jucovy (Eds.), *Generations of the Holocaust* (pp. 183–196). New York: Columbia University Press.
Segal, H. (1979). *Notes on symbol formation.* In E. Bott-Spillius (Ed.), *Melanie Klein today* (Vol. 1, 1988, pp. 160–177). London: Tavistock–Routledge.

Sichrovski, P. (1987). *Schuldig geboren. Kinder aus Nazifamilien.* Köln: Kiepenheuer u. Witsch.

Speier, S. (1987). Der Ges(ch)ichtslose Psychoanalytiker—die ges(ch)ichtslose Pychoanalyse. *Psyche,* 41, 481–491.

Stierlin, H. (1975). *Adolf Hitler: Familienperspektiven.* Frankfurt/M.: Suhrkamp.

Tetlock, P. E. (1979). Identifying victims of groupthink from public statements of decision-makers. *Journal of Personality and Social Psychology, 37,* 1314–1324.

von Westernhagen, D. (1987). *Die Kinder der Täter: Das Dritte Reich und die Generation danach.* München: Kösel.

Winnicott, D. W. (1958). *Collected papers.* New York: Basic Books.

5

"Who Am I in Relation to My Past, in Relation to the Other?"

German and Israeli Students Confront the Holocaust and Each Other

DAN BAR-ON, TAL OSTROVSKY, and DAFNA FROMER

Memory is life, borne by living societies founded in its name. It remains in permanent evolution, open to the dialectics of remembering and forgetting, unconscious to its successive
deformations, vulnerable to manipulation and appropriation, susceptible to being long dormant and periodically revived. History, on the other hand, is the reconstruction, always
problematic and incomplete, of what is no longer. . . . At the heart of history is critical discourse that is antithetical to spontaneous memory. History is perpetually suspicious of
memory and its true mission is to suppress and destroy it.

NORA (1989, pp. 8–9)

INTRODUCTION

The young people of today's Germany and Israel did not experience the Holocaust, not even its
aftereffects as children of survivors (Bergmann & Jucovy, 1982; Danieli, 1980) or perpetrators
(Bar-On, 1989). Though we may still find such aftereffects among the third generation, these
are not clear-cut and extensive (Bar-On, 1994; Segev, 1992). The young can try to ignore its effects or to reconstruct it through history books, the media, or public discourse, thereby expressing the collective memory (Friedlander, 1992). They also may try to make sense of it
through the memory of their parents and grandparents. This is a painful process because of the
dialectical tension within memory and between memory and history, described by Pierre Nora
in the opening quotation. We discussed earlier a group process through which we tried to elaborate the issues of different collective reconstruction of the past and their impact on the present
social and political perspective among German and Israeli students (Bar-On, 1992; Bar-On,
Hare, Brusten, & Beiner, 1993; Brendler, 1994). Since then, many new social and political

DAN BAR-ON, TAL OSTROVSKY, and DAFNA FROMER • Department of Behavioral Sciences, Ben Gurion
University of the Negev, Beer Sheva 84105 Israel.

International Handbook of Multigenerational Legacies of Trauma, edited by Yael Danieli. Plenum Press, New York, 1998.

changes have taken place in both countries as part of the global changes between East and West: the peace process in the Middle East, the Russian immigration to Israel, the unification of Germany, and the rise of the extreme right in Germany. We asked ourselves: What effect did these processes have on the identity-reconstruction and -formation of Israeli and German students and on their relationship to each other?

The idea of identity-formation through group processes is not a new one (Lewin, 1948). Within the more secure group context, members of the group can test, construct, and reconstruct various undiscussable aspects of their identity and memory in relation to themselves and their relevant others (Bion, 1961). However, the group modality was not tried for such purpose in the Israeli–German context until the late 1980s, probably because of the burden and the ongoing rage of Jews toward the Germans, owing to the Holocaust (Bar-On, 1992, 1993). Unicultural German groups, trying to acknowledge and work through the burden of silenced atrocities of family members during the Nazi era, and its ongoing impact, were the exception rather than the rule (Bar-On, 1989; Hardtmann, 1991). So were bicultural attempts (Bar-On, 1992; Staffa & Krondorfer, 1992). Within the Jewish context, groups of second-generation Holocaust survivors who tried to work through the burden of the past became open to the public need in the mid-1970s (Danieli, 1988; Vardi, 1990). Though there were quite a few attempts to bring together German and Jewish or Israeli youth over the years, they more often avoided direct confrontation of the painful past rather than trying to acknowledge and work it through (Segev, 1992).

In our earlier study (Bar-On *et al.,* 1993), we found that German and Israeli students tended to simplify the relevance of past events (especially, the Holocaust) within their present political and social perspectives. While in Germany, students tended to claim that "nothing in the Nazi era was relevant" for their present social perspective, in Israel we found the opposite tendency ("The Holocaust was very relevant for our present social contexts"). We tried to initiate a group process through which we could enhance a more differentiated and meaningful way of acknowledging the Holocaust and relating it to the present social perspective in both groups ("partial relevance").[1] We did that by working with the two groups separately on these issues, bringing them together twice, once in Israel and the second time in Germany (Bar-On, 1992). When evaluating the processes of change within each group, we found that the group processes and, even more so, the encounters between the groups facilitated acknowledgment of the Holocaust and a more differentiated approach of "partial relevance" (Bar-On, Hare, & Chaitin, in press). We saw in this approach a product of the acknowledgment and working-through process.

In parallel, another German–Jewish encounter group was established. First, a self-help group of children of Nazi perpetrators was formed in 1988 as a by-product of the interviews the first author had conducted between 1985 and 1988 (Bar-On, 1989; German edition: Campus Verlag). Then, a group of children of Holocaust survivors from the United States and Israel agreed to meet with the self-help group of the children of Nazi perpetrators. They met four times, starting in June 1992 (Bar-On, 1993). Again, one could observe in this delicate group process in what ways the encounters facilitated individual and collective processes of acknowledgment and working through the aftereffects of the Holocaust, which still had a strong grip on both groups of descendants, 50 years after the events had taken place, when the fathers of one group tried to exterminate the families of the other.

---

[1]We suggested that the Israeli position was the one of "total relevance of the past for the present," while the German position was the one of "no relevance." We were looking for a more differentiated "partial relevance" position in both countries, in which students would say things like "perhaps there is relevance in the Holocaust for what happens here today, but it depends in what respect and how one draws these conclusions." This position would mean to become better informed, both in respect to what had happened in the Holocaust and what is going on today (Bar-On *et al.,* 1993).

At this state we (Brendler, Bar-On, and Ostrovsky, all of whom participated in the German–Jewish encounter group) decided to set up another seminar, similar to the one conducted in 1990 and 1991. Our emphasis was focused on the acknowledgment and working through of the impact of the Holocaust on both groups through different forms of dialogue within each group and between the groups. We assumed that each group must first get involved in an internal dialogue, including its own foreparents, trying to learn about their past through personal accounts. Second, through a group process in which these interviews were presented and discussed, a peer dialogue would evolve, in which the collective memory and identity would be critically examined. Later, an encounter between the two groups should open up a new quality of the dialogue between young Germans and Israelis, who had acknowledged the Holocaust and its ongoing effect on each group separately. Between two such encounters, in Israel and in Germany, there would be an interval in which each group would have a chance to reframe its own agenda and identity- and memory-related issues, based on their initial experience with each other.

We had several questions in mind at the outset of our joint seminar:

1. Will the three forms of dialogue reinforce or antagonize each other? For example, will the discussions around the interviews of the Israeli students with Holocaust survivors and their descendants make it more difficult for them to engage in an open dialogue with their German peers?
2. Will the first encounter between the groups change the quality of the dialogue in each of the groups separately?
3. Will all members of each group be able to take part in each of these dialogues and the transitions between them?
4. Will our seminar only "convince the ones already convinced," or will it draw into the dialogue also students who were less interested in dealing with the aftereffects of the Holocaust in the first place?
5. To what extent did the latest development in each country (the unification and the rise of right-wing extremists in Germany, the peace process in Israel) affect the current dialogues in comparison to the seminar of 1990 and 1991?

We now describe in some detail each one of these stages within the perspective of the Israeli group.

ISRAELI STUDENTS ENCOUNTER THE HOLOCAUST AND ITS AFTEREFFECTS ON THEM

The Israeli Students Interview Holocaust Survivors and Their Descendants

After the first short round of getting acquainted, we asked our 12[2] students, grouped into pairs, to interview one Holocaust survivor and one of their descendants. They were supposed to ask them to tell their life stories, transcribe the interviews, and discuss them in one of the

---

[2]We interviewed all students before the seminar started, to describe the design of the seminar. In 1990, we had the experience that in the seminar that include the encounters with the German students, fewer students subscribed than usually (average, 15 students) even though an almost free trip to Germany was included in the program. No similar difficulties were observed on the German side, who had 15 students also in the present seminar. All the Israeli students were from the Department of Behavioral Sciences, in their last undergraduate year (except Manya, who was an M.A. Anthropology student). Most of these students applied later for graduate studies in psychology.

following sessions. Very few instructions were given as to how to conduct the interviews. We emphasized our interest in the normalization strategies along which the interviewees have constructed their life stories. Interviewers should eliminate leading questions that might impose their own construction on the interviewees (Rosenthal & Bar-On, 1992). Our idea was to let the students experience their interviewees not as professional interviewers, but as human beings, with their genuine reactions to the unfolding stories. We tried to prepare them for the possibility, based on our earlier experiences (Bar-On, 1994), that the descendants of survivors usually would say initially that they do not have an interesting life story to tell, and that the students would have to insist that they have interesting stories to tell in their own right.

Orit[3] was the first one to report about the interview she has conducted with her grandmother. She had heard her stories before but as pieces of an unfinished puzzle, never in such detail and wholeness. Orit approached her with the "task to conduct an interview for a course at the University." Her grandmother first described the life of her extended family in a town in Poland where they all lived. Soon, she spoke of the beginning of the war in 1939, the German occupation, and her first experiences with persecution of Jews in their town, where Jews from other parts of Poland and Germany were transferred. She remembered the German commander, who used to walk around with a huge dog, watching and laughing as the dog attacked Jews. She then described in detail how, in 1941, the SS soldiers entered her home, shot her cousin and, when her father ran away, shot her mother twice and killed her in front of her eyes. Later, she was in hiding and experienced how they heard footsteps of the SS, and women choked their babies who started to cry. The third critical event happened during a year she had spent in an underground bunker, outside the town, where she was hiding with her future husband: Her aunt gave birth in the bunker, and they had to kill the baby immediately after the birth as there was "no way to raise a baby under these circumstances."

Orit told these terrifying stories in detail, readings long sections of the transcribed interview. The opening account of the dialogue around the life stories of survivors was an extremely difficult experience for the group. We were amazed in what detail Orit's grandmother told her about her difficult experiences. We were, however, especially taken by the positive atmosphere that radiated from Orit's grandmother, in spite of the terrible events she had experienced and described, a radiance that one could also sense in Orit while sharing her grandmother's narration.[4] In a way, Orit set a standard in the group that others followed: the personal way of reporting, the detailed interviewing and precise transcriptions. A tender conversation usually followed the reports, in which questions were asked ("How could they endure so much pain and survive? Why did they not talk about it before in such detail?"). A personal and group dialogue slowly emerged, in which students tried to imagine themselves in these situations, to

---

[3]All the students gave their consent for this report. All names have been changed to maintain anonymity.

[4]In the application form, in which the students were asked to write about the connection they saw between the life in Israel today and the Holocaust, Orit wrote:

> For me, as a third generation after the Holocaust, this connections has many sides. The closest to me is my connection to my family and especially to my grandma, as a Holocaust survivor, and to her past. The conversations and stories of that period, the comments about the life in the bunker, the discussions between the adults about memories which have faded away and their feelings about their being survivors, even the question if to accept reparations from Germany, all these are part and parcel of my daily life. It seems as if the wish of her generation to maintain the terrible happenings in consciousness, and the idea that they are the last ones to have experienced these events, has penetrated also into my life, perhaps even more than into the life of my parents' generation, who tried to "save" or avoid the ghost-tales. Today, I feel, it is part of my life to know and to feel this chapter of my family's legend, because of the fear that it may happen again.

envision their aftermath with regard to their own families. All these exceeded by far in scope and intensity what has happened in previous seminars.

We tried now to anticipate: What will the life-story of one of the descendants of Orit's grandmother be like? Will she follow her mother's tales in admiration, or will she distance herself emotionally from them (as Orit wrote in her application form)? Orit did not want her mother to be interviewed. Therefore, it was her mother's sister that Orit interviewed and reported about in the group at a later stage in our seminar. As expected by some students, the life story of the aunt was an "Israeli" life story, unrelated to the life story of her mother. She centered the interview around her father (Orit's grandfather), whom she remembered screaming in his dreams at night. She studied nursing "to learn how to help him in his heart condition" and felt guilty for not saving his life when he finally died of another heart attack.

About her mother's stories, she said, "One could not make sense of them. Four women, each with another version. Only father's ingenuity rescued them." At two points in her narration we observed, however, that Orit's aunt was unconsciously following her mother's stories. First, she reported watching, as a child, a bloody scene of a goat being killed by a train on a railway track. It reminded us of her mother's detailed description of the bloody events at her home in Poland in 1941. Then, when her daughter was born, Orit's aunt believed the baby stopped breathing at nights. She, as a nurse, tried to get physicians to recognize her baby's physical problems. However, they wanted to refer her to a psychiatric clinic, as they could not find anything wrong with the baby. Finally, when one of the physicians "found something and gave the baby a satisfactory treatment," she felt relieved. We saw an association between this experience and the description of her mother in hiding, of mothers choking their babies. Orit's aunt, however, never made these connections, though she must have heard stories from her mother, just as Orit had heard them.

The last interview reported in the group was an exception: Eran, unsuccessful with an earlier interview, decided to interview Orit's cousin, her aunt's son. Avner was the only youngster (18) in the third generation of survivors interviewed by our students. He told a very lively life story, in which he related much more openly and extensively (in comparison to his mother) to the experiences of his grandmother during the Holocaust: "Okay, I feel that my whole education, certain parts of it has to do with her experiences during the Holocaust. All this dealing with food, for example, it certainly comes from there. She had suffered from hunger like everyone else then, so—all the time food, the refrigerator always full and you always buy more 'so it will be there. . . .' To spend money, Okay, but never to waste food. Never take food and leave it in your plate. To throw away food is forbidden!"

Avner went on, associating his family's humanistic political standpoint toward the Arabs to his grandparents' experiences of humiliation and suffering as victims of Nazism. We discussed the different "sides" taken by Avner and his mother, in relation to the grandmother and her stories. We learned from Pierre Nora (1989) cited earlier, how memory can be "unconscious to its successive deformations, vulnerable to manipulation and appropriation, susceptible to being long dormant and periodically revived (pp. 8–9)." We experienced how listening to testimonies challenged the listener: being exposed to the experiences and the pain; feeling the different, conflicting feelings of the interviewee and oneself. We also saw how easy it is to ignore the narration of the storyteller, using a "professional jargon," thereby disassociating ourselves from the more difficult experiences of our interviewees and their effects on us.

We will not be able to go into detail in describing all the interviews. However, we wish to give some taste of the variety of experiences our students have encountered, the variety that enriched the perspective and the dialogue evolving in the group after each interview. There were also serious discussions centered around the different approach of Hedva, who felt antagonized by the way people tried to reflect on the interviews and interviewees. Hedva tended to put herself in the center of the group, leaving aside what the discussion actually tried to clarify or elaborate on. It showed also her difficulty in acknowledging and working through the impact of the Holocaust as a young and proud Israeli woman, who severed herself from that chapter in her own family biography. This occurred, for example, when Yonit told the group about two interviews she had conducted with a survivor and his son. The survivor was a kind of "professional" survivor who used to travel around the country and tell in schools stories of his experiences during the Holocaust. His son (31), experiencing a father who spoke obsessively about the past, told a very sad story: how he tried to construct his independence from the overwhelming presence of his father and did not yet fully succeed in "making it" in life. During the group discussion after Yonit's presentation, Hedva said that she knew the son personally. She felt that he did not tell his story "the right way," according to how "she knew him." This caused a heated discussion: Is there a "right way"? How does Hedva know what he felt about his life, only because she "knew" him in school? Can Hedva's account help us make sense of Yonit's interviewee's self-presentation?

Lena was very quiet during the discussions in the group. She almost had no voice of her own, until she reported on her interview of her uncle, who was a partisan during the war. She actually interviewed him three times, because she felt he had not yet completed his story. The first time he told her "nice" stories about being a soldier in the Polish army during the German invasion, about how he had managed to run away and survive all by himself. During the second interview, she succeeded in getting him to tell of his last minutes with his family, when they were brought to the center of their town and he was excused because he was a good "carpenter," useful for the German police. His sister, still lying on the ground, begged him in Yiddish to try and rescue their mother, but he was afraid and did not say anything. They were all later murdered. This was the only time he showed how helpless he had been in a critical situation, feeling very guilty for not rescuing his family. During the third interview, he told his more well-known, heroic stories among the partisans. Each interview showed a different side of him, a different chapter of his biography. Lena conducted the interviews in a most delicate manner and her report was outstanding. She found herself suddenly in the center of the group, praised for her attentiveness and persistence, her sensitivity and her clever way of getting around her uncle's defensive approach to the more delicate parts of his story.

Yadov is a big man, working in the police, a new Russian immigrant. He comes from a family of officers in the Red Army who used to tell their heroic stories but never told the stories of the family members who had perished during and after World War II. He chose to interview a survivor who had a similar background as his father, in order to see if also that person would follow a similar pattern in his storytelling. His interview was the shortest reported in our group. It included very few facts about the war and some personal stories of the fighting in the Red Army. The interviewee did not want to go into detail concerning his parents and the other members of his family, all killed during the war. Yadov's hypothesis was confirmed. However, members of the group questioned whether he found what he was expecting.

To summarize, the interviewing and reports in the group helped open up undiscussable aspects of personal and family histories. The image, used often, was of a puzzle in which some very important missing parts were found, though perhaps never to be completed. An inner dialogue evolved, of the student interviewers, relating to their interviewees and to themselves, in which they tried to imagine themselves in similar situations. The different ways of remembering the effect on identity were examined. This, in turn, stimulated an examination of personal and collective identity: To what extent is our identity centered around memories of these experiences? Do we still examine current events as if they had happened "then and there" rather than here and now? Do we want them to affect us in this specific way? What other relationships can evolve between memory and identity, once past traumatic events have been worked through? A more open dialogue followed, in which some members of the group could compare and test their private dialogues. This was done carefully, only when the group became supportive enough to let it happen. This was also where we, as facilitators, tried to intervene and help create such an atmosphere, trying to legitimize different personal strategies and sensitivities on the way to reaching this goal.

Through Our Work with the Students, We Developed a Trialogue of Our Own

The three of us (Bar-On, Ostrovsky, and Fromer) met every week for about an hour prior to the seminar. We had by then read the forthcoming interview and would discuss its specific features. We would try to prepare ourselves for the reactions of the student who conducted the interview while reporting it, and for the reactions of other group members. Each of us would report on our contacts between the sessions with group members. This was especially true for Ostrovsky and Fromer, who were closer to the students by age and rank. We would also share our own reactions of not being able to sleep after reading Orit's interview, or dreaming after an exciting discussion in the group. Ostrovsky would reflect on her own experiences as a student, three years earlier: the similarities and differences she found between the group processes and her own two perspectives. Our preseminar work helped us cope with the tremendous emotional burden and to try to stay one step ahead of the group. It presented a kind of model that suggested that, in some cases, pairing or small group discussions were necessary before encountering the whole group.

We had one mishap during the interviewing phase. While interviewing a son of a Holocaust child-survivor, Manya suddenly felt sexually approached by her interviewee. We had never had such an experience with an interviewee before. There was some initial confusion and even an attempt "to blame the victim" for what she had "done" to invite this behavior (Lerner, 1975). However, others gave Manya strong support and refuted such blame as being "an example of what we are trying to acknowledge and work through here in the group." Manya first considered leaving the seminar, because it seemed too much for her. However, after receiving warm support from members of the group, including the three of us, she decided to go on and slowly found her place back in the group discussions. Without the close coordination of the three of us, Manya could have become a "casualty" of the group process, thereby also severely hampering the future working-through capacity of this group.

By the end of January 1994, we had several unexpected problems to address. We had not finished discussing all the interviews in the group but were already supposed to be preparing ourselves for the forthcoming visit of the German group. In addition, a faculty strike at all universities started, threatening the continuation of our planned seminar.

We decided not to let the strike interfere with our work and to continue the group meetings in private settings, outside the university, so that we would be ready for the first encounter with the German group. Members of the group organized a communication system to meet uncertainties stemming from the strike (closing of the campus, students' demonstrations, etc.).

Preparing the First Encounter with the German Students:
The Letters, Booklet, and Video

We corresponded with our German colleague, Dr. Brendler, and heard from him about the parallel group processes in Germany. We found out that only a few of the students had interviewed eyewitnesses of the Nazi era and their descendants, and these interviews had not been reported or discussed in the German group. Instead, they held group discussions, read material, and saw films, trying to inform themselves about the Holocaust and about Israel in general. Toward the end of the semester, the German group prepared a small booklet in which all members of the group presented themselves in photos and in writing describing who they were and their interests. The aim of this booklet was to help the members of the groups form pairs, as every Israeli was going to host at least one German student at his or her home during the forthcoming encounter.

The Israeli group felt challenged by the booklet and decided to prepare a video, as a reply, in which each member of the group would say something about him- or herself and the group work. The visit was now intensively prepared, including a program for almost every day and evening of the visit. We started our joint meetings the next morning, mixing group sessions with formal and informal receptions. We were invited to the Beer Sheva Municipality[5] for lunch, including a tour of the town and an informal dinner later in the evening. We continued our discussions the next morning. The students were supposed to go for the weekend on their own, in pairs or clusters, as they wished.

CONSTRUCTING A DIALOGUE WITH THE "RELEVANT OTHER"

The First Encounter: Obstacles and Accomplishments in Developing a Mutual Dialogue

After a short general session of getting acquainted, two mixed groups were formed. This structure, in different versions, became the main working framework of all the future joint sessions. Students preferred the intimacy of a smaller group, paying the price of being less informed about the second group's processes and its participants. Though groups intermingled during both joint meetings (in Israel and in Germany), there were also competitive feelings of the "better" or the "worse" groups. For example, during the second and the third days, Hedva took a lot of the time of one group, indirectly accusing the German students of their responsibility for lack of interest and involvement in the topic.

Some of the other Israeli students confronted Hedva for being insensitive to the differences among the German students, differences that they could already observe during these first sessions. After a few hours of intensive discussions and emotional outburst, Hedva decided to leave the encounter, and later, also the seminar altogether. She became the first "dropout" of our joint dialogue, though we believe that it had more to do with her conflicts within the Israeli group than with her confrontations with the German students. Still, members of the group in which this conflict has taken place perceived themselves as being the "worse" group, as the other group used this time to get deeper into the process of acknowledgment and working through.

In the "better" group, things took a more personal turn. It started with the open confession of two German students of their efforts to clarify their own family's role during the Nazi era. Mani (G),[6] being an artist himself, had open discussions with his father, whom he appreciated very much. His father had been half a year in jail during the Nazi regime, "accused of being a Communist." Mani could not, however, make sense of the inconsistencies in his father's discourse: His father despised the Nazis, but also described being present at one of Hitler's famous rallies and being fascinated by him. His father also made some anti-Semitic re-

---

[5]The towns of Wuppertal and Beer Sheva are "twinned," as are the local Universities. Therefore, during our joint sessions in one of these places, a formal invitation by the local municipality was received, mostly from the Mayor herself in Wuppertal, and the Mayor or his deputy in Beer Sheva.

[6]German (G) and Israeli (I) students will be identified from now on.

marks, such as: "Jews have been persecuted, but they still control the world," which would provoke Mani.

SIGNA (G): Are you afraid that this will happen to you too?

MANI (G): I try to argue with him but I never can be sure I could control myself.

ERAN (I) [*joining in*]: Perhaps your father had certain anti-Semitic ideas but he rejected others. I guess he would not be able to build camps and gas Jews. Perhaps he had been brainwashed. What can you do about it?

MANI (G): Perhaps I should try to think of this difference. I could also try not to be influenced by his prejudices.

MANYA (I): Do you confront him?

MANI (G): Yes, it is difficult to explain. When he comes to this topic he becomes irrational and then I lose my temper and become aggressive, and this does not help. It is very frustrating.

MANYA (I): So, invite him to the group. [*laughter*]

MANI (G): Yes, I could do that and he may come.

EDNA (I): [*joins in, very aggravated*]: I feel so helpless. Whatever I do, they will always judge me, hate me. Whoever I am will not change their mind, Why?

ERAN (I): I am more optimistic [*turns to Mani (G)*]: You could suggest that your father visit Israel; at least, he should see for himself. You see, my parents also have prejudices which are not easy to change.

Michael (G) is a historian, interested in the Nazi era. His first encounter with Jews was during a visit in England. When he came back and spoke about it at home, he got no answers. His grandmother wanted to talk before her death. His grandfather was still fascinated by Hitler. As a boy, he had watched a movie about the occupation of Holland and the Jews in Auschwitz. "I felt both hurt and ashamed. I felt hurt as the film referred to 'the Germans' and not only to 'the Nazis.' I felt ashamed to be a German under these conditions." Michael found out that his uncle was an SS officer in Norway, became very religious after the war, and never discussed that part of his life. The uncle's brother fled to Switzerland during the war. There were still many tensions between the two brothers during family gatherings. His religious uncle once said, during such an occasion, "The six million Jews died in the Holocaust because that was ascribed to them in the Bible." Michael asked, rhetorically, "How can we construct a positive identity when history has such a negative meaning for us?"

Eran (I) tried to comfort him: "But you have also positive chapters in your history to relate to, don't you?" Michael thoughtfully reacted: "But this would mean denying what I don't like and relating only to what I can see as positive." Others joined in. Manya (I) spoke of the "black hole," which the Holocaust still means for her. Signa (G) described living in a "puzzle" that has so many missing parts in her family and community history: "The Holocaust destroyed our identity. We have to try and reconstruct it, trying to feel what it had been like to live during that era, from both perspectives" (of the victim and the victimizer).

Centering around the self-presentation of Mani (G) and Michael (G), this dialogue introduced a new quality of discourse into the group: not "us" and "them" but a new kind of "we," searching for answers that will break through old schema. But for Edna's (I) painful exclamation ("I cannot do anything to change their prejudices"), most group members tried to sort things out, not to give up, and try make sense of the mixture of emotions and statements of their parents' generation and of their own. While struggling to clarify the "inconsistencies" or "irrationalities" of the concurring prejudices, Jews and the Nazi era, an atmosphere of joint endeavor emerged, to which quite a few members of both groups could contribute.

The next day we asked if it was a new group norm to let the German students present their family biography. This intrigued Malka (I), and she told her family history, which she had not yet shared within the Israeli group context. Her grandfather left Poland as a soldier in Andreas's army,[7] leaving behind his whole family, who later perished in the Holocaust. Originally from Chentochova, he was rescued because he knew all the Catholic prayers by heart and pretended to be a gentile. He had already agreed to be interviewed by Malka but died shortly before she conducted the interview. Her father (his son) never related to this chapter of the family past. Malka remembered having her own nightmares of a wall around her, searching always for a place to hide (in the ground, in the wall) as a child. Borrowing Signa's idiom, she said, "For me, the family past is also like a puzzle with too many missing parts." Signa (G) said, "This hurts. I feel your pain." Eran (I) (turning to Malka) said, "My grandparents came from Morocco, but interestingly, as a child, I had the same fears and the same search for hiding."

Manya (I) and Dorit (I) identified with Malka's fears and fantasies. Two of the German students mentioned that Malka gave them the first opportunity to observe a hidden aspect of Israeli identity that they had never acknowledged before. "We did not know you still have these fears."

The open dialogue about family secrets and conflicts, initiated by Mani (G) and Michael (G), helped Malka (I) come out with her own. Her narration introduced some of the hidden aspects of Jewish or Israeli identity, usually concealed for their relative "weakness." However, other members, German and Israeli, could hardly cope with it. One German student said, "Why do you always ask us to relate to our family members when you discuss this era?" An Israeli member felt very uncomfortable with Malka's opening up "in front of the Germans." One could sense the different undercurrents within each group and how they were supported or confronted by the mutual encounter with "the other" group. Still, the dialogue emerging in this mixed group touched on personal aspects, thereby creating a new space for members of both groups for acknowledgment and working through the burden of the past.

The focus shifted between the past and the present reality in Israel. Two Bedouin faculty members were invited to talk about the Bedouin community in the vicinity of Beer Sheva. The groups traveled to a new Bedouin town nearby and had a chance to see the problems of a cultural shift, being only a small part of the Arab–Israeli conflict. The next morning, we stopped on our way to Jerusalem at Nveh Shalom (the Oasis of Peace), where Palestinians and Jews try to live together and conduct seminars for Arab and Jewish students and pupils. We felt the maturity of most members of both groups, keeping apart the Holocaust from the tensions between Arabs and Jews today, which enabled them to shift from one context to the other, relating to each in its own separate sense.

On the fourth day of the Israeli encounter, the groups planned a trip to Yad Vashem, the Holocaust memorial museum in Jerusalem. The possibility of not going[8] was unanimously turned down. Expectations, fears, and fantasies were discussed. It seemed as if the forthcoming trip was putting members of both groups back behind a hidden, unbridgeable abyss. We tried to legitimate differences in experiencing and reacting to this place of acknowledgment of the Holocaust. This was what actually happened. The next day, some students went in pairs, others in small, mixed groups, while still others preferred to be there on their own. A few wanted to talk after being in the museum, whereas others preferred to keep silent.

[7]A private army of the Polish Government in exile, established by General Sikorsky in 1942 as part of a Polish–Russian agreement. Many of the Jewish soldiers in this army fled during its stay in Palestine and joined Jewish settlements (as Malka's grandfather had done), mainly owing to the anti-Semitic atmosphere in this army.

[8]Proposed by the first author, arguing that it might interfere with the group processes.

The next morning, a collage was created, enabling the expression of feelings after the visit to Yad Vashem. Six girls of both groups planned a mask pantomime: They painted their masks in black and white, put them on and tore them off step by step, throwing the pieces into a box called "HISTORY." It was a strong, nonverbal presentation expressing the painful emotions they were trying to handle during the last few days.

The Intermeeting Phase: Preparations and Fears

The first meeting of the Israeli group after the encounter with the German group was emotional and chaotic. On the one hand, students felt how important this encounter was for them in the context of trying to work through the aftereffects of the Holocaust. On the other, many issues had been addressed or dealt with. Students such as Eran, Yonit, and Ofra (I) reported the very intensive dialogue they were involved in throughout the visit. They also could now better understand how difficult it was for some of the German students to make sense or even inquire about their family history during Nazism. They learned to appreciate the open approach of students such as Signa, Mani, and Michael. But others were disappointed: Yadov did not want to continue his pairing with Bettina (G), because she seemed to him totally uninterested in "our topics." She was only asking "about the pubs and the shopping mall." He asked to be paired with someone else during his visit in Germany. Edna felt very hurt by the pressure being put on her by her partner, Bernd (G), whom she seemed to have liked a lot at the outset. She felt he was immature and talked only about their personal relationship, but not about "the subject." They all asked to be informed further about the German context of the Holocaust, as they felt they got to know only "our side" during the seminar (and probably also before it).

Special meetings were set, with Professor Gabriele Rosenthal, who gave a Colloquium at our Department with a German son of a Gestapo commander, who is member of our group of children of Holocaust survivors and perpetrators (Bar-On, 1993). In addition, we showed a film made by the BBC describing the second encounter of this group at Nveh Shalom in April 1993. We asked the group to take part in an evening session of a conference in Jerusalem, where Dr. Brendler, Michael, and Signa of the German group joined in. During this evening, the students described what they had been doing during the seminar and the special role the first encounter of the two groups had for them.

There were many fears and expectations concerning the following encounter. The two groups communicated intensively by mail, phone calls and E-mail. In the Israeli group, we observed an interesting shift of leadership. Orly and Edna, the initial "in-group," were very disturbed by their experiences during the first encounter. It was Ofra who spoke up now, telling the group how much she had learned, how difficult it was for her to maintain boundaries "because you can be easily flooded by this whole matter." She became a kind of a new leader, waiting impatiently for the next encounter to come. Some of it had to do with the German partners. In comparison to Edna's troublesome experience, Ofra felt that she and Michael had found a way to understand each other, both intellectually and emotionally.

The Second Encounter in Germany: Searching for a Balance between "the Topic" and Me

The second encounter started with a long weekend of socializing back in pairs. Most of the couples were very happy, and the Israelis felt the efforts the German students made to reciprocate their own hospitality. However, there were also "casualties." Edna (I) and Bernd (G) did not get along at all. She again felt under a lot of pressure. We decided to break up this couple, and Bernd responded by leaving the group altogether, as he felt he had "no more interest in our joint group discussions." It was interesting to note that each group had its dropout (Hedva and Bernd), and it happened in both cases at the outset of the encounter in the country of the person who then dropped out.

After the weekend, we resumed our group discussions. Signa, Sabine, and Monika (G) spoke of their efforts to learn of their own family members' participation in the Nazi era. They could describe the immense difficulties but also some of their own sophistication: how to approach this delicate subject anew, without letting the topic be turned down and closed up again. They could now report of experiences as bystanders (while Jews had been deported), of songs in the Hitler Youth (with anti-Semitic flavor), of Nazi indoctrination and children's books with Jewish stereotypes.

> SIGNA (G): They tried all the time to belittle the events. It was awful. I know that my children will ask me questions which I would like to be able to answer. It is so frustrating.

> MONIKA (G): What is difficult for me is not that my mother was a bystander. It is the fact that she feels no remorse even today.

> Eran (I): But perhaps there is no story. Or perhaps it is difficult for them to admit that they enjoyed what was going on, or even were fascinated by Hitler. Your mother was 16. I know how a youth movement can fascinate you at that age. It is a wonderful experience. Only at an older age one learns to say "No!" under certain circumstances, if at all.

> SABINE (G): I feel so helpless, as if I myself am becoming a bystander. I just cannot make my parents talk.

> MALKA (I): I can now see why you had a more difficult time conducting your interviews than we had in ours.

> DAN (I): I am not sure that there is more or less, better or worse, in these matters. Perhaps these are just very different difficulties which cannot be scaled in any form, just as the experiences of the survivors, their suffering, or that of the perpetrators, cannot be scaled.

> ERAN (I): I had difficulties with meeting elder people in the street, here in Wuppertal. I all the time asked myself, where had they been, what had they done?

> MICHAEL (G): I have this difficulty too, though I live here. Usually one has respect for older people. But in their case I cannot feel respectful; I try to imagine what they had been involved in.

> MALKA (I): I remember as a little girl, listening to the Eichmann trial on TV. I was frightened and asked my Dad to sit near me. I had dreams about skeletons. Now I had fears of your parents, how they would relate to me?

> SILKE (G): While you are here, I feel like I walk on thin ice all the time.

> OFRA (I): You came to us to be accepted and we feel we have to defend you. There is too much symbolism in all that we look at. I had my own problems defining who I am, but I felt I had the strength to cope with it until I came here. Now I am, first of all, overwhelmed by your nature and architecture. Everything is so total and rich here. I am not used to it.

The encounter turned to its formal part. Professor Dr. Hoedl, the rector of the University of Wuppertal, hosted a reception and lunch for both groups, with the local press attending. Mrs. Ursula Krauss, the Mayor of the town (well experienced with former students' groups and conferences) held a warm and informal dinner. It helped us take a break we all needed from our very personal and intensive group discussions.

We went to Buchenwald by bus from Wuppertal (a 7 hour trip) and stopped for a short break in Weimar. We walked peacefully in Goethe's and Shiller's hometown, visited Goethe's summer house in the park, enjoying the festive atmosphere of this old and relatively well-preserved East German town. Therefore, reaching Buchenwald was harsh. It took about 8 minutes to reach Buchenwald from Weimar. Michael read to us some facts, and we knew right away that we were approaching another world, the world of persecution and annihilation. To make things worse, upon arrival, we were confronted by a group of German soldiers, who had just finished their visit in the camp, coming out, laughing and shouting. We walked on in silence, looking at the woods, a few birds, some old army barracks used by the local administration, and viewing the original fence, the entrance house, and the gate to the camp, the clock still showing 3:15, the time the camp had been liberated. On the gate, we identified the German words *Yeder in Sein* (meaning "everyone to their own"), to be read from within the camp.

"I never knew how sophisticated they have been, those Nazis," said Eran (I), in Berlin, during the following morning's session. "In Auschwitz they wrote *Arbeit Macht Frei* from the outside, wishing to deceive the newcomers. Here they wrote 'Everyone on Their Own' from within, trying to demoralize those who had already been doomed to become inmates." "One cannot stop wondering what they had known in Weimar, in that wonderful cultured atmosphere, about the planet called Buchenwald. They must have known everything," said Ofra (I), during the same discussion. Utte (G) reacted: "I was shocked by a young woman who came out of the camp in rage and spat on the floor near me. Was she a neo-Nazi or what? Why the hell did she react that way in front of me?"

Michael (G) exclaimed: "I could not stand walking through the museum, reading all these explanations the Communists put there (meaning the old German Democratic Republic (DDR) wording, still present at the museum). They hardly mentioned this camp was full of Jews, only emphasizing resistance fighters all the time. This has been here for years after the war had ended."

Mani (G) said, "And I was put off by this medical device: You entered the physical examination room and they measured your height and then a soldier who was standing in the next room put a bullet in your neck, through a slot, hidden in the measuring scale. They could do it with one bullet by going up and down according to the height of that person. Why did they need this cynical killing method? They could have hanged them or put injections into them. Why were they so creative in their putting people to death methods?" Boaz (I) reacted: "How can I judge them. How can I be sure I would not behave the same way they did, had I been here in their position at that time and context?"

We walked through the open space, almost getting lost in that vastness. A German television company took some "shots" of us walking there. We visited the crematorium and the museum but did not have time for everything, because the local women wanted to close the place and go home. Finally, we gathered around the relatively new Jewish memorial in the middle of the empty space. Some of the Israeli students conducted a short memorial service, in which we all took part: a prayer, a song, a poem written by Orit's grandfather, translated into English; a few memorial candles struggled with the strong wind, a bouquet of flowers was placed, bought an hour earlier in a flower shop in Weimar. The bouquet was bought by both groups together, an act very much appreciated by the German students. They were afraid that the Israelis would not let them participate in the ceremony, or in its expenses. In the previous seminar, 3 years ago, there was a joint bouquet and another Israeli bouquet, and also this, after prolonged discussions (Bar-On, 1992). This time, this was no issue: a tiny symbol of the changing atmosphere?

*   *   *   *

We arrived late that evening at the Jewish Community Center *Adat Yisruel* in Berlin, where we spent the last 3 days of our encounter. The first morning was devoted to reflections, in small groups, on the visit in Buchenwald, but other issues also came up. It became apparent that, this time, the reactions were different on a personal basis much more than on the collective identity basis (Israelis vs. German). Bettina (G) spoke up for the first time: "In Buchenwald it was so quiet, so green, the air so clean. I ate two pieces of bread in Weimar, twice as much as the inmates had for a whole day." Manya (I) reacted: "The silence was difficult in such a place." Yonit (I) asked, "I wonder if they could listen to birds like we did yesterday?"

Bettina then elaborated on her difficulties since the visit in Israel. She was sure, before she came, that "you (the Israelis) wanted me to give up my cheerfulness and liveliness because of what had happened during the Holocaust, and I was not ready to do so." However, she found out that there was no such demand, and she came back to Germany quite mixed up. She then went to see *Schindler's List,* which impressed her very much. Bettina said that for days after, she could not eat or take a shower without thinking of dreadful situations in the film. Now, she understood that she herself did not know where to put the boundaries between getting involved in "our topic" and maintaining her own liveliness. Dan (I) reacted by saying that she formulated in a simple and wonderful way the dilemma we are all having but that most of us cannot state openly: To what extent are we allowed to have a life of our own while getting involved in this difficult topic? The fear some Israeli students expressed during the final gathering in Beer Sheva related actually to Bettina's words: Are we now committed to this process for the rest of our lives? How can we deal with it and live our present life, undisturbed?

Lena (I) spoke after Bettina, very excited. She did not initially plan to come to Germany. She felt helpless and was afraid she could not draw the line between the Germany of then and today. However, now she felt that these days were very important for her and she really could open up, together with the German students. For her, the last intervention with Bettina was a crucial one. She suddenly understood something about her own fears, of which she was not aware. Also Monika (G) spoke up for the first time. She explained how stunned she felt after Yad Vashem, being all alone (which she chose to be), unable to utter a word in the group. Now, after Buchenwald, she felt differently. She could share things with Lena, translating for her the German titles in the museum, as there were no English ones. She felt it was difficult to be a German woman and a human being within this context, but now she could at least talk about her burden, and it made it easier.

*   *   *   *

The two groups went on a bus ride to get to know Berlin from the Jewish historical and contemporary point of view, with the same excellent guide we had 3 years ago. The ride ended at the Wannsee Villa. Dr. Anagred Ehman, leading the educational program of the center, let us first walk around and get a sense of the place, letting everyone choose their own preferred context. A few of us walked out in the garden, near the lake, and we could sense the calm and wealthy atmosphere of the villa, the garden, and the boats on the lake. No one could imagine that in this pleasant atmosphere, the Wannsee Conference took place more than 50 years ago. Within less than an hour, during dinnertime, the annihilation of European Jewry was decided as a technical procedure, to be carried out efficiently.

We visited the exhibition and met for a short first discussion. In the first round, each person could say one sentence about his or her initial impressions of the Wannsee Villa. A few students critiqued the exhibition: Why do they not tell the story of the perpetrators? Why tell also here, in this house, the story of the victims who had never been here? We suggested that during the following morning one of the students' working groups try to design a new exhibition as they would like it to be in this context. About eight students of both groups undertook this mission: One group worked with Anagred on the documents of the Wannsee conference, and another developed a psychohistorical profile of Reinhard Heydrich, the architect of the Final Solution.

During the discussion that followed, the first group presented its sketch of the proposed exhibition: a glass-partitioned double track in which one could follow the development of the participants of the Wannsee Conference (on the right track looking out at the lake), whereas the other (no window) track would describe the simultaneous development of several victims. These tracks would merge in the central round room, where the conference would be activated audiovisually. From there, the tracks would again separate, describing the extermination process. As they entered, visitors would be given names of either victims or perpetrators and would follow their track until arriving at the final "reflection room." There, they would have the option of changing roles and going through the whole exhibit from the second perspective. The glass partition would enable each visitor to look into the other track through a glass painting that would emphasize the perspective of the onlooker's assigned role.

One could learn a lot from this sophisticated proposal that was developed by members of both groups. In a way, it actually simulated the development of our seminar: two groups of people growing up in separate contexts, meeting to acknowledge and work through the aftereffects of the Holocaust, turning back into their own context, and meeting again to reflect on what they have done alone and together. From time to time, they could try to look through "the glass partition" onto the other's context, still very much influenced by their own contextual perspective.

On the way back from Wannsee, Yonit (I) asked Dan, Orit, and Utte (G) to join her in searching for the house where her grandfather used to live in Zelendorf before emigrating in 1938. It was quite an experience to follow directions of an 86-year-old man, not really knowing whether this was the house or not. An old and friendly man let us in after being a bit surprised by our request. He showed us around in a beautiful, old, and well-decorated building. Yonit was excited, took pictures, and tried to absorb as much as she could in order to tell the old man at home what she had experienced.

The stay in Berlin ended with a small Shabbat ceremony, which Eran conducted, explaining the prayers and the rituals while performing them. The next evening, a farewell discussion was held. It was difficult to say good-bye. Everyone tried to say a few words, but they all felt unable to conclude their experiences, thoughts, and feelings. Michael (G), usually the intellectual person in the German group, said, "This is an important experience for me. I feel I went through things in a way I did not expect. The experience itself caused a change in me." The changes in him were unexpected. His words moved many of us. Mani (G) added, "I was glad for the opportunity to take part in the seminar. There are things which are difficult to be explained. This is not necessarily a language problem; it is just those things."

It took time for an Israeli to speak up. Manya was the first: "It is an unfinished process. It was a good experience but perhaps only an opening for something else." Edna cried and Yonit comforted her without words. They were unable to share their feelings with the group. There was an obvious difference between the German students, who expressed gratitude and satisfaction, and the Israelis, who expressed fear, sadness, even anger. Dorit was angry after her visit at the exhibition of the destroyed church in Berlin: "It showed the suffering of the Germans during the war, but it did not mention what preceded, not a word about the Holocaust."

Was it an opening session or a closing one? The jolly atmosphere during the farewell dinner that followed showed another side of the students: their wish to enjoy themselves as youngsters and to say good-bye personally, even if their mission was not yet completed and the "topic" yet undone.

Postscript: Formal Papers and Summary

When the students came back, they were welcomed by many questions from other students, both suspicious and curious. Malka was asked to tell her peers in a Personality course about her experiences. Amcha[9] in Beer Sheva asked Orit, Ofra, Edna, and Yonit to tell a group of child survivors about their experiences in the course. But they also met indifference, even animosity. They were reminded that for quite a few Israeli youngsters, especially those who did not go through a similar process of preparation like our seminar, the idea of an encounter with the Germans was viewed negatively.

Students also had missions to fulfill and papers to present. During our last few sessions in Beer Sheva, we returned to some routine work. Each student presented his or her proposed outline for a final paper. Malka planned to interview Israeli survivors who, like her grandfather, took part in the Andreas army. She would try to understand their motives for joining this endeavor. Eran and Yadov, who had interviewed an Israeli couple who were on Schindler's list, wanted to compare these interviews with older testimonies at Yad Vashem in order to find out to what extent the movie affected their original testimony. Orit, Edna, and Yonit tried to compare the experiences of child survivors hidden by families and in monasteries: How did it effect the reconstruction of their life stories? Dorit and Manya followed the artwork of survivors over the years: Did it change, and if so, owing to what external and internal processes? (Manya's mother, an artist, was going to help them to interpret the artwork). Lena and Boaz wanted to understand the mechanism of silence within families of survivors through microanalysis of family discussions. Ofra was in the process of producing a video reflecting the development of her dialogue with Michael (from the German group).

We met again in August, as there was a strong feeling that we did not finish "our work" at the end of the seminar. We heard also from the German students' group that they had met again, and that some of them decided to go next year, together with their pupils,[10] to Auschwitz, where they would meet with a group of Polish students. Three of them (including Bettina) planned to arrive in October in Israel for a visit. At the beginning of the meeting each of us (Ostrovsky, Fromer, and Bar-On) received a present: a small album with pictures of each of the students and a few words of farewell attached to each picture.

There was not much talking done. There were a few trends of feelings in the room. Some expressed concern about how the Israeli public still reacts to events in Germany. Dorit was still angry: She felt that she was in the middle of something and that, had she had a "better" partner, she would feel more satisfied. Boaz, Lena, Manya, and Edna expressed fears, which Dan interpreted as the fear of being stuck in "a lifelong commitment" that they did not plan to get involved in, especially not in this stage of their lives. They do not know how to continue now that the seminar is over. Ofra, Yonit, Malka, and Eran expressed satisfaction and openness. They were happy with what was achieved, and were also ready to go on dealing with "this subject" in one way or another.

DISCUSSION: FORMING IDENTITY THROUGH DIALOGUE

In this discussion, we concentrate on some of the questions presented in the introduction. Though there are many other perspectives from which such a complex experience can be examined, we felt that these were for us at this time the most important issues to try and address, even if the answers were partial and inconclusive.

[9]Amcha is the Israeli support system for Holocaust survivors and their family members, similar to the Group Project for Holocaust Survivors and their Children in New York. They have just opened a new branch in Beer Sheva.
[10]As part of their practicum for becoming teachers, they will each have at least one pupil next year.

Developing Three Forms of Dialogue: Commitment to the Past and the Present

The Israeli students were presented with a dilemma. The early interviewing phase strengthened their commitment to Holocaust survivors and their descendants. Though such commitment was part of the Israeli culture and collective consciousness before the seminar started ("total relevance"), the interviews helped change it from a myth and symbol to concrete and personal experiences. The encounters with the German students demanded from them an openness to "the other," symbolically representing still the enemy of their recent private heroes. It also demanded a confrontation with the prevalent Israeli norms of prejudice and animosity. How did the members of our group cope with this dilemma? Did one phase help prepare them for the next, or did they interfere with each other?

This dilemma was reinforced by the powerful opening of our seminar. Starting with Orit's report on interviewing her grandmother, this group worked very hard to acknowledge and work through the Holocaust and its long-term effects. One could sense how each interview broadened the scope of what being a survivor or a descendant of a survivor meant to the members of the group. The quality of the discourse that emerged and accumulated with each additional interview helped deepen the understanding of what had happened *there and then* and how it still effects us *here and now*. Moving from being an attentive and empathic interviewer to such difficult stories and storytellers to being a precise and convincing reporter and discussant in the group demanded considerable intellectual capacities as well as emotional involvement. We felt that this experience gave the students a sense of personal and mutual *being* that could support them in their encounter with the German students, but could also interfere with it.

The dropouts, Hedva (I) and Bernd (G), may have found their place in their home group at a later stage had we not engaged the groups with each other at such an early stage. Also, Orit, though participating in the process all along, expressed verbally and nonverbally that she was too absorbed in the earlier phases of the group and had little energy for the dialogue with the German group. In a way, she felt the need to represent her grandmother rather than develop new relationships of her own. Whenever these two roles conflicted, she would choose the first one, consciously or unconsciously. This became very clear during our visit in Buchenwald. Orit took charge of the ceremony, buying the flower bouquet and translating her grandfather's poem.

To some extent, this was also true of Edna, Dina, Manya, and Yadov. In their case, the unsuccessful pairing with Bernd, Susan, Monika, and Bettina may have played some role. But what does "unsuccessful pairing" actually mean? It suggests a lack of personal ripening necessary for acknowledging the other, of one still being too absorbed in one's own earlier phases of the working-through process, feeling committed to the past and its representatives. At least in the case of Yadov and Bettina, one could assume that it was Yadov who contributed more to the "unsuccessful pairing," especially after we heard what Bettina had to say in Berlin (see p. 110).

We had also examples in which the two forms of dialogue (with the past and with the present) reinforced each other. Eran, the only Israeli student of North African origin, presented a more open and accepting approach toward the German students from the outset. One could sense it in his supportive remarks to Mani during the first encounter and to Signa and Monika in the Wuppertal opening session, as well as in his participative approach while Malka was sharing her fears in the first mixed group. This was his role during the earlier phases of discussing the interviews in the group. Ofra presented another version. She was less active while discussing the interviews in the group. To some extent, she identified herself with Hedva's role. However, after Hedva had left the encounter, and owing to her "successful pairing" with Michael, Ofra became much more outspoken. She was searching for her own way to describe what she found in Germany, how she felt there.

The Qualitative Changes between the First and the Second Encounter with the German Group

The groups met twice for an intensive week, 3 months apart, first in Israel and then in Germany. In what aspects did this process "move forward"? In which ways did it not, or even "move backwards"?

There were many external signs for the movement forward. We started with two groups based on strong collective identities, and we ended up by acknowledging the interpersonal differences within each group. Although during the encounter in Israel there were many expressions of "you" or even "they," in Germany, especially after the visit in Buchenwald and Wannsee, there were more expressions of "us" and "we." One could not follow who said what while discussing the design of the exhibition in Wannsee or the reactions to the emptiness of the Museum in Buchenwald. Still, it was like "walking on thin ice," as Signa said in Wuppertal. Whenever a new issue was presented, or a negative reaction was expressed, breaking the "thin ice," it could easily throw some people back to their own initial state of separateness. We felt that the design of the exhibition in Wannsee expressed better than words the delicate equilibrium that has been achieved: looking onto the other through a glass still painted with one's own collective, stereotypical representations of "the other."

The first encounter was also a kind of a mutual test. Bettina expressed it very clearly in Berlin: "I felt that you (the Israelis) wanted me to give up my cheerfulness and liveliness because of what had happened during the Holocaust, and I was not ready to do so." Only when she found out that her expectation was not confirmed did she delve into "the topic" herself, by watching *Schindler's List*. The Israelis wanted to know what the German students could tell about their own families during the Nazi era. They were annoyed with German students who did not feel this to be an important issue. They could open up when students like Mani, Signa, and Michael spoke about their own experiences and concerns in this respect.

Although this was a clear difference between the groups, in which the Israelis had to help the Germans to go ahead and try, Bettina's dilemma, presented in Berlin, was a universal one with which students from both groups (and even we ourselves) could identify as their problem. In this respect, we feel that Bettina was the "hero" of the mutual group process: Michael, Signa, and even Mani, came to the first encounter after achieving a lot in their own personal acknowledgment and working-through process. They could be reinforced to continue by meeting the Israelis, but they could probably achieve it also in other ways. However, Bettina represented for us the typical "uninterested young German girl," who would have never gotten involved in this topic had she not come to this group. This was still true when she came to Israel and looked for pubs and discotheques (according to Yadov's complaints). Once feeling released of "our (imagined) pressures," she looked for her own way into the topic (watching *Schindler's List*) and could express her dilemma in the group in a way that helped others address it, whether Israeli or German.

Comparison to the 1990/1991 Seminar: Issues of Identity and an Openness in Dealing with Them

It is always difficult to compare two such seminars, because so many things have happened simultaneously. Germany has changed (the unification, the emergence of the right-wing extremists), Israel has changed (the peace process, the immigration from Russia) and we, the authors, have changed (Ostrovsky was a student and became a facilitator). Our conceptual framework has changed (from "partial relevance" [Bar-On, 1992] to issues of personal and collective identity, acknowledging and working through the past in relation to the present). Perhaps we also grew older and know better the limited effects of a 1-year seminar in pursuing such complicated and long-standing issues (the aftereffects of the Holocaust on second and third generations) (Bar-On, 1994).

Nonetheless, we did observe some differences. First, it was obvious that the interviews with Holocaust survivors were much more explicit and difficult in their content this time (e.g., see Orit's interview). The survivors spoke more at length (the average interview was 60 pages long, whereas 3 years ago, they averaged 30 pages) and raised issues that had not been mentioned 3 years ago (though probably they had experienced similar ones). Were the survivors this time more ripe to tell, or were our students more ripe to listen? Probably both were true. There are many other signals in Israeli society that point in the same directions (Bar-On, 1994; Segev, 1992).

Second, there was a strange feeling that the first encounter this time started where the last seminar had ended. This we sensed through the openness of Mani's, Signa's, and Michael's self-presentation during the first mutual session, followed by Malka's open self-presentation. Such openness happened only during the latter phase of the previous seminar, and only to a limited extent, during the encounter in Germany. Third, we had a "Bettina" also last time: a young, uninterested German participant, who laughed at Orthodox Jews shortly after walking out of Yad Vashem (Bar-On, 1992). However, then it exploded and created a crisis in the groups, which that student did not comprehend, even a long time after the seminar was over. There were probably different personalities involved, but, symbolically, what was a crisis last time, taking its personal toll, became a positive focal event during this seminar. Did we learn to be more patient and open to personal differences?

Finally, there was also the example of the flower bouquet and ceremony in Bergen Belsen (in 1991) and in Buchenwald (this seminar). Although last time this was an important issue that took a lot of time and energy of the groups, with the Germans first feeling left out by the Israelis but then acknowledging their separate needs (see Bar-On, 1992), it was almost not an issue this time. Such differences can be accounted for by the different personal composition of groups. They can, however, also reflect a change in the atmosphere between the groups: where less value is placed on mere symbolism, and more energy is invested in substance. Only when conducting our next seminar, in a few years, we hope, will we perhaps be able to account for these and other differences. The only way to find answers to such complicated issues is to try again (Lewin, 1948).

ACKNOWLEDGMENTS: This is a report of a project initiated by Professor Dan Bar-On and Dr. Konrad Brendler as part of the collaboration between Ben Gurion University of the Negev and the University of Wuppertal. It was financed mainly by the Ministry of Education, NordRhein Westfallen, Germany, and supported by the Faculty of Humanities and Social Sciences and the Department of Behavioral Sciences at Ben Gurion University of the Negev, Israel.

REFERENCES

Bar-On, D. (1989). *Legacy of silence: Encounters with children of the Third Reich.* Cambridge: Harvard University Press. Paperback edition, 1991. Eshel (in French), 1991, Campus Verlag (in German) in 1993, Jili Tsushin Sha (in Japanese) in 1992.

Bar-On, D. (1992). Israeli students encounter the Holocaust through a group process: "Partial relevance" and "working through." *International Journal of Group Tensions, 22*(2), 81–118.

Bar-On, D. (1993). First encounter between children of survivors and children of perpetrators of the Holocaust. *Journal of Humanistic Psychology, 33*(4), 6–14.

Bar-On, D. (1994). *Fear and hope: Life-stories of five Israeli families of Holocaust survivors, three generations in a family.* Tel Aviv: Lochamei Hagetaot-Hakibbutz Hameuchad. (Hebrew); Cambridge, MA: Harvard University Press (in English), 1993.

Bar-On, D. (1996). Descendants of Nazi perpetrators: Seven years after the first interview. *Journal of Humanistic Psychology, 36*(1), 55–74.

Bar-On, D., & Gil'ad, N. (1994). "To rebuild life": A narrative analysis of three generation of an Israeli Holocaust survivors' family. *Narrative Study of Lives, 2,* 82–112. Also, *Psychosozial* (in German), *51,* 7–21.

Bar-On, D., Hare, P., Brusten, M., & Beiner, F. (1993). "Working through" the Holocaust: Comparing questionnaire results of German and Israeli students. *Holocaust and Genocide Studies, 7*(2), 230–246.

Bar-On, D., Hare, P., & Chaitin, J. (in press). Working through the consequences of the Holocaust: A study of group interaction (Symlog) among Israeli and German students. *Group.*

Bergmann, M. S., & Jucovy, M. E. (1982). *Generations of the Holocaust.* New York: Basic Books.

Bion, W. R. (1961). *Experiences in groups.* London: Tavistock & Routledge.

Brendler, K. (1994, April). Working with German and Israeli students on the after-effects of the Holocaust on the following generations. Paper delivered at the Conference on Identity and Memory among Adolescents, Hebrew University, Jerusalem, Israel.

Danieli, Y. (1980). Countertransference in the treatment and study of Nazi Holocaust survivors and their children. *Victimology, 5,* 3–4.

Danieli, Y. (1988). Confronting the unimaginable: Psychotherapists reactions to victims of the Holocaust. In J. P. Wilson, Z. Harel, & B. Kahana (Eds.), *Human adaptation to extreme stress* (pp. 219–238). New York: Plenum Press.

Friedlander, S. (1992). Trauma, transference and "working through" in writing the history of the Shoah. *History and Memory, 4,* 39–59.

Hardtmann, G. (1991). *Partial Relevance of the Holocaust: Comparing Interviews of German and Israeli Students.* Report to the GIF, Jerusalem, Israel.

Kestenberg, J. S. (1972). Psychoanalytic contributions to the problem of children of survivors from Nazi persecution. *Israeli Annals of Psychiatry and Related Sciences, 10,* 311–325.

Lerner, M. (1975). The justice motive in social behavior. *Journal of Social Issues, 31*(3), 1–19.

Lewin, K. (1948). *Resolving social conflicts.* New York: Harper.

Nora, P. (1989). Between memory and history. *Representations, 26,* 7–25.

Rosenthal, G., & Bar-On, D. (1992). Biographical case study of a victimizer's daughter's strategy: The pseudo-identification with the victims of the Holocaust. *Journal of Narrative and Life History, 2*(2), 105–127.

Segev, T. (1992). *The seventh million.* Jerusalem: Keter. (Hebrew)

Staffa, C., & Krondorfer, B. (1992). The third generation after the Shoah: Between remembering, repressing, and commemorating. Attempts of a common time in Philadelphia, Berlin, and Auschwitz. Berlin: Evangelische Akademie Bildungswerk, Documentation 88/92.

Vardi, D. (1990). *The memorial candles: Dialogues with children of Holocaust survivors.* Jerusalem: Keter. (Hebrew)

II

World War II

6

Conflicts in Adjustment
World War II Prisoners of War and Their Families

MURRAY M. BERNSTEIN

Regardless of its cause, trauma impacts upon the victim's self-image. Professionals in mental health have identified various patterns of coping with forms of trauma that range from denial of the severity of the event to overcompensation (deWind, 1984; LaCoursierre, Godfrey, & Ruby, 1986; Tanaka, 1988). Various stages of Posttraumatic stress disorder (PTSD) have been identified as a function of the types of defenses engaged by the individual (Fairbanks & Nicholson, 1986). For example, loss of control relating to trauma leads to intrusive thoughts and the repetition of traumatic events. A "dominate" continual coping mechanism for trauma has been attributed to denial and emotional numbing. The result for the victim is a state of denial of one aspect of the traumatic event and the experience of intrusive thoughts regarding another aspect of the same event.

In a study by Lazarus and Folkman (1984), three veterans' groups were examined. The first group was considered well adjusted. The second carried the diagnosis of PTSD, and a third group as a control was used to assess coping responses to present difficulties (financial, retirement, etc.) and past coping strategies with events of World War II. The result demonstrated that veterans with a diagnosis of PTSD were found to have more maladaptive coping strategies, whereas those who were more adjusted demonstrated strategies that utilized their experience in a positive manner. Dent, Tennant, and Goulston (1987) studied World War II combat veterans and former prisoners of war (POWs), who presented their symptoms as a form of anxiety, and assessed their moods by using direct interviews and the self-administered Beck Depression Inventory. Results showed a direct connection from wartime nervous illness to postwar and present-day depression. Another study of returning POWs examined mood states, relationships, and communication (Hall & Malone, 1976). They found that a POW's tendency toward emotional withdrawal was attributed to feeling guilty for being captured. Their study also showed that, occasionally, the wives of these men were unaware of such feelings.

MURRAY M. BERNSTEIN • Department of Social Work, Zablocki Veterans Administration Medical Center, Milwaukee, Wisconsin 53295.

International Handbook of Multigenerational Legacies of Trauma, edited by Yael Danieli. Plenum Press, New York, 1998.

For many, readjustment problems seemed to manifest themselves within family relationships. In the "war on the home front," families (parents, spouses, etc.) also underwent stress. The worries could be about those in combat, not heard from, missing in action, or prisoners. The constant anticipation was of loss, with feelings perpetually changing from hope to despair and back to hope. Role changes for compensation were necessary for survival. Members of the family took on dual roles relating to various responsibilities from child-rising to financial survival. Children also had to assume greater levels of responsibility. Stress and coping were daily struggles.

Upon returning from war, POWs' homecoming brought on new problems. Tensions rose as family members needed to negotiate and redistribute roles and responsibilities (Hogancamp & Figley, 1983). Marital conflicts developed as family members were seen as more independent and assertive. Among the greatest sources of conflict were the feeling that families did not understand the experience of war. This led to periods of acting out, such as violent outbursts toward the family. Spouses unable to display their feelings tended to take things out on themselves in the form of guilt and depression. Divorce was frequently viewed as a solution to the interpersonal difficulties (Hall & Malone, 1976), with veterans often unable to perceive the difficulties that were attributed to their emotional detachment. The children often experienced the return of their father in yet another way, sharing the nightmares, low self-esteem, and vulnerability of their fathers—a concept later called secondary traumatization (Figley, 1985). This has been noted with both children of the Holocaust and offspring of POWs (Danieli, 1985; Figley, 1985; Rosenheck, 1986; Sigal, 1976). Sons were found to become more sensitive to criticism and daughters to manifest greater degrees of depression then control groups.

For most POWs, imprisonment was their first encounter with total loss of freedom. These experiences were extremely difficult for the American POWs, who were accustomed to interpersonal expression and validation from others. The result was often a sense of despondency. The sight and sound of pain were followed by the silence of death. For those captured on the field of battle, transportation to prison was by foot, truck, or by being crammed into boxcars or ships. For many men whose planes had been shot down, this was their first parachute jump. Surrounded by enemy fighters or ground fire (an experience different from that of ground troops), the pilot was usually separated from his crew members and left alone without support. For all prisoners, anxiety and depression were apparent. Starvation, interrogation, slave labor, torture, and in some cases, execution, were common. The marches from camp to camp lasted months in all weather. The food and medical care were poor, resulting in dysentery, pneumonia, fever, malnutrition, and frostbite. Bayonetings, clubbings, and shootings were frequent. After the initial shock, the prisoners typically would report a heightened sense of alertness, with their status and surroundings constantly evaluated in terms of their survival. In general, the primary focus was on their physical health and its maintenance.

For many, once freed from captivity, the only treatment received was for physical injuries. The need to leave the military seemed more important than any need for seeking psychological care. This has been substantiated through reports of POWs who left their hospital beds soon after receiving their discharge notice (Veterans Administration Office of Planning and Program Evaluation, 1979). Another factor was the strong feeling of elation most experienced upon being set free and the tendency to minimize their previous situation. Finally, many men experienced a powerful sense of guilt that stifled any attempts to communicate the experience with the military. This reflects a mind-set (often mutually held by the POW and the military) that associates captured lacked courage or acted in a cowardly fashion. Figley (1985), in his study of trauma, notes that those who were captured usually had been in severe and hopeless combat situations and were ordered to surrender by their superior officer.

Attention was drawn to the "survivor's response," a term coined by Figley (1978) to describe the mentality of soldiers while on tour. This involved a sense of alienation from others and depersonalization as a coping device to manage their experiences and feelings of isolation. Thus, survivors's responses prevented emotional involvement with others and also reduced the fear of loss, since family and friends were often perceived as not interested in hearing about their experiences. The veteran relied upon denial, suppression, and repression as his coping mechanisms. As a result many generally paint their experiences in the best possible light. For some, however, feelings of guilt and anger are frequent and become worse with time. How does all this impact on returning veterans and their families? In our interviews with World War II POWs, it was noted that compulsive work habits (extending beyond 8 hours per day/40 hours per week) were a common form of behavior. As a result, many POWs avoided close emotional relationships with their spouses and children, and lacked social interaction in their community. Fear of closeness was related to wartime loss of friends, thoughts, and nightmares of combat, deaths, beatings, starvation, and isolation. These symptoms are outlined in the fourth edition of the *Diagnostic and Statistical Manual of Mental Disorders* (American Psychiatric Association, 1994) under the diagnosis of Posttraumatic stress disorder. Included are the areas of sleep disturbance, recurrent dreams of traumatic events, feelings of detachment, diminished interest, guilt, and avoidance of social activities. Now in retirement, these World War II POWs are no longer able to escape into work. Fears of illness and death of family members emerge, leading to feelings of abandonment. The result may intensify such behaviors as withdrawal, depression, alcoholism, and marital conflicts.

To examine these concepts further, information was gathered through both personal interviews and correspondence with POWs. Questionnaires were completed that assessed their patterns of behavior since discharge from the military. These included communication within the family regarding community and social activities, as well as a self-report of nightmares, intrusive thoughts, and outbursts of anger. Additional interviews were completed with spouses and children. Fifty World War II POWs were randomly selected from a list of 150. Of these, 31 responded. In addition, 21 spouses and 24 children volunteered information.

An examination of the data for demographic information revealed that the ages of the POWs ranged from 67 to 76 years. Spouses' ages ranged from 67 to 73, and the average for the children was 42 years. The range of years of marriage extended from 14 to 30 years. Educational statistics indicated that 4 of the veterans completed grade school, 13 completed high school, 5 had 1–2 years of college, 2 had associate degrees from a trade school, 13 had completed 4 years of college, and 3 had completed graduate school. Eleven of the veterans were in professional employment, 13 were in technical employment, and 7 were in service employment.

The results of the interviews indicated agreement among family members regarding the POWs' emotional anxiety and mood changes. The POWs and their spouses showed emotional distance within relationships. Forty-eight percent of the spouses and 63% of the POWs identified sustained difficulties in the POW's response to physical illness of friends and family, as well as fears of management should the POW be left widowed. The issue of mood swings (sudden shifts in the POW's mood without appreciable precipitant) was reported by 73% of the POWs and confirmed by 70% of the spouses. Sudden anger outbursts were noted by 67% of the POWs and 70% of the spouses. The children's responses were split on issues of both mood swings and anger outbursts.

The POWs' responses showed that 38% engaged in social activities outside the home. Sixty-one percent were involved in community services organizations, such as the Disabled American Veterans, Veterans of Foreign Wars, or a Prisoner of War chapter. Fifty-one percent stated that they were comfortable within their community, and 53% of the spouses concurred.

Involvement outside of veterans groups was found to be infrequent. Seventy-three percent of the veterans and 81% of the spouses agreed that there was little or no military discussion by the veterans when engaged in outside activities.

Regarding retirement, 55% felt that their retirement had been unexpected (cutback, illness, or behavioral). About half (51%) described themselves as more irritable, and 49% had concerns regarding their role change after retirement. Seventy-two percent identified extended work hours prior to retirement (which included weekends) as a method of prolonging their absence. Spouses and children agreed with the importance that work held in the POW's life, with 58% and 68% affirming, respectively.

Areas of discrepancies included discussion of war experiences within the family, with 44% of POWs reporting open discussion of their capture, and 83% of spouses denying that this was discussed, as did 72% of the children. Regrettably, 90% of the children reported they were tired of hearing the POW's war stories, even though 86% identified a lack of knowledge regarding personal experience of the POW.

In the area of dependency, 76% of the POWs identified a dependency on their wives for support, whereas 70% of the wives disputed this matter. In like manner, 67% of the POWs reported engaging in most activities with their spouse, and 70% of the spouses responded negatively to the question regarding whether they were an active part of their husbands' social lives. When closeness was defined as knowing the whereabouts of the family, POWs agreed they were aware of family activity, but 59% responded that they purposely kept a distance emotionally from the family and preferred to be alone. Sixty percent of the POWs reported experiencing recurring thoughts and nightmares of war, whereas an equal percentage of the spouses and 50% of the children reported being unaware of any manifestation of these events. Suicidal ideation was reported by only 3% of the POWs.

The findings of this study indicate a high prevalence of psychiatric morbidity for POWs. Most of the subjects reported some form of difficulty at home, work, and in the community. Social problems appeared most pronounced, particularly in the area of communications as seen by the families but not the POWs. These POWs reported discomfort when among nonmilitary, non-POW social groups. Emotional problems were present in this group, particularly mood changes. In response to a list of overall feelings, the following emotions were identified as of major concern: discouragement, worthlessness, helplessness, loneliness, unworthiness, hopelessness, and annoyance. Sleep disturbance (nightmares and increased awakenings, often with startle reactions) continued, as did intrusive thoughts regarding the war and captivity. These affected both social and family roles.

Children reported estranged relationships with their fathers, and identified some carryover effects into their own lives. The spouses and children split in their views as to the dependency of the veteran, with children viewing him as in need of care in the event of loss of spouse, and wives viewing the POW as dependent. The former importance of long work hours appeared to have increased the stress among family members further. Retirement, for many, caused an increase in withdrawal and hostile behavior. Such behaviors were noted in a later study of Vietnam POWs (Hall & Malone, 1976). Their cognitive functioning and ability to discuss emotional issues often evolved only after significant family crisis occurred and treatment was obtained. For the families of World War II POWs, interventions were not available. These families have survived under emotionally trying circumstances.

It has been demonstrated (Keating & Cole, 1980; Mutrian & Reitzes, 1980) that in the general population, relationships, socialization, and satisfaction with self were largely predicated by prior level of functioning. In addition, well-being was associated less with visiting friends than with socializing, as defined by community activities. Within such a context, the retired POW faces a rather isolated existence, based on few relationships outside the family and little community involvement. There continues a fear of abandonment, alienation, guilt, rejection, and loss of respect. For many, anger, hostility, anxiety, lack of commitment, poor communication, depression, dependency, and fear of intimacy continue. Intrusive, painful memories plague many, thereby denying the POWs a normal retirement. Many POWs may be seen as living in the past *and* the present at the same time, trying to survive in the present, and struggling to separate themselves from the grief, guilt, anger, and fear of war. For many spouses and children, there may be an emotional emptiness. The impact of war continues to live within the minds and bodies of each veteran. Although very little may come from pain, the fact of these soldiers' survival is a living example of overcoming man's inhumanity to man, as well as of man's overcoming and emerging from this inhumanity.

Only recently, through the Former POW Act of 1982, have these soldiers received the recognition and treatment they deserve. Since the passage of this Act, many POWs have come forward with their stories, which were held inside for over 40 years. For many, it was the fear of rejection that caused this containment. POWs were and do remain survivors, representing the strength of a country engaged in war, and never giving up, even in the enemy's hands. Their courage has been passed on to their children and grandchildren as a symbol of what can be endured under life-threatening stress. Special conventions held annually (state and national) provide opportunities for POWs to gather together, along with their families, military groups, and community leaders to support, honor, and teach each experience as a symbol of remembering the price of freedom. During these occasions, many grandchildren have written and presented poems and essays about their grandparents' experiences and the impact they had upon them. Children and spouses are willing to share feelings with others, many for the first time.

Duty, honor, and country remain an ongoing symbol for all POWs interviewed in this research. Love and respect hold a high position within the family value system.

In conclusion, POWs are people who survived the battles of war and have moved beyond the field of combat. They carry with them the trauma of the past and the hope of the future.

ACKNOWLEDGMENTS: This author wishes to express his thanks to Ms. Mary R. Rust, MSW, and Ms. Eve Roland, MSW, who, as students, aided in the research of this project.

REFERENCES

American Psychiatric Association. (1994). *Diagnostic and Statistical Manual of Mental Disorders* 4th ed. Washington, DC: Author.

Center for POW Studies. (1976). *Medical Care Repatriated Prisoners of War: Manual for Physicians.* San Diego: Navy Medical Network Unit.

Dent, O. P., Tennant, C. C., & Goulston, K. J. (1987). Precursors of depression in World War II veterans 40 years after the war. *Journal of Nervous and Mental Disease, 175*(8), 486–490.

deWind, E. (1984). Some implications of former massive traumatization upon the actual analytic process. *International Journal of Psychoanalysis, 65*(3), 273–281.

Danieli, Y. (1985). In the treatment and prevention of long-term effects and intergenerational transmission of victimization: A lesson from Holocaust survivors and their children. In C. R. Figley (Ed.), *Trauma and its wake* (pp. 309–313) New York, Brunner/Mazel.

Fairbank, J. A., & Nicholson, R. A. (1987). Theoretical and empirical issues in the treatment of post-traumatic stress disorder in Vietnam vet. *Journal of Clinical Psychology, 43*(1), 44–45.

Figley, Charles R. (Ed.) (1978). *Stress disorders among Vietnam veterans: Theory, research, and treatment.* New York: Brunner/Mazel.

Figley, Charles R. (Ed.) (1985). *Trauma and its wake: The study and treatment of post-traumatic stress disorder.* New York: Brunner/Mazel.

Hall, J. M. (1981). The aging survivor of the Holocaust: Father hurt and father hunger. The effect of a survivor father's waning years on his son. *Journal of Geriatric Psychiatry, 14*(2), 211–223.

Hall, R. C., & Malone, P. T. (1976). Psychiatric effect of prolonged Asian captivity: A two year follow-up study. *American Journal of Psychiatry, 133*(7), 786–790.

Hogancamp, V. E., & Figley, C. R. (1983). *War: Bringing the battle home.* New York: Brunner/Mazel.

Keating, N. C., & Cole, L. (1980). Changes in the housewife role after retirement. *Gerontologist, 20*(1), 84–88.

LaCoursierre, R. B., Godfrey, K. E., & Ruby, L. M. (1986). Traumatic neurosis in the etiology of alcoholism: Vietnam combat and other trauma. *American Journal of Psychiatry, 137*(8), 966–968.

Mullis, M. R. (1984). Vietnam: The human fallout. *Journal of Psychosocial Nursing, 22*(2), 22–26.

Mutran, E., & Reitzes, D. C. (1980). Retirement identity and well-being: Realignment of role relationships. *Journal of Gerontology, 36*(6), 733–740.

Rosenheck, R. (1986). Impact of post-traumatic stress disorder of World War II on the next generation. *Journal of Nervous and Mental Disease, 174*(6), 319–327.

Scaturo, D. J., & Hardoby, W. J. (1988). Psychotherapy with traumatized Vietnam combatants: An overview of individual, group and family treatment modalities. *Military Medicine, 153*(5), 262–269.

Sigal, J. D. (1976). Effects of paternal exposure to prolonged stress on the mental health of the spouse and children. *Canadian Psychiatric Association, 21*(3), 169–172.

Tanaka, K. (1988). Development of a tool for assessing post-trauma response. *Archives of Psychiatric Nursing, 11*(1), 350–356.

Veterans Administration Office of Planning and Program Evaluation (1983). *POW: Study of former prisoners of war.* Washington, DC:

7

Intergenerational Effects of the Japanese American Internment

DONNA K. NAGATA

February 19 is called the Day of Remembrance for Japanese Americans throughout the United States. On that date in 1942, just 10 weeks after Japan attacked Pearl Harbor, President Franklin D. Roosevelt signed Executive Order 9066 authorizing the exclusion of all persons of Japanese ancestry from "prescribed military areas." The order led to the removal and incarceration of more than 110,000 individuals, over 90% of the Japanese American mainland population. The military considered the action necessary. Internment was presumably a precaution against the actions of any potentially disloyal Japanese near the Pacific. As a result, Japanese Americans living along the West Coast and portions of Arizona were ordered to leave their homes and move to concentration camps in desolate areas of the interior. Neither citizenship nor demonstrated loyalty mattered. Two-thirds of the interned were U.S. citizens. Surrounded by barbed wire and armed guards, the Japanese Americans were held in camps for an average of 2–3 years. The intergenerational effects of their ordeal are the focus of this chapter.

THE INTERNMENT AS TRAUMA

Japanese Americans underwent numerous traumata during their internment. Under the conditions of forced relocation, they feared for their safety and suffered severe economic losses and sudden unemployment. Many also experienced the destruction of social and family networks (Loo, 1993). The internment represented a significant trauma in other critical ways as well. First and foremost, it was based on racism. Although Germany and Italy were also at war with the United States, neither German Americans nor Italian Americans were subjected to such drastic measures as an entire group. Japanese Americans, easily identifiable and already the target of discrimination, were singled out for mass internment. The fact that the internment was a culturally based trauma has particular significance for the study of intergenerational processes since culturally based traumata "potentially serve as the axial point for group and generational self-understanding. . . . [T]hey define the parameters of communal

DONNA K. NAGATA • Department of Psychology, University of Michigan, Ann Arbor, Michigan 48109.

International Handbook of Multigenerational Legacies of Trauma, edited by Yael Danieli. Plenum Press, New York, 1998.

conversations, thus providing the components from which collective identity is built" (Miller & Miller, 1991, p. 36).

Also significant is the fact that the internment resulted from intentional human design (Loo, 1993). The treatment of the Japanese Americans was deliberate and planned. Such traumata of human design can lead to more severe and prolonged posttraumatic stress disorder than trauma resulting from natural or accidental design (American Psychiatric Association, 1987). The forced nature of the uprooting, in combination with their minority status, placed Japanese Americans at risk. O'Sullivan and Handal (1988) note that while studies have shown any form of relocation, voluntary or compulsory, to be a significant stressor, the effects of compulsory relocation are significantly more detrimental to psychological functioning and social support. They also cite literature indicating that minority groups and community-oriented cultural groups are at particularly high risk for such negative effects under forced relocation, and that relocations that affect entire communities have more "profound and enduring effects" (p. 4).

The injustice of the internment can be seen as another aspect of trauma. Edward Ennis of the American Civil Liberties Union (ACLU) referred to the internment as "the greatest deprivation of civil liberties by government in this country since slavery" (cited in Irons, 1983, p. 349). The rights of Japanese Americans were blatantly ignored in the move to intern. No charges were brought against them, nor were they granted the right to a trial, and the U.S. Supreme Court held that the exclusion was constitutionally permissible in the context of war (Commission on Wartime Relocation and Internment of Civilians [CWRIC], 1997). Fear, prejudice, and political motivations overrode facts that contradicted the justifications underlying internment decision (CWRIC, 1997). For example, although West Coast Japanese Americans were targeted for internment because of their proximity to Japan, barely 1% of Hawaiian Japanese were interned (Ogawa & Fox, 1986). In addition, intelligence reports from the Federal Bureau of Investigation and naval intelligence did not consider mass incarceration of Japanese Americans a military necessity (CWRIC, 1997). A formal investigation of the events surrounding the internment by the CWRIC concluded that there was no basis for the detention and that "a grave injustice was done to American citizens and resident aliens of Japanese ancestry" (p. 18). In fact, "not a single documented act of espionage, sabotage or fifth column activity was committed by an American citizen of Japanese ancestry or by a resident Japanese alien on the West Coast" (p. 3).

PREINTERNMENT CONDITIONS

The attack on Pearl Harbor provided a catalyst for the internment of Japanese Americans. However, preinternment social conditions set the stage for their removal, including a long-standing history of anti-Asian prejudice and discrimination. The Japanese were initially welcomed in the mid-1800s as a source of cheap labor on Hawaiian sugar plantations, following the Chinese, who had been recruited earlier for the same purpose (Daniels, 1988). By the 1900s, the Japanese were reruited from Hawaii to work on the mainland. But, as had been the case with the Chinese before them, the rise in the Japanese population was met with increased prejudice and fear from non-Asians. Anti-Japanese activist groups such as the Japanese Exclusion League (Asiatic Exclusion League) fought for school segregation and the boycotting of Japanese businesses, while anti-Asian legislation significantly restricted immigration from Japan (CWRIC, 1997). Additional laws prohibited the Japanese from intermarrying with whites, and the Alien Land Law of California (where most mainland Japanese

Americans lived) barred alien Japanese from purchasing land and owning property (CWRIC, 1997). Japanese immigrants were also barred from citizenship until 1952. Economic competition along the West Coast contributed to anti-Japanese tensions, as the success of Japanese American farmers threatened many white American groups (Daniels, 1988). Much of the anti-Japanese sentiment stemmed from the fear of the "yellow peril," that Asians would overrun California and the Pacific Coast, and claims of grossly overestimated birthrates among people of Japanese ancestry ran rampant (CWRIC, 1997).

The prohibition against naturalization of the first-generation Japanese immigrants (Issei) as well as Japanese customs, language, and an emphasis upon group cohesion contributed to political as well as social exclusion. As noted by the CWRIC (1997):

> The Japanese were a major focus of California politics in the fifty years before World War II. Their small numbers, their political impotence and the racial feelings of many Californians frequently combined with resentment at the immigrants' willingness to labor for low pay to make them a convenient target for demagogues or agitators. (p. 31)

THE INTERNMENT PROCESS

Although Executive Order 9066 was issued in February 1942, steps taken against the Japanese began immediately after the attack on Pearl Harbor. On the night of the attack, the FBI arrested some 1,500 Japanese (Daniels, 1988). Fathers and husbands were abruptly taken from their homes, with no information as to their destination or how long they would be gone. Most were Issei leaders of the Japanese American communities, and protest against the government's actions was difficult since the second-generation children, Nisei, were significantly younger and less politically experienced (CWRIC, 1997). Japanese Americans lived in the post–Pearl Harbor weeks fearful about their families, communities, and future. Worried that possession of Japanese items would be viewed as evidence of disloyalty, many burned or buried any belongings that could be linked with Japan or its emperor. Irreplaceable heirlooms and mementos were destroyed as they anxiously awaited their fate.

The mass evacuation of Japanese Americans began soon after Executive Order 9066 was issued. Evacuees often had only a week's notice of their removal, giving them little time to dispose of their belongings. They took only what could be carried. Many prized possessions were sold for a fraction of their worth or had to be abandoned altogether. In addition, relocation was made even more difficult because the government would not provide information as to their future: Evacuees did not know what type of climate to expect or how long they would be gone from their homes.

The vast majority did not actively protest the evacuation orders. Japanese cultural values stressed deference to authority, and, for most, it would have been unthinkable to question a mandate from the U.S. Army. These values, combined with a void in community leadership, lack of political power, and an absence of information about the future made it unlikely that most Japanese Americans would resist. Also, having already been a population subjected to Anglo domination for years prior to the war, Japanese Americans were much more likely to respond in a conforming manner (Kitano, 1986). Nonetheless, it should be noted that a few individuals did challenge the internment (Irons, 1983), and there was disagreement within the community between those who advocated full compliance as a means of proving one's citizenship and patriotism and those who opposed this position (CWRIC, 1997; Spickard, 1983).

Most Japanese Americans endured two relocations; first, from their homes to a temporary "assembly center," and second, to one of the permanent "relocation centers." Each family was identified by an impersonal, numbered tag in preparation for the evacuation. With the number, stated one former internee, "I lost my identity. . . . I lost my privacy and my dignity" (CWRIC, 1997, p. 135). Travel to the assembly centers, and later from assembly centers to the camps, often took place in buses or trains with shades drawn, adding further to fears and anxieties. The assembly centers were located primarily in California, at fairgrounds or racetracks hastily converted to house thousands of evacuees under communal conditions with little to no privacy. Many facilities still smelled of animal manure. There, under guard, Japanese Americans lived for an average of 3 months before being transferred to the more permanent internment camps (CWRIC, 1997).

The 10 permanent internment camps, euphemistically termed "relocation centers" by the government, were constructed in desolate areas of the interior, including the deserts of California, Arizona, and Utah, and the swamplands of Arkansas. Japanese Americans were prisoners behind barbed wire and armed guard towers. This time, they lived in barrack-style housing with communal mess halls, toilets, and bath facilities. The smallest camp housed 7,000, the largest, 18,000. Each family was assigned to a single room, ranging in size from 20 by 8 feet to 20 by 24 feet, depending upon family size (Daniels, 1988). In many of the camps, temperatures ranged from below zero in winter to 115 degrees in the summer (CWRIC, 1997). Internees spent up to 4 years living under these harsh conditions.

LITERATURE ON THE EFFECTS OF THE INTERNMENT

Literature on the internment's effects spans several disciplines, including historical (e.g., Daniels, 1989, 1993; tenBroek, Barnhart, & Matson, 1968; Thomas & Nishimoto, 1969; Weglyn, 1976) and judicial analyses (Irons, 1983). Insights into the psychological impact of the camps and evacuation emerge from powerful autobiographical accounts of former internees (e.g., Hanson & Mitson, 1974; Tateishi, 1984) testimonies from the CWRIC (CWRIC, 1997; Rite of Passage, 1981), and Asian American writers (e.g., Inada, 1992; Mirikitani, 1987; Okada, 1976; Uchida, 1989). Recent books also cover the range of historical, sociological, economic, and psychological issues related to the internment (CWRIC, 1997; Daniels, Kitano, & Taylor, 1986). A key reference in this regard is the CWRIC's final report entitled *Personal Justice Denied,* originally published in 1982, and recently republished in 1997.

Mass (1986) has stated that "the psychological impact of the forced evacuation and detention was deep and devastating" (p. 160). Cramped conditions within the single-room barracks made privacy within the family nearly impossible, while shared toileting and bathing facilities made privacy equally difficult outside the barracks. At the same time, communal meals in the mess halls replaced mealtimes with the nuclear family and contributed to a breakdown in the traditional Japanese family structure (Kitano, 1986; Morishima, 1973). Parental authority diminished as children spent more time with peers, outside the confines of the families' room. Gender roles changed as Issei men lost their role as providers for their families and Issei women were relieved of previous obligations.

Events within the camps had critical psychological impact as well. One of the most significant was the government-imposed "loyalty oath" that required all internees, male and female, citizen and alien, 17 years or older, to declare complete loyalty to the United States and a willingness to serve in its armed forces. Those who did not answer affirmatively to the loyalty questions were segregated from other internees and sent to the Tule Lake camp. Answering the loyalty oath created tremendous conflict. In the words of one internee:

The resulting infighting, beatings, and verbal abuses left families torn apart, parents against children, brothers against sisters, relatives against relatives, and friends against friends. So bitter was all this that even to this day, there are many amongst us who do not speak about that period for fear that the same harsh feelings might arise up again to the surface. (CWRIC, 1997, pp. 14–15)

Divisions stemming from the loyalty oath can still be observed within Japanese American communities today.

Many of the psychological effects of the internment varied depending on generational status. The Issei lost all that they had worked so hard to establish (Mass, 1986). Inside the camps, it was the Nisei, not the Issei, who were allowed positions of authority, reversing the power roles of children and parents. And already in their late 50s or 60s after the camps closed, most Issei never reestablished their prewar status. Many became dependent upon their children for the remainder of their lives (CWRIC, 1997). The Nisei, whose median age was 21 in 1942 (Daniels, 1993), suffered a different psychological blow. For them, the internment was a direct "assault on their expectations and identity" as citizens of the United States (CWRIC, 1997), a rejection by their own nation (Mass, 1986). Even as they left the camps to resettle, their ethnic identity was denigrated as they were advised not to live next to other Japanese Americans or to congregate in public with other former internees (CWRIC, 1997). Nisei reactions to this assault varied after the war. Many responded by avoiding discussion of their camp experiences. Others developed a mistrust of white America and associated only with other Japanese Americans, whereas some identified with the aggressor by refusing to be associated with anything Japanese or Japanese American (Mass, 1986). Feelings of shame and guilt were also observed. Like the victims of rape, Nisei felt somehow responsible for their fate, even though they had done nothing wrong, and internalized their anger (CWRIC, 1997; Hanson & Mitson, 1974; Mass, 1986). The response of many was compliance, noted Mass (1986), who suggested that "like the abused child who still wants his parents to love him and hopes by acting correctly he will be accepted, Japanese Americans chose the cooperative, obedient, quiet American facade to cope with an overly hostile, racist America during World War II" (p. 161). Even the identity and self-concept of the earliest members of the third generation (Sansei) who were either very young or born in camp were affected, as Sansei born in camp have reported a sense of shame associated with their birthplace (Mass, 1986; Nagata, 1993; Tomine, 1991).

EXPLORING THE INTERGENERATIONAL EFFECTS OF INTERNMENT: THE SANSEI RESEARCH PROJECT

Clearly, the internment had important consequences for those who directly experienced the camps. The challenges to identity, as well as the disruption of parental, gender, and generational roles, affected entire families, indeed whole communities. But would these effects also be evident intergenerationally, in the third-generation Sansei offspring born after the war to former internees? If so, in what ways? These were the primary questions that guided the Sansei Research Project.

The pioneering work of Nobu Miyoshi (1980) provided an important basis for the project. Using the family systems theory of Boszormenyi-Nagy and Sparks (1973), Miyoshi was among the first to document how the camp experiences of the Nisei were transmitted to their Sansei offspring. The theory postulated that family relationships are accountable to the standards of loyalty and justice from previous generations. Family rules, credits for merits in fulfilling obligations, and debits for unfilfilled obligations are passed on from one generation to the next (Miyoshi, 1980). Other family therapists have also discussed the process of intergenerational familial transmission with respect to family myths, loyalties, secrets, and expectations, noting that the uncompleted actions of past generations may impinge on relationships within the new generation (Hoopes, 1987; Kramer, 1985). Miyoshi hypothesized that "the Sansei are heir to ethnic values that have been passed down to them from their Issei grandparents through their Nisei parents" (p. 41). The internment-camp experience represented an important part of that legacy, and the lack of communication about the internment between the Nisei and Sansei (the majority of whom were born after the war), she theorized, "represents a symbol of an intergeneration ethnic and personal gap" (p. 41).

In addition to family systems theory, life-span development theory provided a useful framework for the Sansei Project. Therefore, project questions asked about perceptions of both the present and the past. Researchers such as Elder (1974) and Stewart and Healy (1989) have also noted the importance of individual differences within generational cohorts and the need to consider the age at which significant life events occur when evaluating the impact of such events. According to Stewart and Healy (1989), "The experience of psychologically significant social events at different stages of adulthood will have different consequences not only for the individual personally, but also for his or her children" (p. 33). This developmental perspective suggested that the project should also explore whether the age of a Nisei parent in camp mediated any intergenerational effects.

The empirical framework for the Sansei Research Project came from previous studies on the children of Holocaust survivors. These investigations have examined multiple aspects of the Holocaust trauma, including the transmission of disrupted family patterns, separation and individuation issues among children of survivors, patterns of family communication about the Holocaust experience, and ethnic identity among the children of survivors. Although studies on children of Holocaust survivors vary widely in terms of their methodological strength (see Solkoff, 1992, for an overview), they helped to identify key areas of exploration for the Sansei Project. In addition, they delineated a model for comparing individuals whose parents experienced a trauma with same-cohort individuals whose parents did not. One study specifically hypothesized a link between the intergenerational effects of the Holocaust and the internment. Heller (1981) reported that the stressful experiences of Holocaust survivors led to a heightened sensitivity to culture and ancestry among their children. He speculated that other victimized cultural groups who emphasize traditional ideals might reflect a similar posttrauma heightening of ethnic identity and noted that "the responses of the Japanese to internment resemble quite closely the responses of survivor children to the Jewish Holocaust" (p. 259). However, he did not empirically explore this observation.

Design and Methodology

Given the literature on the intergenerational effects of the Holocaust, it seemed likely that the internment might also have affected postwar Japanese Americans. Yet there were no empirical studies directly exploring the intergenerational effects of the internment. Therefore, the Sansei Research Project investigated the impact of the internment on Sansei born after the war whose parents had been interned. The project surveyed over 700 Sansei from across the United States and included semistructured, in-depth interviews with over 40 Sansei. Major findings from the study are summarized here. However, the reader is encouraged to refer to the book *Legacy of Injustice: Exploring the Cross-Generational Impact of the Japanese American In-*

ternment (Nagata, 1993) and Nagata (1990a) for a more extensive accounting of the project and its results.

Participants for the Sansei Project were recruited in 1987 with assistance from the Japanese American Citizens League (JACL), directories of the Young Buddhists Association, and by word of mouth within the Japanese American community. Of the 1,250 surveys initially sent, 740 were returned, yielding an approximately 60% return rate. Seven of these were eventually excluded due to incompleteness or were returned too late for inclusion into the data analysis. Surveys from another 137 were excluded because the respondents were Sansei who were either born in a camp or had been interned at a young age. The data from Sansei who directly experienced the internment were analyzed as a separate study (Nagata, Trierweiler, & Talbot, 1997). Therefore, the survey data reported here are based on a sample of 596 Sansei respondents.

Survey participants fell into one of three groups: (1) those who had both parents interned (Two-Parent Sansei, $N = 323$), (2) those who had only one parent interned (One-Parent Sansei, $N = 168$), and (3) those who had neither parent interned (No-Camp Sansei, $N = 105$). Interviewees also fell into either the Two-Parent ($N = 26$), One-Parent ($N = 10$), or No-Camp ($N = 6$) groups. Comparisons between these groups provided a way to study how the effects of parental internment on the Sansei varied as a function of extensiveness of family contact with that experience. It should be noted that the use of the term *effects* in this research study suggests the identification of a causal relationship. However, it is, in reality, impossible to assess the specific effects of internment upon the Japanese Americans (Kitano, 1986), and caution should be used in interpreting the Sansei Project results.

Survey participants responded to a range of fixed-choice questions regarding family communication about the internment, level of interest and knowledge about the internment, sense of security about their rights, ethnic socialization and outmarriage, membership in Japanese American community groups, ability to understand the Japanese language, and anticipated reaction to a future internment. Interview questions covered similar areas of interest in an open-ended format. In addition, broader interview questions asked participants to describe what ways, if any, they felt their parent's internment had affected their own lives as well as their parents' lives. The survey data were analyzed using a variety of quantitative statistical techniques, whereas the interview questions were summarized using qualitative analyses.

Intergenerational Project Findings

Survey data from the Sansei project indicated that Sansei who had one or both parents interned did not differ significantly from Sansei with noninterned parents with respect to their rate of outmarriage, current level of interest in the internment, reported level of comfort in discussing the internment with parents, membership in Japanese American community groups, or their anticipated reaction to a future internment. Two-Parent Sansei did not report significantly more negative internment effects than One-Parent Sansei, and Sansei gender differences were few. In addition, contrary to expectations, parental age during internment and the length of their incarceration were generally uncorrelated with the Sanseis' survey responses.

However, the data revealed significant group differences in other areas of interest. One major area of interesting results occurred with respect to familial communication. Not surprisingly, Sansei who had one or both parents interned had significantly more frequent and longer conversations about the internment than did the Sansei who had neither parent interned. However, even those who had had a parent in camp indicated that there had actually been very little familial discussion about the internment. Most reported having only about 10 such conversations in their lifetime with their parents, and the average length of these conversation was approximately 15–30 minutes. In addition, Sansei in the Two- and One-Parent groups indicated that the style in which their parents talked about the internment did not differ significantly from the style reported by the No-Camp group: Only one-third of all respondents felt that the camps had been the central topic of the discussion, compared with approximately 70% of each group who felt the camps were an incidental topic or merely a reference point in time. Interviewee comments also indicated a striking absence of conversation about the internment, referring to conversations with their parents as "cryptic," "oblique," "left-handed," "evasive," and "superficial." As one person stated, this absence became increasingly noticeable as they grew older:

> A lot of times you assume that your parents do not have a past when you're little and because you live in the present so much. The older I got . . . I would ask more and more about their lives—how they got married and how they met. Through those discussions, . . . discussion of camp were conspicuously absent. . . . So I really didn't learn about the camps through my parents. I got bits and pieces, . . . never a coherent story. (Nagata, 1993, p. 82).

The absence of knowledge about their parents' camp years led Sansei to feel sadness and a sense of incompleteness. As one interviewee revealed, it felt as if there was a "void in my personal history." Many experienced a shroud of secrecy surrounding the topic, and sensed they should not push their parents to discuss more. As another interviewee noted, "It's like a secret or maybe more like a skeleton in the closet—like a relative who's retarded or alcoholic. Everyone tiptoes around it, discussing it only when someone else brings it up, like a family scandal" (Nagata, 1993, p. vii). Other individuals were struck by the fact that their parents seemed more able to discuss their camp experience with Caucasian American acquaintances than with their own children, and One-Parent Sansei frequently reported that it was the noninterned parent who talked most about the camps.

When previously interned parents did speak, they often shared only positive aspects of their camp experience. Also striking was the lack of expressed bitterness. "When I've asked his feelings about the whole internment experience," stated one individual about his father, "he says he is not bitter. . . . The memories will always be with them, and I don't think I will ever really know the pain and degradation felt by my family" (Nagata, 1993, p. 87). The overall absence of communication may perhaps explain an additional finding. When asked 11 objective historical questions about the internment (e.g., the name of the President who signed Executive Order 9066, the number of people interned, and the proportion of U.S. citizens interned), Sansei whose parents were interned did not necessarily have more factual information about the internment than the No-Camp group.

Although it was relatively rare that parents raised the topic of the internment as a central focus for family discussion, brief exchanges between the Sansei and their parents were triggered by specific stimuli in their environment. Certain foods such as apple butter, gelatin, and Spam were reminders of camp and could spontaneously elicit comments by the Nisei. In other families, discussions were sparked by driving by the site of a former camp or assembly center.

The absence of direct conversations about the internment did not diminish the Sanseis' level of interest in that event. Survey data showed that respondents from all of the study's groups expressed a high degree of current interest in the internment. In addition, the Two- and One-Parent Sansei reported significantly higher levels of interest than the No-Camp Sansei from the elementary school years through their young adulthood. Comments from interviewees suggested that the void in family conversations about the camps signaled the presence of something too painful to discuss rather than the absence of something to talk about. In fact, interviewee and survey-respondent comments showed that many Sansei feel they carry an unspoken sense of sadness and anger for their parents.

From a life-span developmental perspective, it is interesting to note that Sansei within each of the three study groups reported increasing levels of interest in the internment over time. In addition, interview data showed that, over time, Sansei whose parents were in camp often had changed their own views about the lack of communication. Several individuals stated that they had moved from feeling angry and frustrated in their early 20s, to feeling an increased respect for their parents' silence today.

The communication findings revealed that even though there had been little overt communication about camp, the Sansei nonetheless felt affected by their parents' experience. This was reflected in their sense of security as well: Two- and One-Parent Sansei who were surveyed rated themselves as being significantly less confident in their rights in this country than the No-Camp Sansei, and although all respondents were split in the opinion of whether an internment of Japanese Americans could occur again, Two-Parent Sansei were most likely to see this as possible. Interviewee comments supported the survey results. Nearly half of those whose parents were interned believed an internment could happen again. As one stated, "I think it (the internment) has made me aware of the immense injustices that can occur in this society. It's made me cynical about government. . . . It's made me distrust power" (Nagata, 1993, p. 130).

The internment appeared to affect the Sanseis' self-esteem and ethnic identity. Survey respondents reported generally little understanding of the Japanese language, regardless of whether their parent was interned, and interviewees felt that the internment led to an accelerated loss of the Japanese language and culture. Many perceived their parents as minimizing their own and their children's Japanese identity, while at the same time emphasizing the importance of blending in and "acculturating" so as not to stick out and draw attention to themselves. For some, this resulted in feelings of shame and inferiority about their "Japaneseness." One interviewee commented, "I assume they (Caucasian Americans) are going to reject me because I'm Japanese since there was such rejection of my parents" (Nagata, 1993, p. 139). Such sensitivities may have contributed to survey findings that showed Two-Parent Sansei expressed a stronger preference for associating with other Japanese Americans than either the One-Parent or No-Camp Sansei. This preference did not, however, extend into outmarriage rates, which were similar between the three groups.

The concept of shame within Japanese culture is noteworthy in relation to the Sansei findings. Shame has a central role in traditional Japanese society, significantly shaping individual behavior (Benedict, 1946). "Failure to follow . . . explicit signposts of good behavior, a failure to balance obligations or to foresee contingencies is a shame (*haji*)" and public judgment of one's deeds is critical (p. 224). Hence, the shame generated by the unjust imprisonment and public degradation of internment was especially intense for Japanese Americans, whose culture emphasized the significance of shame and humiliation. And, although the third-generation Sansei have not lived in a traditional Japanese environment, they nonetheless retain remnants of their ethnic culture. Despite the absence of explicit instruction in traditional cultural values, "some values, such as respect for elders, *enryo* (reservation), *haji* (shame), and diligence, were passed on to the Sansei" (Takezawa, 1995, pp. 129–130). The fact that some Sansei feel the continued effects of shame from the internment is, in this context, not surprising.

The rich interview data yielded additional ways in which Sansei see their lives as being affected by the internment. Several chose a particular educational institution or career to finish the uncompleted goals of a parent whose dreams were disrupted during the war. For others, the internment was a primary factor in choosing careers dedicated to community activism, the ministry, or law—careers that focused on concerns of justice. Many felt a special pressure from their parents to achieve and "prove" themselves to society. Some families, however, emphasized achievement for a different reason. Education was important because, although others may take away your freedom, they can never take away your ideas.

Furutani (1981) hypothesized that yet another effect of the internment was its impact on the interned Niseis' physical health. Preliminary data from the Sansei Research Project supported this hypothesis with respect to males. Although mothers did not differ significantly in early deaths, more than twice as many Sansei whose fathers were in camp died before the age of 60, compared to Sansei whose fathers were not interned. Interviewees whose fathers died early also speculated that the internment experience might have created unusual stressors that contributed to the premature deaths. "I really strongly believe that the trauma of incarceration had a physiological effect on them," commented one. "Most of my Japanese American friends' fathers have died before age 60" (Nagata, 1993, p. 141). The present data are based on a small sample and therefore are limited. However, one might speculate that there is a link between the early deaths of the Nisei fathers and their general reluctance to discuss the internment. Pennebaker, Barger, and Tiebout's (1989) research suggests that avoidance of discussing one's traumatic experience may negatively affect physical health, and Sansei in the present study reported that their Nisei fathers were much less likely to bring up the topic of internment than their mothers.

Sansei whose fathers died early wonder how their futures might have been if their fathers were still alive. At the same time, both they and other Sansei wonder how their entire lives and the postwar lives of their parents might have been different without the internment. Interviewees questioned whether their parents might have been more assertive, more confident, or more expressive if they had never been in camp. How, also, might their life course have differed without the severe economic losses and lost careers? These "what if" questions haunt the Sansei long after the war.

The previous examples suggest a variety of negative postinternment consequences for the Sansei. However, although the Sansei saw the internment as unjust and traumatic, they were also able to identify some positive outcomes in their lives. They admire the postwar resilience of the Nisei and see them as valuable role models. Ironically, many also recognized that since their parents met in camp, they would never have been born had it not been for the internment. Others saw the internment as having sensitized them to issues of injustice for all groups whose rights are threatened. Several interviewees, for example, expressed concern upon hearing that proposals had been made to round up "suspicious" Iranian Americans during times of tension between Iran and the United States.

At the time of the Sansei Project, the movement to seek a governmental apology and monetary redress for surviving internees was strong but had not yet succeeded. Hence, the injustice of the internment was highly salient for most Japanese Americans. Survey results showed that although approximately equal percentages of Sansei (close to 80%) favored seeking redress, regardless of whether they had a parent interned, Two- and One-Parent Sansei expressed a significantly stronger level of agreement with the redress movement than the No-Camp Sansei. Interviewees who supported redress were clear that no amount of money could compensate for the injustice, loss, and hardships related to internment. However, they noted, "money talks" in the United States. Redress payments, in their eyes, symbolized one form of public recognition of significant wrongdoing on the part of the government. Substantial monetary payment, suggested several Sansei, might also deter the government from repeating such injustices in the future.

The redress legislation was successfully passed in 1988, resulting in a one-time payment of $20,000 to each surviving internee and an official governmental apology. Preliminary analyses of data from a subset of the original Sansei Project participants suggest that, on the average, Sansei felt that the success of the redress movement created some feeling of relief and moderately increased their faith in the U.S. government. However, these actions had only a slight impact in reducing the negative feelings the Sansei held about the internment itself. Such initial data indicate that individual Sansei reactions to the success of the redress movement may not necessarily reflect a sense of closure. Other researchers, however, point out that the passage of the redress legislation has had significant positive effects for Japanese Americans as a larger group by lifting the psychological burden of distrust that had been carried for decades (Danieli, 1992; Takezawa, 1995). In addition, Takezawa (1995) observed that the redress movement strengthened intergenerational ties. "Because of the movement, the Nisei and Sansei began a true dialogue concerning the family and community history" (p. 173). One important benefit of the redress movement for the Sansei, in particular, was that it "triggered an appreciation and recognition of their ethnic history and a consciousness of racism in American society . . . (as well as) a positive reinterpretation of the past which enhances their ethnic pride" (Takezawa, 1995, p. 197).

LIMITATIONS AND IMPLICATIONS

The Sansei Research Project findings provide useful information in exploring the cross-generational impact of the internment. This research demonstrates the importance of assessing a wide range of potential intergenerational effects since some areas of interest revealed significant between group differences, while others did not. The combination of survey and in-depth interview methodologies was particularly useful in uncovering such a range. At the same time, several limitations of the research deserve mention. First, the results have limited generalizability to the general Sansei population. Most Sansei are not members of the Japanese American Citizens League, whereas many of those included in the project survey reported membership in this organization. Results are also limited by the fact that they are based upon data from only those who agreed to participate. Other sampling-related issues concern the No-Camp group. Although they were included as an approximation of a "control group" because they had neither parent in camp, they may have had "exposure" to internment effects through aunts or uncles who were interned. In a somewhat similar vein, it should be noted that although the Sansei Project focused upon the effects of parental internment, in almost all cases where a parent was interned, the grandparents were in camp as well. This means that the observed findings reflect Sanseis' status as both the children *and* grandchildren of internees.

As mentioned previously, one also cannot assume that the reported "effects" from the study are causal since no true experimental design could possibly be applied to an investigation of this kind. Kitano (1986) aptly noted that

> the problem of measuring the results of an event that occurred over forty years ago is complicated by intervening years, a lack of relevant material, a complexity of the many interacting variables that affect behavior, the vagaries of memory, and the near impossibility of reconstructing an event not designed for evaluative purposes. (p. 152)

It is perhaps most useful to consider the Sansei Project data as reflecting Sanseis' perceived impact of the internment; that is, while we cannot directly measure an effect of a parent's internment, we can assess the ways in which the Sansei view the impact of that event on their current lives and their past. An additional limitation stems from the fact that, given the racial basis underlying the internment, all Japanese Americans were psychologically affected by its occurrence, even if they escaped incarceration during the war. In this sense, the term *No-Camp* is inaccurate (Nagata, 1993).

Given a life-span developmental framework, it is also likely that the perceptions shared by the Sansei in this research will change over time as both they, and their Nisei parents, move on to different stages of life. The Sansei are now parents themselves, and the Nisei are grandparents. In addition, many Nisei are in their final years. Danieli (1994a) notes that the aging process can interact with past trauma experiences to present uniquely challenging issues. Many Holocaust survivors, for example, "experience the normal phenomenon of old age as a recapitulation of Holocaust experiences" (p. 3). Feelings of abandonment, loneliness, and isolation that often accompany old age can be experienced as "a repetition of being shunned and dehumanized during and right after the Holocaust" (Danieli, 1994a, p. 3). Danieli (1994b) cites additional research documenting the implications of aging for other trauma populations, such as war veterans. How the Nisei negotiate the aging process and the degree to which the changes accompanying this process affect their postinternment lives are important questions that deserve attention. Similarly, an understanding of the ways in which the internment experience and the impact of redress are processed within and between the Nisei and Sansei generations will require ongoing research, sensitive to developmental processes.

The Sansei Project was not designed to tap psychopathology or clinical functioning. Nonetheless, several survey respondents and interviewees noted ways in which they perceived either themselves, other Sansei, or their interned parent to have suffered emotionally from the internment. One woman saw a correlation between Sansei who overdosed on drugs and their low self-esteem, which she believed stemmed from the negativity attached to their Japanese ancestry. Another described having had a recurring nightmare of being interned. In addition, a separate paper (Nagata, 1991) presents case studies in which the intergenerational impact of a parent's internment emerged. The paper also suggests factors to consider when exploring the potential impact of parental internment with Sansei clients. Family communication patterns (in particular, the role of silence about a parent's past), self-esteem, ethnic identity, and vocational choices may be related to a parent's internment experiences. In addition, Sansei concerns regarding assertiveness, independence, acceptance by others, and being uprooted or displaced (physically, socially, or psychologically) may also be linked to the internment.

Individual psychotherapy can provide one useful way for Sansei to understand the legacy of the internment. However, other forums for expression have also been therapeutic. These include group therapy (Tomine, 1991), the testimonies of Sansei who appeared before the CWRIC hearings in the early 1980s (CWRIC, 1997), and Sansei-focused and intergenerational support groups that encourage interchange around issues related to the internment. Research itself can also have a positive clinical impact by providing an outlet for unspoken feelings and concerns, and by legitimizing respondents' perceptions. Over half of the respondents in the Sansei Project wrote additional comments. Many of these were lengthy, extending for several pages, and shared personal stories and reactions. Their comments expressed gratitude to the author for conducting the study. The research let them know that they were not alone in the experience of silence or in their perceptions that their lives, too, were affected by the camps. This was not only affirming for the Sansei who participated but also demonstrated how research can be a tool for building a sense of community by linking the personal stories of individuals (Fine, 1983).

SUMMARY AND CONCLUSIONS

The Sansei Project supports the importance of investigating the internment's intergenerational impact. At the same time, it raises important methodological issues and additional areas for explorations (Nagata, 1990b, 1995). Many questions remain to be answered. How, for example, does sociohistorical context affect Sansei perceptions of the internment's significance? Economic friction between Japan and the United States, and conflict surrounding the Smithsonian Institute's exhibit of the atomic bomb, represent recent situations that generated tension and resulting anti-Japanese sentiments. To what extent do these dynamics reraise the internment legacy? Also, how has the success of the redress movement affected the place of the internment in the lives of the Nisei and the Sansei? Finally, as we look to the future, what cross-generational internment effects might emerge in the fourth- (Yonsei) and fifth-generation (Gosei) Japanese Americans, and to what extent will ongoing acculturative processes influence the positive and negative consequences of these effects? I hope that further research will study these and other issues to understand more fully the intergenerational consequences of the internment trauma.

REFERENCES

American Psychiatric Association. (1987). *Diagnostic and statistical manual of mental disorders* (3rd ed., rev.) Washington, DC: Author.

Benedict, R. (1946). *The chrysanthemum and the sword: Patterns of Japanese culture.* New York: New American Library.

Boszormenyi-Nagy, I., & Sparks, G. M. (1973). *Invisible loyalties: Reciprocity in intergenerational family therapy.* New York: Basic Books.

Commission on the Wartime Relocation and Internment of Civilians. (1982). *Personal justice denied.* Washington, DC: U.S. Government Printing Office.

Commission on the Wartime Relocation and Internment of Civilians. (1997). *Personal justice denied.* Washington, DC: Civil Liberties Public Education Fund, & Seattle: University of Washington Press.

Danieli, Y. (1992). Preliminary reflections from a psychological perspective. In T. van Boven, C. Flinterman, F. Grunfeld, & I. Westendorp (Eds.), *Seminar on the right to restitution, compensation and rehabilitation for victims of gross violations of human rights and fundamental freedoms* (pp. 196–213). Maastricht, The Netherlands: University of Limburg.

Danieli, Y. (1994a). As survivors age: Part I. *National Center for Post-Traumatic Stress Disorder Clinical Quarterly, 4*(1), 3–7.

Danieli, Y. (1994b). As survivors age: Part II. *National Center for Post-Traumatic Stress Disorder Clinical Quarterly, 4,* 20–24.

Daniels, R. (1988). *Asian America: Chinese and Japanese in the United States since 1850.* Seattle: University of Washington Press.

Daniels, R. (1989). *American concentration camps: A documentary history of the relocation and incarceration of Japanese Americans: 1942–1945.* New York: Garland.

Daniels, R. (1993). *Prisoners without trial: Japanese Americans in World War II.* New York: Hill & Wang.

Daniels, R., Kitano, H. H. L., & Taylor, S. (1986, 1991 Rev. ed.). *Japanese Americans: From relocation to redress.* Salt Lake City: University of Utah Press.

Dunham, C. C., & Bengtson, V. L. (1986). Conceptual and theoretical perspectives on generational relations. In N. Datan, A. L. Greene, & H. W. Reese (Eds.), *Life-span developmental psychology: Intergenerational relations* (pp. 1–27). Hillsdale, NJ: Erlbaum.

Elder, G. H. Jr. (1974). *Children of the Great Depression.* Chicago: University of Chicago Press.

Fine, M. (1983). The social context and a sense of injustice: The option to challenge. *Representative Research in Social Psychology, 13,* 15–33.

Furutani, W. (1981). The Commission on Wartime Relocation and Internment of Civilians: Selected testimonies from the Los Angeles and San Francisco hearings. *Amerasia Journal, 8,* 101–105.

Hanson, A. A., & Mitson, B. E. (1974). *Voices long silent: An oral inquiry into the Japanese American evacuation.* Fullerton: California State University Oral History Program.

Heller, D. (1981). Themes of culture and ancestry among children of concentration camp survivors. *Psychiatry, 45,* 247–261.

Hoopes, M. H. (1987). Multigenerational systems: Basic assumptions. *American Journal of Family Therapy, 15,* 195–205.

Inada, L. F. (1992). *Legends from camp.* Minneapolis, MN: Coffee House.

Irons, P. (1983). *Justice at war: The story of Japanese American internment cases.* New York: Oxford University Press.

Kitano, H. H. L. (1986). The effects of the evacuation on Japanese Americans. In R. Daniels, H. H. L. Kitano, & S. Taylor (Eds.), *Japanese Americans: From relocation to redress* (pp. 151–158). Salt Lake City: University of Utah Press.

Kramer, J. R. (1985). *Family interfaces: Transgenerational patterns.* New York: Brunner/Mazel.

Loo, C. M. (1993). An integrative–sequential treatment model for posttraumatic stress disorder: A case study of the Japanese American internment and redress. *Clinical Psychology Review, 13,* 89–117.

Mass, A. I. (1986). Psychological effects of the camps on the Japanese Americans. In R. Daniels, H. H. L. Kitano, & S. Taylor (Eds.), *Japanese Americans: From relocation to redress* (pp. 159–162). Salt Lake City: University of Utah Press.

Miller, D. E., & Miller, L. T. (1991). Memory and identity across generations: A case study of Armenian survivors and their progeny. *Qualitative Sociology, 14,* 13–38.

Mirikitani, J. (1987). *Shedding silence.* Berkeley, CA: Celestial Arts.

Miyoshi, N. (1980, December 19–26). Identity crisis of the Sansei and the American concentration camp. *Pacific Citizen, 91,* 41–42, 50, 55.

Morishima, J. K. (1973). The evacuation: Impact on the family. In S. Sue & N. N. Wagner (Eds.), *Asian Americans: Psychological perspectives* (pp. 13–19). Palo Alto, CA: Science and Behavior Books.

Nagata, D. K. (1990a). The Japanese American internment: Exploring the transgenerational consequences of traumatic stress. *Journal of Traumatic Stress, 3,* 47–69.

Nagata, D. K. (1990b). The limitations of traditional research paradigms: A case example. *Focus: Newsletter of the Society for the Psychological Study of Ethnic Minority Issues, 4,* 5–6.

Nagata, D. K. (1991). The transgenerational impact of the Japanese American internment: Clinical issues in working with the children of former internees. *Psychotherapy, 28,* 121–128.

Nagata, D. K. (1993). *Legacy of injustice: Exploring the cross-generational impact of the Japanese American internment.* New York: Plenum Press.

Nagata, D. K. (1995). Studying the legacy of injustice: Psychological research on the Japanese American internment. In J. Fong (Ed.), *Proceedings of the Asian American Psychological Association Annual Convention, August 11, 1994* (pp. 67–73). Atascadero, CA: Rogers and Associates Consultants to Management.

Nagata, D. K., Trierweiler, S. J., & Talbot, R. (1997). Long-term effects of internment during early childhood among third-generation Japanese Americans.

Ogawa, D. M., & Fox, E. C., Jr. (1986). Japanese American internment and relocation: The Hawaii experience. In R. Daniels, S. C. Taylor, & H. H. L. Kitano (Eds.), *Japanese Americans: From relocation to redress* (pp. 135–138). Salt Lake City: University of Utah Press.

Okada, J. (1976). *No-no boy.* Seattle: University of Washington Press.

O'Sullivan, M. J., & Handal, P. J. (1988). Medical and psychological effects of the threat of compulsory relocation for an American Indian tribe. *American Indian and Alaska Native Mental Health Research, 2,* 3–19.

Pennebaker, J. W., Barger, S. D., & Tiebout, J. (1989). Disclosure of trauma and health among Holocaust survivors. *Psychosomatic Medicine, 51,* 577–589.

Rite of passage: The Commission Hearings 1981. (1981). *Amerasia, 8,* 54–105.

Solkoff, N. (1992). Children of survivors of the Nazi Holocaust: A critical review of the literature. *American Journal of Orthopsychiatry, 62,* 342–358.

Spickard, P. R. (1983). The Nisei assume power: The Japanese American Citizens League, 1941–1942. *Pacific Historical Review, 52,* 147–174.

Stewart, A. J., & Healy, J. M. (1989). Linking individual development and social changes. *American Psychologist, 44,* 30–42.

Takezawa, Y. I. (1995). *Breaking the silence: Redress and Japanese American ethnicity.* Ithaca, NY: Cornell University Press.

Tateishi, J. (1984). *And justice for all: An oral history of the Japanese American detention camps.* New York: Random House.

tenBroek, J., Barnhart, E. N., & Matson, F. W. (1968). *Prejudice, war, and the constitution.* Berkeley: University of California Press.

Thomas, D. S., & Nishimoto, R. (1969). *The spoilage: Japanese American evacuation and resettlement during World War II.* Berkeley: University of California Press.

Tomine, S. I. (1991). Counseling Japanese Americans: From internment to reparations. In C. Lee & B. L. Richardson (Eds.), *Multicultural issues in counseling: New approaches to diversity* (pp. 91–105). Alexandria, VA: American Association for Counseling and Development.

Uchida, Y. (1989). *Desert exile.* Seattle: University of Washington Press.

Weglyn, M. (1976). *Years of infamy: The untold story of America's concentration camps.* New York: William Morrow.

8

The Second Generation of Hibakusha, Atomic Bomb Survivors
A Psychologist's View

MIKIHACHIRO TATARA

> Ah, What a fool I am
> Twenty years ago
> A shining and burning A-bomb
> Heat of more than thousands centigrade
> Speared my skin
> Fifteen years later
> My son was born
> Already speared and burnt
> NAGOSHI (1972, pp. 98–99)

Fifty years ago, two atomic bombs were dropped on the cities of Hiroshima and Nagasaki, Japan, instantly killing close to 70,000 people. Some were evaporated. Their shapes remained as shadows, like negatives from exposed film, on the stone walls and steps. Another 20,000 died within 2 weeks. In all, more than 100,000 people died from the blast and the radiation released by the bombs.

Causes of death attributable to the bomb have been multiple, including burning, hematesis, pneumonia, multiple types of cancer, and diseases of the inner organs. Physical disorders and symptoms include keloid disorders of eyesight such as cataracts, low blood pressure, and general weakness and disability.

The atomic bomb was massive and nonselective. Everybody in the immediate area where it fell was killed, without exception. Death was instantaneous. In adjacent areas, assistance was impossible, because since everyone nearby was dead or fatally wounded. The trauma of the bomb has been described as extensive:

1. It was a massive happening.
2. It was an instantaneous happening.

MIKIHACHIRO TATARA • Department of Psychology, Hiroshima University, Hiroshima, Japan 739.

International Handbook of Multigenerational Legacies of Trauma, edited by Yael Danieli. Plenum Press, New York, 1998.

3. The cause of death after the bombing was invisible.
4. There has been long-lasting physical and psychological suffering.
5. There are many still unknown areas to explore regarding the effects of radiation on the human body, even 50 years later (Hiroshima and Nagasaki Committee, 1979).

Yuzaki (1978) has shown the massive destruction from the atomic bomb in schematic form. Figure 1 illustrates the totality of the bomb's impact, including the destruction of hu-

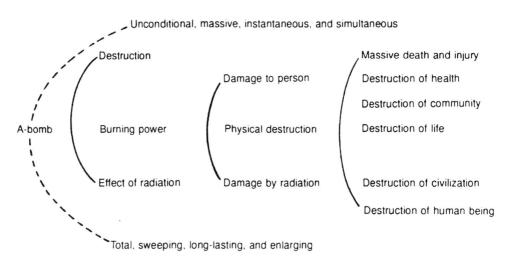

Figure 1. The characteristics of destruction of A-bomb (Yuzaki, 1978, p. 255).

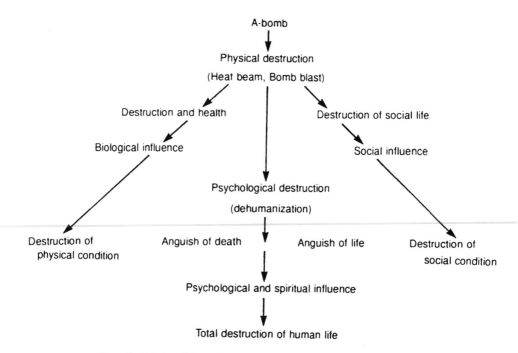

Figure 2. Relation of destruction and psychosocial life (Yuzaki, 1978, p. 256).

man life, and the destruction of communities and civilization. However, as shown in Figure 2, traumatic consequences from the bomb extended beyond physical destruction and into the psychosocial life of those who survived. The combination of effects from Yuzaki's two diagrams demonstrates the enormity of the devastation.

THE HIBAKUSHA: SURVIVORS OF THE ATOMIC BOMB

Those who lived through the atomic bomb are referred to as Hibakusha. Their offspring are referred to as second-generation Hibakusha (or Hibakusha Nisei). Relatively little has been written about the Hibakusha, and there is even less written about the Hibakusha Nisei. The reasons for this lack of attention can be tied to a range of factors. This chapter reviews these factors and, in doing so, illustrates how the intergenerational consequences of the atomic bomb must be seen in the context of sociopolitical, cultural, and biological issues, all of which have had important psychological effects upon the Hibakusha and Hibakusha Nisei.

Sociopolitical and Cultural Factors

Part of the lack of attention to the Hibakusha and Hibakusha Nisei may be understood in the context of broad sociopolitical factors. Although there is a strong antinuclear armament movement in the world today, there remain many strong supporters of nuclear weapons. For nations who favor them, these weapons are a justifiable means of defense against threats from enemies. Nuclear advocates tend to minimize the disasters of Hiroshima and Nagasaki and, as a result, the suffering of those who survived the atomic bombs in those cities.

In addition, many Asian countries that were occupied by Japan during the war still believe that their countries were liberated by the atomic bomb, that the use of the bomb on Hiroshima and Nagasaki was necessary in order to defeat Japan. In this view, Japan should express an apology to each of these nations for her occupation rather than emphasize the disaster and tragedy of the bomb.

Within Japan itself, the government covers payments for the medical care of individual Hibakusha, but provides no social or economic support for their families. Because of the physical weakness that is a lasting effect of radiation from the bomb, Hibakushas frequently cannot keep a steady job and tend to drop out of employment. Most of them have below-average incomes and cannot afford the expenses for their children's schooling in an educationally conscious society. This leads to a vicious cycle, with the low economic status of the Hibakusha leading to the low educational level of the Hibakusha Nisei, who then also remain at a low economic level.

A variation of the vicious cycle leading to socioeconomic disadvantage is illustrated in the following description of one 75-year-old Hibakusha mother: When the atomic bomb fell, she was 25, married, and had a 1-year-old baby. The mother survived but was badly burned, and the baby died. Massive keloid scarring that resulted from her burns made it physically difficult for her to move in day-to-day life after her recovery and limited her employability. The physical disability also created difficulties in her relationship with her husband, and her marriage eventually ended in divorce in 1945. The woman remarried in 1947. After 2 years, she gave birth to a baby, who died 10 days later. Over the next 4 years, she had two other babies. Although her fears that these babies would die did not materialize, one baby, a daughter, was mentally retarded. Then, following the birth of another baby, a son, the mother had to be hospitalized for heart disease and stomach problems. The hospitalization created significant financial hardship for her family. Her second husband eventually deserted her, leaving her to support herself and the children on welfare. When the son reached 15, he ran away from home. The mother had been living with her daughter, with aid from a social worker (Yamada, 1995).

Biological Factors

Scientific evidence about the long-range effects on the human body of radiation from the atomic bomb, particularly with regard to the genetic and hereditary aspects of radiation, is currently inconclusive. However, there is some research documenting the aftereffects of atomic radiation on heredity (Hiroshima and Nagasaki Committee, 1979), and there have been reports of damaging radiation effects among the Hibakusha Nisei (Plummer, 1952; Neal *et al.*, 1953; Russell *et al.*, 1973; United Nations Scientific Committee, 1969). Journalists in the 1970s gave considerable attention to these ill-effects, noting cases of physical malformation, brain damage, microcephalus, and mental retardation in babies born to pregnant women who had been exposed to the bomb. The Japanese government also recognized the defects in these children as one of the effects of the atomic bomb (Wakabayashi, 1995).

One incident was widely publicized as demonstrating the ill-effects of radiation from the atomic bomb. Mrs. Nagoshi, a Hibakusha mother, had one boy who was healthy and active until junior high school. However, when he became 15, he developed leukemia and eventually died from it. Mrs. Nagoshi attributed her son's death to the aftereffects of radiation. Journalists reported this incident as evidence of the continuing effect of the atomic bomb, raising the level of public fears about such effects.

Social and Psychological Factors

Such reports on the genetic transmission of the radiation's ill-effects generate lingering fears among the Hibakusha and Hibakusha Nisei, and the consequences of these fears have extended well beyond the period of recovery from physical wounds and trauma. As one Hibakusha Nisei stated, "In ordinary life, we forget the effect of the radiation. But when we have any kind of physical symptom which does not disappear over a period of time, we cannot but connect it with the radiation from the A-bomb" (Anonymous man in Nagasaki, 1972, p. 113). Many Hibakusha and their offspring also worry that they should not marry or have children for fear that they would be responsible for transmitting radiation-related physical disorders. As one Hibakusha mother noted, "If I have transferred genes contaminated by radiation to children, I cannot imagine how these children would hate us for it" (Fukazawa, 1972, p. 100).

Fears of genetic and chromosomal effects also exist among the people surrounding the Hibakusha, creating a stigma for the Hibakusha and their families. Arranged marriages and preservation of the family name through children remain important in Japan. Knowledge that an individual comes from a Hibakusha family raises the specter that there may be "bad blood" (i.e., blood contaminated by radiation). As result, the Hibakusha Nisei may be socially rejected out of fear that their genes will taint marriages and families.

The social stigma stemming from fears of continued radiation effects among subsequent generations engenders additional psychological consequences. For example, the Hibakusha and their families tend to avoid being open about their history as atomic-bomb survivors, aware of the potential rejection that might result from such a disclosure. This further increases their feelings of isolation within the community and creates an additional burden of trying to maintain secrecy and silence about their suffering. One Hibakusha mother revealed the strain of this burden:

When people talk about Hibakusha Nisei, the second generation of Hibakusha, this makes me nervous that my children cannot marry, because people want to avoid the possibility of an unhealthy baby. However, I know that I cannot keep the fact of being a Hibakusha from people's attention forever. (Esuko, 1972, p. 101)

Interestingly, this press for silence can extend even to those who research and/or advocate for the Hibakusha. One of the leading figures in the antinuclear movement in Hiroshima, Professor Moritaki (1972), noted,

I know this (the problem of Hibakusha Nisei) is important and must be discussed openly. But I have a mixed feeling. You know, I could not figure out how to treat them. My friend, a professor at the university, said to me, "Please don't talk about it openly. I have a daughter myself. You must understand this!" If I think about the feeling of the family of Hibakusha, it is hard for me to talk about this openly, even though it is important. (p. 106)

SUMMARY: UNDERSTANDING THE HIBAKUSHA IN CONTEXT

Many of the scientific investigations on the consequences of atomic bomb have focused on the biological transmission of long-term effects of radiation. Such research is clearly important. However, the points raised in this chapter suggest that if we wish to understand the psychological experience of the Hibakusha and the second generation of atomic-bomb survivors, we must look at their lives in a broader context, one that extends beyond the question of whether there are definitive data on questions of biological transmission. The case examples cited here revealed that it is the *perceptions* of possible ill-effects from radiation that play a critical role in the psychological experience of Hibakusha and their families. The fear of having and transmitting genetic effects or illnesses is a burden that must be carried throughout their lives; it is a fear that can create significant social isolation and stress. When such fears are shared by those in the community, the Hibakusha and Hibakusha Nisei feel socially stigmatized as well, and may be blocked from marital and social opportunities that are open to non-Hibakusha.

The Hibakusha also carry a burden of silence about their experience. Part of this silence has been defined by the previously noted fears of biological aftereffects and by social stigma within Japan. However, part of the silence has also been defined within the context of sociopolitical and cultural factors. The views of other countries that supported the use of the atomic bomb during the war, as well as the views of countries that currently favor nuclear arms, can create a climate that discourages focusing upon the Hibakusha and their suffering. Without a supportive sociopolitical context, these survivors are even less likely to discuss their concerns.

Adopting a broader view also required a recognition of the interplay between multiple levels of factors affecting the Hibakusha experience. The vicious cycle by which the physical disabilities stemming from the bomb can affect the employment and subsequent socioeconomic status of Hibakusha and their families illustrates the "domino" effect of trauma. As a result, the second-generation Hibakusha are prevented from gaining the credentials and skills necessary to raise their own socioeconomic status. Such limits on educational and economic resources are exacerbated by the social stigma discussed previously, because families of high socioeconomic background would likely reject the option of marrying into families of Hibakusha. Hence, physical, socioeconomic, cultural, and social factors can interact to affect the Hibakusha and Hibakusha Nisei decades after the atomic bombs were dropped.

Given the range of factors described in this chapter, we see that there is still a great deal to be learned about those who survived the atomic bomb, and about their children. Future attempts to develop a psychological understanding of the Hibakusha and the Hibakusha Nisei would benefit from examining the relationships between the individual and the broader sociopolitical, economic, and cultural contexts presented here.

REFERENCES

Esuko, S. (1972). Appeal for Hibaku Nisei. In S. Ienaga, H. Odagiri, & K. Kuroko (Eds.), *Hibaku Nisei* (p. 101). Tokyo: Jiji-Tushin Co.

Fukazawa, K. (1972). Appeal for Hibaku Nisei. In S. Ienaga, H. Odagiri, & K. Kuroko (Eds.), *Hibaku Nisei* (p. 100). Tokyo: Jiji-Tushin Co.

Hiroshima and Nagasaki Committee on A-bomb Disaster. (1979). *Report on A-bomb disasters of Hiroshima and Nagasaki.* Tokyo: Iwanami Shoten Publishers.

Anonymous man in Nagasaki. (1972). In Fear of People. In S. Ienaga, S. H. Odagiri, H. & K. Kuroko, K. (Eds.). (1972). *Hibaku Nisei* (p. 4). Tokyo: Jiji-Tushin Co.

Moritaki, I. (1972). An intricate experience. In S. Ienaga, H. Odagiri, & K. Kuroko (Eds.), *Hibaku Nisei* (p. 106). Tokyo: Jiji-Tushin Co.

Nagoshi, M. (1972). Fumiki, my son. In S. Ienaga, H. Odagiri, & K. Kuroko (Eds.), *Nibaku Nisei* (pp. 98–99). Tokyo: Jiji-Tushin Co.

Neal, J. V., Morton, N. E., Schell, W. J., McDonald, J. D., Kondani, M., Takeshima, K., Suzuki, M., & Kitamura, S. (1953). The effect of exposure of parents to the atomic bomb on the first generation offspring in Hiroshima and Nagasaki. *Japanese Journal of Genetics, 28,* 211–216.

Plummer, G. (1952). Anomalies occurring in children exposed in utero. *Hiroshima Pediatrics, 10,* 687–692.

Russell, W. J., Keehn, R. J., Ihno, Y., Hattori, F., Kigura, T., & Imamura, K. (1973). Bone maturation in children exposed to the atomic bomb in utero. *Radiology, 108,* 367–370.

United Nations Scientific Committee. (1969). *Report on the effects of atomic radiation-induced chromosome aberrations in human cells.* New York: United Nations Publications Office.

Wakabayashi, S. (1995). Microcephaly: Children exposed to the atomic bomb *in utero.* In T. Suzuki & Atomic Bomb Sufferers and Counselors Groups (Eds.), *With Hibakusha* (pp. 63–79). Hiroshima: Chugoku Shinbun Newspaper Co.

Yamada, S. (1995). Holding Hibaku Nisei. In T. Suzuki & Atomic Bomb Sufferers and Counselors Group (Eds.), *With Hibakusha* (pp. 141–145). Hiroshima: Chugoku Shinbun Newspaper Co.

Yuzaki, M. (1978). Atomic bomb disaster in Hiroshima. *Historical Review, 12,* 255–256.

9

Children of Dutch War Sailors and Civilian Resistance Veterans

WYBRAND OP DEN VELDE

Nowadays it is generally acknowledged that the Nazi persecution, as well as other extreme experiences during World War II, left deep mental scars. There is also a growing realization that children of traumatized parents can struggle with more or less severe psychological problems. Albeit initially piecemeal, around the end of the 1960s, (auto)biographical and scientific publications about the "second generation" began to appear. The majority of the publications relates to survivors of Nazi concentration camps, in particular to Jewish survivors (Chapters 1–3). The literature is considerably less voluminous about the offspring of war sailors and former civilian Resistance fighters. Nevertheless, physicians, psychologists, psychiatrists, and social workers come in contact with these now adult children regularly. Their general impression is that the problems and complaints of these "children" are closely associated with the experiences of their parents during World War II.

The extant literature reflects a growing awareness of the heterogeneity within the group of "victims of war and persecution" and the "second generation." Another important conclusion from the literature about the offspring of war victims is that they do not constitute a separate diagnostic entity. Also, the problems of these children cannot be exclusively expressed in psychopathological terms. What possible makes the second generation a separate category is the complex psychodynamics of their problems and complaints, and their relationship to their parental traumatic experiences. Despite the absence of evidence for a "second generation syndrome," a number of complaints and symptoms are frequently observed. These symptoms are diverse and include social isolation, authority conflicts, and work and relationship problems, as well as delinquent behavior and psychoses.

The family dynamics described shows a number of characteristics, such as reversal of the parent–child roles (parentification), and separation and identification problems (Coopmans, 1993). It seems that a "family secret" often is connected with loyalty demands and conflicts. The family secret is directly linked to the pattern and quality of the communication about parental war experiences inside the family. The conflict between wanting to know and not

WYBRAND OP DEN VELDE • Department of Psychiatry, Saint Lucas Andreas Hospital, P.O. Box 9243, 1006 AE Amsterdam, The Netherlands.

International Handbook of Multigenerational Legacies of Trauma, edited by Yael Danieli. Plenum Press, New York, 1998.

wanting to or being allowed to know, in other words, the quality of communication or the lack of it, may have major consequences for the inner and interpersonal life of the children. In some cases, this is a demonstrable cause of pathological development.

In order to gain insight into the problems of the offspring of war sailors and Resistance veterans, it is necessary to understand the way in which the war has affected their parents. Not only the war traumas, but also the way in which the parents have coped with them, have proved to be of importance to the psychosocial development of the children. The following describes the stress war sailors and participants of the Resistance were exposed to during World War II, the late effects of these war traumas, including the disturbed family dynamics, and the effects on the development of the children.

THE PARENTS

War Sailors

The sailors of the merchant navy during World War II may be categorized as a "forgotten group" of war victims in Holland. According to Dutch law, merchant sailors who were disabled during the war, like military veterans, are eligible for a disability pension. In 1980, around 475 sailors received such a pension. Former war seafarers are not formally organized.

The Stress on War Sailors.   The stress the sailors were exposed to during the 5 years of war was characterized by a constant threat to their lives and frequent, or even continuous, interruption of sleep. The principal dangers were enemy submarines and airplanes. The freight carried by the ships consisted mainly of highly explosive materials, such as gasoline and ammunition. In contrast to concentration camp survivors, sailors experienced primarily psychological stress that consisted of continuous and long-lasting confrontation with danger, without the ability or possibility to fight back or escape—a particularly vicious kind of helplessness. In addition, the sailors were separated from their families for years and deprived of knowing the fate of their relatives in the occupied homeland. Many of them lost brothers, a father, or close friends in the same convoy, without having any opportunity to rescue them (Weisaeth & Eitiner, 1993).

The Number of War Sailors.   Six hundred and forty merchant vessels and 200 coasters sailed under the Dutch flag during World War II. These ships were manned by 12,000 Dutch and 6,500 foreign sailors. Of these ships, 46% were lost, mainly due to submarine attacks. Twenty-one hundred Dutch sailors did not survive.

Studies of War Sailors.   Askevold (1980) studied a group of Norwegian war sailors and compared them to Norwegian concentration camp survivors. Of the 35,000 Norwegian sailors in the merchant navy who sailed for the Allied forces, 6,000 were killed at sea. Askevold recognized in both groups a similar symptom complex, consisting of fatigue, irritability, lack of initiative, emotional incontinence, disturbed sleep, and recurrent dreams. For the sailors, these dreams were typically filled with alarm bells, torpedo hits, explosions, and burning ships. The description of the aging Norwegian war sailors is strikingly similar to our observations of Dutch Resistance veterans (Op den Velde *et al.,* 1993).

Participation in the Resistance

The participants in active civilian Resistance against the German occupation during World War II were a rather heterogeneous group of people. What these people had in common was that they served the same cause and took the same dangerous, sometimes fatal, risks. One part of the Resistance engaged in the "large," more "noticeable" activities, such as raids on distribution and registry offices, sabotage, espionage, liquidations, courier services, and organization of strikes. However, a much larger group occupied itself with less conspicuous, but surely not less risky, activities, such as helping persons in hiding, mostly Jews; providing for shelter, food and ration tickets; counterfeiting; and delivering identity cards.

Motives for Resistance Participation.   The motives for active participation in the Resistance were diverse. In some cases, strong political or ideological beliefs were the dominating factors, but more often, one became involved as a result of the spontaneous and growing disgust with the enemy, or sympathy with the people threatened with death or deportation. In several cases, lust for adventure and excitement or coincidental, circumstantial factors played an important role.

The Number of Resistance Veterans.   After the liberation in 1945, no registration of Resistance participants took place. These veterans, who had operated in secrecy, opposed any formal registration. Therefore, the exact number of Resistance participants is unknown. Bastiaans (1957) estimated the number of Resistance veterans to be 76,000 (less than 1% of the adult population of Holland during World War II); of these, 2,000 took part in armed Resistance. Of the 16,000 Resistance participants deported between 1940 and 1945, only 4,000 survived the war.

Stress as a Consequence of Resistance Participation.   The various stresses to which the members of the Resistance were exposed during the German occupation may be outlined as follows (Op den Velde, Frey-Wouters, & Pelser, 1994):

- The participation in the Resistance, no matter in what form, meant a period of permanent stress that could exceed the limits of personal endurance. There was a continuous fear of loss of life and the stress of responsibility for the lives and well-being of family members and the Resistance group.
- It was often necessary to keep information from even close family members. This could easily lead to a drifting apart and having to lead a double life. In addition, there was the constant fear of betrayal or being arrested. People of Christian or humanistic denominations found themselves confronting immense moral conflicts. It was sometimes "out of necessity" that they did things and made choices that were contrary to their deepest beliefs, such as planning for or participating in liquidations.
- Arrests, interrogation, and torture are obviously traumatic. Added to this must be the fear of "talking," the thought of actually having endangered the lives of comrades or having betrayed them, and being imprisoned or on death row, with the associated passivity, uncertainty, and mock executions. Some Resistance fighters were interned for months or years in prisons or concentration camps. Undernourished and exhausted, they were forced to carry out heavy labor under very difficult, often cold, and wet circumstances, knowing full well that weakness or illness could mean death. They had to survive without any privacy, in dreadful hygienic conditions, in the face of hunger, humiliation, and helplessness.

- Many have, while in prison or concentration camps, suffered severely from the power-lessness with which they had to watch fellow prisoners—comrades from the Resistance, Jews, Poles, and prisoners of war—tortured and murdered before their eyes.

The war situation of Dutch Resistance fighters differed from those of World War II military combat veterans. Military combat during World War II was generally characterized by the alternation of periods of fighting and danger with periods of rest and the absence of imminent threat. Participants in the Resistance were exposed to continual fear and stress. However, the sailors of the allied merchant marines were in a situation that could be said to resemble that of the Resistance fighters (Op den Velde *et al.,* 1993).

They were deprived of understanding, appreciation, and the necessary care for their physical and mental sufferings. The encounter with war victims may elicit strong emotional reactions in family members, relatives, significant others, and professional helpers. These reactions range from disbelief to pity and overinvolvement, and go hand in hand with distress, anxiety, and denial, often leading to the tendency to avoid confrontation with the memories of the traumatized individual.

The Late Effects of War Trauma

Most Dutch people experienced the liberation as a victory of good over evil. Those who had actively fought against the Nazi occupiers had every reason to be proud of their personal contribution to the victory and might have expected to be treated and appreciated as heroes. However, they often experienced exactly the opposite, for example, indifference, or even hostility and rejection (Op den Velde, Koerselman, & Aarts, 1994).

After the liberation in 1945, the disorganized and plundered country immediately claimed all its energies for reconstruction. In a way, every citizen considered him- or herself a victim of war. Collectively, as well as individually, the people tried to forget the five frightening years of Nazi occupation. The vast majority of the Dutch population had strongly disapproved of the behavior of the Nazis, yet only a few openly expressed it or offered active Resistance. Most people simply lacked the courage to risk their lives for ideals such as freedom and a just society. Members of this silent majority did not appreciate being reminded of their own lack of courage and their guilt feelings. Thus, the social appreciation of war victims as well as war heroes became beset with ambivalence. The result was that the war sailors and participants in the Resistance, as a special group of people in need of support and care, were largely ignored. As a consequence, many of them stifled their emotions, enhancing their feelings of neglect and rejection by society in general.

On top of that, some members of the Resistance suffered an additional disappointment. Typically, they had expected a much better postwar society, one with more justice, "civil courage," and mutual responsibility. They often responded to their disappointment with disillusionment, bitterness, or an apathetic and depressive-like mood. On the other hand, many participants in the Resistance themselves wanted to forget the past. They joined with the larger society's focus on recovery and rebuilding. They, too, wanted to start a new life and shake off the past by working hard and achieving as much as possible.

In actual fact, survivors of severe war stress may display the following symptoms and ailments:

- They are, even many years after the liberation, still quite often (involuntary) reminded of painful events from the war years.

- Hyperarousal, leading to increased startle reactions, feelings of fear, stress, and agitation, are continuously present.
- Sleeping problems, often accompanied by terrifying dreams or nightmares in which war experiences are relived, are frequent.
- There is a desire to keep silent about scary and life-threatening experiences, and to put up a brave front.
- The connection on the one hand between the psychological and physical problems and, on the other, the war experiences, is often denied.
- Many have difficulty with noticing and expressing emotions.
- There may be either excessive activity or serious passivity, the later often accompanied by depression of affect and vitality.
- By association through a stimulus from the environment (pictures, scents, sounds, anniversary dates, of important events during the war) or from within their own minds, they relive some traumatic experiences over and over.
- Avoidance behavior is often present, for they wish, as much as possible, not to be reminded of the war (no television, no newspapers, etc.). But sometimes there is, in contrast, an opposite need to dwell continually on, or talk about, the past.
- There may be a strong or overdeveloped need for self-justification, and/or a strong sense of justice, which can lead to placing great demands and rigid requirements on the surroundings and family members.
- Although, after the liberation, many Resistance veterans and war sailors, in contrast with Jewish survivors, found their families and social surroundings intact, among them there is quite often talk of "survival guilt." This guilt may be related to the powerlessness they experienced and to the death during the war of comrades with whom they felt a very close relationship, or because of their own behavior in order to survive.
- Regardless of the fact that looking back at the war is difficult and arduous, there is, sometimes, also a strong pull toward that period of intense mutual involvement and comradeship. After the liberation, it has proven very difficult, for some, to go on living without the familiar framework of good and bad characteristics of wartime. Owing to the lack of usually intense, comradeship, friendship, and purposiveness, postwar life seems to have lost color and meaning.

Many of these features, especially those that focus on alternating between reliving and denying traumatic experiences, fit the syndrome of posttraumatic stress disorder (PTSD). The prevalence of current PTSD in these now elderly Dutch Resistance veterans is between 25% and 50% (Op den Velde *et al.,* 1996). Many former Resistance fighters, however, must struggle with problems of a psychosomatic and/or characterological nature, which are not included in the concept of PTSD (Op den Velde, 1985). Another characteristic is the period of latency, a (seemingly) symptomless interval. In about half of the veterans, PTSD only became manifest more than 20 years after the end of the war (Op den Velde *et al.,* 1993, 1996). Already, in 1946, Tas, himself a survivor, predicted the possibility of a delayed onset of posttraumatic reactions in survivors of Nazi persecution. A latency period in World War II survivors has been described by various authors (Bastiaans, 1957; Krystal, 1968). It is a matter of ongoing debate whether this latency phase, or so-called symptom-free interval, is indeed typified by the absence of disturbances. Bastiaans (1957) studied Dutch Resistance veterans who had survived the concentration camps. He characterized the latency period as pathological adaptation to so-called normality and repression of traumatic war experiences. In this phase, neurotic overactivity combined with tenseness and irritability were present, as well as psychosomatic syndromes such as hypertension, myocardial infarction, asthma, and gastric ulcers in high frequency. The period of latency typically coincides with the period in which their children grow up.

The Third Traumatic Sequence.   The "third traumatic sequence," an expression coined by Keilson (1992), refers to a period following the actual traumatization. Research by Keilson has shown that conditions or circumstances under which young survivors grew up after 1945 are of great significance to the nature and severity of subsequent complaints. Understanding and empathy for the traumas of the children often turned out to be, independent of the nature of the war traumas, essential for rehabilitation. Conversely, the lack of psychosocial support had a negative influence on their ability to cope. The third traumatic sequence refers not only to the possibility to cope within the personal realm but also to a general social interest. When understanding and support are adequate, the postwar period does not have to be, by definition, a traumatic sequence.

FAMILIES OF WAR SAILORS AND RESISTANCE PARTICIPANTS

The Family Secret

Many of the conflicts between parents and their children, in cases where these manifest themselves, reflect the psychological and social problems of the parents. In principle, two opposite forms of communication are seen: on the one hand, keeping quiet, and on the other, talking excessively about war experiences and traumas. However, the reality is always more complex. Keeping quiet can be revealing, and speaking can be obscuring. We can state that communications about traumatic experiences—verbal or nonverbal—are always present in the family realm.

In many families of war sailors and participants in the Resistance, we observed that the traumatized parent had difficulty discussing his or her war experiences with the children. Many of these parents stated as a motive for remaining silent the "vulnerability" of children. They hoped to protect their children from their own burdening war memories by painstakingly avoiding the theme of war. But in many cases, feelings of guilt and shame played a role in this keeping silent. The intent to suppress their war experiences, which comes through in the parents' decision, concerns both negative experiences such as fear, sadness, the feeling to have failed, powerlessness, and humiliation, and positive ones such as mutual solidarity and shared hope. In some cases, the negative experiences were so dominating that they rendered the parent unable to remember the pleasant experiences. They made sure, however, not to tell most shocking experiences to the children. The tragedy is that the intention not to share war traumas with the children had the opposite effect. The aversion of the parents to acknowledge and deal with their traumas, together with the fear of injuring and burdening their children, often made the communication diffuse, confusing, and ambivalent. A child, dependent as he or she is on the parent(s), registers what he or she sees and feels with the parent. The parent weeps, is depressed or emotionally inaccessible, enraged or wakes up screaming, and has nightmares. In everyday life, sudden emotional outbursts may occur, from the child's point of view, without an apparent or actual reason. Or the parent may not react at all to disobedient or provocative actions of the child. Children receive and register messages and hints about their parents' past, even where no "open" communication takes place or is even intended. The children may respond to the loaded silence and the partial and indirect telling by withdrawing in fear or, sometimes obsessionally, trying to plug the holes in the fragmented knowledge of the family history.

The effect on the child who experiences the echo of (war) traumas without knowing or being allowed to know can be damaging. Knowledge of the traumatic history of the parents, however brief and deficient, can lead its own life in the fantasy of a child, in the form of un- or subconscious fantasies that fill the child with fear and shame. The child, in turn, may keep quiet, yet remain agitated. Threatening and burdening impressions about the parents' behavior may develop, however without the possibility of testing them against reality. The parents' silence about (part of) their experiences and their demeanor keep the children from asking questions. Their fear of what they possibly might learn is another reason to remain silent. We know of cases where the child walked around nursing a more or less suppressed suspicion that the parent had been "on the wrong side" during the war (Op den Velde & De Graaf, 1985). Only through the stories of others, after the parent's death, did the child found out what really happened.

By now, many of the children have reached middle age and developed the need to learn about their parent's history only to test their own thoughts and feelings against reality. The initiative may come even from the grandchildren. But often there is much uncertainty about the effect of this "search." They do not know whether they do harm or good by asking the parents about their experiences. They often have a need to help and understand their parents, and they are afraid that their questions may actually reopen old wounds. Usually, the fear to break through family secrets stems from strong feelings of loyalty toward the parents.

Even when the war experiences, at least on the surface, are no secret within the family, the family "secret" may play a role with regard to the outside world. Daily life with traumas from the war period, stimulated by parents or not, can trigger in the children a feeling of being different from other children, albeit to a lesser degree than observed with the Jewish second generation. This can produce a feeling of social isolation. The world within the family appears to be different from the world outside the family sphere. But responsibility and loyalty count also at a mature age, especially to the (former) family and their own parents.

The Loyalty Conflict

Taken literally, loyalty means "true to the law." Here, however, it concerns a personal and mutually preserved standard. The parents conscious and subconscious wishes and desires, ambitions, fears, and guilt feelings always influence the way they relate to the children. In this way, some war victims unintentionally pass on to their children the fact that the outside world is untrustworthy, dangerous, and hostile. When the children feel that one of the parents has suffered considerably during the war, they may develop a strong sense of loyalty. Their behavior is also predominantly geared to accommodate the desires and needs of the parents. And parents expect their children to be spared further suffering and, through the children, for their own lives to become "meaningful" again. The children are prepared to make themselves available for the emotional care of the parents. However, this encroaches on the room for the development of personal identity of the children. During the growth toward independence, a child—unpunished—must be able to establish distance from the parents. This is a sometimes difficult task for children of war sailors and participants in the Resistance.

The conflict between the need to break away and the obligation of loyalty can reach sizable proportions. Faced with this situation, the child can turn in two directions:

1. The child can forego and deny the need to become independent, remaining largely involved with the family, even when not living "at home" anymore. Parents and children thus continue to live in a state of mutual dependency and restrict their contacts outside the family to superficial and business relations.

2. When the child does not relinquish his or her need for independence, breaking away can be accomplished only after a hard battle. Mounting conflicts with the parents are often the result. The feelings of loyalty diminish due to the emergence of strong, negative emotions toward the parents that had been previously suppressed. It is understandable that severe inner conflicts and guilt feelings are the price paid for this "breaking away." Manifest or latent puberty, or authority conflicts are therefore often present in the life story of children of war victims.

Therapeutic contacts with these children reveal that they have great difficulty expressing criticism toward the parents, and that they cannot bear it when an outsider tries to make them aware of their, understandably, negative feelings toward their parents. Simultaneously, the suppressed guilt feelings about severing the loyalty, and the associated fantasies about the hurt they caused their parents, are being relived. In their minds, their parents already suffered so much, even when the realistic picture of the true dimensions of the suffering is missing. Many times, the actual relationship of the grown-up children and the now elderly parents has a distinctly compromising character. Seemingly, there is an acceptance of the status quo and the limited nature of their contacts. Both parties try to have a "good" relationship, electing to have common standards as a base: Children are obligated to visit their parents; adults do not quarrel; parents are happy when their children are socially successful. Therefore, current relationships are often characterized by obligation, lack of spontaneity and intimacy, and persevere only due to an avoidance of frankness and sincerity.

These children's history of providing emotional care and accommodating the desires and needs of the parents are sometimes generated so that as adults, they may be especially altruistic and engaged in humanistic activities. Many of them choose a social or helping profession (Op den Velde, Aarts, & De Graaf, 1991; Major, 1993).

The problems of children of participants in the Resistance differ in an important dimension from those of children of Jewish survivors. The suffering of the Jews was caused by others, without their having had any choice in the matter. Their children cannot blame their parents for their ancestry. However, there often exists in these children a lack of understanding for, in their eyes, the severe defenselessness and complacency of their parents during the attempt by the Nazis at genocide, which causes them to feel great fear and (self-)reproach.

Children of members of the Resistance, however, must regard their parents as heroes who dared face danger. It is difficult to blame or criticize a hero, even if you experience yourself as a victim of his or her choices. In both situations, that of condemning the parents for being weak or of honoring them as a heroes, the identity development of the child is burdened. The development of their own personality on the basis of identification with the parents is rather difficult: In the first case the identification with a weak and defenseless parent is very unattractive; in the second, a meaningful competition with a "hero" is impossible (Op den Velde et al., 1991).

Psychodynamic Considerations

To understand "intergenerational transmission of trauma," it is necessary to explore the underlying psychodynamics. By repression and somatization, the traumatized parent may attempt to release his or her consciousness from tortured memories and emotions. Fear of return of persecution, blocked aggression, feelings of guilt, shame, and a damaged self-image become split off: One is not capable of personally experiencing these feelings and characteristics as an integral part of the self. When such a person becomes a parent, his or her child is inevitably confronted with the split-off memories and emotions. One of the hazards is that the split-off part of the parent is projected onto the child.

In the course of treatment of persons whose (one or both) parents, during the war, as war sailors or participants in the Resistance, had been exposed to severe stress and mortal danger, it is necessary to take the previously described mechanism into account when reconstructing the past and family dynamics. The complexity of these dynamics may well be apparent from the face that the relationship between parent and child is hardly ever a simple, unidimensional (e.g., hostile) demeanor. Love and hate are often easily suffused with each other. It is, however, typical that the original intrapsychic struggle of the war victim–parent with weakness and power, and good and bad, is continued in the relation with the child, and sometimes also with the partner.

CHILDREN OF WAR SAILORS AND RESISTANCE VETERANS

Studies of Children of War Sailors and Resistance Veterans

Haenen, Van den Hout, and Merckelbach (1994) examined children of Dutch war sailors 0–18 years of age at the time of the war. Complete questionnaires were obtained from 191 subjects (74%) and compared to standard controls. In 78 cases (41%), the father died during the war. On the Symptom Checklist (SCL-90), the children of war sailors had significantly elevated scores for phobia, hostility, and insomnia. Age was not related to their SCL-90 scores, nor was whether or not their father had survived the war. Fourteen percent of the children matched the *Diagnostic and Statistical Manual of Mental Disorders* criteria for PTSD. There was a positive relationship between PTSD and problems in raising their own children. A study of Dutch postwar children born to war sailors has not been conducted.

Major (1993) studied 288 children of Norwegian male Resistance fighters. Few of the participants in the Resistance reported that their offspring had any problems, but they believed that their war experiences may have had some impact on their children. The majority of the children have experienced their upbringing as positive. Former concentration camp prisoners among the Resistance fathers communicated with restrained openness about their war experiences. However, even in those families where the father rarely or never spoke about his ordeals, most children felt they were always aware the father's imprisonment. Many children of camp survivors mentioned their father's special behavior with regard to food and eating. The fear of not having enough to eat is still prevalent among several of them. The children often reported a strict prohibition against throwing away food, especially bread. Major concluded that the children of the Norwegian Resistance veterans seem to be quite healthy. Nevertheless, some of the offspring really feel that they have suffered because of their father's parental behavior. Children reporting that their fathers' war experiences made a deep impression scored significantly higher on depression and anxiety (Hopkins Symptom Checklist) than children reporting less impression. Furthermore, children with fathers avoiding communication had significantly higher scores on the Hopkins Symptom Checklist than those with fathers who talked openly. Significantly higher scores also were found for children with depressed or hot-tempered fathers, and for children growing up in families where the mother had to "excuse" the father's behavior, attributing it to his war experiences (Major, 1993).

Schreuder, Van der Ploeg, Van Tiel-Kadiks, Van Mook, and Bramsen (1993) studied children of Dutch war victims, including Resistance veterans, who applied for treatment at a specialized institute for World War II victims. Their symptoms did not differ from those of average patients of a psychiatric outpatient clinic. No significant differences were found between the mean values of the group with one traumatized parent as compared to the group with two traumatized parents.

Six of 46 children of war victims under study displayed reexperiencing symptoms that contain the psychotraumatic experiences of the parents (Schreuder & Van Tiel-Kadiks, 1994). In all cases, these concerned nightmares and flashbacks with extraordinary clarity. Their avoidance symptoms were related to situations that are associated with the traumatic experiences of the parent. These 6 exhibited a complete clinical picture of PTSD, without having had war experiences themselves. Much attention was paid to the traumatic war experiences of the parents in all six families. The vivid impressions that appear in their dreams and flashbacks, and awarded a high reality content, led the researchers to speculate that these patients must have been inundated with the traumatic experiences of the parents already at a young age. Similar observations in children of Holocaust survivors have been described by Barocas and Barocas (1979).

Intergenerational Traumatization

We would like to stress that there are families of war sailors and participants in the Resistance in which the above mentioned problems are surmountable or seem to be of little consequence. This may mean that war experiences were and are freely discussed in these families. Good communication is, after all, an indication of an adequate coping process. Obviously, not every survivor of severe war stress is mentally damaged.

At first glance, many problems of children of war sailors and members of the Resistance appear to be not much different from problems of peers whose parents have been severely traumatized in other ways. After exploration, however, it frequently becomes apparent that the current issue ties in with the special situation in the family, where the family rules and the communication and interaction patterns were largely determined by war experiences of the parent(s). Only rarely did the children who entered psychotherapy spontaneously tell about the war experiences of the father and/or mother. Even during the documentation of the life history, this important fact quite frequently did not emerge. Mostly, this became apparent only during the course of the psychotherapeutic treatment. When the war history ultimately became a theme in the therapy, it caused great confusion for these children. The family secret was in danger of being disclosed.

That traumatized parents can directly stimulate the continued existence of the war in their children can be illustrated through the following cases:

D. is a 32-year-old unmarried woman. She is an only child. She came for treatment after a suicide attempt. She suffers from strong feelings of uncertainty, culminating in a forced apprehension, phobias, and contact disorders. During the initial period of her treatment, she suffered from hallucinations, which caused her to refuse to eat cooked food. D.'s father was the youngest son of a farmer's family. Together with three brothers, he helped care for Jews who were in hiding and helped with the concealment of weapons, obtained from airdrops, for the local Resistance group. Often, he served as a lookout when his brothers took part in an action. During a raid on the farm, in early 1945, one of his brothers was shot and killed on the spot. His father, two other brothers, and seven of the people in hiding were arrested and subsequently deported to a concentration camp. His mother, who had been arrested as well, was released after a few days. D.'s father did not dare use his weapon during the raid. Instead, he fled and hid in the woods for several weeks. After a while, he managed to go into hiding with friends, where he stayed until liberation. His father was the only one to return. Emaciated, sickly, and broken, he died a few years later. D.'s father suffered from intestinal disorders and severe attacks of stomach pains. He maintained that this was due to the bad, uncooked food that he ate while hiding in the woods. D.'s father considered getting her "ready" for war an important part of raising his daughter. He forced D. to eat uncooked food in order to condition her stomach and intestines, and he stressed that this was her only chance to survive the next war. As part of the "survival training," she was forced to go camping under the most primitive and dreadful conditions during her vacations. During the one and only discussion we could arrange with D.'s father, it became apparent that he was suffering from a chronic paranoid disorder. This had not previously been recognized. He never came to grips with his severe feelings of guilt toward his deceased brothers. When he spoke about his brothers, he became very emotional and frightened. Central to his experience stood the failing of his father, who had neglected adequately to prepare him and his brothers for the war. D., as well as her mother, adopted by induction the father's world of thoughts and feelings. Socially, the family was very isolated. (This might well be a repeat of the father's flight and the subsequent isolation in the woods.) The father managed to maintain himself as a bookkeeper after the war. D.'s mother lacked initiative and acted submissively and obediently with regard to D. as well as her husband. D.'s treatment had little success. She discontinued it in order to be able to care for her father. We managed to keep seeing her on an outpatient basis, but the impossibility of discussing her relationship with her father prevented actual change. Attempts to involve both parents in the treatment failed (Op den Velde & De Graaf, 1985).

K. was born in 1952. During the war, his father served as a commander of a merchant vessel. Twice he survived the loss of his ship due to a torpedo attack and witnessed the loss of many of the crew members, for which he felt responsible, during the sinking of the ships, and during a tormenting period in a damaged lifeboat, with increasing exhaustion, hunger, and, in particular, thirst. It took 3 weeks before they were discovered by an Allied airplane and subsequently rescued. On his last voyage, he was severely injured by machine-gun fire. After the war, the father was granted a disability pension. K.'s mother was employed as an editor. The father was responsible for the housekeeping and daily care of the children. He often spoke about his dreadful time as a war sailor. To correct his son, he always brought up the courageous behavior of a teenage sailor in the lifeboat, who died without complaining in sight of rescue. At the age of 12, K. began to suffer from nightmares in which he perished in a lifeboat. He had spells in which he experienced severe pain and thirst, like in his nightmares and also during waking states. His school performance dropped, and he underwent repeated medical examinations that failed to disclose the origin of his pain attacks. He never dared tell his parents about his dreams. When he was seen for psychiatric examination at the age of 27, he lived a very restricted life in the parental home and had the full picture of PTSD.

Authority Problems

Authority conflicts may develop when parents treat their children in a rigid, authoritarian, and demanding manner, and, in doing so, neglect their emotional needs. The child cannot compete with a parent who has "proven" his or her moral and mental superiority during the war. We can understand an authority conflict as a reaction to such an authoritarian parent. Also, when a child avoids an open conflict with the parent(s), it is possible that the child is looking for a confrontation outside the home. The children's defiance toward authorities, whether directed at police, teachers, employers, or even their own partner, may be regarded as an attempt to continue the "Resistance" of the parents, or to experience it themselves.

Also, problems in school or at work are often a display of Resistance against the demanding parent. The emotional vacuum in which some of these children were raised renders them helpless and lonely. Poor performance in relation to intellectual opportunities is often a subliminal revenge against the emotional shortcomings and the demanding behavior of the parents.

Mainly because of this unconscious aspect, the child, as well as the parents, can suffer immensely. The result can be additional uncertainty and lack of self-confidence. However, in some cases, the basis for this problem is the identification with the "failing parent." The continuous tension in a family may result in concentration problems that may also cause (relatively) poor performance in school or at work. But the children will only infrequently resist the expectations of the parents. Their achievements in school and career are often good to excellent but still do not provide the children emotional peace. The need for acceptance by the parents, both as children and as persons, may stay unsatisfied and bring about a paradoxical feeling of failure.

Separation and Individuation

The difficulties with developing or maintaining relations other than with the parents are often related to mutual expectations of loyalty. When the parents are emotionally dependent on their children's care and attention, the children may feel guilty about their desire for a life with others. Also, there may develop problems with partners, because their first loyalty is to their parents. The family secret may be a reason for unsatisfactory relationships as well. Part of the personality of the child, namely, the part that is related to the war and the parents' traumas, cannot, or can only with great difficulty, be shared with others. Frequently we established that (un)conscious conflicts with the parents are being repeated or agitated in other relations.

The basis for the issues described previously is a number of intrapsychic conflicts often connected with separation, identity, and affective problems. The special family interactions are the driving force. Separation–individuation problems may display themselves at various levels. When the parent is emotionally dependent on the love and attention of the still-young child or is not able to support the child's growth and development, the necessary separation and individuation processes can become problematic. The child, then, can build an identity independent of the parent only under penalty of loss of love and appreciation from the parent. When the child reaches the age at which he or she feels the urge to leave the parental home, separation problems may manifest themselves (again) in demands of loyalty and feelings of guilt.

Separation–individuation problems are often regarded as characteristic in children of Holocaust survivors. They exist as well in children of members of the Resistance. We are of the opinion, however, that the psychodynamics of these problems in the two groups are quite different. After all, unlike former members of the Resistance, Jewish survivors often suffer from the destruction of large segments of their family. In most cases, their children are for them the most important, sometimes even the only, reason for living and a source of (emotional) security. The onset of separation–individuation problems with the children in the Jewish group therefore tends to take place at a very early stage. We have the impression that separation–individuation issues with children of participants in the Resistance become important mainly during the Oedipal phase. Especially during this phase, the child can easily become a weapon in conflicts between the parents. Such an Oedipal collusion can dominate the life of a child for a long time and considerably influence the development of his or her identity. The depressed, scared, and self-estranged parent is hardly an ideal identification object for a child, not just because he or she is a joyless, negative object, but also because the parent often displays such strong ambivalence in his or her own attachment behavior. Fearful of losing the parent's love, the child may, nonetheless, identify with the parent, and therefore also with his or her depression, fears, and traumatic memories. But even when the child resists or defends against such an identification, he or she may consider him- or herself bad and guilty, because of abandoning the parent and leaving the parental home.

The identification process may also be problematic when the parent derives pride and self-esteem from wartime experiences and exhibits this as an act of heroism with which the child is unable to compete. Thus, the child will develop a feeling of always falling short. He or she may attempt to compensate for this feeling of failure by fantasies of grandeur and pretentious behavior. However, these fantasies and associated behaviors may be created to compensate for the parent's failure. The children identify themselves (partly) with the emotions and behavior of their parents, be they depression, guilt feelings, fear, bitterness, self-discipline, pride, or self-control. Consequently, the response of the parents to their traumatic conflicts influences the identity of the child. Some acquire a philosophy of life that is based on their parents' historical dramas. For these children World War II thus has become "a history of today."

Emotional Constriction

Inability to express emotions and fear of intimacy are quite noticeable in children of war sailors and participants in the Resistance. The awareness and expression of aggressive feelings are especially problematic. These children also often have difficulty dealing with guilt, fear, and grief. In many cases, traumatized parents are not, or are only with difficulty, capable of dealing with their emotions. Suppression or concealment of feelings occurs often, combined, sometimes, with severe and sudden emotional outbursts. The affect intolerance of the parents is one of the reasons the children react with suspicion and apprehension toward their own and other people's emotions. But these affective problems can develop also in situations where the child becomes the one who takes care of the parents. The child, after all, must suppress his or her own needs and desires in order not to be a burden to the parent. There is clinical evidence for the presumption that affect intolerance of the traumatized parent results in problems with affect tolerance in their children. The need to care for the well-being of the parents is in many cases considerably exacerbated due to the frequent suffering of the parent who participated in the Resistance from more or less severe physical illnesses, such as gastric ulcers, heart infarction, rheumatic afflictions, or diabetes.

The problems within families of war sailors and Resistance veterans can form the basis for sometimes genuinely serious psychiatric disorders, such as psychoses and serious personality disorders. During our work in psychiatric institutions, we were confronted with disorders of children of war victims that were difficult to treat and, initially, hard to grasp. However, as soon as the traumatic background of the parent(s) became clear, the children's symptomatology became much more understandable.

CONCLUSIONS AND RECOMMENDATIONS

The few scientific studies conducted do not indicate that, as a group, children of war sailors and Resistance veterans are less healthy or have a particularly high prevalence of mental disorders. However, because no relevant control groups were systematically examined, the question of the actual mental health of these groups cannot be answered unequivocally. The symptoms of children of war victims, in fact, are not different from those of the average clients of mental health services. There appears to be no notion of specific diagnostic categories. Case analysis does, however, show a number of regularities: The psychosocial issues of the offspring of war sailors and participants in the Resistance seems to center around authority conflicts, problems with study and work, and relational problems.

1. It is advisable, during the recording of the life history, always to determine whether the parents of the patient were exposed to traumatic circumstances during the war. When this is the case, it is important to request detailed information.

2. With regard to the nature of the problems, especially when they are the result of a disrupted or burdened family interaction, a psychotherapeutic approach is indicated. Considerable attention must be given to contending with problems within the parental family. When exploratory psychotherapy is decided upon, managing the transference relationship is often found to produce great problems. This is associated with anxiety surrounding independence, loyalty conflicts, and the fear of being manipulated by the therapist.

3. As soon as the war experiences can be discussed with the parents in the form of a meaningful and honest exchange of experiences and feelings, a noticeable improvement is usually observed. A word of caution is in order here. Remaining silent with regard to their traumatic experiences must be considered a part of war victims' defense patterns. This defense must not be automatically appraised as "Resistance against treatment." We consider it to be a mistake to demand of former war sailors, Resistance fighters, and survivors of concentration camps that they discuss their experiences, just because "once in a while it is good to get it off your chest." We are of the opinion that the objections of war victims against becoming involved with the therapy of their child must be respected. The necessity to create an atmosphere of security and trust is paramount. In the course of treatment of a second-generation child, it is advisable first to attempt to engage him or her in a discussion with their parent(s) about the war years. Only then, after several attempts have failed, should consideration be given to inviting the parent in question, possibly accompanied by the partner or the child, for a discussion in the psychotherapy session.

ACKNOWLEDGMENT: This chapter is based in part on the translation from the original Dutch version and the revision of two earlier publications (Op den Velde, Aarts, & De Graaf, 1991; Op den Velde & De Graaf, 1985).

REFERENCES

Askevold, F. (1980). The war sailor syndrome. *Danish Medical Bulletin, 27,* 220–224.

Barocas, H. A., Barocas, C. B. (1979). Wounds of fathers: the next generation of Holocaust victims. *International Review of Psychoanalysis, 6,* 331–341.

Bastiaans, J. (1957). *Psychosomatische gevolgen van onderdrukking en verzet* [Psychosomatic aftereffects of oppression and resistance]. Amsterdam, the Netherlands: Noordhollandse Uitgeversmaatschappij.

Coopmans, M. J. A. M. (1993). *Separatie-individuatie-problematiek van een naoorlogse generatie oorlogsslachtoffers* [Separation-individuation problems in the second generation of war-victims]. Delft, the Netherlands: Eburon.

Haenen, M. A., Van den Hout, M. A., & Merckelbach, H. (1994). *Psychische probleman bij kinderen van oorlogsgetroffenen* [Psychological problems in children of war victims]. Unpublished manuscript, Heerlen, the Netherlands: Buitengewone Pensioenraad.

Hartvig, P. (1977). Krigsseilersyndromet [The war sailor syndrome]. *Nordisk Psykiatrisk Tidsskrif, 29,* 302–12.

Keilson, H. (1992). *Sequential traumatization in children.* Jerusalem: Magnus Press.

Krystal, H. (Ed.) (1968). *Massive psychic trauma.* New York: Little, Brown.

Major, E. F. (1993, June). *Transgenerational effects of different war experiences.* Paper, presented at the Third European Conference on Traumatic Stress, Bergen, Norway, 1993.

Op den Velde, W. (1985). Posttraumatische stressstoornis als laat gevolg van verzetsdeelname [Posttraumatic stress disorder as a late effect of resistance participation]. *Nederlands Tijdschrift voor Geneeskunde, 129,* 834–838.

Op den Velde, W., Aarts, P. G. H., & De Graaf, T. K. (1991). Kinderen van verzetsdeelnemers [Children of resistance participants]. In W. Wolters (Ed.), *Posttraumatische stress bij kinderen en adolescenten* [Posttraumatic stress in children and adolescents] (pp. 157–178). Baarn, the Netherlands: Ambo.

Op den Velde, W. & De Graaf, T. K. (1985). Psychische problemen bij kinderen van voormalige verzetsdeelnemers [Psychological problems in children of former resistance participants]. *ICODO-info, 2*, 39–51.

Op den Velde, W., Hovens, J. E., Aarts, P. G. H., Frey-Wouters, E., Falger, P. R. J., Van Duijn, H., & De Groen, J. H. M. (1996). The prevalence and course of posttraumatic stress disorder in Dutch veterans of the civilian Resistance during World War II: An overview. *Psychological Reports, 78*, 519–529.

Op den Velde, W., Frey-Woutrs, E., & Pelser, H. E. (1994). The price of heroism: Veterans from the Dutch Resistance to the Nazi occupation of the Netherlands in World War II. *Holocaust and Genocide Studies 8*, 335–348.

Op den Velde, W., Hovens, J. E., Falger, P. R. J., De Groen, J. H. M. Van Duijn, H., Lasschuit, L. J., & Schouten, E. G. W. (1993). PTSD in Dutch Resistance veterans from World War II. In J. P. Wilson & B. Rafael (Eds.), *International handbook of traumatic stress syndromes* (pp. 219–230). New York: Plenum Press.

Op den Velde, W., Koerselman, G. F. & Aarts, P. G. H. (1994). Countertransference and World War II Resistance fighters: Issues in diagnosis and assessment. In J. P. Wilson & J. D. Lindy (Eds.), *Countertransference in the treatment of posttraumatic stress disorder* (pp. 308–327). New York: Guilford Press.

Schreuder, J. N., Van der Ploeg, H. M., Van Tiel-Kadiks, G. W., Van Mook, J., & Bramsen, I. (1993). Psychische klachten en kenmerken bij poliklinische patiënten van de naoorlogse generatie [Psychological complaints and characteristics of outpatients of the postwar generation]. *Tijdschrift voor psychiatrie, 4*, 227–241.

Schreuder, J. N., & Van Tiel-Kadiks, G. W. (1994). Psychopathologische klachten bij kinderen van oorlogsslachtoffers [Psychopathological complaints in children of war victims]. *Nederlands Tijdschrift voor Geneeskunde, 138*, 641–644.

Tas, J. (1946). Psychische stoornissen in concentratiekampen en bij teruggekeerden [Psychical disorders among inmates of concentration camps and repatriates]. Maandblad voor de Geestelijke Volksgezondheid, 1, 143–150. Reprinted in A. Ladan, H. Groen-Prakken, & A. Stufkens (Eds.), *Traumatisation and war. The Dutch annual of psychoanalysis, 1995–1996* (pp. 16–24). Lisse, the Netherlands, Swets & Zeitlinger.

Weisaeth, L., & Eitinger, L. (1993). Posttraumatic stress phenomena: common themes across wars, disasters, and traumatic events. In J. P. Wilson & B. Rafael (Eds.), *International handbook of traumatic stress syndromes* (pp. 69–77). New York: Plenum Press.

10

Children of Collaborators

From Isolation toward Integration

MARTIJN W. J. LINDT

Germany had its collaborators in all the countries it occupied during World War II. These collaborators were called *quislings* after the best-known among them, the Norwegian Vidkun Quisling. Many of them were arrested and put on trial after the German defeat and the liberation of the occupied countries. In some countries (e.g., France), many of them were killed without a trial, while others escaped, either by leaving their country or by hiding their past. These historical facts are well known. Particularly in The Netherlands, a number of extensive studies about the trials have appeared in the last decades (Belinfante, 1978; Groen, 1984; Romijn, 1989).

What happened after this? What was the fate of the quislings and that of their families and children? This is an unwritten page of history.

Interest in the fate of children of collaborators is growing rapidly. The amount of attention paid to this subject by the media testifies to this. On the occasion of the fiftieth commemoration of the end of World War II in Europe this year, in The Netherlands alone there were more than 20 interviews with children of collaborators on radio and television or in various newspapers (Donkersloot, 1995). Scientific publications had begun to appear in modest numbers since the 1980s. Most of the existing research was carried out in The Netherlands. Therefore, the subject of this chapter is the situation of children of collaborators in this country.

The German regime in The Netherlands was particularly severe. Austrian Nazis were in charge, and they had to prove their good "German" Nazi mentality.

The well-organized Dutch bureaucracy was a reliable instrument in the hands of the occupier, and this contributed greatly to the efficacy of the extermination of Dutch Jews (De Jong, 1988; Scheffel-Baars, 1988).

This left Dutch society with an enormous trauma. Without any doubt, the deepest chasm in The Netherlands is the one caused by World War II between people who sided with the Germans and those who did not. This trauma and this chasm make the subject of the fate of the collaborators' families and their children a very sensitive one. The first authors of scientific publications on the subject were attacked as if they spoke on behalf of criminals (Montessori, 1987).

MARTIJN W. J. LINDT • Faculty of Educational Sciences, University of Amsterdam, 1091 GM Amsterdam, The Netherlands

International Handbook of Multigenerational Legacies of Trauma, edited by Yael Danieli. Plenum Press, New York, 1998.

Researchers on this subject are confronted with difficulties in access to data. Dutch collaborators were and are, when they are still alive, absolute outcasts, and their shame has extended to their children. Children of collaborators tend to hide their background in public as well as in clinical situations. Their situation is a part of the "conspiracy of silence" resulting from World War II, described by Danieli (1985).

In this chapter, I first describe the sources of data on the subject, and then I discuss some methodological issues. Subsequently, I present the information under the headings of "isolation" and "integration."

SOURCES AND ISSUES OF DESCRIPTION

In 1981, Hofman wrote his dissertation on the sociopsychological backgrounds of the collaborators. This started a new period in The Netherlands, in which it became possible to write more objectively about the war. The dissertation attracted the attention of the press to the situation of children of collaborators. Hofman, several professionals from helping professions, a journalist, and a radio minister took the initiative to create opportunities for children of collaborators to react to publicity. The radio minister, Reverend A. Klamer, responded to the reactions. These contacts led to the creation of a working group composed of children of collaborators and several professionals. It was baptized *Herkenning* (Recognition). Its goal was to offer support to these children and break the taboo of their situation in society. The children of collaborators participating in this group were born before, during, and after the war. The group made very clear that any person who might have fascist sympathies and might wish to participate in the self-help group would be excluded. The youngest such child to contact the self-help group was born in 1963.

All the authors (nine so far) of scientific studies published on the subject profited from the existence of this self-help group in obtaining their data. The first to publish about the children were Montessori (Psychoanalytisch Instituut, 1981) and Hofman (1984), both professional helpers engaged in the self-help group and clinical practitioners offering children of collaborators a safe setting. They both base their descriptions on interviews with 40 children of collaborators.

From 1984 on, other leading personalities from the self-help group began to publish: Scheffel-Baars (1984), Donkersloot (1988), and Blom (1988). These authors had received historical (Scheffel-Baars), sociological (Donkersloot) and psychiatric (Blom) training. All of them based their work on contacts with the members of the self-help group, which extended to 3,500 people in 1995. This comprised counseling, regular meetings, and telephonic first aid.

In 1986, Willemse did a study on the fate of children of collaborators in the period immediately after the war, using government archives as sources. This kind of research was continued by Reuling-Schappin (1993).

Extensive studies of qualitative research have been done by Vorst-Thijssen & de Boer (1993) and Lindt (1993). Vorst-Thijssen and de Boer interviewed 13 children of collaborators and 19 professional helpers who had experience with these clients. Lindt reviewed the earlier studies and interviewed 40 children of collaborators, among them the leading personalities of the self-help group. Among his interviewees were children of collaborators who had made their backgrounds public without having any links to the self-help group. This latter study also placed the material in a theoretical perspective. It explored the way in which existing theories may clarify the results and proposed several hypotheses and amended theories.

To what extent is the information gathered about these children of collaborators representative for the whole population of children of collaborators? In The Netherlands, their number is estimated between 150,000 and 250,000 such children. As already mentioned, these individuals are rather secretive about their backgrounds. Therefore, overall surveys seem possible only far in the future. Nothing is known about the range of generalizability of the characteristics found in studies concerning the persons who contacted the self-help group.

There is also a particularly tricky aspect to generalization. Treating children of collaborators as a population means grouping them under their only common feature, namely, being the child of a collaborator. But it is precisely this feature that causes them pain and fear. When their backgrounds became known, they were subjected to a great deal of prejudice, stereotypes, projections, and outright rejection.

The description in this chapter is based on induction, and any generalization should be read in a tentative manner where it has not been written in that way for reasons of readability.

Interested researchers and clinicians are very much prone to countertransference. The work on countertransference with Holocaust survivors done by Danieli (1980) can also be applied to the work done with children of collaborators. Dutch society knows a wide range of perspectives on this subject and the individuals involved. These perspectives run from suspicion and fear of recurrence of the Holocaust by recruiting new perpetrators from among the children of Nazi sympathizers, to acceptance of these children in their own right.

The terms used in presenting the results reflect an important source of bias, which requires further discussion. It is interesting to consider the terminology for *collaborator* in The Netherlands. The Dutch counterpart of the word *collaborator* is not used very often in Dutch publications concerned with the subject, apart from the work of Hofman (1981, 1985, 1988). The term *quisling* is not used at all. The term most often used, symbolic for the Dutch way of looking at this subject, is that of *wrong*.

Dutch people are classified in accordance with their attitude during the war as either "right" or "wrong." Although many authors point to the fact that in reality there were many shades in between these attitudes, until now, no other terms have been coined. This is the Dutch semantic expression to connote coming to "terms" with World War II. Thus, one of the phrases used for children of collaborators in The Netherlands is that of "children of wrong parents." This phrase causes difficulties for the individuals involved, as it is stigmatizing and does not leave room for conflicts of loyalty.

Another frequently used term is that of *NSB children*. The national socialist movement in The Netherlands was the NSB (Nationaal-Socialistische Beweging). This term has some disadvantages, too. Strictly speaking, it does not cover all the population of children of collaborators involved. Many more Dutch people had opted for the occupier than those who were actual members of the NSB. Still, as Hofman (1988) remarks, the terms *NSB* and *NSB children* have become dominant in naming all the people who had collaborated with the Germans, and also their children.

From an international point of view, the term *children of collaborators* seems the most objective for this specific population.

This chapter groups the psychological histories of children of collaborators under the contrasting categories of "isolation" and "integration," which appeared to describe and structure best in the long iterative process of research. The first to use the concept of isolation to characterize the situation of children of collaborators was Montessori (1987). The concept of integration is the result of a process that elaborated upon Bar-On's (1988) psychological concept of "working through." I have extended the concept to the social integration of children of collaborators both in the second generation after World War II and, in a broader sense, in society (Lindt, 1993).

ISOLATION

Before and during the War

Before the war, children of members of the Dutch Nazi party were already seen as outcasts (Spruit, 1983). During the war, the isolation of these children in school and neighborhood was growing. Out of contempt and fear, "right" parents were forbidding their children to mingle with "wrong" children (Willemse, 1986).

On "Crazy Tuesday" (September 5, 1944), at the moment when the German defeat in The Netherlands seemed imminent, about 65,000 collaborators, most of them, together with their families (De Jong, 1980), fled from The Netherlands to Germany. Many of them took their children with them. They traveled through Germany and lived in camps. Montessori (1987) writes:

> This was a shocking, confusing and terrifying experience. There was cold, hunger, contempt from the German population, there were bombings and artillery attacks. Children experienced maltreatment and kidnapping (p. 50, author's translation).

These children felt unprotected, homeless, unwelcome, and powerless.

Arrest, Internment, and Conviction

After the German capitulation, the collaborators who remained in The Netherlands were arrested. This started immediately after the "Crazy Tuesday" in the south, when this part of the country was liberated by the Allied forces. In the rest of The Netherlands, it occurred in April and May. After the German capitulation, the collaborators who had fled to Germany gradually returned to The Netherlands and were arrested there. According to Hofman (1988), nearly 100,000 persons were arrested, 23,000 of whom were women. The number of suspects was much larger. By the end of 1947, 450,000 files were opened. The courts passed sentences in 90,000 cases (Romijn, 1989).

There were 141 death sentences, of which 40 have been carried out. The other collaborators were put into internment camps. The situation in these camps was described by Belinfante (1978), Groen (1984), and de Jong (1980), the Dutch official World War II historian. The situation in the camps was bad. There was a lack of food and sanitary facilities, rules were severe, and there was forced labor. Individual camp guards committed excesses of violence and maltreatment. This has been reported in 69 of the 130 internment camps. In many cases, it was hard to distinguish the behavior and the methods of the guards from those of the Nazis.

The possessions of the collaborators were confiscated. They also lost several civil rights for many years after internment, for example, the right to leave the country and the right to vote. All this followed the message sent from London by the Dutch government stating that "there will be no place for collaborators in The Netherlands." In most cases, after internment they remained unemployed.

Children in Camps, Children's Homes, and Foster Homes

It is not know how many children born before 1945 were involved. There must have been well over 100,000. The arrest of the parents brought along much violence and humiliation for the children. The families were forced to abandon their homes. According to Reuling-Schappin (1993). 50,000 children were left behind because both parents had been arrested.

Many of them were interned in camps. Children were anxious about their parents. According to De Jong (1980), many children died during internment.

In October 1944, the Dutch military government issued an order that prohibited the arrest of wives and children together with the collaborating father. Wives and children were to be supported and taken care of. As the majority of the population wanted revenge (Belinfante, 1978), this order was disregarded. The Dutch government (in exile in London) did not pay attention to the families of collaborators.

During the war, child care institutions disappeared. In 1945, the institution of Special Youth Care was organized. About 25,000 children were placed in children's homes and about 8,000 in foster homes (Reuling-Schappin, 1993).

In children's homes, conditions were pretty bad. Often, there was no heating; medical and social care were hard to find, and the personnel were not qualified. The children were provided with little guidance. Contacts with parents were almost completely broken off. Children were humiliated and sometimes maltreated, with little attention given to their needs.

In foster homes, children were forced to show gratitude. Often, they were severely punished for behavior that could easily be explained by the tension they were going through. Sometimes, those that took care of the children were vindictive to them.

The Families and Children in Society

The families of collaborators were cast out of Dutch society; they were surrounded by hatred. Children who stayed with the mothers or returned to their families, and those who were newly born, lived in poverty because of confiscation of property and lack of income. Children born after the war numbered approximately 100,000.

Their families were disrupted. In many cases, the father's return from internment added to the already existing tensions. His children no longer accepted his authority. Material poverty, demoralization, difference of opinion between marital partners, and long periods of separation contributed to marital problems. There were many divorces and extramarital children. Thus, these families lacked the material and social conditions for bringing up their children as secure members of the society. The fathers were embittered and discouraged by their experiences. The parents were preoccupied with their own emotions, and little energy was left for providing the children with attention and protection.

Hofman (1988) remarks that in The Netherlands, children of collaborators were identified by others with their parents. He finds it understandable that the misery of the occupation resulted in an intensely emotional and nondiscriminantly critical attitude. When the atrocities done by the Nazis were made public, collaborators were regarded and treated as fully responsible (De Jong, 1988). There was little willingness to improve the image of the "wrong."

By identifying the children with their parents, Dutch society has complicated greatly their attempts to find their own place in society. Children of collaborators feel that they are not entitled to be treated as equals, regardless of the choices made by their parents. They are alienated by Dutch society because of mistakes for which they are not guilty.

Several investigations (Groen, 1984; Hofman, 1988; Lindt, 1993; Montessori 1987; Scheffel-Baars, 1988) mention the scapegoat mechanism that works against children of collaborators. These authors attribute it to feelings of shame and guilt existing among a great part of the Dutch population about their halfhearted attitude toward the Germans.

Children of collaborators were scolded, sometimes maltreated, and excluded from social activities. They suffered from stigma in school, in examination situations, and in job applications. In some work situations, they were fired because of their background. They experienced discrimination even in situations of professional assistance. Vorst-Thijssen and de Boer (1993) quote a helper who refused to give aid to children of collaborators because he "detested NSB-people" (p. 17).

These situations continue to the present. Children of collaborators are confronted with mistrust and prejudice when their backgrounds are revealed. In many respects, Dutch people do not live according to the principles of antidiscrimination codified in the first article of the Dutch Constitution and specified in the United Nations Convention on the Rights of the Child, that is, not to be discriminated against for the political convictions and political past of the parents (Cohn, 1991).

Family Dynamics

In most families, discussing the history of the family during and after the war was a complete taboo. It remained a secret for children born after the war. They learned to avoid embarrassing questions. The consequences of growing up with a family secret are well known in the literature (Pincus & Dare, 1980). They hamper the development of the children, contributing to feelings of insecurity and social anxiety.

The discovery of the family secret at a later age forced these children to struggle to come to terms with their parents' choice during the war. The discovery meant a conflict with the parents, sometimes manifest, sometimes latent. Many of the children, particularly those born after 1943, broke their relationship with their parents.

> Jessica discovered her father's war history when she was 12. She felt compelled to be his judge, yet she despised herself for judging him. She wanted to defend her father, and then felt guilty about that.

Boszormenyi-Nagy and Spark (1984) made clear that the loyalty of children toward their parents is always a reality. For children of collaborators, this loyalty conflict is particularly violent. In this conflict, children of collaborators struggle with substitute guilt feelings toward Nazi victims. Also they wrestle with the realization that their parents have become social outcasts because of their choice, and all this has made their own youth an agony (Montessori, 1987).

Developing an identity in these families was very difficult. The common phrase "I got that from my parents" is an impossible utterance for children of collaborators. They have to check carefully everything they have received at home.

Taboo

The background of children of collaborators is a taboo subject in the Netherlands. A "dear" neighbor of a collaborator's daughter refused to participate in a television program in which the collaborator's daughter was interviewed, stating: "I don't want to be associated with children of collaborators." The society has remained silent for a long time. It has not recognized these children's problems. It has not recognized freedom of speech for children of collaborators. It has not even recognized their existence.

What are the forces that maintain this silence? From the children's youth, their families exert pressure to be silent. Parents are afraid to be exposed. Once exposed, they go through hard times. Their children are willing to spare them new agonies in their old age. The constant vigilance to prevent a revival of fascism also contributes to silence about children of collaborators. However, this vigilance does not justify the taboo. In fact, this contributes precisely to what one wishes to fight against. Modern individualism notwithstanding, the tendency to judge children by their parents operates in all of us. Sometimes the subject "children of collaborators" is avoided to protect Nazi victims against renewed pain. As mentioned before, some Dutch camp guards had engaged in behavior that rivaled that of Nazi guards. They were never brought to trial for their behavior. Silence was substituted for justice. The subject of the collaborators is so embarrassing that people become silent when it is mentioned directly by "representatives" of "the other side."

Finally, remaining silent has become second nature for children of collaborators themselves. Most children of collaborators hide their backgrounds for fear of rejection. Conforming with the general taboo on the subject seems to be their only way of coping with the danger of stigmatization. As stated before, Montessori (1987) writes that this group of people finds itself in isolation.

Even those who decided to make their backgrounds public still doubt whether they have taken the right step, given the high emotional costs and the fears and disappointments they meet in their lives. Children of collaborators who hope to make a successful career must avoid appearing on television to discuss their predicament.

Having been silent for such a long time makes it increasingly difficult to speak openly. When bottled-up emotions come to the surface, they scare off potential conversation partners, and this experience reinforces the silence.

The commemoration of the liberation and the judgment of "right" and "wrong" are at the core of postwar Dutch culture. Children of collaborators are outsiders in this core culture. To advance their viewpoints means to risk being misunderstood, mistrusted, and rejected. Saying that your parents were not just "wrong," but that they were also "right," is against the national "right–wrong scheme."

In the context of the commemoration, children of collaborators, like the rest of the population, are happy that the values of the civil order have been restored. They are as sad as many other Dutch people about the losses and pains of the past. But they also feel depressed to live in a country that for them is not completely liberated, a country in which they are afraid to speak about their background, a country in which they have to stay out of conversations about the war. To be silent about your background means to be silent about the war. To be silent about one of the most important and most emotional topics in Dutch memory means not to belong.

Being silent about such an essential topic as one's own background, which can be a daily topic, ends all spontaneity. It causes difficulties with self-disclosure even in the most intimate relationships. On the other hand, many children of collaborators have become good listeners (Donkersloot, 1988).

Lack of Social Support

Children of collaborators go through many difficulties with their partners, which, in turn, engender guilt feelings (Scheffel-Baars, 1988). They feel guilt because it is their background that seems to cause the difficulties. The relationships with their own children are hampered as well. Many children of collaborators do not dare to reveal their backgrounds to their own children. A national advertising campaign for libraries in 1994 seemed to depart from this fact. On the billboards the posters read: "Was grandfather wrong? Look it up in the library."

So social support was absent, and research indicates that social support is the most important factor in coping with traumatic stress. The reference group offered no support until 1981. The group cohesion was nil because each member (child of collaborators) was an isolated individual.

Consequences

The past has left many tormenting memories for children of collaborators (Hofman, 1988). Events that seem of little impact to bystanders can trigger heavy emotional reactions because they are experienced as if past events are being revived. Problems that occur frequently among the population of children of collaborators include depression, suicide, incapacity for work, alcoholism, and psychosomatic conditions.

Their constant feelings of guilt and shame cause social defenselessness. When something goes wrong, children of collaborators automatically assume guilt. They are frequently unable to express adequately aggressive impulses (Horman, 1988).

According to Montessori (1987), the long-term effects of the children's experiences are dissociation of emotions and repression of hatred. This blocks their ability to understand themselves. Scheffel-Baars (1988) points to the resulting feeling of inferiority, the feeling that one has no right to be there.

According to Donkersloot (1988) the main component of the personality of children of collaborators is anxiety and a vague feeling of being "different" and "wrong." They live in a world they experience as threatening. They are constantly alert, always preparing for disaster. They feel more comfortable with people who also know the experience of being threatened. Children of collaborators try to avoid any possible mistakes (Donkersloot, 1988). They are particularly alert and try consistently to be politically correct.

As a result, they feel a constant fear of failure. Although they have developed leadership qualities in their long struggle for survival, a leading role provokes too much anxiety because it contradicts remaining silent and trying to avoid any mistakes.

They have developed very critical attitudes that lead to a great sensitivity to issues of abuse of any kind. They consider their choices thoroughly and are aware of the relativity of "good" and "bad" in many situations. Children of collaborators have cultivated an acute intuition. Having no other framework for orientation, intuition has gradually become the basis for their judgments (Donkersloot, 1988).

According to Blom, the core of the problem is not to feel allowed to be there, to have to hide. "I have to adjust at any price" (Blom 1988, p. 1). They dare not be who they are, but not just because of their background. They also do not dare to ask for help for problems for which one normally would not be ashamed to seek help.

Children of collaborators find it hard to accept love and support. Being uprooted undermines their self-esteem. Seldom to they realize the consequences of societal attitudes and their interaction with the handicap of their family backgrounds. Instead, they usually experience their problems as personal failure (Scheffel-Baars, 1988). They fear and suspect that they are accused of not living up to ideals and norms, and that they are excluded (Lindt, 1993).

There are some differences between children of collaborators who lived through the war period and those who were born after 1942. Nevertheless, similarities outnumber the differences (Lindt, 1993). Factors in which the aforementioned differences are manifest include war experiences, loyalty conflicts, direct rejection after the war, and relationships with their own children. Children of collaborators born before 1942 are more often plagued by conscious memories of war events and they have experienced direct rejection more often. For children born after 1942, the loyalty conflict with the parents is more outspoken. They have relatively more fear of being rejected by their own children. They also fear the rejection of their parents by their children. The other characteristics of children of collaborators mentioned in this chapter do not differ between the two groups.

INTEGRATION

Changes

The churches formed an exception to the prevailing attitude in The Netherlands of ignoring the existence of children of collaborators (Lindt, 1993). They requested their parishioners to look after the families of collaborators. They pointed to the suffering of children in these isolated families. But it appears that this request has only partially been answered. The life stories of children of collaborators in my dissertation study included not only incidences of pastoral care but also of exclusion emanating from the pulpit (Lindt, 1993).

The thawing of the isolation actually began in 1981, when Hofman (1981) wrote his dissertation about the sociopsychological backgrounds of the collaborators. This led to the creation of a self-help group of children of collaborators. The goals of this self-help group are to survey the existing problems, educate the helping institutions, and break the existing taboo. Apart from that, several self-help groups have been formed in order to exchange thoughts and ideas about the burdening past.

In these groups, many children of collaborators dared to reveal their background for the first time in their lives. Here, they could receive understanding from each other, more understanding than anyone else can give (Scheffel-Baars, 1988).

Integration of the Second Generation

From 1988 on, several initiatives were taken to break through what is called the "compartmentalization of suffering." Individuals from all categories of second-generation, war-affected groups were brought together in congresses and meetings. Children of collaborators were emphatically included. From now on, the term *children of war* refers to war-affected children from any background. In 1991, a University chair was created for "transgenerational consequences of war," including all background categories. Much opposition had to be overcome. The pioneer role of well-known Jews and resistance fighters in this process was outstanding.

After long hesitation, in 1995, the Dutch government decided to subsidize some of the work done by the self-help group for children of collaborators.

Outcomes of Help

In several research studies (Lindt, 1993; Vorst-Thijssen & de Boer, 1993), children of collaborators reported positive experiences with the helping professions, along with the negative experiences reported earlier. Over and over again, the crucial factors reported by children of collaborators were the trustworthiness of helpers, not being blamed for their parents' past, unconditional acceptance, unprejudiced listening, and other unspecific factors of psychotherapy. Essential in experiencing the liberation so many years after 1945 is to be allowed to be there with one's story. Telling this story engenders insight and the capacity to come to terms and cope with a hindering past, a toilsome present, and an insecure future.

Self-Acceptance

Insights that contribute to self-acceptance are important. Among these, identifying unfounded guilt feelings and weakening them by reinforcing self-esteem and laying the foundation for the conviction that one has the right to be there are paramount:

For Ella, the key in her therapy was one sentence that she had to repeat many times: "I am I, and they are they."

Anna learned that she had the right to be who she was, and that making mistakes and falling short are part of being human.

After a long struggle over "good" and "bad," Jessica concluded that they are *both* present in every person, including her father and herself.

Titia, whose father was killed by the liberators, accepts her inability to belong to any group because she is so sensitive to totalitarian traits which, she feels, always appear in groups.

Children of collaborators have tried to speak with their parents about the past. This succeeded only in very few cases. But many of them were able to reach a less emotional attitude toward their parents. The sharpness of the loyalty conflict was lessened. Jessica, having discovered good and bad in her parents and in herself, is no longer judging her father.

Attitude of the Public

The attitude of the public in The Netherlands has changed. Nowadays, children of collaborators meet rejection less frequently than in the past. Most reactions to publicity about children of collaborators are positive. Still, there are also angry reactions of people who either are unable or unwilling to see people in their own right, regardless of the political past of their parents.

Also, recognition of children of collaborators is often conditional. In a reaction to the government subsidy, the spokesman of the major political party in The Netherlands declared that he did not like to subsidize these people, but he argued for it because subsidizing a self-help group was the cheapest way of solving the problem. A famous psychiatrist argued for help because it would be politically dangerous to neglect this group. The recognition of the existence of problems among children of collaborators is almost unanimous but, for the most part, the cause of these problems is seen in the behavior of the parents during the war, rather than in the postwar reaction to this behavior. The size of the subsidy granted to children of collaborators is not proportionate to the subsidies granted to other "children of the war."

On the other hand, for the first time (1995), the self-help group of children of collaborators was officially invited to be present at the commemoration of the liberation of The Netherlands from the Germans 50 years ago.

Out of the 200,000 to 300,000 children of collaborators living in The Netherlands, less than 4,000 have made themselves known to the self-help group. Of the latter group, only very few have taken the step to make themselves known in the media. Most reactions to media programs on the subject are positive. However, children of collaborators who have revealed their backgrounds in public report much lack of understanding. In particular, people find it difficult to understand that children of collaborators can also have positive feelings toward their parents, that for these children, their parents were not only "wrong" parents, but also "right" parents.

Giving Meaning

A last important factor for the integration of children of collaborators in society is the inspiration they received to give meaning to their experiences. Many report that this inspiration came from people who represent philosophical and religious traditions. It helped them to accept their own life histories, face the negative aspects, and try to distill positive insights from them. They were inspired to cope with the enormous issues of guilt, suffering and, evil, and, in particular, that of belonging. Many searched for information about the past and struggled to give this information meaning.

Many have matured from unfounded guilt feelings to a sense of responsibility and the desire to contribute to the community. It is likely that they will always stand out in their critical attitude toward discrimination and exclusion of people, toward projecting evil onto others.

CONCLUSION

This chapter is based on findings that have been confirmed by means of "member check" within the group of children of collaborators who participated in the self-help group formed in The Netherlands. The judgments of clinicians and researchers have also been taken into account in the description. However, much more work remains to be done.

One aim for further research could be to check a particular implication of the findings: the importance of nonspecific therapy factors for this group of individuals. Another aim could be to elaborate scapegoat theories in order to clarify the reactions war-affected people encounter in everyday life. Focusing on the societal aspects of the continuing trauma described herein might be of help for the work of the self-help group in corroborating self-esteem.

The descriptions in this chapter can serve several purposes. For example, they can be used as a framework for further research in that they provide rich material for formulating new hypotheses and questionnaires. They can also be used to develop educational material for training and retraining psychotherapists, pastoral workers, and other professionals.

The insights into the life conditions of children of collaborators constitute an appeal to the citizens of this country to become informed about this uneasy subject, face this aspect of the heritage of World War II, and confront the many questions that arise. This can enhance the full integration of the consequences of the war.

Far more work is needed to extend the information contained herein to the people not attending the self-help group. The challenging question of how to inquire into the life stories of people who are silent about their backgrounds must be tackled.

The findings and tentative generalizations may also suggest a framework for studying the situation of children of collaborators in other countries occupied during World War II, as well as that of people involved in today's conflicts, such as that in former Yugoslavia.

REFERENCES

Bar-On, D. (1988). Children of perpetrators of the Holocaust: Working through one's own moral self. In D. Bar-On, F. Beiner, & M. Brusten (Eds.), *Der Holocaust* (pp. 33–56). University of Wuppertal, Wuppertal, Germany.

Bar-On, D. (1989). *Legacy of silence.* Cambridge, MA: Harvard University Press.

Bar-On, D., Beiner, F., & Brusten, M. (Eds.). (1988). *Der Holocaust.* University of Wuppertal, Wuppertal, Germany.

Belinfante, A. D. (1978). *In plaats van bijltjesdag, de geschiedenis van de bijzondere rechtspleging na de Tweede Wereldoorlog* [Instead of a day of reckoning, the history of the special jurisdiction after the Second World War]. Assen: Van Gorcum.

Blom, P. C. (1988). Interview in *Noord-Hollands Dagblad,* August 27, 1988, p. 1.

Boszormenyi-Nagy, I., & Spark, G. M. (1984). *Invisible loyalties.* New York: Brunner/Mazel.

Cohn, I. (1991). *The Convention on the Rights of the Child: What it means for children in war. International Journal of Refugee Law, 3*(1), 100–109.

Danieli, Y. (1980). Countertransference in the treatment and study of Nazi Holocaust survivors and their children. *Victimology: An International Journal, 3,* 345–363.

Danieli, Y. (1985). The treatment and prevention of long-term effects and intergenerational transmission of victim-ization: A lesson from Holocaust survivors and their children. In C. Figley (Ed.), *Trauma and its wake* (Vol 1, pp. 295–313). New York, Burnner/Mazel.

De Jong, L. (1980). *Het koninkrijk der Nederlanden in de Tweede Wereldoorlog, deel 10a, het laatste jaar, de tweede helft* [The kingdom of The Netherlands in the Second World War, the last year, the second half]. Den Haag: Nihoff.

De Jong, L. (1988). *Het Koninkrijk der Nederlanden in Oorlogstijd,* deel 12, Epiloog (The kingdom of The Nether-lands in war time, part 12, Epilogue). Den Haag: Nijhof.

Donkersloot, H. (1988). Psychological aspects of children of Dutch national socialists. In D. Bar-On, F. Beiner, & M. Brusten (Eds.), *Der Holocaust* (pp. 106–110). University of Wuppertal, Wuppertal, Germany.

Donkersloot, H. (1995). De vijftigste mei [The fiftieth of May] *Bulletin Stichting Werkgroep Herkenning 10,* 3–4.

Groen, K. (1984). *Landverraad, de berechting van collaborateurs in Nederland* [High-treason, the trial of collabora-tors in The Netherlands]. Weesp: Unieboek.

Hofman, J. (1981). *De collaborateur: Een sociaal-psychologisch onderzoek naar misdadig gedrag in dienst van de Duitse bezetter* [The Collaborator: A sociopsychological study of criminal behavior in the service of the German occupier]. Meppel: Boom.

Hofman, J. (1984). Het lot van de N.S.B.-kinderen [The fate of the NSB-children]. *Maandblad voor de Geestelijke Volksgezondheid, 3,* 243–254.

Hofman, J. (1985). *The fate of the children of Dutch quislings.* Paper presented at the 8th Annual Convention of the In-ternational Psychohistorical Association, New York, NY.

Hofman, J. (1988). Dutch collaborators and the problems of their children. In D. Bar-On, F. Beiner, & M. Brusten (Eds.), *Der Holocaust* (pp. 95–105). University of Wuppertal, Wuppertal, Germany.

Lindt, M. W. J. (1993). *Als je wortels taboe zijn: Verwerking van levensproblemen van kinderen van Nederlandse na-tionaal-socialistein* [When roots are taboo: Children of Dutch national-socialists coming to terms with life prob-lems]. Kampen: Kok.

Montessori, M. M. (1987). N.S.B.-kinderen, tweede generatie [NSB-children, second generation]. In R. Beunderman & J. Dane (Eds.), *Kinderen van de oorlog* [Children of war]. Utrecht: ICODO.

Pincus, L., & Dare, C. (1980). *Secrets in the family.* New York: Harper & Row.

Psycho Analytisch Instituut. (1981). *Psychoanalyse en Psychotherapie op psychoanalytische basis aan oorlogs-slachtoffers, verzetsdeelnemers en hun kinderen* [Psychoanalysis and psychotherapy on analytic lines for war vic-tims, resistance fighters and their children]. Amsterdam: Psycho Analytisch Instituut.

Reuling-Schappin, M. (1993). Kinderen in gevaar of gevaarlijke kinderen? Politieke heropvoeding van NSB-kinderen in tehuizen 9145–1950 [Children in danger or dangerous children? Political Reeducation of NSB-children in children's homes 1945–1950]. *Pedagogisch Tijdschrift, 18,* 147–153.

Romijn, P. (1989). *Snel, streng en rechtvaardig: Politiek beleid inzake de bestraffing en reclassering van "foute" Ne-derlanders* [Fast, severe and righteous: Politics of punishment and after-care of 'wrong' Dutch]. Bussum: De Haan.

Scheffel-Baars, G. (1984). *Kind van foute ouders* [Child of wrong parents]. Schiedam: Werkgroep Herkenning.

Scheffel-Baars, G. (1988). Self-help group for children of collaborators with Nazi's in Holland. In D. Bar-On, F. Beiner, & M. Brusten (Eds.), *Der Holocaust* (pp. 80–94). University of Wuppertal, Wuppertal, Germany.

Spruit, I. P. (1983). *Onder de vleugels van de partij* [Under the wings of the party]. Bussum: Wereldvenster.

Vorst-Thijssen, T., & de Boer, N. (1993). *Daar praat je niet over! Kinderen van foute ouders en de hulpverlening* [We don't talk about that! Children of wrong parents and professional help]. Utrecht: Nederlands Instituut voor Zorg en Welzijn.

Willemse, T. (1986). Kinderen van N.S.B.-ers tussen 1944–1949 [Children of NSB-members 1944–1949] *Maandblad voor Geestelijke Volksgezondheid, 41*(4), 367–382.

11

Intergenerational Effects in Families of World War II Survivors from the Dutch East Indies

Aftermath of Another Dutch War

PETRA G. H. AARTS

INTRODUCTION

It is generally know that The Netherlands, along with many other European countries, was occupied by Nazi Germany during World War II. It is less known that many Dutch, civilians and military alike, also suffered as a consequence of the war in the Far East. For three centuries, The Netherlands dominated a beautiful and exotic archipelago, presently known as the Republic of Indonesia. In 1942, the Japanese occupied the Dutch East Indies and terrorized those of European descent until the end of the war. In the years following World War II, most war victims who had special ties with the Dutch moved to The Netherlands. However, upon arrival, little or no attention was paid to the survivors from this former Dutch colony. Approximately halfway into the 1980s, it became clear that some children of East Indian war victims displayed symptoms and problems similar to those of, for instance, children of Holocaust survivors.

In the 1970s, along with their American and Israeli colleagues, Dutch mental health professionals were among the first to publish on intergenerational traumatization. In those early days, studies were mainly focused on children of the few surviving Dutch Jews (de Graaf, 1975; Musaph, 1978). In The Netherlands, a distinction is made between various groups of children of World War II survivors. First of all, but by no means the most numerable, are the offspring of Jewish survivors of Nazi persecution. Second are children of participants of the resistance against the German oppressor (Op den Velde, Chapter 9, this volume). The third and most ignored group are children of so-called Dutch quislings (Lindt, Chapter 10, this volume). The last, but likely the most sizeable group, are the sons and daughters of survivors of World War II from the former Dutch Indies. Very little has been published on the latter.

PETRA G. H. AARTS • Aarts Psychotrauma Research, Consultancy and Training, Rozenstraat 55, 1016 NN Amsterdam, The Netherlands.

International Handbook of Multigenerational Legacies of Trauma, edited by Yael Danieli. Plenum Press, New York, 1998.

The effects of the occupation of the former Dutch Indies by the Japanese and the Indonesian War of Independence have only recently become open to public reflection and debate in The Netherlands. For more than four decades, the warfare in the former Dutch Indies seemed forgotten. This chapter will elaborate upon

1. The reasons for this forgetfulness within Dutch society. Society as a whole plays a significant role in the individual's mastery of traumatic experiences, particularly when the traumas are of man-made origin.
2. Mechanisms and expressions of intergenerational traumatization in children of survivors from the Dutch Indies, with an emphasis on projective identification.
3. Presentation and discussion of some brief vignettes and a case presentation to exemplify the concepts used to illuminate different expressions of intergenerational traumatization.
4. The results of studies on the second generation of survivors from the Dutch Indies.

The chapter begins, however, with a brief overview of relevant historical processes and events of this "other" Dutch war.

THE DUTCH INDIES DURING WORLD WAR II

The prosperity of the Dutch Republic in the seventeenth century, commonly called its Golden Age, was to an important extent obtained from the trade with the islands that are now known as Indonesia. The small seafaring nation benefited from the rich variety of exotic spices, which yielded high profits in the West. Soon this trade developed into straightforward colonization by the Dutch. Over the centuries, large agricultural estates and trade centers developed and generated considerable revenue and status not only for the Netherlands but also for the individuals that ruled them on site. The bulk of the hard work required for the returns was provided by the indigenous population. The upper class consisted of the Dutch rulers and their families. In reality, of course, the social structure developed into a much more complex system. The native population of the Dutch Indies was culturally and ethnically highly diverse, with its own standards for prerogatives. Furthermore, ever since the first European sailors had set foot ashore, children were born that showed conclusive signs of mixed origin. Once the Dutch began to settle, their numbers increased. In particular, families that had lived in the Dutch Indies for several generations were often partly of inland blood. As a rule, however, ethnic descent and wealth determined ones authority and status: the whiter and richer, the better.

Late in December 1941, some 3 weeks after the attack on Pearl Harbor, the Japanese army invaded the Dutch Indies. Resistance from the military proved futile, and in March 1942, the Dutch Indian army surrendered. By then, the Indian islands were practically occupied. It was estimated that on the eve of the Japanese invasion nearly 250,000 Europeans lived in the Dutch Indies. Some 210,000 were of Dutch origin. Approximately 134,000 were Indo-European families that had lived in the Dutch Indies for several generations (Stevens, 1991). As part of the policy to free Eastern Asia from Western domination and influence, the Japanese isolated the European inhabitants and began to stir the resistance of the native population against the "white oppressors" by means of intensive, anti-imperialistic propaganda.

All Europeans and Indo-Europeans were forced to demonstrate openly their subservience to the Japanese. For instance, they had to bow deeply while passing by the Japanese. Brutal punishment would follow any sign of insolence or disobedience. Men were separated from their wives, mothers, and children, and young and old were forced to work under deplorable circumstances on the many projects the Japanese initiated. Probably due to the popular film

The Bridge over the River Kwai, the construction of the railroad through Burma and Siam is the most notorious. Exhaustion, famine, and infectious diseases in the work camps were life threatening. Some 41,000 Dutch men, military and civilian alike, were imprisoned in work camps. Nearly one-fourth did not survive the war.

Women and children, too, were confined, first in restricted urban areas and later, when the interned population grew more and more dense, also in specially built camps. By the end of the war, there was a large number of concentration camps scattered throughout the Indian islands. Approximately 100,000 Dutch women and children were interned in civilian camps. Some 16,000–18,000 American men, women, and children were also trapped in Japanese internment camps in the Pacific war theater (Potts, 1994). Although conditions varied among camps, by and large the situation and regime worsened over time. Famine was one of the greatest predicaments, but also the numerous, lengthy, sometimes unscheduled roll calls caused immense suffering. The internees had to wait for hours, heads up, shoulders straight, unprotected from the burning sun. Most camps were overpopulated, and deportations from one camp to another occurred frequently. The hygienic circumstances in the concentration camps were abominable and, when combined with famine and exhaustion, were a short cut to death.

Life in the camps was hard for other reasons as well: Families had been torn apart. The uncertainty of the whereabouts and fate of loved ones was agonizing. Children, however, usually stayed with their mothers. For most children and women, the Japanese guards were the only men they were to see for years. The relation with fathers, sons, and husbands could only survive in often idealized fantasies. Fervent competition between groups of prisoners was frequent, although bravery and altruistic behavior also evolved. Education of children was strictly forbidden and had to be organized by the women in secrecy. Each individual was repeatedly confronted with severe illness and death. Medical care in the camps was primitive. Depending on the policy of each particular camp, boys at the age of 10, 11 or 12, far too young to be separated from their mothers and siblings, were sent to prison camps for men, where the conditions were even worse.

Contrary to the Nazi concentration camps in Europe, the Japanese internment camps were not designed to annihilate the captives. Their main purposes were the isolation, exploitation, and humiliation of Europeans: Western influence in Eastern Asia had to be eliminated and replaced by Japanese hegemony. The mortality rate in Japanese civilian concentration camps was 12.8%, contagious infectious diseases and starvation being the main causes of death. In the European concentration camps, close to 70% did not survive the war (Van Waterford, 1994). Not all the Dutch were interned in the Japanese concentration camps. Analogous to the Nazis' Nuremberg Law, the number of Indian grandparents determined to some extent whether one became interned. Those who had enough Indian grandparents escaped internment. Again, the color of the skin proved crucial for one's position. The situation outside the camps was rather different but by no means less complicated. The anti-Western propaganda of the Japanese in the Dutch Indies proved successful. Some of the Indonesians turned fiercely against those who were related to the former Dutch rulers. Therefore, the Indo-Europeans had to fear not only the Japanese but also the adherents of Indonesian independence. Many of those who were not in the camps were forced to live in strict isolation or hiding and feared for their lives. Food in the internment camps was, however limited, at least provided regularly by the Japanese. The Indo-Europeans outside the camps had to obtain their own food by trading whatever they possessed. During their daily ventures for nourishment, they had to be extremely careful, since trading with the inlanders was strictly forbidden. Their situation during World War II could best be characterized as completely outlawed. Furthermore, with regard to their identity, they had to perform a complicated psychological twist: Having always been proud of the status derived from their relation with the Dutch, they now had to deny any such association.

Apart from the Soviet army in 1945, there is only indirect evidence of sexual torture in Europe during World War II. There are only a few testimonies of women who were forced into prostitution or fell victim to sexual torment in German concentration camps (Krystal, 1968, see also Brownmiller, 1975). It is unlikely that the incidence of sexual assaults in Nazi Germany and concentration camps will ever be known. However, there is ample evidence of sexual exploitation by the Japanese during World War II. So-called "comfort women" were forced to satisfy the sexual urges of Japanese soldiers on a large and well-organized scale, an average of 1 woman to 50 soldiers. These women were not "volunteering" Japanese prostitutes, but were young women from occupied territories, abducted in raids especially designed for this purpose (Hicks, 1995). Some years ago, a now middle-aged Dutch woman publicly told of having been sexually abused by the Japanese in the former Dutch Indies. A few more Dutch women have recently dared to tell of their distressing sexual harassment by the Japanese. However, in the former Dutch Indies, the victims were more often East Asian than European women and girls, and there is no indication that a high proportion of European women became sex slaves of the Japanese army. The Japanese, apparently, did not prefer blondes.

The surrender of the Japanese in August 1945, however, did not bring and end to the misery of the survivors in the Dutch Indies. Instead of being able to return to their homes and families and resume their previous occupations and positions, they were confronted with a serious threat from the Indonesian nationalists. World War II marked the finale of centuries of imperialism. Strong movements for national independence had evolved and reached a climax at precisely the time the oppressing nations were preoccupied with conflicts among themselves and with the recovery from World War II. The English soon lost most of their empire and ceased to "rule the waves." France, Germany, and Belgium gradually lost control over their African colonies. In the Dutch Indies, a war of independence immediately broke out after the proclamation of the Republic of Indonesia, only 2 days after the capitulation of Japan. In a way, this was more painful for the Dutch survivors than the oppression by the Japanese, for many had survived, hoping to restore their "normal" prewar lives. Instead of the usual compliance of the inlanders, they met overt animosity. Many survivors experienced this as yet another injury to their pride: Humiliation was their turn again. Many had to remain in, or return to, the internment camps, only this time, paradoxically, to be defended by the Japanese against the aggression of the Indonesians.

In order to preserve the Indies, the Dutch government immediately sent the military overseas to fight the Indonesian revolt. So soon after the liberation from Nazi Germany, many Dutch people feared that the economy could not recover without the revenues derived from their former colony. Without the necessary economic growth, many feared social disintegration as a consequence of a communist revolution. Until the end of 1949, several military efforts to preserve Dutch rule were undertaken. However, they failed, and Indonesian independence was firmly established. From the beginning, all critical voices concerning the goal of the military actions in Indonesia, and atrocities committed by the Dutch military, were stifled. Only recently has the policy of the Dutch in Indonesia been somewhat open for public debate. Simultaneously, a growing awareness developed that many Dutch civilians and military suffered the sequelae of this distant war.

MIGRATION TO THE NETHERLANDS

Shortly after World War II, the majority of Dutch survivors from the Indies, who still had ties with The Netherlands, returned. Later, many Indo-Europeans also moved to the small country, which most of them knew only from stories. For them, leaving the Indies was mainly motivated by Indonesian violence. Over the years, some 300,000 men, women, and children, migrated to The Netherlands (Van der Velde, Eland, & Kleber, 1994). The loss of their homeland and the necessity of adapting to a new country, however, caused severe strain. Migration, in general, is known to be a significant stressor (Grinberg & Grinberg, 1989). Indeed, for the survivors from the Dutch Indies, there were three distinctive stages that were potentially traumatizing.

- World War II, including the eventual internment in Japanese camps.
- The war for Indonesian independence.
- The return or migration to The Netherlands.

At some point after the war, families were reunited. Surviving husbands and wives, sons, and daughters needed to reestablish their bonds, which was particularly difficult after having been separated for so long. Like many trauma survivors, they often scarcely spoke about their predicaments during the war. Of course, not all spouses, parents, and children were able to bridge the gaps easily. Especially younger children hardly remembered or even knew their fathers. The atrocities each individual had survived had changed many beyond recognition, and fantasies concerning each other, cherished throughout the war, often proved false. The initial estrangement between family members sometimes persisted.

The migration to The Netherlands presented additional challenges to their ability to adapt to new circumstances. As it is in psychic trauma, loss is crucial in migration too, especially when the migration is coerced by adverse circumstances. Also, the contrast between the small, Northern European country and the exotic islands in the Pacific was enormous. The climate, colors, language, smells, even daily life itself, could not have been more dissimilar, and many survivors yearned for their lost homeland. Furthermore, many men had to accept jobs that were far below their former occupations in both wages and status. Women had to get used to keeping house themselves, or adapt to living with relatives or in lodgings during the first years after their migration. There was yet an additional problem for the Indo-European migrants. Their fine features and dark complexions revealed their (partially) foreign descent. Children especially, but also adults, sometimes faced discrimination by the Dutch. Most survivors did not articulate their difficulties or openly mourn their losses, but concentrated as much as they could on the present and future.

There were also external reasons to remain silent over the decades following their traumatic experiences. What made migration particularly difficult was the Dutch indifference to their situation. The survivors were given some material support. Not unlike the reactions to Jewish survivors, almost no one was interested in what they had gone through in a war that was fought and suffered so far away. Underlying this indifference was a new but strong ambivalence on the part of the Dutch population about the military involvement in the young Indonesian Republic, particularly intensified by harsh criticism from the United Nations. Not many Dutch were prepared to question the policy and warfare against the Indonesians. This reciprocal silence reduced the survivors' opportunities for recovery from their traumatic experiences.

Social and political circumstances can also partly explain why various groups of World War II survivors and their offspring were mainly studied separately. In order to get society in general, and politicians in particular to address individual and collective needs of war victims, the barriers of silence needed to be removed. Thus, the various Dutch indemnification laws for war victims were passed only at those points in time when society as a whole was willing to face the historic events that shaped the life of each particular group of war victims. The first compensation law for veterans of the Dutch resistance was passed in 1947; the second, for survivors of persecution, was passed in 1973. During its first decade, this law was mainly used on behalf of Jewish survivors. Lately, the majority of applicants are survivors from the Dutch Indies. Children of Dutch quislings had to wait until 1994 for some governmental financial support. Indeed, it took a social movement to interest not only policy makers, but also most mental health professionals (Herman, 1992). This may also explain the tendency of some clinicians, themselves often belonging to the particular victim group, to generalize clinical findings to the victim population, thereby exaggerating the incidence of severe pathology, and, as a result, neglecting evidence of resilience and health in trauma survivors and their children.

FAMILIES OF SURVIVORS FROM THE DUTCH INDIES

There are no grounds to assume that the majority of Dutch Indian war survivors developed serious and lasting complaints. However, it is clinically well established that unresolved posttraumatic conflicts may interfere with parental functioning. Over the years, it has become apparent that some children of Indian war survivors developed symptoms and complaints similar to those of children of Holocaust survivors. Problems related to affect regulation, diffuse ego boundaries, extreme loyalty and overattachment to the parents, self-deprecation, repetition, compulsion, guilt feelings, acting-out behavior, and depression, for example, have been reported by various clinicians (Dorelijers & Donovan, 1990; Filet, 1987). In themselves, such phenomena are by no means typical of offspring of trauma survivors. They often can be observed in any group of patients in Western society. What makes the problems and symptoms of children of World War II survivors distinctive is not so much the group of diagnostic characteristics but the underlying pathogenesis. Family dynamics, in combination with personal susceptibility, appear to be crucial to the process of intergenerational traumatization.

A conspiracy of silence is generally understood to be at the core of the dynamics that may lead to more or less serious symptomatology in the second generation. Silence about the parents' experiences was often motivated by a sincere wish to spare the children such devastating knowledge. But, at the same time, it served to protect the parents themselves from confronting their memories and helped to stifle their emotions. However, the conspiracy of silence is truly mutual, as all parties involved are well aware of the themes that are governed by silence and share in the efforts to maintain their suppression. As mentioned earlier, the conspiracy of silence was not limited to the families. Repression was encouraged by the society, and silent adjustment was, therefore, typical of the postwar adaptation of Indian war victims in The Netherlands. One general survival strategy was the avoidance of any display of conspicuous behavior. War experiences, or problems related to their immigration, were hardly ever mentioned. Children soon learned to share in this conspiracy. Even in families where parents did speak about the war, children refrained from asking particular details. As a consequence, children tended to fantasize, not always consciously, about their parents' experiences. Furthermore, the secrecy of one's deepest thoughts, images, and emotions sometimes transcended the realm of traumatic war experiences to cover other aspects of the personality as well. Emotions such as pain, loneliness, anger, and fear became associated with a sense of imminent danger. Loyalty toward parents often hindered children from rebelling against this restriction on their vitality and needs. Overadaptation to "normality," which is generally regarded as characteristic of families of survivors of the Dutch Indies, could lead to a pathogenic breach of inner world and outer reality.

Donna was referred to a psychotherapist at the age of 38. She appeared to suffer from dysthymia and had trouble falling asleep. Her mother, who had survived Japanese internment camps, had previously been married. Her infant son had not survived the war. After returning to The Netherlands, she divorced her first husband and, some years later, married Donna's father. Her mother always claimed that it was not a marriage of love but of reason: He was a good and quiet man who took good care of her and Donna. She neither spoke about the war nor about Donna's deceased half-brother. She was very depressed and isolated. The essence of her identity was of being a powerless victim in an evil world. As an only child, Donna never managed to separate from her symbiotic relationship with her mother. Her father was emotionally unavailable to her. Donna recalls suffering from nightmares and panic attacks from a very young age, and frequently fantasizing about the cruelties she imagined her mother to have gone through. In treatment, she was not only secretive about these fantasies but also about the life she led as a fairly gifted and mature woman. Secrecy had become second nature to her, while splitting enabled her to escape partially from her mother's symbiotic demands.

The interference of unmetabolized traumata or posttraumatic changes of the personality of the parent(s) with the development of their children is very complex and unique in each case. However, typical patterns of divergent family dynamics have been described by Danieli (1981). Although she referred to families of Jewish Holocaust survivors, many of the (ideal–typical) characteristics she described can be recognized in families of other groups of war victims. Overvaluation and overprotection on the one hand, and neglect or overt aggression toward children on the other, are parental inadequacies that may well harm the child's development. Sometimes parents envy their children's "unburdened" youth. Jealousy of parents toward a child may manifest itself in a restrictive and humiliating control over his or her life, while at the same time demanding unconditional loyalty and love.

> During the war, Peter was incarcerated by the Japanese and worked on the Burma railroad. After the war, he repeatedly claimed to be totally unaffected by it. On the contrary, it had taught him how to survive. He was always strong and healthy, and would never give in to any emotion. Once, upon breaking his leg, he could hardly be persuaded to go to a hospital. But because his professional career was not what he had expected, he became a very embittered man. He saw it as his responsibility to teach his two children the lessons that he found so valuable in Burma: They should never complain; they should never be ill; they should never be demanding or wish for anything; they had better not be heard or seen too often. Shortly after his fiftieth birthday, he broke down.
>
> His youngest child, a daughter, sought psychotherapy not long before her expected graduation from the university. She was unable to concentrate on her studies, and she suffered from anxiety attacks. She progressively isolated herself. Only after several sessions was she willing to discuss her father's lessons and the little she knew about his war experiences. She was unable to feel any resentment toward him, and she refused to criticize the regime that dominated her childhood. She did not complete her education. Her older brother also failed to pass his final exams. The children's breakdown during late adolescence was perhaps due to their effort at bringing to the surface some of the never-articulated pain of their father. They may also have been afraid that their own potential educational achievements would confront their father with his own unsuccessful career. Their failure proved their loyalty.

THEORIES ON THE TRANSMISSION OF TRAUMA
TO SUCCEEDING GENERATIONS

Various psychological schools have contributed significantly to our understanding of intergenerational transmission of trauma. Indeed, most of the earlier studies on the second generation were reported by psychoanalysts. *Drive theory,* for instance, helped us understand how the traumatized parents' confrontation with the wide range of emotions in a young dependent child can reactivate the struggle between conflicting affects and self-images. Combined with the suppression of affects, regression is crucial to surviving life-threatening persecution. However, once the threat is over, and such survival strategies and defenses have outlived their usefulness, they may nevertheless persist. The normal developmental stage related to preoccupation of children with food, excrement, birth, death, and omnipotent monsters confronts the parent(s) with traumatic images out of their past and makes it hard for them to respond in a comforting, understanding, and playful manner. The result may well be a subsequent lack of basic trust and feelings of shame, guilt and anger in the children.

Many clinicians recognized that fantasies concerning the parents' past experiences play an important role in the symptom formation of second-generation patients. These fantasies are not only determined by the parents' actual communication, but also by the particular developmental stage of the child (Bergman & Jucovy, 1982; Grubrich-Simitis, 1979; Kestenberg, 1972). The relationship between parental trauma and the nature of sexual(ized) problems and conflicts in World War II survivors' offspring has been a mostly neglected theme in the literature. The children's sexuality could be expected to be affected, especially when the parent has been sexually molested during the war. The sexual violence and abuse of victims themselves has been commonly neglected as well.

Psychoanalytic *object relation theory,* especially Mahler's work on the separation–individuation process in children (Mahler, 1975), also amplified the understanding of family dynamics underlying pathology in the second generation. The special meaning of having children for survivors of massive traumatization could lead to excessive overprotection and symbiotic demands, or to rage and powerlessness, thereby burdening the separation and individuation of their children. The quest of the individual to maintain continuity of relationships with the self and others in the presence of contradictory pleasurable and distressing, loving and hateful feelings, is central in object relations theory. This theory's concept of *projective identification* proved fruitful in deepening the insight into the transmission of parental trauma and the pathogeneses in the second generation. Unbearably conflicting and, therefore, split off parts of the parents' posttraumatic imagery can induce behaviors or feelings in their children. These could be the acting out of parental conflicts, or the projection onto the child of feelings of shame, despair, rage, or worthlessness. Some children became tormented by aggressive fantasies, mostly, but not always, emotionally associated with hurting the parents like the oppressor did. Others engaged in unacceptable aggressive and even delinquent behavior.

Feelings of shame, despair, rage, or worthlessness can be split off and subsequently projected onto the child. For example, the parent can induce the feeling in the child that his or her anger is evil, sometimes even by verbally comparing the child with the Japanese oppressor. The child is at risk of internalizing this image of badness, and the interaction between the parent and the child can become a repetition of an aggressor–victim dyad from the traumatic past, that first became an intrapsychic conflict, and subsequently, through projective identification, sought outlet in object relations. The concept of projective identification may also clarify phenomena such as anniversary reactions, observed in some children of survivors when a child becomes hard to handle, ill, or even psychotic at precisely the same developmental stage in which the parent was traumatized.

Yet another significant issue emanating from the latter is the so-called core identity as (potential) victim or aggressor. Thus, the ambiguity between good and bad self-representations is mainly an intrapsychic force; it may also bear on external relations. Gratification may be found in the acting out of a victim role, thereby evading confrontation with inner conflicts and avoiding self-responsibility. Moreover, a supreme victim identity compensates for the narcissistic blow of originating from a group of victims but may just as well derive from jealousy of the "special" victim parent(s). However, such a pseudoidentity, gratifying as it may be, places the individual outside the community until this conflict is faced and resolved (Aarts & De Graaf, 1990).

Jonathan, a 20-year-old man, was referred to a psychiatrist in a state of manic excitement and displaying ideas of grandiosity. In the first session, although denying the need for professional care, he shared that he was very afraid of his father, who, according to him, was aggressive. The following sessions were with Jonathan and his father.

Previously a conscientious and timid student, at age 15, Jonathan had suddenly begun to cause serious problems at school. He disturbed his classes and refused to do his homework. He claimed to be a genius, capable of effortless and complete comprehension. After he was dismissed by one school, his father sent him to another. His misconduct, however, persisted. Jonathan's parents responded with utter helplessness. His father explained in one session that he gave in to Jonathan's demands for money because he might otherwise steal it, which, eventually, he did.

Both Jonathan's parents had been interned in Japanese concentration camps as young children. At the age of 5, Jonathan's father, here named Paul, was caught stealing some sugar cane by a female inmate of the camp. The woman severely battered and nearly suffocated Paul by forcing a wooden stick into his throat. He remembers his mother watching the scene from nearby without trying to interfere.

After the Japanese capitulation, Paul's father, whom he could hardly remember, joined the family but was soon recruited by the Dutch army to fight the Indonesian independence movement. The family emigrated to The Netherlands when Paul was 15 years old. Paul's father, like many migrants from the Dutch Indies, had to accept a job much below his former standards. Feeling humiliated, he loudly and frequently complained about his fate. For reasons Paul never quite understood, his father also felt disappointed with, and betrayed by, the Dutch military command. He left the care of Paul and his siblings entirely to his wife, completely yielding to her wishes. He showed no recognition of Paul's achievements at school. Instead, he sometimes seemed jealous of Paul's progress at school.

As a husband and father himself, Paul has always done his best to hide his feelings from both his wife and Jonathan, for fear of burdening them with his problems, as his own father did to him. However, unlike his own father, Paul was strongly involved with Jonathan's education. He could neither eat nor sleep when Jonathan had to take a test at school. Although Paul clearly overvalued Jonathan, he could not help feeling that his son took advantage of his dedication and made a fool out of him.

In therapy, quite unexpectedly, Jonathan's condition improved impressively. The advancement was apparently caused by Paul's sudden and furious reaction to his son's grandiloquence. His outburst happened upon coming home from therapy, finding the living room a complete mess, and feeling an overwhelming resentment for having to see a psychiatrist for his son's benefit, while Jonathan continued his misconduct with utter indifference to his parents' worries and sacrifices. For the first time, thereafter, Jonathan showed some understanding for his father's concerns.

A careful scrutiny of the psychodynamics and particular symptom formation of offspring of World War II survivors from the former Dutch Indies and their antipodes of the European war theater do not reveal that mechanisms of intergenerational traumatization are unique to any group of offspring of World War II survivors. Some features that can be directly understood from the unique historical and geographic circumstances are nevertheless typical for the progeny of survivors of the war in the Far East. Just like the Jewish second generation, they, somehow, need to come to terms with their particular sociocultural identity, their historical inheritance, and their relation toward the Dutch.

STUDIES ON CHILDREN OF WORLD WAR II SURVIVORS IN THE DUTCH EAST INDIES

As stated earlier, only very little has been published specifically on the offspring of survivors from the Dutch East Indies. Dorelijers and Donovan (1990) reported that their search of international databases yielded only one publication concerning Dutch Indian camp survivors. They concluded that "these individuals and their families are clearly the forgotten souls of the

1940's" (p. 435). Furthermore, the few existing reports are all clinical and, as such, reflect a selected fraction of the population only. In most cases, the war in the former Dutch Indies was part of the clinicians' own family history. Two recent Dutch studies, however, are worth mentioning. The first is a small study based on semistructured interviews with experienced clinicians concerning problems and treatment of children of Dutch Indian survivors (Aarts, 1994). The second is an extensive, controlled, empirical study involving the same group (Van der Velden *et al.*, 1994). The latter was initiated and financed by the Dutch Ministry of Welfare, Health, and Culture, and focused specifically on the prevalence and nature of problems in a representative sample of Indian survivors' offspring born after 1945.

In the first study, Aarts (1994) interviewed 6 psychotherapists concerning their experiences with children of survivors from the Dutch Indies. They were selected from a list of expert psychotherapists, compiled by the Dutch National Institute for Victims of War (ICODO). Although their actual work experience with children of survivors from the Dutch Indies proved highly variable (ranging from 1 to nearly 50 patients), all 6 had considerable expertise with second-generation patients in particular, and with treating average Dutch patients in general. The interviews, therefore, included questions concerning possible differences between the second-generation and non-war-affected Dutch patients.

There was a consensus among all 6 therapists that children of parents who were not able to master their (war-related) traumas run a higher risk of developing complaints and pathology. To the interviewed clinicians, it was obvious that themes that are bound to become pivotal in each child's development, such as aggression, shame, guilt, attachment, and loss, intensify the parents' posttraumatic struggles. As a response, according to the therapists, the parents were often either too permissive or too strict, or even sadistic with their child. Parents sought to avoid confronting these complex emotions or actively engaging in them. In various, subtle ways, the parent also may have lured the child into acting out ambivalent behavior or emotions in an effort to externalize their own inner conflicts. It was, in fact, "the return of the repressed" within the family, whose impact depended on the severity of the parents conflicts and the individual susceptibility of the child.

The interviewed therapists described the underlying family dynamics of their second-generation patients as shrouded in a potentially pathogenetic "conspiracy of silence," which, in turn, caused disregulation of strong affects such as aggression and attachment. Most second-generation patients entered treatment with unspecific complaints such as dysthymia and a low self-esteem, which was often manifested in self-destructive behavior. Many expressed problems concerning separation, individuation, and autonomy. Loyalty conflicts, insufficient basic trust, identity diffusion, and difficulties in expressing and/or regulating strong emotions were mentioned as the core complaints of second-generation patients. Interestingly, one therapist mentioned a marked discrepancy between these complaints on the one hand, and the high level of occupational functioning on the other.

Most of the therapists' conclusions and opinions in the study were in concert with the ones cited in the mainstream literature on the second generation. Moreover, all 6 therapists stated that, in general, their second-generation patients were more difficult to treat than their average patients. This relative difficulty concerned both the intensity and duration of the therapy. In their view, this was not so much caused by the severity of pathology as by the rigidity of defense mechanisms and intense loyalty toward the traumatized parent(s). It is important to note that the opinions of these expert psychotherapists do not principally contradict the results of the empirical study reported below. The two analyses are based on populations that are not comparable. The results of neither study can be, or should be, generalized from one group to the other.

Comparing characteristics of children of survivors from the Dutch Indies with those of other second-generation groups, the clinicians mentioned shame and lack of assertiveness. Shame, especially in children of Indo-Europeans, may be related to the "typical" Asian shame-culture, whereas their subaggressive attitude or "inconspicuousness" can be viewed as a survival strategy during the war, and as a postwar adaptation. Transference was especially burdened. Time and again, the therapists felt subtly tested for their loyalty toward these patients. Sudden aggressive outbursts from these otherwise timid and compliant patients seemed typical. It was particularly difficult when sadomasochistic patterns were reenacted in transference, while aggression within the relationship with the parents was passionately denied. Some patients indirectly endeavored to humiliate the therapist, as they themselves had felt humiliated, while demanding unconditional loyalty at the same time. Therapists often had to struggle not to become overwhelmed by the complexity of such transference. Establishing a balance between the fear of pushing the patient away while interpreting his or her attitude, and of getting caught in a protective narcissistic collusion, proved crucial for the success of the therapy (see also Op den Velde, Koerselman, & Aarts, 1994).

The results of the controlled empirical study concerning the well-being and health of children of World War II survivors from the Dutch Indies were published in 1994. Both the randomly selected sample and the sociodemographically matched comparison group contained 266 respondents. The subjects of the target group were divided into two groups of approximately the same size. The first group included children whose ancestors had lived in the Dutch Indies for several generations, the Indo-Europeans. The second group encompassed the (white) offspring of parents who stayed there for a relatively short period and still felt strongly attached to The Netherlands. (In the Dutch Indies, the latter group were called *Totoks*).

Although the data collection and statistical analyses were comprehensive, hardly any significant or near-significant differences between the two target groups and the comparison group were found. The only differences were that the older children of Totoks, born between 1945 and 1955, had sought professional help for their problems in the past more frequently, while the older Indo-Europeans displayed more psychic complaints. Furthermore, children whose parents had been imprisoned in Japanese internment camps had more often consulted professional help in the past. But this fact had no bearing on their current well-being and health. Yet another, but not very surprising, difference was that the Indo-Europeans, in their tender years, had more often been confronted with discrimination by the Dutch. At present, they were also more involved with questions concerning their sociocultural identity. The former experiences with discrimination and present concentration with identity, however, were not related to their general health and well-being. In conclusion, there appeared to be no differences in the nature and number of complaints. Yet an alarmingly high proportion of 16% in both target and comparison groups gave evidence of serious health problems.

The negative results of this study are in accordance with the outcomes of many other empirical studies on the second generation (Felsen & Erlich, 1990; Last & Klein, 1984; Leon, Butcher, Kleinman, Goldberg & Almagor, 1981; Sigal & Weinfeld, 1989). The failure of most empirical studies to give proof of a high(er) incidence of problems or of distinctive pathology in children of trauma survivors was frequently attributed to the use of inadequate diagnostic measures, concepts, and/or research methods (Aarts, Eland, Kleber, & Weerts, 1991; Felsen & Erlich, 1990). Strikingly, the same arguments were used when affirmative results were presented (Harel, 1983; Solkoff, 1981).

The study under scrutiny, however, was of a sufficiently sophisticated design. It combined various relevant, standardized (diagnostic) instruments, with questionnaires particularly tailored for the target group, and with semistructured additional clinical interviews with 57 out of a total of 532 respondents, who completed the data collection. Notwithstanding the extensiveness of the study, the results are not beyond debate. It is arguable that selection bias has played a role. The response rate in the target group was rather low (approximately 35%), with only a very limited analysis of the nonresponse. The sampling of the comparison group may also have been biased, since quite a number of the controls reported serious war experiences of their parents during World War II (Aarts, 1995).

SUMMARY

During World War II, a Dutch colony, presently known as Indonesia, was occupied by the Japanese. Most Dutch civilians suffered from persecution, and a large number were interned in concentration camps and work camps. In the first decade after the war, many Dutch victims migrated to The Netherlands. A general lack of interest regarding their ordeal in The Netherlands reinforced the tendency to repress and deny their traumatic experiences. A conspiracy of silence ruled society and the families raised by these survivors. Although pathology is not a necessary outcome of growing up with traumatized parents, some clinical reports on the offspring of survivors from the Dutch East Indies reveal mild to severe complaints, which are understood to be related to not having worked through traumatic experiences of the parent(s).

Studies reveal that problems of the second generation may not be found in special diagnostic classifications, but in the psychodynamics that led to each individual's problems. The parents' traumatic imagery can play a pivotal role in various patterns of family dynamics. Overprotection and overvaluation on the one hand, and jealousy and sadomasochism on the other, may dominate the relationship with the children. The traumatic experiences of the parents become the focus of the children's fantasies and grow attached to a variety of complaints and problems. The complaints and problems are not always severe and disabling. The palette on which pathology and health are the extremes appears to be richly shaded.

Neither clinical reports nor research results give evidence that problems of children of Dutch Indian survivors are different from those of offspring of other war victims. However, it is obvious that children who grow up with parents who suffered massive or prolonged traumatization as a consequence of violence and cruelty may be at risk. A maturing understanding of the vulnerability of parents and children might enable us to provide better support for trauma survivors.

ACKNOWLEDGMENTS: I would like to thank the six psychotherapists who permitted me to interview them for a previous study and provided me with the clinical vignettes presented in this chapter. I especially wish to express my gratitude to Dr. Th. K. de Graaf for allowing me to present the case of Jonathan.

REFERENCES

Aarts, P. G. H. (1993). Kind in oorlogstijd: Enige overwegingen over behandeling en begeleiding van jong-vervolgden [Children in times of war: On their problems and treatment]. In W. Visser (Ed.), *Kind in Indië: Oorlogservaringen en hun gevolgen* (pp. 128–153). Utrecht, The Netherlands: ICODO-Uitgeverji.
Aarts, P. G. H. (1994, June 15). *In behandeling: De Indische naoorlogse generatie bij de RIAAG* [In treatment: Children of Dutch East Indies survivors in out patient health institutions]. Paper read at a training course for mental health professionals, Utrecht, The Netherlands.

Aarts, P. G. H. (1995). De Indische naoorlogse generatie gezond verklaard! Van kille feiten tot verhitte gemoederen [A health certificate for children of survivors from the Dutch East Indies! Book review]. *ICODO-Info, 12*(1), 54–61.

Aarts, P. G. H., & de Graaf, T. K. (1990, September 23–27). *Family dynamics in transgenerational traumatization: Projective identification.* Paper read at the Second European Conference on Traumatic Stress, Noordwijkerhout, The Netherlands.

Aarts, P. G. H., Eland, J., Kleber, R. J., & Weerts, J. M. P. (1991). *De joodse naoorlogse generatie. Onuitwisbare sporen?* [The Jewish second generation. Ineffaceable traces?]. Houten, The Netherlands: Bohn Stafleu Van Loghum.

Arnoldus, M. P. E. (1984). Tussen twee werelden: De Indische naoorlogse generatie [Between two worlds: The Dutch East Indian second generation] *ICODO-Info, 1*(2), 5–9.

Bergmann, M. S., & Jucovy, M. A. (Eds.). (1982). *Generations of the Holocaust.* New York: Basic Books.

Brownmiller, S. (1975). *Against our will: Men, women, and rape.* New York: Bantam Books.

Danieli, Y. (1981). Differing adaption styles in families of survivors of the Nazi Holocausts. *Children Today, 10,* 6–10, 34–35.

de Graaf, T. K. (1975). Pathological patterns of identification in families of survivors of the Holocaust. *Israel Annals of Psychiatry and Related Disciplines, 13,* 335–363.

Dorelijers, T. A. H., & Donovan, D. M. (1990). Transgenerational traumatization in children of parents interned in Japanese civil internment camps in the Dutch East Indies during WW II. *Journal of Psychohistory, 17,* 435–447.

Ellemers, J. E., & Vaillant, R. E. F. (1985). *Indische Nederlanders en gerepatrieerden* [Dutch Indians and immigrants]. Muiderberg, The Netherlands: Dick Coutinho.

Felsen, I., & Erlich, S. (1990). Identification patterns of offspring of Holocaust survivors with the parents. *American Journal of Orthopsychiatry, 60,* 506–520.

Filet, B. C. (1987). Indische kampkinderen en hun kinderen [Interned Indian children and their offspring]. In R. Beunderman & J. Dane (Eds.), *Kinderen van de oorlog* (pp. 31–45). Utrecht, The Netherlands: ICODO.

Grinberg, L., & Grinberg, R. (1989). *A psychoanalytic study of migration: Its normal and pathological aspects.* Paper presented at the 36th International Psychoanalysts Association Conference, Rome.

Grubrich-Simitis, I. (1979). Extremtraumatisierung als kumulatives Trauma [Massive traumatization as cumulative trauma]. *Psyche, 33,* 991–1023.

Harel, Z. (1983). Coping with stress and adaptation: The impact of the Holocaust on survivors. *Society and Welfare, 5,* 221–230.

Herman, J. L. (1992). *Trauma and recovery.* New York: Basic Books.

Hicks, G. (1995). *The comfort women: Sex slaves of the Japanese Imperial forces.* London: Souvenirs Press.

Kestenberg, J. S. (1972). Psychoanalytic contributions to the problems of children of survivors from Nazi-persecution. *Israel Journal of Psychiatry and Related Disciplines, 10,* 310–325.

Krystal, H. (Ed.) (1968). *Massive Psychic Trauma.* New York: International Universities Press.

Last, U., & Klein, H. (1984). Impact of parental Holocaust traumatization of offsprings' reports of parental child-rearing practices. *Journal of Youth and Adolescence, 13*(4), 267–283.

Leon, G. R., Butcher, J. N., Kleinman, M., Goldberg, A., & Almagor, M. (1981). Survivors of the Holocaust and their children: Current status and adjustment. *Journal of Personality and Social Psychology, 41,* 503–516.

Mahler, M. S. (1975). *The psychological birth of the human infant.* New York: Basic Books.

Musaph, H. (1978). De tweede generatie oorlogsslachtoffers: Psychopathologische problemen [The second generation war victims: Psychopathologic problems]. *Maandblad Geestelijke Volksgezondheid, 33*(12), 847–859.

Op den Velde, W., Koerselman, G. F., & Aarts, P. G. H. (1994). Countertransference and Dutch war victims. J. P. Wilson & J. D. Lindy (Eds.), *Countertransference in the treatment of PTSD* (pp. 308–327). New York: Guilford.

Potts, M. K. (1994). Long-term effects of trauma: Post-traumatic stress among civilian internees of the Japanese during World War II. *Journal of Clinical Psychology, 50,* 681–698.

Sigal, J. J., & Weinfield, M. (1989). *Trauma and rebirth.* New York: Praeger.

Solkoff, N. (1981). Children of survivors of the Nazi Holocaust: A critical review of the literature. *American Journal of Orthopsychiatry, 51,* 29–41.

Stevens, T. (1991). Indo-Europeanen in Nederlans-Indië: Sociale positie en welvaarts ontwikkeling [Indo-Europeans in the Dutch East Indies]. In P. J. Drooglever (Ed.), *Indisch Intermezzo: Geschiedenis van de Nederlanders in Indonesië* (pp. 33–46). Amsterdam: De Bataafse Leeuw.

Van der Velden, P. G., Eland, J., & Kleber, R. J. (1994). *De Indische na-oorlogse generatie* [The Indian second generation]. Houten: Bohn Stafleu Van Loghum.

Van Waterford, W. F. (1994). *Prisoners of the Japanese in World War II.* Jefferson, NC, London: McFarland & Company.

III

Genocide

12

The Turkish Genocide of the Armenians

Continuing Effects on Survivors and Their Families Eight Decades after Massive Trauma

DIANE KUPELIAN, ANIE SANENTZ KALAYJIAN,
and ALICE KASSABIAN

INTRODUCTION

This chapter will introduce to the psychological literature a traumatized group that is little known, although its story is 80 years old. When this group, the Armenians, first emerged from its catastrophic trauma after World War I, psychology was in its infancy. Moreover, there was no impetus for collecting this group's personal data, in contrast to the reparations requirements that produced much of the early literature on Holocaust survivors.

The story of the Armenians is not well known and will be summarized here. The descendants of the survivors have only recently turned to conducting studies relevant to understanding intergenerational issues. Two such studies are presented here, followed by two illustrative case studies.

THE HISTORY OF PERSECUTION

Eight decades ago, the Turkish government decided to kill or expel all members of an indigenous minority group. In 1915, under cover of World War I, Turkish armed forces systematically moved to exterminate Turkey's Armenian population.[1] By 1916, German officials

[1] For scholarly and historical discussions, see, for example, Boyajian (1972), Dadrian (1995), Hovannisian (1967), Kuper (1981), Melson (1992), and Simpson (1993). For collections of official papers and eyewitness reports from the World War I era, see, for example, Adalian (1985, 1991–1993), Bryce (1916), Dadrian (1991), Davis (1989), Morganthau (1975a), Toynbee (1916), and Sarafian (1993).

DIANE KUPELIAN • 1545 18th Street, N.W., Washington, D.C. 20036   ANIE SANENTZ KALAYJIAN • Department of Psychology, Fordham University, 113 West 60th Street, New York, New York 10023-7472; Private Practice, 130 West 79th Street, New York, NY 10024   ALICE KASSABIAN • School of Social Work, Virginia Commonwealth University, Arlington, Virginia 22201; Private Practice, 133 Maple Avenue East, Suite 306, Vienna, Virginia 22180.

International Handbook of Multigenerational Legacies of Trauma, edited by Yael Danieli. Plenum Press, New York, 1998.

191

stationed in Turkey reported that the campaign had killed 1.5 million Armenians, including 98% of the Armenian male population and 80–90% of the total Armenian population of Turkey (compiled in English in Dadrian, 1994a). These estimates did not count survivors driven out of Turkey or the victims of further massacres that occurred up to 1923 under the founders of the current Turkish government (Horowitz, 1980).

The Turkish government of that time hid this genocide as much as possible, and its successor has steadily denied it since, with a disinformation effort that has grown progressively more forceful, sophisticated, and public in recent years.[2] Lacking an accounting akin to the Nuremburg trials, the genocide and its continuing nonacknowledgment have become double assaults confronting Armenian survivors and their descendants.

Historical Background

Armenia is an ancient nation. Armenians continually occupied the region of historic Armenia, including what is now northeastern Turkey, from before 500 B.C. until their virtual annihilation in 1915 (Walker, 1991). Armenia was the first nation to accept Christianity as its state religion in A.D. 301.

Conquered by Turkic invaders from the east, Armenia was one of many nations made subject by what was eventually consolidated as the Ottoman Empire. The Turks considered this non-Muslim minority of Armenians as second-class citizens and for centuries subjected them to legal repression. For example, Armenians and other Christians had to pay special taxes, including child levies (Housepian, 1971; Hovannisian, 1985; Reid, 1984), and had to give Muslims and their herds free room and board for up to 6 months under the "hospitality taxes" (Housepian, 1971). In some areas, Armenians were barred from speaking Armenian except when praying (Hovannisian, 1985), and some localities punished public Armenian speaking by cutting out tongues (Housepian, 1971).[3] Armenians were subject to forced migration, enslavement (Reid, 1984), and repeated massacres (e.g., Dadrian, 1995; Lidgett, 1897). Armenians were also barred from giving legal testimony or bearing arms, leaving them no legal recourse or self-defense against gun-bearing Muslim neighbors (Hovannisian, 1985; Kalfaian, 1982).

Ottoman imperial expansion led to periods of relative peace and prosperity for the subject populations. But as the empire began to decline, persecutions of all the various minorities increased. A particularly severe series of massacres occurred during 1895–1896, in which 100,000–200,000 Armenians were killed or driven out of the Armenian provinces (Dadrian, 1995; Lidgett, 1897). In 1909, there were renewed massacres of approximately 30,000 Armenians and other Christians (Boyajian, 1972; Dadrian, 1995).

The Ottoman Empire shrank rapidly as scores of independent nations broke free. The Turkish government was determined to unify the empire's remnants, which they now considered Turkish heartland, as a homogeneous, Turkish-speaking population of Turkic peoples.[4] They decided to eliminate the Armenians (Dadrian, 1994b) and began doing so in April 1915.

---

[2]For a typology and annotated bibliography of Turkish historical revisionism, see Adalian (1992); for discussions of Turkish patterns of denial, see, for example, Charny (1993), Dobkin (1984), Gunter (1993), Guroian (1988), Hovannisian (1988), Melson (1992), Minasian (1986–1987), Papazian (1993), and Simpson (1993); for instances of Turkish governmental pressure, see, for example, Boven (1985), Charny (1983), Cohen (1983), Miller (1990), and Smith, Markusen, and Lifton (1995).

[3]When the first author interviewed elderly Armenians in 1992, several spontaneously mentioned that as children in pregenocide Turkey, they had known Armenian men in their villages whose tongues had been so cut out.

[4]See, for example, Dekmejian (1988), Hovannisian (1985), Libaridian (1985), and Melson (1992).

The regime carefully controlled the effort.[5] It removed any possibility of defense or leadership from the Armenian population by disarming and killing all Armenian men in the Turkish army and arresting and killing all current or potential community leaders, including the intelligentsia, religious leaders, merchants, and civil servants. The remaining men were then rounded up and killed.

The women, children, and elderly were either forced into slavery or onto death marches, and they were frequently attacked by specially organized gangs. They were often held without food for days before the march began, so that they would be too weak to escape (German missionary quoted in Morganthau, 1975b), and forced to march on the most circuitous, difficult paths, to maximize attrition through exhaustion (e.g., German eyewitness report in Hoffman, 1985). They were deliberately refused water (e.g., Barton, 1918) and had to buy or scrounge food. Many subsisted on grass. In some areas, Greeks, Jews, and other non-Turkic groups were also forced onto death marches along with the Armenians (Simpson, 1993).

A German missionary in Turkey recorded typical eyewitness reports of German railway engineers (Hoffman, 1985, p. 77). One reported "corpses of violated women, lying about naked in heaps on railway embankment[s] . . . with clubs pushed up their anus." Another saw "Turks tie Armenian men together, fire several volleys of small shot . . . and go off laughing, while their victims perished. . . . Other men had their hands tied behind their backs and were rolled down steep cliffs" to be slashed at by women with knives. He added that a German Consul told him that he had seen so many severed children's hands lying on a road that he could have paved the road with them. At the German hospital at Urfa, he knew of a little girl who had both her hands hacked off.

Survival rates from the marches were very low. For example, German eyewitnesses reported that out of 19,900 Armenians from the three towns of Sivas, Kharput, and Erzerum, only 361 reached the last stop before being driven into the desert, with unknown result (Dobkin, 1984). Writing in 1988, Kuper states, "Thus ends the Armenian presence in Turkey, reduced from a population of about 2 million to less than 25,000 at the present time" (p. 52).[6]

ARMENIANS IN DIASPORA

The remnants of the Armenians were scattered throughout the globe after World War I, to whatever countries would accept refugees. Outside the Middle East or Russian Armenia, these refugees were often the first and only Armenians, and even there, the preexisting community's resources were vastly overwhelmed by the survivors' extraordinary destitution. The severely traumatized, utterly impoverished refugees were on their own in foreign lands, among people who often knew nothing about them.

In the United States, these new immigrants frequently settled in tight-knit ethnic urban communities (Mirak, 1983). Their world was starkly split between the outside world of strangers and their inner, shared world of intimate community. Social gatherings often concluded with the survivor generation's talk of the genocide, accompanied by quiet weeping and consoling. This central emotional fact of life was essentially unknown by outsiders.

[5]This overview is taken largely from the summary in Kuper (1981, pp. 101–119).
[6]This number does not, however, account for the descendants of the thousands of Armenian women, girls, and small children forced into Turkish households as slaves or family members. Many thousands of their descendants are now passing as Turks in Turkey. It is a question whether they know, or are willing to disclose, their identity. The effect on them is unknown, and it may not ever be possible to learn what it has been like for these part-Armenian people to live as members of the group that exterminated their mothers' forebears.

The traumatized remnants of the Armenian people were swept up with everyone else by the Great Depression and the new horrors of World War II, which relegated the Armenian genocide to historical obscurity. Frequent nonrecognition of their plight surrounded Armenians with an experience of indifference and disregard.

TRAUMATIC AFTEREFFECTS

The historical situations culminating in the genocide of the Armenians and the destruction of the Jews resemble one another (Melson, 1992). So do the reactions of the survivors (Boyajian & Grigorian, 1982, 1988; Salerian, 1982).[7] Although some details differ, both groups were targeted because of their birth membership in a despised group. The level of obliterating massive trauma and the deeply personal nature of the persecutors' hatred has made for parallels in the reaction of survivors and their families.

Boyajian and Grigorian (1982), in their study of psychosocial sequelae of the genocide, found symptoms among Armenian survivors that are similar to those of Holocaust survivors, including anxiety, depression, compulsive associations to trauma-related material, guilt, nightmares, irritability, anhedonia, emptiness, and a fear of loving. Salerian (1982) adds phobias, psychosomatic disorders, and severe personality changes. Boyajian and Grigorian's subsequent (1988) study of Armenian survivors, their second-generation children, and third-generation grandchildren, concludes that most participants experienced anxiety, anger, frustration, and guilt. Second-generation participants reported manifestations of anxiety in association with extreme parental overprotectiveness. Anger and frustration for all generations were associated with modern Turkey's denial of the genocide and other governments' tolerance of that denial. One participant, a self-described pacifist, was concerned because his 11-year-old son verbalized angry, militant ideas, and vengeful feelings.

Cultural differences, however, may give rise to some varied responses in the two victim groups. For example, survivor guilt has been described as a major manifestation of the survivor syndrome among Jewish Holocaust survivors (Krystal & Niederland, 1968; Niederland, 1981). Danieli (1988) has described various defensive and coping functions of survivor guilt for this population, including a commemorative function. In this function, guilt serves to maintain a connection and a bridge of loyalty to those who perished and to metaphorically provide the respectful regard of a cemetery that these victims were denied.

However, this guilt experience may not have a parallel among Armenians. For example, a comparison of Armenian and Jewish literary responses to these two genocides noted that the sense of remorseful guilt in some Jewish writings is largely absent from Armenian literature (Peroomian, 1993). In Boyajian and Grigorian's sample, the respondents' guilt was associated with duties to the living (i.e., not having done enough for the Armenian community) and, among the second generation, not having done enough for their survivor parents. The commemorative function of guilt may not be as imperative or culturally supported among Armenians on a personal level because of their Christian belief in the afterlife. The psychological function of commemoration may be adequately served on a community level by the Church service of commemoration for the genocide victims. Also, Turkey's active, ongoing denial of

---

[7]The authors know of only four other psychological studies of Armenian genocide survivors in the English language: Kalayjian *et al.* (1996), and Sarkissian (1984), two studies of coping in Armenian survivors; Kupelian (1993), an assessment of PTSD symptomatology and general adjustment in Armenian survivors; and Miller and Miller (1993), an oral-history project based on 100 survivor interviews, which offers a very thoughtful and sensitively described typology of responses by the authors who are not mental health professionals.

their victimization may have created an abiding anger that overshadows any experience of guilt for surviving and prospering.

However, another factor may be parallel on the individual level but different on the community level. Regarding Jewish Holocaust survivors, Danieli (1982, 1984, 1989) has described the effect of the "conspiracy of silence" between survivors and those who did not go through the Holocaust: the tacit but strongly motivated agreement to avoid acknowledging the Holocaust experience because it was simply too overwhelming to face. Such avoidance left Holocaust survivors profoundly rebuffed, alienated, and mistrustful. It sustained their silence, and impeded their ability to mourn, integrate, and heal; it helped to isolate them from others, including other Jews who had not shared their experience.

The silence for the Armenians differed in one important regard. It came from outside the community. The silence did not tend to create a chasm within the Armenian community, because the genocide had affected virtually all Armenians. The silence, particularly as time passed, existed because the story had simply faded for most non-Armenians, not because of any tacit agreement to avoid a known source of overwhelming pain.

Nonetheless, the effect of nonacknowledgment from the outside world on individual Armenian genocide survivors was very similar; they felt alienated and dishonored, their sufferings pointless. The effect of silence from outside sustained an additional sense of obliterating invalidation for survivors and the entire Armenian community. It was not only the survivors' ability to mourn, integrate, and heal that was impeded, but it was also impeded for their progeny. Some Armenians clung more tenaciously to their brethren in the face of this external lack of acknowledgment; others melted into assimilation. However they reacted to the silence, all Armenians were faced with an additional emotional and psychological burden.

Boyajian and Grigorian speculate that the major divergence in the experience of Holocaust and Armenian genocide survivors—the fact that the world is well aware of one and largely oblivious to the other—has intruded on the experience of an Armenian identity for all Armenians since the genocide. This intrusion has forced Armenians to cope with Turkish hatred not only in the form of the genocide, but also in the form of trivializing and denigrating the survivors and their families by denying their victimization. They view the Turkish denial of the historical fact of the genocide as a psychological continuation of the genocide, and a second, continuing victimization. The purpose of genocide is to eradicate a people and a culture from the face of the earth; to deny their pain is to deny their humanity, and it psychologically serves the genocidal purpose.

THE ARMENIAN FAMILY IN THE POSTGENOCIDE AMERICAN DIASPORA

While Boyajian and Grigorian recognized the potential destructive power of the invalidating nonrecognition of trauma from without on the individual's experience of Armenianness, the potential supportive power from within the Armenian community and family was recognized and investigated in another study.

In 1987, Kassabian completed a three-generation exploratory study of survivor families that focused primarily on Armenian ethnic identity. It included grandparents who survived the genocide as children before coming to the United States and their U.S.-born adult children and grandchildren. The objective was to study, in the context of the massive loss of the survivor generation, the level of Armenian ethnic identity for each generation (the independent variable) and to relate that level to the dependent variables of Armenian family structure, family congruence (degree of agreement on perceived family environment), and Armenian community cohesion.

The Measured Constructs

Armenian Ethnic Identity.   The concept of Armenian ethnic identity should be understood in the context of centuries of repression. The sense of ethnic identity, formed over centuries and internalized by the survivors, formed the basis of what they transmitted to their progeny.

Several factors historically supported a coherent and persistent sense of Armenian ethnic identity within the Ottoman context. First, the Armenians' ancient origins and the preservation of their historic territory until World War I gave them a sense that they knew who they were in their own homeland. Second, the Armenian language, a unique early branch from the Indo-European root, is distinct from that of surrounding peoples. Third, the unique Armenian church, the first to separate theologically, has remained a central cultural unifying factor for almost 2,000 years. Fourth, the Millet system, the Ottoman administrative system of classifying non-Muslim communities by their religion, created a social distance between the subject minorities and the ruling Ottoman and strengthened the ethnocentrism of the various minority ethnic groups, ultimately supporting the effects of the three aforementioned factors on Armenian ethnic identity (Atamian, 1955).

Armenian Family Structure.   The historical forces that maintained the sense of Armenian ethnic identity also affected the pregenocide Armenian family structure, which was formed through generations of family interactions in adaptation to historical conditions of oppression. This structure was internalized in the person through family relationships and came with the survivors into the diaspora.

Ackerman posits that "[a] family is intensely affected by either a friendly and supportive environment or by a hostile and dangerous one. . . . A social environment that imposes danger may cause a family to either crumble or react by strengthening its solidarity" (1958, p. 15). From research based on the recall of Armenian survivors, we learn that the Armenian family was organized into multigenerational communal groups of often more than 30 people living under one roof (Atamian, 1949; Kalfaian, 1982; Mazian, 1983; Villa & Matossian, 1982). These groupings were patriarchal, patrilineal, and patrilocal, and provided the individual's central core of values. Each individual received protection and definition from the patriarch's leadership and authority, for which he or she returned loyalty and cooperation. The individual's interest was subordinated to the common family goal (Atamian, 1955; Villa & Matossian, 1982).

The organization of the patriarchal *gerdastan* (extended family) was necessary for the Armenian family's survival. It provided some shielding against periodic raids and persecutions, and assured that some family group would remain. The Armenian family structure was also necessary for the Armenian individual's survival, as these communal groups were the only available method to maximize the likelihood of a given individual's surviving. Chaliand and Ternon (1983) describe the Armenian family as a "closed cell" that made survival possible in the presence of a permanent lack of security. In the wake of massacres, the family would withdraw into itself and heal as best it could. The periodic massacres amplified the social distance from the Turks, and this very social distance maintained the unique Armenian identity and family organization.

Armenian Family Congruence. The pregenocide Armenian *gerdastan* reflected the family's perception of the social environment: For Armenian families to have survived in the hostile environment, they needed a close-knit network of kin in which there was a high level of compliance regarding values and norms. They had to share fundamental beliefs and values that would translate into cooperation regarding basic family survival and life. This expectation of family interdependence, cohesion, and primacy of the family group is the template survivors brought to the New World.

Community Cohesion. Upon reaching the United States, Armenians quickly established formal and informal means for transmitting ethnic identity (Atamian, 1955; Kernaklian, 1967; Malcolm, 1919; Tashjian, 1947; Warner & Srole, 1945). Informal means included ethnically oriented family socialization (e.g., food, stories, songs, friends, and speaking Armenian). Formal means included founding organizations that are educational, religious, political, cultural, and charitable. The Armenian church was central: "[it] linked the widely scattered Armenians to their long and troubled past, their homeland, their language, their literature and their faith. It provided the Armenian-Americans with the centuries-long function of the church: the preservation of the culture from assimilation" (Mirak, 1983, p. 180).

The Measurements

Kassabian used six instruments. She constructed three for the interviews,[8] adapting much from studies of Holocaust survivors and other ethnic groups. To confirm trauma level, she used the Massive Traumatic Loss Scale, a structured interview with the survivor generation. To measure Armenian ethnic identity, she used the Armenian Identity Scale, a measure of attitude, to assess the centrality of social and family relationships and language maintenance to a sense of Armenian identity, and the Armenian Activities Scale, a behavioral scale, to assess the frequency of selected ethnically oriented activities. She assessed the level of participation in both American and Armenian formal organizations (religious, educational, professional, social service, cultural, social, and political) by a self-report of participation.

The final two instruments were standardized scales. The Family Adaptability Cohesion Evaluation Scale, FACES II (Olson, Portner, & Bell, 1982), measures family adaptability, defined as the degree to which the family system is flexible and able to accommodate change, ranging from rigid to chaotic. The moderate or balanced range, a dimension of adaptability termed flexible–structured, depicts a viable range of healthy family structure. It also measures the family cohesion, defined as the emotional bonding between family members and the degree to which individuals are connected to or separated from their families, ranging from enmeshed to disengaged. As with adaptability, scores in the moderate balanced range of cohesion indicate the viable levels of family functioning.

The last scale, the Family Environment Scale (FES; Moos & Moos, 1981), measures the three primary dimensions of relationship, personal growth, and system maintenance within the family. It assesses the extent to which the family members of each generation perceive the family's social environment in similar terms.

Kassabian collected data from the survivors in face-to-face interviews. She hand-delivered or mailed self-report questionnaires to the second and third generations, which were filled out and returned via mail.

---

[8]The instruments, their development, and psychometric properties are available in Kassabian (1987). An additional instrument was constructed but not found useful, and is not reported on here.

Description of the Participants

The criteria for a family's inclusion were (1) that the survivor's child and grandchild were born and reared in the United States and (2) that there was at least one participant from each of three generations in one family. First, a survivor was located who would participate. The second-generation participant was usually the caretaking child, and then a third-generation family member who was willing to cooperate and at least 15 years old was included.

There were 22 survivors, 5 males and 17 females; 6 were married, 14 were widows, and 2 were widowers. Most (95.5%) were Armenian Apostolic, and 4.5% were Catholic. Their ages ranged from 72 to 88 years, with a mean of 78.7 years. In 1915, their ages had ranged from 3 to 19, with most (73%) between ages 6 and 13.

There were also 22 American-born second-generation respondents, 5 males and 17 females; 77.4% had married other adult children of survivors. A total of 86.4% had married within the ethnic group, while 13.5% had married non-Armenian spouses, and none were widowed or divorced. Their ages ranged from 43 to 62, with a mean of 51 years. Like their parents, 95.5% were Armenian Apostolic.

There were 28 third-generation respondents, 21 females and 7 males. Their ages ranged from 15 to 31, with a mean age of 22 years. Only 14.3% were married, 2 to Armenian spouses and 2 to non-Armenians. In this generation, 92.9% were Armenian Apostolic, 3.6% were American Protestant, and 3.6% indicated no religious affiliations.

Eleven other families were approached. Eight declined because the survivor did not want to discuss the genocide experience, one declined because the adult child of the survivor found the questionnaires intrusive, and one family declined without explanation. One family was disqualified because the grandchild would not cooperate.

Major Findings

Armenian Ethnic Identity. Armenian ethnic identity was operationalized by the Armenian Identity Scale and the Armenian Activities Scale, both of which were item-analyzed, emphasizing a qualitative analysis.

The three generations did not significantly differ in most attitudinal measures. These included the desire to maintain social contact in the Armenian community; to teach their children Armenian history, culture, and traditions; and, even among the third generation that largely had lost the Armenian language, to give their children Armenian language lessons. These results suggest that all three generations had a strong investment in their Armenian heritage.

However, the third generation differed from the older two generations on two items of the attitudinal measure. It reported a lower sense of belonging when in contact with other Armenians and a lower level of self-perceived Armenian identity than the two older generations. These results suggested that the third generation is more assimilated and may thus experience some sense of separation and loss.

The attitudinal measures indicate that the third generation feels a strong commitment to an Armenian ethnic identity. However, this generation's behavioral expression is different, as indicated by significant differences on virtually all items on the Armenian Activities Scale between the grandchildren and their older family members. The older generations' more traditional ethnic activities (cooking, listening to Armenian music, Armenian language activities, and regularly attending church services) are not part of the grandchildren's behavior. However, the three generations did not differ significantly in attending educational and cultural activities and certain particularly significant Church services. Although it did not worship regularly on

Sundays, Christmas, or Easter, the third generation marked important community life events with the most significant church rituals (baptisms, weddings, funerals, the annual church service commemorating the genocide, and an annual ritual mourning and memorial service for family and community members called the *Hokehankist*). This generation's greater commitment to the church's community function than to its theological, faith function suggests a deep commitment to the Armenian community.[9]

Family structure is conceptualized as having two central dimensions: adaptability and cohesion. The analyses indicated that the three generations were very similar in family structure.

Each of the three generations was in the structured–flexible range of adaptability, depicting a structured but flexible family functioning style. This style denotes a healthy functioning range. The scores reflect a moderate level of cohesion in each of the three generations. The moderate levels are the central balanced areas of cohesion hypothesized as the most viable for healthy family functioning, reflecting a balance of independence from families and connection to families. These findings indicate that the three generations have enough cohesion to develop a continuing attachment to their family of origin and to continue both a sense of ethnic identity and family structure. At the same time, cohesion must be moderate enough so that family members are not enmeshed in their family of origin and have enough energy for development of self and establishing their own families.

Family Congruence.   The degree of family congruence is an assessment of the extent to which the family members of each generation perceive the family's social environment in similar terms. No significant differences were found in the mean scores for family perception across the three generations, indicating that the three generations perceive the family environment similarly.

Armenian Community Cohesion.   Armenian community cohesion was defined as the level of participation in Armenian organizations. The first generation participated actively and exclusively in Armenian organizations. Those in the second generation met their expressive needs by participating in Armenian religious, social service, and cultural organizations more than American organizations serving the same purposes. Understandably, second-generation Armenians met their instrumental needs through American professional, educational, and political organizations, not Armenian ones.

Like their parents, the third generation followed the expected pattern of meeting expressive needs through Armenian organizations and meeting instrumental needs through American organizations. Surprisingly, their political activity differed. They were more active in Armenian political organizations than American ones. Responses to open-ended questions reveal that the impetus for this difference was largely due to the grandchildren's concern with addressing Turkey's continuing denial of the genocide and their expressed desire to "right the wrong."

Interpretation of Findings

A clear commitment to an Armenian ethnic identity continued throughout the generations, suggesting the family was able to protect and transmit that identity. The three generations shared a similar perception of the family environment, as indicated by the similar family congruence scores, suggesting that they share a mutual sense of values. The family structure

---

[9]Studies of American-born Armenian high school students, a cohort similar to Kassabian's third generation, have found similar trends of high self-reports of Armenian ethnic identity associated with frequent Armenian church and Armenian political activities, and low involvement in other traditional ethnic activities (Der-Karabetian, 1980).

scores indicate a balance of adaptability and cohesion. The adaptability affords the family the flexibility to accommodate extraordinary changes over the three generations, with optimal cohesion for keeping the family together. The sampled families were able to weather the genocide and acclimate to a new country. The community cohesion levels indicate that the community offered adequate support and responsiveness to sufficiently strengthen the family in transmitting a coherent Armenian ethnic identity.

While close-knit families are expected in ethnic family structure, the three generations' high degree of similarity was surprising. Their consistency in both the adaptability and the cohesion scores of the family structure measure stood out. It is congruent with historical descriptions of Armenian family coping strategies within the context of five centuries of Turkic persecutions. This hostile external environment reinforced close intra- and interfamily relationships conducive to survival, both physically and as a distinct people. The family structure maintained closeness and structured flexibility, a combination that offered stability and the capacity to integrate the genocide's catastrophic changes and to adapt to the immediate postgenocide period and beyond.

Theoretical hypotheses offered by Olson *et al.* (1982) and others (Beavers, 1977; Bowen, 1978; Lidz, 1960; Lidz, Cornelison, Fleck, & Terry, 1957; Minuchin, Montalvo, Guerney, Rossman, & Schumer, 1967; Reiss, 1971; Stierlin, 1974; Wynne, Ryckoff, Day, & Hirsch, 1958) conceptualized these constructs of adaptability and cohesion necessary for variable family functioning. Historical descriptions of the Armenian family's functioning throughout its turbulent existence indicate its survival strategies of "closing up" to the outside world to regroup and then "opening up" temporarily when the acute danger passed. These phenomena fit the conceptualizations proposed by the aforementioned theorists of healthy family functioning and show the balance of adaptability and stability needed for survival and growth.

To survive, the Armenian family had to have relied on its experience of what constituted danger or safety. When acting against hostile events, it recognized what was hopeless, reacted with a realistic appraisal of powerlessness, shut down affectively with an experience of depression, and withdrew. By the same token, it had the potential to renew interest in the world and act on opportunities when hostile events abated, as demonstrated in the third generation. The changed outward circumstance (the nonhostile U.S. environment) has removed its need for a depressed communal response.

The difference between the second and third generations in how the painful history is regarded is shown in the response to the open-ended question, "Do you feel different from other people because of the genocide experience of your parents/grandparents?" The second and third generation both answered "yes." One third-generation participant typified the determination "to identify in history the Turkish government of 1915 as the perpetrators of the Armenian genocide and the present Turkish government as an accomplice to the crime because of that government's refusal to admit the occurrence of the genocide and accept the responsibility for the brutal acts of its predecessor" (Kassabian, 1987, p. 143).

The second generation's responses lacked this insistence on Turkish accountability. Second-generation respondents expressed feelings of anger, loss for their homeland and family, immense pride that Armenian culture could not be extinguished, and determination to perpetuate Armenian heritage and culture. The first and second generations of the sample put a lifetime of effort into maintaining their group cohesion and thereby making it possible to transmit the sense of ethnic identity to younger generations. The third generation's effort is more externalized and differs from the second generation's more internalized response, which focused primarily on keeping the Armenian culture alive and strong. The reactions of the older generations reflected a historical paradigm of overt limitation by Ottoman society and the postgenocide chaos, eliciting an intensely private communal opposition and consolidation. The youngest generation's response is to a newer paradigm of American freedom and respect for human rights that allows for a more open appeal for redress of injustices.

Spicer (1971) has suggested that opposition is a primary factor in a persistent ethnic identity. Armenians perpetuated a distinct identity for centuries by adapting their family structure to a persecutory context. Functionally, the persecutory oppositional pressure (the recurring massacres up to the genocide) became an integral part of Armenian family structure and identity. Each generation in its own way opposed the intended effects of annihilation and unified the Armenian community to withstand those effects. By existing with an Armenian self-awareness, each family has transmitted this opposition from generation to generation. Ironically, the psychological continuation of the genocide, the active Turkish denial, has provided the psychological oppositional pressure that has maintained the effect of a persistent ethnic identity.

THIRD-GENERATION EFFECTS IN AN OLDER COHORT

Kassabian's third-generation cohort was two generations away from the 1915 genocide. A different starting point defined the third-generation cohort in the following study (Kupelian, 1993), when it was two generations away from massacres of the mid-1800s. Kupelian's study of Armenian genocide survivors[10] produced an unexpected finding within the control group concerning a subgroup of grandchildren of survivors of pregenocide massacres.

Description of Participants

In Kupelian's study, all subjects were Armenians born during the genocide period, (1923 or before) and were from a nonclinical, community population. When interviewed in 1992, the control group ranged between 70 and 90 years of age, with a mean of 75.75. While the control group (the only group discussed here) was of the same age range as the genocide survivors, they did not go through the genocide. Most came from families who had fled Turkey in the 1800s, after earlier massacres. There were 34 participants in the control group, 22 females and 12 males. They were 1 to 20 years old in 1923, at the end of the genocide.

Method and Analysis

Kupelian recorded the number of generations separating each control subject from their ancestor's direct experience of massacres in Turkey. Thirteen were one generation away (second-generation children), 10 were two generations away (third-generation grandchildren), and 11 were three or more generations away from massacres.

All participants were assessed for symptoms of posttraumatic stress disorder (PTSD) via the clinician-administered Structured Clinical Interview for DSM-III-R (SCID) PTSD module (Spitzer, Williams, Gibbon, & First, 1989). In addition, the following self-report measures were used to assess current adaptation: the Tennessee Self-Concept Scale (TSCS; Roid & Fitts, 1989), the Life Satisfaction Scale (LSI; Neugaraten, Havighurst, & Tobin, 1961), and the Brief Symptom Inventory (BSI; Derogatis & Melisaratos, 1983), which also screened for psychopathology.

A series of one-way analyses of variance (ANOVA) were conducted for each assessment scale listed here, using as the subject grouping factor the generational distance from massacres

[10]Due to space limitations, only those findings of this study relevant to intergenerational issues are presented here.

(one, two, or three or more generations removed). In all cases, where the ANOVA was significant, appropriate contrasts were used to examine the difference in means.

Results and Discussion

The 10 grandchildren of survivors from pregenocide massacres scored significantly higher on several measures than other control subjects (those one generation away, and those three or more generations away). They scored significantly higher on the following: all three of the global BSI scales (the Positive Symptom Total indicating the number of symptoms endorsed, the Positive Symptom Distress Index indicating the degree of distress reported, and the General Severity Index indicating the overall pathology score), and also on the items of the SCID assessing symptoms of increased arousal. They also registered the highest self-esteem on the TSCS global measure.

The third generation's BSI scores indicate that they self-report an experience of more distress from a greater number of symptoms, and their SCID scores may suggest somatization. This nonclinical population also scored higher on the self-esteem measure, indicating that although they endorse and were observed to exhibit more symptomatology, they nonetheless indicate they feel better about themselves.

The third generation unexpectedly registered more pathology than the second generation. A potential explanation for this counterintutitional finding may involve two important situational factors: (1) the relatively small amount of social support available to the grandparents who left Turkey, and to the families they had in the new country; and most importantly (2) the occurrence of the genocide during the childhood of the third generation in this study, a historical fact that must have been a devastating emotional blow to every Armenian already in diaspora. Virtually all of them still had family in Turkey.

When the grandparents arrived in the United States in the late 1800s, the very few other Armenians in America tended to congregate in small communities. The devastating traumas the grandparents had endured were generally unknown by non-Armenians outside of Turkey. These immigrants may have found trusting non-Armenians difficult after so many generations of crushing persecution from a majority culture. The small Armenian communities would probably have provided any validating support and solace the immigrants could have received.

The third-generation Armenians in this study were children during the time of the Armenian genocide and observed that cataclysm from safety. What must it have been like for those children and their families to watch helplessly the virtual destruction of their kind in their homeland? For all Armenians, the certainty that every single person in their ethnic group was despised and desired dead may have been a significant narcissistic blow. Their parents, especially, would have confronted several difficult pressures. The parents would certainly have been acutely sensitive to this catastrophic repetition of their own parents' experience. The genocide may have exacerbated whatever past painful experience the parents had or knew about in their own family history. They may have lost their last hopes of returning to the homeland. Most painfully, they probably knew relatives were going through the death marches.

The presumably intense reactions to these pressures, whatever form those reactions took, may have affected family interactions and the ability of the stressed parents to cushion the children's emotional distress. The hypothesized emotional pressures on the entire family observing the genocide during the childhood of this third-generation cohort may be related to their observed scores. The presumed emotional pressures experienced during their childhood may have left this group more vulnerable and reactive to pain, reflected in their higher pathology scores. If they drew meaning from this pain and took pride in their continued existence as Armenians, then that may be related to their higher self-esteem scores. Ongoing research is investigating whether this unexpected finding in a small sample replicates in a larger sample of the same cohort. As the generations proceed from the 1915–1923 genocide and earlier massacres, many changes, both inside and outside the Armenian community and family, affect the manifestation of the elder generation's trauma in its children and grandchildren.

INTERGENERATIONAL EFFECTS OF TRAUMA

Some, but not all, children of severely traumatized Holocaust survivors suffer pathological consequences (e.g., Davidson, 1980; Kestenberg, 1972; Klein, 1971; Krell, 1982; Steinberg, 1989). Intergenerational consequences may be the most accurate term (Albeck, 1994), recognizing the widely varying situational factors, survivor reactions, and the responses of succeeding generations to their family history. For survivors' children, a crucial factor is the degree to which the meaning of the trauma has been integrated into the family's emotional life.* Lifton (1969) has suggested using a structured, psychohistorical interview with this population to elicit information it might not otherwise perceive as salient. Kalayjian, Shahinian, Gergerian, and Saraydarian (1996) found two variables unique to the Armenian survivor community: (1) the meaning construed by the individual of the profoundly invalidating experience of the denial of the genocide by Turkey, and (2) the degree of the family's involvement in the Armenian community.

For those survivor's children who do suffer pathological consequences, a heuristic explanation of intergenerational effects in the cause of Holocaust survivor's children describes behaviors of these children as (1) originating dynamically either in symbolic relationship to their parents' trauma, or (2) as shaped by their parents' trauma-related pathogenic behaviors (Danieli, 1988). The two following cases reported by Kalayjian, illustrate these points in relation to Armenian families.

CASE STUDIES OF AMERICAN-BORN
SECOND-GENERATION ARMENIANS

The first case study demonstrates that in a family where catastrophic loss has been suffered with very little apparent integration of the trauma, separation–individuation would be experienced as a crisis and another overwhelming loss, resulting in an enmeshed family. This is an example of a child's reaction to the parent's trauma-related pathogenic behavior (Danieli, 1988).

Ms. S., a 44-year-old U.S.-born only child, had a masters degree and a responsible position. She came for treatment after suffering intolerable rejection when her boyfriend excluded her from a professional activity. She had moved out of her parents' home in her late 30s to live with him, and although deeply wounded by his autonomy, did not break off the relationship. The treatment quickly focused on her difficulty separating from her parents.

It took several sessions to elicit the fact that her father was a death march survivor, because she viewed events of nearly eight decades before as irrelevant to her life. This suggests a difficulty in her family in recognizing, articulating, and tolerating affects.

Ms. S. described her father, aged 83 and a shoemaker, as a workaholic who refused to retire, and who never stopped. Her father was 12 when the genocide began. Turkish gendarmes arrested

---

*After the manuscript of this chapter was completed, a chapter by Dagirmanjian (1996) came to our attention that offers a psychocultural description of the Armenian community, and further illustrates the importance of the construed meaning of the trauma in the family's life.

his father in the middle of the night, and he never returned. Ms. S.'s father and his family of eight were forced onto a death march, from which only he and his mother survived. Ms. S. knew little of his genocide experience because he rarely talked about it without becoming tearful and overwhelmed by emotion, which he found intolerable.

Ms. S.'s mother, age 69, was born in a Syrian refugee camp to parents who had survived months of forced marches through the desert. She told her daughter few details of her parents' genocide story. When Ms. S. entered puberty, her mother had begun to suffer asthma attacks when distressed. Like her husband, Ms. S.'s mother was extremely involved in the social network of the local Armenian community.

Ms. S.'s mother was the eldest child. Clinical reports indicate that the eldest child born to Holocaust survivor parents shortly after the trauma in displaced persons camps was often severely affected (Danieli, 1982; Freyberg, 1980; Grubrich-Simitis, 1981; Russell, 1974). In this case, the mother's somaticized style suggests that she had difficulty perceiving her own affect consciously and in the verbal realm, her feelings did not become symbolically articulated (Krystal, 1988; Stolorow & Atwood, 1992). She may have lacked early validating responsiveness, which is very possible with two recently highly traumatized parents. If she never learned to translate affect experienced first as physical sensation into the cognitive and verbal realm, she cannot be expected to have helped her daughter make this translation successfully.

Her father's obsessive defense warded off intolerable affect. His manifest reaction to his own genocide story, avoiding it or being overwhelmed by it, suggests that he communicated an inability to tolerate the range of affect he needed to confront in order to integrate his trauma. A child who perceives that a parent cannot tolerate certain affects will stop experiencing and expressing those affects to protect the bond with that parent. In a family with a tenuous translation of affect from the physical to the verbal realm, the alienating effects of this translation will further attenuate it for that child (Stolorow & Atwood, 1992). Ms. S. would thus be unable to know or regulate her feelings.

Based on Ms. S.'s description, her family resembled the closed system with few internal boundaries of the *victim family* (Danieli, 1985). For example, her mother freely went through Ms. S.'s personal mail and belongings, and whenever Ms. S. objected, her mother acted surprised and hurt. This engendered anger and guilt in Ms. S., in a stable pattern of intrusion and ineffectual resentment. Her mother's constant worry, depression, and clinging exemplified the family atmosphere.

The norm that "No one outside the family could be trusted" had ingrained a distrust into Ms. S., which maintained a strong familial overinvolvement and impeded her from establishing meaningful outside relationships. Ms. S. had long reciprocated overinvolvement and overprotectiveness. Her parents' mediator, she often came home from school early as an adolescent to ensure that her parents did not fight and that her mother did not have what the daughter feared might be a potentially fatal asthma attack.

Ms. S. worked obsessively like her father to "get ahead" and somaticized like her mother (emotional distress triggered severe menstrual cramps and migraines, with no apparent medical cause). She did not have the insight to recognize parallels with her parents' defensive styles.

When Ms. S. tried to separate, her mother reacted with asthma attacks and guilt-inducing remarks. Her father tried to shame her into compliance by asking, "What would the Armenian community, our relatives, and friends say?" Ms. S. responded with immobilizing guilt, and the family's enmeshment was effectively maintained, a dynamic she brought to her relationship with her boyfriend.

The second case illustrates the sensitivity to invalidation in a case of PTSD, which echoes the ultimate invalidation the survivor parent suffers from Turkish denial. This case, in which the daughter echoes in her symptom picture the repeating affront of profoundly devaluing denial that all Armenians struggle against, is an example of a child manifesting symptomatology that is in symbolic relationship to the parents' traumatic experience (Danieli, 1988).

Ms. M. was a 42-year-old U.S.-born woman with a graduate degree and professional occupation. Ms. M. came for treatment after being severely traumatized in a car accident. She had nightmares that she could not recall and woke up with symptoms of a panic attack. She also had flashbacks, difficulty concentrating, and angry emotional outbursts that were uncharacteristic of her premorbid functioning. Her appetite decreased markedly, and she lost 10 pounds in less than 2 weeks.

Ms. M. had suffered another traumatic car accident 5 years earlier, which she said "was just like this one," although the situations were quite different. The similarity she perceived was in the lack of validation. According to Ms. M., she had not been at fault in either incident. However, her accounts of the events were disputed by the other drivers; therefore the police and insurance agents also challenged her accounts of both incidents. While she had not been clearly ruled against in either case, the authorities had divided the responsibility and settlements to avoid protracted investigation.

She believed the other drivers' claims were inaccurate and felt wronged by what she interpreted as a lack of vindication. Undoubtedly suffering from PTSD, she nonetheless reported that the most painful aspect was the indifference of and invalidation by the insurance agents and police officers who were traumatizing her "all over again." She saw parallels with a robbery 10 years earlier, when she interrupted a thief in her apartment. Although he stole her heirloom jewelry, the trauma to her was the indifference of the police. As she repeatedly went through mug shots, she experienced their jaded lack of sympathy as intolerable invalidation and an uncaring abandonment of her.

Ms. M. believed it was critical that the fact of victimization be confronted and the story be known, understood, and honored. This belief echoed her interest in her mother's extreme genocide experience and reaction to the Turkish denial. Ms. M.'s maternal grandfather was one of the first intellectuals rounded up in 1915. Her mother's 40-person *gerdastan* was forced onto a death march. Ms. M.'s mother, then a 10-year-old girl, saw most of them murdered, including her pregnant mother, who had collapsed and had told her daughter to leave her there and to take care of her six younger siblings. Turkish gendarmes then cut out and killed the infant before murdering the mother, while cursing her with racial epithets. Mrs. M.'s mother continued the march but could not save her siblings. Four died. Two were taken by Kurdish villagers. At the end of the death march, American missionaries took Ms. M.'s mother to an orphanage in Lebanon.

Ms. M.'s father had come to the United States before World War I. When he learned his second cousin (Ms. M.'s mother-to-be) had survived the genocide, he offered to marry her. He felt fortunate to have escaped the genocide but also guilty for not staying behind to help his relatives.

Although her mother rarely spoke of her experience, Ms. M. concentrated on reconstructing her mother's genocide story from her mother's notes in the family Bible, and stories told by other relatives. Her mother confirmed her research, but did not add much. Ms. M. also became extremely knowledgeable about the genocide and conducted surveys on that topic in the Armenian community.

A critical motivating theme that ran through Ms. M.'s family was the painful issue of coping with the Turkish denial. The entire family was active in the Armenian community and participated in all genocide commemorations. Ms. M.'s need to learn and validate the story was in the context of that story's intentional denial.

Ms. M. associated the Turkish denial, perceived as a second and continuing attempt at obliteration, to her experiences of invalidation respecting the car accidents and robbery. Invalidation meant that someone had gotten away with a horrendous act, and that the victim's survival was not valued, respected, cared about, or even much noticed. She felt such invalidation repudiated the victims' right to exist. Ms. M. clung to an underlying fantasy of a just world and emotionally railed at injustice and at nonacknowledgment of victimization. Her reactions were deeply rooted in her parents' experience of invalidation by the world for the devastating traumas they endured.

CONCLUSION

A history of persecution, genocide, and exile reverberates in the Armenian family. Much of what has been found in the literature on Holocaust survivors applies also to Armenian survivors, despite some cultural and situational differences (e.g., as noted earlier regarding the experience of survivor guilt). Clearly, more research, beyond the exploratory work presented here, is needed to more fully delineate the unique qualities of the Armenian experience. More studies would help not only in understanding the Armenian experience, but also in better understanding how differing cultural and situational factors affect traumatic responses.

The Armenian family adapted its structure to an ever-present oppositional pressure over centuries of persecution, and this oppositional pressure has become a habitual presence in the formation of the individual Armenian's ethnic identity. Currently, Turkish denial of the genocide psychologically continues the historic persecutions.

The rage and stress created by Turkey's denial, and the widespread acquiescence to that denial, has interfered with the ability of the survivors, their children, and grandchildren to mourn, process, and integrate their deeply painful history. According to Sullivan (1953), validation of a traumatic experience is an essential step toward resolution and closure. In addition, a perpetrator's explicit expression of acknowledgment and remorse has enormous value in healing the victim (Montville, 1987). Obviously, such healing has not taken place for these survivors.

The struggle for victims and the generations who proceed from them is to defy the dominance of evil and find a way to restore a sense of justice and compassion to the world. It adds to the pain, to know that so much more pain came after the Armenian genocide, and could have been stopped, but was not. It was not stopped because justice was not done for the Armenians, and Hitler saw that and learned the lesson of audacity and the permission of indifference. Survivors of great injustices feel a need to bear witness, to speak the truth, to keep it from happening again. But Armenians cannot say "never again" because it did happen again, and when it did, it was modeled on the Armenian genocide. Hitler has been quoted twice (Bardakjian, 1985; Loftus, 1993) as noting how effectively, with what impunity, and with what universal indifference the Armenians were exterminated. When the extermination of the Armenians was made negligible, the exterminations of the Holocaust were made possible.

ACKNOWLEDGMENTS: The first author is deeply grateful to Ms. Sonia Crowe, Mr. Pierre Richard, to Drs. Rouben Adalian, Levon Boyajian, Kenneth Lutterman, and Alen Salarian for their close reading of drafts of this chapter and their many insightful and helpful comments.

REFERENCES

Ackerman, N. (1958). *Dynamics of family life.* New York: Basic Books.

Adalian, R. (Ed.). (1985). *The Armenian genocide and America's outcry: A compilation of U.S. documents, 1890–1923.* Washington, DC: Armenian Assembly of America.

Adalian, R. (Ed.). (1991–1993). *The Armenian Genocide in the U.S. Archives, 1915–1918.* Alexandria, VA: Chadwyck–Healey Microfiche.

Adalian, R. (1992). The Armenian genocide: Revisionism and denial. In M. N. Dobkowski & I. Wallimann (Eds.), *Genocide in our time: An annotated bibliography with analytical introductions* (pp. 85–106). Ann Arbor, MI: Pierian Press.

Albeck, J. H. (1994). Intergenerational consequences of trauma: Reframing traps in treatment theory—a second-generation perspective. In M. B. Williams & J. F. Sommer (Eds.), *Handbook of post-traumatic therapy* (pp. 106–125). Westport, CT: Greenwood Press.

Atamian, S. (1949, October 13). Traditional Armenian family of Turkish Armenia. *Hairenik Weekly,* pp. 4–5.

Atamian, S. (1955). *The Armenian community.* New York: Philosophical Library.

Bardakjian, K. (1985). *Hitler and the Armenian genocide.* Cambridge, MA: Zoryan Institute.

Barton, J. L. (1918). U.S. Inquiry Document No. 808. Atrocities, Turkish: American Board of Commissioners for Foreign Missions. Reprinted Spring 1984 in *Armenian Review, 37,* 164–202.

Beavers, W. (1977). *Psychotherapy and growth: A family systems perspective.* New York: Brunner/Mazel.

Boven, T. V. (1985). Paragraph 30: Note on the deleted reference to the massacre of the Armenians in the study on the question of the prevention and the punishment of the crime of genocide. In G. Libaridian (English language ed.), *A crime of silence: The Armenian genocide* (pp. 168–172). Bath, UK: Pitman Press.

Bowen, M. (1978). *Family therapy in clinical practice.* New York: Aronson.

Boyajian, D. H. (1972). *Armenia: The case for a forgotten genocide.* Westwood, NJ: Educational Book Crafters.

Boyajian, K., & Grigorian, H. (1982, June 20–24). *Sequelae of the Armenian genocide on survivors.* Paper presented at the International Conference on the Holocaust and Genocide, Tel Aviv, Israel.

Boyajian, K., & Grigorian, H. (1988). Psychological sequelae of the Armenian genocide. In R. G. Hovannisian (Ed.), *The Armenian genocide in perspective* (pp. 177–185). New Brunswick, NJ: Transaction Publishers.

Bryce, V. (1916). *The treatment of Armenians in the Ottoman Empire 1915–1916.* London: Sir Joseph Causton & Sons.

Chaliand, G., & Ternon, Y. (1983). *The Armenians: From genocide to resistance* (T. Benett, Trans.). London: Zed Press.

Charny, I. (1983). The Turks, Armenians, and Jews. In I. W. Charny & S. Davidson (Eds.), *The Book of the International Conference on the Holocaust and Genocide: Book One. The Conference Program and Crisis* (pp. 269–316). Tel Aviv: Institute of the International Conference on the Holocaust and Genocide.

Charny, I. (1993). A contribution to the psychology of denial of genocide: Denial as a celebration of destructiveness, an attempt to dominate the minds of men, and a "killing" of history. In *Genocide and human rights: Lessons from the Armenian experience* (pp. 289–306). Belmont, MA: Armenian Heritage Press. (A special issue of the *Journal of Armenian Studies, 4*(1 and 2).)

Cohen R. (1983, May 31). Killing truth. *Washington Post,* p. B1.

Dadrian, V. N. (1991). The documentation of the World War I Armenian massacres in the proceedings of the Turkish military tribunal. *International Journal of Middle East Studies, 23,* 549–576.

Dadrian, V. N. (1994a). Documentation of the Armenian genocide in German and Austrian sources. In I. W. Charny (Ed.), *The widening circle of genocide: A critical bibliographic review* (Vol. 3, pp. 77–125). New Brunswick, NJ: Transaction Publishers.

Dadrian, V. N. (1994b). The secret Young-Turk Ittihadist conference and the decision for the World War I genocide of the Armenians. *Journal of Political and Military Sociology, 22*(1), 173–202.

Dadrian, V. N. (1995). *The history of the Armenian genocide: Ethnic conflict from the Balkans to Anatolia to the Caucasus.* Providence, RI: Berghahn Books.

Dagirmanjian, S. (1996). Armenian families. In M. McGoldrick, J. Giordano, & J. K. Pearce (Eds.), *Ethnicity and Family Therapy* (2nd ed., pp. 376–391). New York: Guilford Press.

Danieli, Y. (1982). Families of survivors of the Nazi Holocaust: Some short- and long-term effects. In C. D. Spielberger & I. G. Sarason (Eds.), *Stress and anxiety* (Vol. 8, pp. 405–421). New York: Wiley.

Danieli, Y. (1983). Psychotherapists' participation in the conspiracy of silence about the Holocaust. *Psychoanalytic Psychology, 1*(1), 23–42.

Danieli, Y. (1985). The treatment and prevention of long-term effects and intergenerational transmission of victimization: A lesson from Holocaust survivors and their children. In C. R. Figley (Ed.), *Trauma and its wake: The study and treatment of post-traumatic stress disorder* (pp. 295–313). New York: Brunner/Mazel.

Danieli, Y. (1988). Treating survivors and children of survivors of the Nazi Holocaust. In F. M. Ochberg (Ed.), *Posttraumatic therapy and victims of violence* (pp. 278–294). New York: Brunner/Mazel.

Danieli, Y. (1989). Mourning in survivors and children of survivors of the Nazi Holocaust: The role of group and community modalities. In D. R. Dietrich and P. C. Shabad (Eds.), *The problem of loss and mourning: Psychoanalytic perspectives* (pp. 427–460). Madison, CT: International Universities Press.

Davidson, S. (1980). Transgenerational transmission in the families of Holocaust survivors. *International Journal of Family Psychiatry, 1*(1), 95–112.

Davis, L. (1989). *The slaughterhouse province: An American diplomat's report on the Armenian genocide, 1915–1917.* S. Blair (Ed.). New Rochelle, NY: Aristide D. Caratzas.

Dekmejian, R. H. (1988). Determinants of genocide: Armenians and Jews as case studies. In R. G. Hovannissian (Ed.), *The Armenian genocide in perspective* (pp. 85–96). New Brunswick, NJ: Transaction Publishers.

Der-Karabetian, A. (1980). Relation of two cultural identities of Armenian-Americans. *Psychological Reports, 47,* 123–128.

Der-Karabetian, A. (1981). Armenian identity: Comparative and context-bound. *Armenian Review, 34,* 25–31.

Derogatis, L., & Melisaratos, N. (1983). The Brief Symptom Inventory: An introductory report. *Psychological Medicine, 10,* 125–132.

Dobkin, M. (1984). *What genocide? What holocaust? News from Turkey, 1915–23: A case study.* In I. W. Charny (Ed.), *Toward the understanding and prevention of genocide: Proceedings of the International Conference on the Holocaust and Genocide* (pp. 100–112). Boulder, CO: Westview Press.

Freyberg, J. T. (1980). Difficulties in separation–individuation as experienced by offspring of Nazi holocaust survivors. *American Journal of Orthopsychiatry, 50*(1), 87–95.

Grubrich-Simitis, I. (1981). Extreme traumatization as cumulative trauma: Psychoanalytic investigations of the effects of concentration camp experiences on survivors and their children. *Psychoanalytic Study of the Child, 36,* 415–450.

Gunter, M. M. (1992). Historical origins of Armenian-Turkish enmity. In *Genocide and human rights: Lessons from the Armenian experience* (pp. 257–288). Belmont, MA: Armenian Heritage Press. (A special issue of the *Journal of Armenian Studies, 4*(1 and 2).)

Guroian V. (1988). Collective responsibility and official excuse making: The case of the Turkish genocide of the Armenians. In R. G. Hovannissian (Ed.), *The Armenian genocide in perspective* (pp. 135–152). New Brunswick, NJ: Transaction Publishers.

Hoffmann, T. (1985). *German eyewitness reports of the genocide of the Armenians, 1915–16.* In G. Libaridian (English lang. Ed.), *A crime of silence: The Armenian genocide* (pp. 61–92). Bath, UK: Pitman Press.

Horowitz, I. L. (1980). *Taking lives: Genocide and state power.* New Brunswick, NJ: Transaction Books.

Housepian, M. (1971). *The Smyrna affair: The first comprehensive account of the burning of the city and the expulsion of the Christians from Turkey in 1922.* New York: Harcourt Brace Jovanovich.

Hovannisian, R. (1967). *Armenia on the road to independence 1918.* Berkeley: University California Press.

Hovannisian, R. (1985). The Armenian Question, 1878–1923. In G. Libaridian (English lang. Ed.), *A Crime of Silence: The Armenian Genocide* (pp. 11–33). Bath, UK: Pitman Press.

Hovannisian, R. (1988). The Armenian Genocide and patterns of denial. In R. Hovannissian (Ed.), *The Armenian Genocide in Perspective* (pp. 111–134). New Brunswick, NJ: Transaction Publishers.

Kalayjian, A., Shahinian, D., Gergerian, E., & Saraydarian, L. (1996). Coping with Ottoman Turkish genocide: An exploration of the experience of Armenian survivors. *Journal of Traumatic Stress, 9*(1), 87–97.

Kalfaian, A. (1982). *Chomaklou: The history of an Armenian village* (Trans. K. Asadourian). New York: Chomaklou Compatriotic Society.

Kassabian, A. (1987). *A three generational study of Armenian family structure as it correlates to Armenian ethnic identity within the context of traumatic loss.* The Catholic University of America, No. 87-13,571, University Microfilms International, *48* (04A).

Kernaklian, P. (1967). *The Armenian-American personality structure and its relationship to various states of ethnicity.* Syracuse University No. 67-12,068, University Microfilms International, *28* (04A).

Kestenberg, J. S. (1972). Psychoanalytic contributions to the problem of children of survivors from Nazi persecution. *Israel Annals of Psychiatry and Related Disciplines, 10,* 311–325.

Klein, H. (1971). Families of Holocaust survivors in the kibbutz: Psychological studies. In H. Krystal & W. G. Niederland (Eds.), *Psychic traumatization: Aftereffects in individuals and communities* (pp. 67–92). Boston: Little, Brown.

Krell, R. (1982). Family therapy with children of concentration camp survivors. *American Journal of Psychotherapy, 36*(4), 513–522.

Krystal, H. (1988). *Integration and self-healing: Affect, trauma, alexithymia.* Hillsdale, NJ: Analytic Press.

Krystal, H., & Niederland, W. (1968). Clinical observations on the survivor syndrome. In H. Krystal (Ed.), *Massive psychic trauma* (pp. 327–348). New York: International Universities Press.

Kupelian, D. (1993). *Armenian genocide survivors: Adaptation and adjustment eight decades after massive trauma.* American University, No. 94-22,771, University Microfilms International, *55* (04B).

Kuper, L. (1981). *Genocide.* Suffolk, UK: Penguin Books.

Kuper, L. (1988). The Turkish genocide of Armenians, 1915–1917. In Richard Hovanissian (Ed.), *The Armenian genocide in perspective* (pp. 43–59). New Brunswick, NJ: Transaction Publishers.

Libaridian, G. (1985). The ideology of the Young Turk Movement. In G. Libaridian (English lang. Ed.), *A crime of silence: The Armenian genocide* (pp. 37–49). Bath, UK: Pitman Press.

Lidgett, E. (1987). *The ancient people.* London: James Nisbetter.

Lidz, T. (1960). Schism and skew in the families of schizophrenics. In N. W. Bell & E. F. Vogel (Eds.), *A modern introduction to the family* (pp. 595–607). Glencoe, IL: Free Press.

Lidz, T., Cornelison, A. R., Fleck, S., & Terry, D. (1957). The interfamily environment of schizophrenic patients. *American Journal of Psychiatry, 114,* 24–248.

Lifton, R. (1969). *Death in life: Survivors of Hiroshima.* New York: Vintage Press.

Loftus, J. (1993). Genocide and deterrence. In *Genocide and human rights: Lessons from the Armenian experience* (pp. 363–371). Belmont, MA: Armenian Heritage Press. (A special issue of the *Journal of Armenian Studies, 4*(1 and 2).)

Malcolm, V. M. (1919). *The Armenians in America.* Boston: Pilgrim Press.

Mazian, F. (1983, Winter). The patriarchal Armenian family: 1914. *Armenian Review, 36*(4), 14–66.

Melson, R. (1992). *Revolution and genocide: On the origins of the Armenian Genocide and the Holocaust.* Chicago: University of Chicago Press.

Miller, J. (1990, April 22). Holocaust museum: A troubled start. *New York Times Magazine,* sec. 6, p. 34.

Miller, D., & Miller, L. (1993). *Survivors: An oral history of the Armenian Genocide.* Berkeley: University of California Press.

Minasian, E. (1986–1987). The forty years of Musa Dagh: The film that was denied. *Journal of Armenian Studies, 3,* 121–132.

Minuchin, S., Montalvo, B., Guerney, B., Rossman, B., & Schumer, F. (1967). *Families of the slums.* New York: Basic Books.

Mirak, R. (1983). *Torn between two lands: Armenians in America, 1890 to World War I.* Cambridge, MA: Harvard University Press.

Montville, J. V. (1987). Psychoanalytical enlightenment and the greening of diplomacy. *Journal of the American Psychoanalytic Association, 37,* 297–318.

Moos, R. H., & Moos, B. S. (1981). *Family environment manual.* Palo Alto, CA: Consulting Psychologists Press.

Morganthau, H. (1975a). *Ambassador Morgenthau's story* (2nd ed.). Plandome, NY: New Age Publishers. Original published 1918, Garden City, NY: Doubleday, Page.

Morganthau, H. (1975b). *The tragedy of Armenia* (2nd ed.). Plandome, NY: New Age Publishers. Original published 1918, London: Spottiswoode, Ballantyne & Co.

Neugarten, B. L. Havighurst, R. J., & Tobin, S. S. (1961). The measurement of life satisfaction. *Journal of Gerontology, 16,* 134–143).

Niederland, W. (1981). The survivor syndrome: Further observations and dimensions. *Journal of the American Psychoanalytic Association, 29*(2), 413–425.

Olson, D. H., Portner, J., & Bell, R. Q. (1982). Clinical rating scale for the circumplex model of marital and family systems. St. Paul: University of Minnesota Press.

Papazian, D. R. (1933). Misplaced credulity: Contemporary Turkish attempts to refute the Armenian genocide. In *Genocide and human rights: Lessons from the Armenian experience* (pp. 227–256). Belmont, MA: Armenian Heritage Press. (A special issue of the *Journal of Armenian Studies, 4*(1 and 2).)

Peroomian, R. (1993). *Literary responses to catastrophe: A comparison of the Armenian and the Jewish experience.* Atlanta: Scholars Press.

Reid, J. (1984). The Armenian massacres in Ottoman and Turkish historiography. *Armenian Review, 37,* 22–40.

Reiss, D. (1971). Varieties of consensual experience I: A theory for relating family interactions to individual thinking. *Family Process, 10,* 1–26.

Roid, G. H., & Fitts, W. H. (1989). *Tennessee Self-Concept Scale (TSCS): Revised manual.* Los Angeles: Western Psychological Services.

Russell, A. (1974). Late psychosocial consequences in concentration camp survivor families. *American Journal of Orthopsychiatry, 44,* 611–619.

Salerian, A. (1982, June 20–24). *A psychological report: Armenian genocide survivors—67 years later.* Paper presented at the International Conference on the Holocaust and Genocide, Tel Aviv, Israel.

Sarafian, A. (Ed.). (1993). *Archival collections on the Armenian genocide: United States official documents on the Armenian genocide. Vol. I: The Lower Euphrates.* Watertown, MA: Armenian Review.

Sarkissian, Z. (1984). Coping with massive stressful life events: The impact of the Armenian genocide of 1915 on the present day health and morale of a group of women survivors. *Armenian Review, 37,* 33–44.

Simpson, C. (1993). *The splendid blond beast, Money law, and genocide in the twentieth century.* New York: Grove Press.

Smith, R. W., Markusen, E., & Lifton, R. J. (1995). Professional ethics and the denial of the Armenian Genocide. *Holocaust and Genocide Studies, 9*(1), 1–22.

Spicer, D. (1971). Persistent identity systems. *Science, 174,* 795–800.

Spitzer, R., Williams, J., Gibbon, M., & First, M. (1989). *Instruction manual for the Structured Clinical Interview for DSM-III-R (SCID, 5/1/89 revision).* New York: Biometrics Research.

Steinberg, A. (1989). Holocaust survivors and their children: A review of the clinical literature. In P. Marcus & A. Rosenberg (Eds.), *Healing their wounds: Psychotherapy with Holocaust survivors and their families* (pp. 23–48). New York: Praeger.

Stierlin, H. (1974). *Separating parents and adolescents.* New York: Quadrangle.

Stolorow, R. D., & Atwood, G. E. (1992). *Contexts of being: The intersubjective foundations of psychological life.* Hillsdale, NJ: Analytic Press.

Sullivan, H. S. (1953). *The interpersonal theory of psychiatry.* New York: W. W. Norton.

Tashjian, J. (1947). *The Armenians of the United States and Canada.* Boston: Hairenik Publications.

Toynbee, A. J. (1916). *The treatment of the Armenians in the Ottoman Empire.* London: Sir Joseph Causton and Sons.

Villa, S. H., & Matossian, M. K. (1982). *Armenian village life before 1914.* Detroit: Wayne State University Press.

Walker, C. J. (1991). *Armenia and Karabagh: The struggle for unity.* London: Minority Rights Publications.

Warner, L., & Srole, L. (1945). *The social system of American ethnic groups.* New Haven, CT: Yale University Press.

Wynne, L. C., Ryckoff, I., Day, J., & Hirsch, S. I. (1958). Pseudomutuality in family relations of schizophrenics. *Psychiatry, 21,* 205–222.

13

The Effects of Massive Trauma on Cambodian Parents and Children

J. DAVID KINZIE, J. BOEHNLEIN, and WILLIAM H. SACK

The goal of this chapter is to describe the effects of the Pol Pot trauma on two generations of Cambodians and their families. The time since the end of the Pol Pot era (1979) is still too short to document a second-generation effect, but we now have some data on the psychiatric effects this trauma has inflicted on young and old Cambodians, and the impact refugee status has had on Cambodian family life.

HISTORY OF THE CAMBODIAN TRAUMA

Cambodia, a poor but peaceful country, became involved in the Vietnam War in 1970. It was taken over by radical Khmer Rouge Communists under Pol Pot in 1975, which resulted in an unexpected, massive catastrophe. This brutal regime attempted to isolate the country and replace all Western and traditional influences with a poorly planned agrarian work–concentration camp program. Doctors, teachers, government leaders, Buddhist monks, Chinese, and military leaders as well as their family members were singled out for execution. All other influences were regarded as enemies of the regime and were eliminated. Almost all urban people were moved to tightly controlled country areas and forced into labor. As the list of "enemies" grew when the expected increase in rice production did not occur, the number of executions increased. Disease and starvation killed many more. During the 4 years of Pol Pot, between 1 and 3 million of the 7 million population died (Becker, 1986; Hawk, 1982). The killing ended only with the invasion by the Vietnamese in 1979.

The Cambodian tragedy not only killed individuals but also destroyed the very fabric of Cambodian life and society (i.e., the Buddhist monks, teachers, and government leaders). No one was left untouched by these events, and many became refugees, first in Thailand, then later in a third country (usually the United States, France, or Australia). Our experience over the past 15 years involves those who came to the state of Oregon, in the United States and became

J. DAVID KINZIE, J. BOEHNLEIN, and WILLIAM H. SACK • Department of Psychiatry, Oregon Health Sciences University, Portland, Oregon 97201.

International Handbook of Multigenerational Legacies of Trauma, edited by Yael Danieli. Plenum Press, New York, 1998.

patients in our Indochinese Clinic. We have also studied a group of young students in the community who did not become our patients.

We began treating primarily Indochinese refugees in 1978 (Kinzie and Manson, 1983). Two years later, we saw the first Cambodians, who seemed different from other refugees; they were more withdrawn, more frightened and affectively numb. Our clinical experience showed that they did not improve with standard treatment for depression, and it took some time before we realized that we were dealing with a severe form of posttraumatic stress disorder (PTSD; Kinzie, Fredrickson, Ben, Fleck, & Karls, 1984). Follow-up study showed that many had improved in 1 year (Boehnlein, Kenzie, Ben, & Fleck, 1985), but all suffered relapses during the next few years. The chronic course of the disorder—with remission, exacerbation of the intrusive symptoms, and marked vulnerability to stress—has been well established (Kinzie, 1988). Continuity of care and medication have been crucial in reducing some major intrusive symptoms. Socialization group experiences also help reduce the social and cultural isolation by focusing on problems these refugees have in adapting to their new country (Kinzie *et al.*, 1988). We have continued to find a very high prevalence of PTSD in Cambodian patients, and also a moderately high level in the Vietnamese (Kinzie *et al.*, 1990).

CULTURE, TRAUMA, MIGRATION, AND FAMILY LIFE

Heller (1982) described how the stressful experience of the Jewish concentration camp survivors greatly influenced their children, who felt an increased sensitivity to culture and ancestry, and to the primacy of ethnic survival.

The family is the primary social unit in all Southeast Asian cultures, with individual identity frequently inseparable from that of the family. Traditional Southeast Asian values include a strong family identity as the foundation of personal identity and self-worth. Elders are placed in roles of authority and are treated with great respect. Their decisions traditionally have gone unquestioned. It was the child's duty (even after reaching adulthood) to follow parents' recommendations. Moreover, elders traditionally were also the first to consult healers when a family member became ill. Attentive, indulgently child rearing from multiple parental figures encourages children to be interdependent, with increasingly strict expectations imposed as they mature (Sack, Angell, Kinzie, & Rath, 1986). The sense of self is defined by the family and the community within which a child lives. Severe trauma, with its symptoms of PTSD and severe depression, although experienced by individuals, has a broad ripple effect on the person's family and social network.

Important precepts of Buddhism strongly influence familial and social norms of communication and behavior in Cambodia. These include correct intent for specific actions, good conduct, honesty, honest effort, and a correct understanding of the sources of unhappiness (Zadrozny, 1955). Religious beliefs also serve as the source of conceptions about the world, the self, and their interrelationship (Geertz, 1973). Basic religious concepts must be considered when attempting to understand the chronic grief of many Southeast Asian families. Ritual mourning of the loss of family members and friends has not been possible for many traumatized refugees (Boehnlein, 1987).

The effects of trauma on individuals—depression, startle reaction, hypervigilance, nightmares, and irritability—greatly affect the way individuals function within the family. Numbness, avoidance, and vulnerability to stress often lead parents to be frightened, confused, or simply uninvested in the basic care of their children.

The effects of trauma (migration and resettlement) on the individual and his or her parents have placed great burdens on family units as a whole and on specific generations within the family. Elders have had to endure diminished status within the family, as well as in society at large, because of a lack of language proficiency, little or no formal education, and no vocational experience transferable to a Western economy. Combined with financial difficulties, these problems have reduced the importance of elders in some "made-up"[1] Southeast Asian refugee families. Cultural conflict regarding what is considered to be retirement ages have a also complicated family matters. In Southeast Asian cultures, elders traditionally are placed in roles of authority because of their age and experience, and reach this status at a relatively early age. They then expect their children to support them financially. Due to greater financial pressure on middle generations in resettlement countries, this has been difficult.

Another significant source of conflict in the refugee family is the relationship between parents and children. Because of the high prevalence of male deaths during the Cambodian trauma, the family unit most often consists of a single parents in a position of authority, most commonly a single mother. For children, the normal developmental struggles of adolescence are heightened by a single parent's diminished authority role. This is further exacerbated when the parents are emotionally disconnected from the children because of psychiatric disorders (PTSD). The children's greater proficiency with the language of the host country and greater access to educational opportunities often lead to a reversal of generational roles within families, with children becoming the cultural brokers and communication facilitators between the nuclear family and the mainstream culture. This transfers much of the authority from elders to the young.

Even the normal life-cycle separation of young adults from the nuclear family represents unique conflicts for refugees. Parents and children have frequently suffered the loss of numerous family members during the war and the process of migration. Surviving family members need to remain particularly close to each other for emotional and physical survival. Anything affecting that closeness may be seen as a threat that can reawaken frighteningly vivid memories of prior losses. This threat may be perceived even in positive transitions, such as marriage, or the move to another city for a better job opportunity. Depression and PTSD, although successfully treated previously, often are exacerbated by these family life-cycle transitions. Dating and marriage may represent additional cultural challenges for young Cambodian adults, because many parents continue to expect to give their approval before their offspring can marry. Interethnic marriages, even among Southeast Asian ethnic groups, frequently are looked upon with displeasure by traditional parents.

Another source of stress for young adult refugees involves separation from the family for educational and career opportunities. Often, the child is faced with choosing between educational opportunities in other locales and traditional loyalties toward the nuclear or extended family. This conflict can be particularly formidable for young women who have been the major care providers for their younger siblings when a single parent has been impaired by illness. Young adults are also saddled with a great deal of emotional pressure because of the enormous expectations for educational performance and financial success their families place on them in the hopes of raising the socioeconomic level of the nuclear family. Drug use, gang activities, and unintended pregnancies may be responses to some young Cambodians' attempts both to acculturate and to improve their family's standard of living. In summary, the

---

[1]The phrase "made-up" families connotes a family structure often of non-blood-related members, created to substitute for families that were destroyed (Danieli, personal communication, 1997).

individual's psychosocial development is affected by life's transactions, the ongoing stresses of ethnic group acculturation, and family dynamics (Boehnlein, 1987).

Although scant literature exists on longitudinal Southeast Asian refugee family functioning, some studies have examined adjustments by specific generations. Among Vietnamese, for example, parents strongly endorse traditional family values regardless of the amount of time they have lived in the United States, and are ambivalent about privileges for adolescent children (Nguyen & Williams, 1989). A nostalgic orientation to country of origin in adults most likely relates to the severity of stress after resettlement (Beiser, 1987; Beiser, Turner, & Ganesan, 1989). In a recent study, Vietnamese parents reported significantly more difficulties with and problems in their adolescent children than Cambodian parents (Boehnlein *et al.,* 1995). Moreover, Vietnamese were more likely than Cambodians to state that these difficulties and problems adversely affected their health, and that their family life would have been better had they stayed in Southeast Asia. Parents' relationships with their adolescent children had a significant impact on their perceptions of their own health, producing both cognitive and somatic symptoms. This concern existed both with and without evidence of socially disruptive adolescent behavior. A recent longitudinal study of Vietnamese refugees in Norway underscored the significant impact of family factors on long-term adjustment by demonstrating that chronic family separation was a major predictor of long-term psychopathology in resettled refugees (Hauff & Vaglum, 1995). In this study, self-rated distress correlated more closely with chronic separation from a spouse or child than with the severity of a psychiatric disorder.

Clinically, many of the Cambodian families we treated seemed to be "numb" in Danieli's classification (1985). Warmth is lacking and the parents display avoidance and withdrawal behavior, with periodic agitation and irritability. The unrest and tension may lead to domestic violence with spousal and child abuse, alcohol abuse, and dropping out of school.

LONG-TERM EFFECTS OF TRAUMA ON CAMBODIAN CHILDREN

The Cambodian genocide was clearly designed to destroy the basic family structure by separating children from their parents before the ages of 6 to 8, turning young people into informants, forming early teen cadres of armed guards, and publicly and brutally denouncing "crimes" of the older generation. After 4 years of forced labor, starvation, witnessing executions and deaths, and separation from family, many spent several years as refugees in Thailand before migrating to America, France, or Australia. Children arrived in small family groups, very often with no adult males (they had been killed), and almost always had other "missing" family members whose whereabouts had been unknown for years. The following describes our observations of the effects of this trauma and refugee status on Cambodian culture and family.

In 1984, we began to study 40 Cambodian high school students to determine the effects of their experiences, and followed up by interviewing them 3 and 6 years later. Their descriptions of trauma were extremely sad and graphic. Forty-six percent were separated from their family for more than 2 years; 60% of the subjects or their relatives were beaten by cadres; 63% had a parent killed or lost; 63% witnessed killings; 83% suffered malnutrition; 38% were threatened with death (Kinzie, Sack, Angell, Manson, & Ben, 1986).

The average age of the 40 subjects in our original study was 17. They had been in the United States between 1 and 2 years (Kinzie *et al.,* 1986). Interviews were conducted by psychiatrists aided by a Cambodian mental health worker. Fifty percent of the students met the full diagnostic criteria for PTSD, 50% for depression; and 8% for anxiety disorder. Follow-up interviews 3 years later, conducted by the same psychiatrists, revealed that 48% had PTSD, 47% depression, and only one individual (i.e., 4%) had anxiety disorder. A 6-year follow-up using trained lay interviewers demonstrated 38% with PTSD; depression had dropped to 6%. No conduct disorders were found throughout the study. The PTSD diagnosis did not necessarily affect the same subjects (i.e., some cases resolved over time) and a few new ones arose between the first and second study. This confirmed our clinical findings that the course of PTSD will wax and wane over time. At first, we thought that PTSD and depression might be comorbid conditions. In this group, however, depression greatly decreased over time, while PTSD remitted only slightly. Thus, they do have separate clinical courses (Sack et al., 1993).

The family continued to be a source of stress for these young Cambodians. In the 6-year study (average age 23 now), 72% were worried about family left in Cambodia; 31% reported family conflict and family fights over American versus Cambodian ways of doing things. Despite this, our first study (but not subsequent studies) showed that living with family instead of in a foster home afforded some protection against developing PTSD (Kinzie et al., 1986).

COMPARISON OF PTSD AND DEPRESSION IN TWO GENERATIONS OF CAMBODIAN REFUGEES

Rates of PTSD and depression in two generations of Cambodian refugees were examined as part of a large epidemiological study of Cambodian refugees (Sack et al., 1994, 1995). A sample of 209 Khmer adolescents, ages 13 to 25, in two western U.S. communities, Portland and Salt Lake City, was randomly selected to undergo psychiatric assessment. When available, one of the parents, usually the mother, was also interviewed separately. Interviews were conducted in English by a master's level clinician and a Khmer interpreter. The diagnostic portion of the interview was based on the PTSD section of the Diagnostic Instrument for Children and Adolescents (DICA; Welner et al., 1987), as well as sections from the Schedule of Affective Disorders and Schizophrenia for School-Age Children, epidemiological version (Kiddie-SADS-E, Ed. III, Puig-Antich, 1983; Puig-Antich, Orvaschel, Tabrinzi, & Chambers, 1980). The same version of the adolescent interview was also given to the parents, and the results were compared. Four groups were created to compare potential mediating factors of family PTSD concordance: (1 no family or youth PTSD; (2) family only PTSD; (3) youth only PTSD; and (4) parent and youth PTSD. PTSD rates in the mothers were high, 55%, compared with the fathers, 30%, as was depression (20% vs. 14%). The relationship between PTSD in a parent (mother, father, or both) and PTSD in an adolescent was consistently significant. In contrast, the relationship between parent and adolescent diagnoses of major depression and depressive disorder was not found to be significant, although there was a trend in this direction.

A trend for higher PTSD rates among adolescents when both parents were diagnosed with PTSD was also established. When neither parent had PTSD, only 12.9% of youth received the diagnosis. When one parent had PTSD, the adolescent prevalence rate increased to 23.3%. With both parents diagnosed, the rate increased to 41.2% (Sack et al., 1995).

The following case history illustrates the multiple problems that can occur in Cambodian family life due to trauma and refugee experience.

Pham is a 25-year-old married woman first seen in the clinic 10 years ago. Her husband was also being seen at that time. She was referred because of ongoing depressive symptoms, but her symptoms also included nightmares three or four times a week, along with intrusive thoughts about the past. She lost interest in many things, experienced guilt about the brother she had to leave behind in Cambodia, was angry and irritable, and lost 20 pounds. She had no education and had worked to help support her family. At age 15, when Pol Pot came to power, she was separated from her family, began forced labor, and faced starvation. She tells of being tied up and severely beaten on the face and hands. Two years later, her father, who had held a minor official position, was executed. Shortly thereafter, her brothers, ages 12 and 9, were killed. Another younger brother starved to death. She remembers the horror she felt in the Pol Pot camp, alone and weak, with no one to care for her. In 1979, she escaped with her younger brother and mother, and went to Thailand. In the Thai camp, she married another Cambodian and gave birth to three children. She arrived in the United States a year before she was seen at the clinic. At that time, she denied any problems with her marriage other than those due to her own irritability.

She was withdrawn, affect constricted, and her expression rarely changed. She shed no tears, even when describing her traumatic events, and displayed no evidence of a thought disorder. She was diagnosed with PTSD and major affective disorder, depressed type. Individual therapy and medication, including imipramine and clonidine, proved helpful, and she also took part in socialization group therapy.

Her husband, Dom, was 31 when first seen. He was very depressed, felt hopeless about trying to fit into this modern country, and expressed some suicidal ideation. He also had been in Pol Pot concentration camps for 4 years, subjected to severe physical harassment, constant starvation, and threats of execution. His parents and six siblings had been executed. Like his wife, Dom was diagnosed with depression and PTSD, and was followed in the clinic, placed on medication, and enrolled in socialization group therapy.

Pham's mother, Chan, came to the clinic 2 years later. She was a depressed 44-year-old woman who had experienced multiple somatic complaints over the past several years. Her symptoms had worsened recently while feeling pressured to search for a job. She felt dizzy, had difficulty concentrating, lost interest in her normal activities, and began having nightmares for the first time. Over and over again, in vivid dreams she would see her husband being tied up and forced underwater as he screamed out her name, but she could not help him. Chan graphically relived the scenario of her children being beaten to death; they, too, called out her name, and she could do nothing to save them. Intrusive thoughts throughout the day made her feel increasingly irritable, and she had a strong startle response to noises. Her future seemed more and more hopeless when she could not force these memories out of her mind.

Augmenting the history given by her daughter, she said that she had borne seven children and was separated from her family in 1975. Apparently, two children died of disease after Pol Pot came to power, and two, as mentioned earlier, were executed. She was cruelly and deliberately told that they had called out her name as they were beaten to death. Her 3-year-old died of starvation. Chan's mother also died of starvation, and her husband was executed in 1976. Chan said that she heard he was shot so many times that his head fell off. Her nightmares centered around her inability to help her family; however, she was not with them when they were killed. She also related how she, her one remaining daughter, Pham, and a son, escaped by going to another part of the country and then survived the trip to Thailand.

A sedate and attractive Cambodian woman, Chan was controlled during the interview but began crying when she talked about her husband's death and the fatal beatings of her two children. Her anguish was appropriate, and she was diagnosed with PTSD and severe depression.

The entire family lived together: the grandmother, Chan, the daughter, Pham, and her husband, Dom, their three children, and Chan's younger son. All three patients remained in treatment for several years, repeatedly denying any stressors at home, yet exhibiting multiple symptoms of PTSD and depression.

About 5 years into the treatment, it became clear that Dom and Pham were having several major marital problems. Abuse was not noted until much later, after a separation, when both Pham and Chan reported that Dom had beaten them. Pham had a brief affair during this time and became very preoccupied with working and earning money. The grandmother and the uncle had become the primary caretakers for the three young children. Subsequently, Dom left the area and did not contest the divorce. Seven years later, Pham terminated treatment and then was able to get a job. However, 1 year ago, Pham had recurrence of her symptoms, quit her job, and restarted treatment. Chan has continued in treatment for almost 10 years, and has been the primary support for the family. Her posttraumatic stress symptoms have persisted, and she also has developed hypertension. The younger son married outside the culture but continued to live at home and later fathered a child.

Dom recently remarried and lives in another state. He rarely has contact with his children and provides very little financial assistance to them. Pham has a boyfriend and spends the nights with him, but spends afternoons and evenings with her children. The primary family unit consists of Pham, her three children, Chan (who is effectively the mother), Chan's son, the children's uncle (who is effectively the father), and her son's wife and baby.

Pham's three children, Gom, 15-year-old girl, Loo, a 13-year-old boy, and Ann, an 11-year-old girl, were interviewed together, without the other family members present. All had heard about the Pol Pot experience and knew of the deaths of relatives. They had received from their grandmother most of the details, which were consistent with the history we obtained. The only effect, they said, from the story, was that they felt sad about it. They all had seen the film *The Killing Fields,* which made them feel sad about Cambodia. The only current effect that they know of the Pol Pot era is hearing their grandmother scream at night. They, themselves, feel that they are halfway between the Cambodian and American way of life, although they report speaking much more English than Cambodian.

All the children described the previous fighting between their mother and their father, and how much it bothered them. Gom had actually been beaten by the father, who stopped only when she reported it at school. They felt sad when their father left, even though they admitted that they were frightened of him. However, they felt even more afraid when their mother left for a time with a boyfriend. They all felt that "no one loved us," in spite of the fact that the grandmother and uncle stayed. They gave much more personal credit to the family discord than they did to any past effects of the Cambodian experience.

Individually, Gom, who is now a freshman in high school, is very unhappy. A recent disagreement with the grandmother over using the phone and going out with friends had caused her to be profoundly sad. Her school grades have suffered and she began, for the first time, failing some classes. She spent much time in her room alone crying. She sleeps poorly, is tired, and has poor concentration and little energy. She even says she has lost hope fulfilling her dream of becoming a nurse and now is unsure if she will ever even complete high school. She has thought about leaving home and living with her father. Even in the presence of the others, she becomes tearful upon describing her current situation.

Loo, a seventh grader, has a goal of being a basketball player. Recently, his grades also have dropped, and school has become very difficult for him. He says he does not understand it very well. His uncle has offered to help him. He spends much time with his Asian friends and wonders if he will be able to resist group pressure and continue school. He is not sad now, but sees his future as very uncertain.

Only Ann, a sixth grader, who does not have much memory of the family fights, seems bright and happy. She gets excellent grades and plans to be a doctor. She expressed and nonverbally showed confidence in her future.

Comment

It is apparent that at least three of the four people traumatized in Cambodia suffered severely for many years. In addition, Dom and Pham found it impossible to maintain their relationship and, as a result of the abuse, divorce seemed inevitable and necessary. Pham became more concerned about being established in her new country and earning a living than about raising her own family; indeed, at times, she seemed to be totally indifferent to her children's well-being. Fortunately, the grandmother was able to intervene and become involved in this semiextended family and provide both parenting and continuity of culture for them. However, this has added an ongoing problem for the adolescent children. She is seen as very restrictive. Treatment reduced both the mother's and daughter's symptoms and may also have increased greatly the tolerability of family life.

The effects on the survivors, grandmother, parents, and children are complicated. The events of Pol Pot era have been discussed, and all the children are aware of their country's history and culture. They express a sense of sadness and probably of loss. However, the children do not identify their current problems with that of the effect of Pol Pot but more directly to the fighting between the parents who left them and, most recently, to the conflicts with the grandmother. The latter probably represent a culture and generation difference. The problems for the children are very significant. The oldest girl suffers from clinical depression and sees no way out, and no future for herself. The boy, beginning adolescence, is also finding school difficult and is beginning to identify with peer groups, and he, likewise, is beginning to question his future. Only the younger girl seems unaffected at this time. Whether she will remain so, as adolescence develops, is uncertain.

Although the children do not identify the traumatic events of Pol Pot with their current problems, it is probable that they are a great source of difficulty. The parents' behavior, increased irritability, physical abuse and abandonment, permanently by the father and partially by the mother, is very unlike traditional Cambodian behavior. The posttraumatic symptoms of irritability and numbing of the parents, along with the effects of refugee status in a foreign country, seem to have left a powerful legacy on the growing children.

DISCUSSION

The Cambodian agony is one of the recent reminders of man's inhumanity to man. The severe trauma certainly produced many symptoms of PTSD and, to a lesser extent, depression in victims. Even more than a decade after the Pol Pot regime ended, a large segment of the U.S. Cambodian community still exhibits the full PTSD constellation of symptoms: more than 50% of adult women, 30% of adult men, and 20–30% of adolescents. These very high rates illustrate both the prevalence and the chronicity of this disorder. Of the 150 Cambodians treated in the Indochinese Psychiatric Clinic, more than 80% are in treatment for over 3 years. About 70% of all who began treatment have continued. Patients remain vulnerable to stress despite marked reduction in intrusive symptoms, and life stressors often produce an acute exacerbation of symptoms.

Young Cambodian adults tend to have lower rates, later onset, and less persistence of symptoms over time than do the older adults. Their impairment is also rarely as severe. Despite being separated from parents at an important developmental age, and exposed to (and in some cases, having participated in) violence, they display more resilience than their parents. Early data suggest that they also handle stress in a more private and quiet way, not antisocial acting-out behavior, as is common with other young people in the United States. However, their school dropout rate indicates that academic life is particularly difficult for them.

Adult parents present a more complicated picture, however, because they tend to have more symptoms and more diagnoses. They are more socially and vocationally impaired, and have more trouble learning English and acquiring the skills necessary to adapt to a complicated Western culture. Their children, especially adolescents, remain their major source of worry and contribute greatly to their symptoms. But parents are very poor sources of information on how their children are doing psychologically, since they seem unable to connect emotionally with them and therefore usually underestimate their suffering.

The older generation of Cambodians displays the social effects of this disorder. Wife abuse and divorce, as indicated by the case example, are becoming more common. Although such events occurred rarely in traditional Khmer families in Cambodia, now, even our own small Cambodian community of 5,000 people, experiences domestic violence, and there are reports of physical and sexual abuse of children. Today, both mothers and fathers abandon their families with apparent indifference. Alcoholism is evidence in both sexes and accelerates the breakup of families.

The pressure on Cambodian refugee families is intense and unremitting. Not only are individual members often psychiatrically impaired but also they have suffered numerous socio-cultural losses. Most painful for many has been loss of the sense of shared values and continuity inherent in a stable, traditional Buddhist culture, where elders and leaders are respected, duties and responsibilities are delineated and accepted, and the extended family provides safety and support. This cultural framework was solid, and a shared acceptance of Buddhism (along with its local folk beliefs) provided a coherent, peaceful worldview. The pervasive violence, wanton destruction, and widespread death of family members and Cambodian leaders shattered this security and rendered life incoherent and devoid of meaning for many. Completely demoralized and traumatized, they came from unstable refugee life in Thailand to the shores of the United States. Here, their isolation was compounded by living among "foreigners," since they usually did not live among many other Cambodians. Confused parents were thrust into new roles. Values, behavior, religion, and basic institutions such as education were much different from what they had ever experienced before. Since children generally learned English faster, they also had new roles, often serving as guides and interpreters. Often unable to find or maintain employment, fathers lost status. Neither parent could help children with such basic activities as homework or take part in afterschool events. Family members often seemed withdrawn, numb, or unresponsive, and became violent periodically.

Our studies demonstrate that PTSD clusters in families. The rate of PTSD among children increases when one parent has PTSD, and greatly increases if PTSD is present in both. Irritability, poor sleep, avoidance, startle reaction, and nightmares are symptoms of PTSD that can greatly impair parents directly, through aggression and avoidance, or indirectly, through being totally exhausted and preoccupied, which, in turn, impacts the children. Vulnerable, these children can and often do develop or maintain the symptoms of PTSD.

Earlier onset of PTSD symptoms in the majority of adult patients suggests that parents suffer more severe forms of PTSD syndrome than do their offspring. Adult sufferers, but not their adolescent children, functioned at a lower level and had lower income levels when they had PTSD (Sact et al., 1995). Likewise, they reported recurrence of traumatic dreams more frequently than did the adolescent group (Sack et al., 1993). Acculturation in the adolescent group appears to proceed relatively smoothly despite underlying PTSD symptoms (Kinzie et al., 1995; Sack et al., 1995).

Disaster research (Three-Mile Island, nuclear accidents, industrial fires, lightning strikes, and the Buffalo Creek Flood) provides some empirical evidence for the intergenerational effects trauma has on children. All of these studies demonstrate that family factors—parental distress, fears, and mental health, and an irritable family atmosphere—have a high correlation with PTSD symptoms following significant trauma (Bromet, Hough, & Connell, 1984; Dollinger, O'Donnell, & Staley, 1984; Green et al., 1991). Green et al.'s Buffalo Creek Dam study showed that both the severity of a parent's PTSD symptoms as well as irritability and depressed family atmosphere independently contribute to PTSD symptoms in children. Data were collected $1^{1}/_{2}$–2 years following the disaster (Green *et al.,* 1994). Such studies are compatible with clinical experience and echo Anna Freud's written report from World War II (Freud & Burlingham, 1943).

The Cambodian tragedy provides yet another experience of the effect of severe trauma on individuals and their families. Our studies indicate that younger people and children seem to have fewer symptoms than their parents. However, adults with PTSD in addition to personal symptoms are having severe problems with their parenting roles. These problems may be caused by irritability and numbing from PTSD itself or other social disruption such as divorce, violence, or alcohol abuse. The result is certainly more stress on the children. It is as if Pol Pot won. He destroyed the fabric of Cambodian culture and family life, and left the survivors without a sense of continuity of existence itself. We can hope that young Cambodians can find meaning for themselves and their families, and that the transmission of traumatic anguish ends.

REFERENCES

Becker, E. (1986). *When the war was over.* New York: Simon & Schuster.

Beiser, M. (1987). Changing time perspective and mental health among Southeast Asian refugees. *Culture, Medicine, and Psychiatry, 11,* 437–464.

Beiser, M., Turner, R. H., & Ganesan, S. (1989). Catastrophic stress and factors affecting its consequences among Southeast Asian refugees. *Social Science and Medicine, 28,* 183–195.

Boehnlein, J. K. (1987). Culture and society in posttraumatic stress disorder: Implications for psychotherapy. *American Journal of Psychotherapy, 41,* 519–530.

Boehnlein, J. K., Kinzie, J. D., Ben, R., & Fleck, J. (1985). One-year follow-up study of posttraumatic stress disorder among survivors of Cambodian concentration camps. *American Journal of Psychiatry, 142,* 956–959.

Boehnlein, J. K., Tran, H. D., Riley, C., Vu, K., Tan, S., & Leung, P. K. (1995). A comparative study of family functioning among Vietnamese and Cambodian refugees. *Journal of Nervous Mental Disorders, 183,* 510–515.

Bromet, E. J., Hough, L., & Connell, M. (1984). Mental health of children near the Three Mile Island reactor. *Journal of Preventive Psychiatry, 2,* 275–301.

Danieli, Y. (1985). The treatment and prevention of long-term effects and intergenerational transmission of victimization: A lesson from holocaust survivors and their children. In C. R. Figley (Ed.), *Trauma and its wake: The study and treatment of post-traumatic stress disorder.* New York: Brunner/Mazel.

Dollinger, S. J., O'Donnell, J. P., & Staley, A A. (1984). Lightning-strike disaster: Effects on children's fears and worries. *Journal of Consulting and Clinical Psychology, 52,* 1028–1038.

Freud, A., & Burlingham, D. (1943). *Children and war.* New York: Ernst Willard.

Geertz, C. (1973). *The interpretation of cultures.* New York: Basic Books.

Green, B. L., Karol, M., & Grace, M. C. (1994). Children and disaster: Age, gender and parental effects on PTSD symptoms. *Journal of the American Academy of Child and Adolescent Psychiatry, 30,* 945–951.

Green, B., L., Karol, M., Grace, M., Vary, G., Leonard, H., Glesser, G., & Smitson-Cohen, S. (1991). Children and disaster: Age, gender, parental effects on PTSD symptoms. *Journal of the American Academy of Child and Adolescent Psychiatry, 30,* 945–951.

Hauff, E., & Vaglum, P. (1995). Organized violence and the stress of exile: Predictors of mental health in a community cohort of Vietnamese refugees three years after settlement. *British Journal of Psychiatry, 166,* 360–367.

Hawk, D. (1982). The killing of Cambodia. *New Republic, 187,* 17–21.

Heller, D. (1982). Themes of culture and ancestry among children of concentration camp survivors. *Psychiatry 45,* 247–261.

Kinzie, J. D. (1988). The psychiatric effects of massive trauma on Cambodian refugees. In J. P. Wilson, Z. Harel, & B. Kahana (Eds.), *Human adaptation to extreme stress.* New York: Plenum Press.

Kinzie, J. D., Boehnlein, J. K., Leung, P. K., Moore, L., Riley, C., & Smith, D. (1990). The prevalence of posttraumatic stress disorder and its clinical significance among Southeast Asian refugees. *American Journal of Psychiatry, 147,* 913–917.

Kinzie, J. D., Fredrickson, R. H., Ben, R., Fleck, J., & Karls, W. (1984). Posttraumatic stress disorder among survivors of Cambodian concentration camps. *American Journal of Psychiatry, 141,* 645–650.

Kinzie, J. D., Leung, P., Bui, A., Ben, R., Keopraseuth, K. O., Riley, C., Fleck, J., & Ades, M. (1988). Group therapy with Southeast Asian refugees. *Community Mental Health Journal, 24,* 157–166.

Kinzie, J. D., & Manson, S. M. (1983). Five years' experience with Indochinese refugee patients. *Journal of Operational Psychiatry, 14,* 105–111.

Kinzie, J. D., Sack, W. H., Angell, R. H., Manson, S., & Ben, R. (1986). The psychiatric effects of massive trauma on Cambodian children: I. The children. *Journal of the American Academy of Child and Adolescent Psychiatry, 25,* 370–376.

Nguyen, N. A., & Williams, H. L. (1989). Transitions from East to West: Vietnamese adolescents and their parents. *Journal of the American Academy of Child and Adolescent Psychiatry, 28,* 505–515.

Puig-Antich, J. (1983). *A report on the KIDDIE-SADS (K-SADS).* Paper presented at the research forum of the American Academy of Child Psychiatry, San Francisco, CA.

Puig-Antich, J., Orvaschel H., Tabrinzi, M. A., & Chambers, W. (1980). *The Schedule of Affective Disorders and Schizophrenia for School-Age Children—Epidemiologic version (KIDDIE-SADS).* New York: New York State Psychiatric Institute and Yale University School of Medicine.

Sack, W. H., Angell, R., Kinzie, J. D., & Rath, B. (1986). The psychiatric effects of massive trauma on Cambodian children: II. The family, the home, and the school. *Journal of the American Academy of Child and Adolescent Psychiatry, 25*(3), 377–383.

Sack, W. H., Clarke, G., Him, C., Dickason, D., Goff, B., Lantham, K., & Kinzie, J. D. (1993). A six-year follow up of Cambodian youth traumatized as children. *Journal of the American Academy of Child and Adolescent Psychiatry, 32,* 431–437.

Sack, W. H., Clarke, G. N., Kinney, R., Belestos, G., Him, C. D., & Seeley, J. (1995). The Khmer adolescent project: II. Functional capacities in two generations of Cambodian refugees. *Journal of Nervous Mental Disorders, 183,* 177–181.

Sack, W. H., McSharry, S., Clarke, G. N., Kinney, R., Seeley, J., & Lewinsohn, P. (1994). The Khmer adolescent project: I. Epidemiologic findings in two generations of Cambodian refugees. *Journal of Nervous Mental Disorders, 182,* 387–395.

Welner, Z., Reich W., Herjanic, B., Jung, K. G., & Amado, H. (1987). Reliability, validity, and parent–child agreement studies of the Diagnostic Interview for Children and Adolescents (DICA). *American Journal of Child and Adolescent Psychiatry, 26*(5), 649–653.

Zadrozny, M. G. (Ed.). (1955). *Area handbook on Cambodia.* New Haven, CT: Human Relations Area Files Press.

IV

The Vietnam War

14

Warrior Fathers and Warrior Sons
Intergenerational Aspects of Trauma

ROBERT ROSENHECK and ALAN FONTANA

This chapter considers whether Vietnam veterans *whose fathers served in combat* have an increased risk of posttraumatic stress disorder and other postwar adjustment problems when compared with other Vietnam veterans. Samples are Vietnam veterans who participated in the National Vietnam Veterans Readjustment Study (NVVRS) and veterans seeking treatment for PTSD from the Department of Veterans Affairs (VA). In the total NVVRS sample there were no differences between these two groups. However, *within the subgroup of veterans who met criteria for PTSD,* those whose fathers had been exposed to combat had more severe problems on several measures. In the VA sample, too, veterans whose fathers served in combat scored higher in PTSD symptoms, suicidality, guilt, and loss of religious faith. We conclude that intergenerational effects of trauma emerge when the second generation itself has PTSD, and show that these transgenerational effects are related to intergenerational processes during the homecoming period rather than to differences in premilitary experience.

The role of intergenerational processes in the development and perpetuation of posttraumatic psychological distress has attracted increasing attention from both clinicians and researchers in recent years (Danieli, 1985; Kulka *et al.,* 1990a; Sigal & Weinfeld, 1989). The traumatic experiences of parents have been widely hypothesized to have a continuing effect on the well-being of the next generation, either directly through traumatization of the children by their parents' behavior (Egeland, Jacobvitz, Papataola, 1987; Harkness, 1994; Hunter, Kilstrom, & Kraybill, 1978), through identification of the children with their parents (Danieli, 1985; Felsen & Erlich, 1990), or more indirectly as a result of nonspecific strains or dysfunction in the family that impair child development (Schwartz, Dohrenwend, & Levav, 1994). In this chapter, we review previously published literature and present data from two new studies to examine the specific conditions under which traumatic war-zone experiences of American combat veterans appear to have a significant impact on the psychological status of their children.

The exploration of intergenerational effects of trauma was initiated by reports from psychodynamically oriented clinicians on their treatment of children of Holocaust survivors

ROBERT ROSENHECK and ALAN FONTANA • Department of Veterans Affairs, Northeast Program Evaluation Center, Veterans Affairs Medical Center, West Haven, Connecticut 06516.

International Handbook of Multigenerational Legacies of Trauma, edited by Yael Danieli. Plenum Press, New York, 1998.

(Bergmann & Jucovy, 1982; Rakoff, Sigal, & Epstein, 1966; Sigal, 1971). Additional insights came from detailed autobiographical accounts of children of survivors themselves (Epstein, 1979). These studies suggested that many children of Holocaust survivors grew up in seriously strained environments. In some case, they were emotionally frozen in a conspiracy of silence, numbing, and grief about wartime horror (Danieli, 1981, 1985, 1993; Davidson, 1980; Kestenberg, 1982), while in others, families were observed to be stiflingly close, with poorly maintained intergenerational boundaries (Barocas & Barocas, 1973; Fryberg, 1980; Trossman, 1968). Children of survivors were described in some accounts as bearing the awesome responsibility of making up to their parents the unimaginable losses they had experienced at the hands of the Nazis.

Echoing these reports, clinical studies identified similar processes in the families of traumatized combat veterans of both World War II (Rosenheck, 1986) and Vietnam (Rosenheck & Nathan, 1985). For the most part, these veterans were seeking treatment for posttraumatic stress disorder (PTSD) from the Department of Veterans Affairs (VA). Like the families of Holocaust survivors, the families of American combat veterans with PTSD were observed to manifest a diversity of interactive patterns ranging from remote detachment to intensive symbiotic involvement (Rosenheck, 1986). In one especially troubled group of Vietnam veterans, veterans whose severe PTSD was accompanied by self-destructive behavior and intense self-loathing (Rosenheck, 1985a, 1985b), a large proportion of their fathers were found to have served in combat in World War II. Clinical exploration suggested that the exposure of these veterans to the brutal realities of the war in Vietnam resulted in an especially devastating loss of patriotic and military idealism—an idealism that developed, originally, out of their childhood images of their fathers as war heroes. Unlike the second-generation Holocaust survivors who were not exposed to catastrophic trauma of their own, the problems faced by these veterans were based on their own personal traumatic experiences, which seemed to have been exacerbated by features of their relationship with their veteran fathers.

Clinical reports, even when based on detailed observation of numerous cases over many years, are of limited value in determining whether a clinical phenomenon is widespread or rare, or whether the association between current problems and the experiences of previous generations is real or spurious. To address these questions, surveys using standardized measures must be conducted, first on clinical samples, which are more readily accessible, and then on representative community samples. Only through such formal research efforts can hypothesized lines of influence be put to a serious empirical test.

A recent literature review reported that 11 published studies have investigated the effect of surviving the Holocaust on the second generation (Schwartz *et al.,* 1994). In most of these studies, survivor children were compared with children of Jewish immigrants who did not experience the Holocaust, and/or with children of nonimmigrant Jewish families. In contrast to the clinical reports, the majority of these studies (8 of the 11 covered in the review and a ninth presented by the reviewers themselves) found little or no relationship between the children's psychiatric symptoms and either the parents' survival of the Holocaust or their exposure to the environment of the concentration camps (e.g., Leon, Butcher, Kleinman, Goldberg, & Almagor, 1981; Schwartz *et al.,* 1994; Sigal & Weinfeld, 1989; Weiss, O'Connell, & Siiter, 1986).

Examples of nonsymptomatic consequences, however, were noted in several papers. One study found a relationship between survival in a concentration camp and an especially great need for personal support, feelings of low self-esteem, and conflicted family relationships (Last & Klein, 1981). Another study found second-generation survivors less likely to externalize aggression (Nadler, Kav-Venaki, & Gleitman, 1985). One of the more methodologically sound studies (Sigal & Weinfeld, 1989) found no differences between groups in clinical status or social adjustment. However, that study did note more liberal political attitudes, a greater sense of political activism, and greater knowledge of the Holocaust among children of survivors than in comparison groups. A fourth study of a large sample of Israeli adults also found no current effects on the second generation, but significantly more frequent reports of psychopathology in the *past* (Schwartz *et al.,* 1994). Another study showed that 3 years after the war ended, Israeli soldiers who suffered from acute combat stress reactions during the Lebanon War, and who were children of Holocaust survivors, had more severe and more prolonged PTSD than other soldiers (Solomon, Kotler, & Mikulciner, 1988). Although findings are not consistent across studies and do not typically suggest significant psychopathology, there is *some* empirical evidence of intergenerational effects on offspring of Holocaust survivors.

Several empirical studies of the children of American combat veterans have also appeared in recent years. The first, conducted in a predominantly VA clinical sample of Vietnam veterans suffering from PTSD, found no relationship between the severity of the veterans' PTSD and their children's adjustment (Harkness, 1994). A significant relationship was observed, however, between violent behavior by the veteran and maladaptive behavior of children living at home. Several clinic-based studies (Davidson, Smith & Kudler, 1989; Matsakis, 1988) and a rigorous community-based epidemiological study of Vietnam veterans, the National Vietnam Veterans Readjustment Study (NVVRS; Jordan *et al.,* 1992; Kulka *et al.,* 1990a), describe clear and consistent relationships between war-related PTSD and disruptive family environments, marital instability, familial psychopathology, and behavioral maladjustment in veterans' children. The apparent discrepancy between the Harkness study and the NVVRS may be attributable to the fact that the Harkness clinic-based study examined the impact of different *degrees* of PTSD on child behavior, whereas the NVVRS compared children of veterans with PTSD to children of all other Vietnam era veterans, most of whom suffered from no psychiatric disorder.

Finally, a recent empirical study of the causes of PTSD in a sample of Vietnam combat veterans treated in VA noted a significant relationship between having a father who had served in combat and symptoms of both war-related PTSD and general psychological distress (Fontana & Rosenheck, 1993). The reasons for this relationship, however, were not a focus of that study.

Empirical studies thus lend some support to clinical observations of intergenerational effects of trauma, although such confirmation has been more consistent in studies of war veterans' children than in studies of the children of Holocaust survivors. Studies of combat veterans may show stronger intergenerational effects than studies of second-generation Holocaust survivors because (1) they have typically focused on those veterans whose war-zone service resulted in PTSD, rather than on the larger group who were exposed to trauma, and (2) less time elapsed between the time of the trauma and the initiation of intergenerational data collection. Studies of Holocaust survivors have focused more generally on the effect of living through the Nazi period in Europe or of having been incarcerated in an concentration camp. They have not focused directly on those with psychiatric difficulties, since information on whether parents manifest "the Survivor Syndrome" (Niederland, 1961; Krystal & Neiderland, 1968) or PTSD has been lacking in most studies.

Another possible reason for the apparent inconsistencies among intergenerational trauma studies is that there has been a lack of clarity or consistency in defining the traumatic status of both the first and the second generation under study. As indicated earlier, some studies focus on parents who were exposed to trauma (i.e., in concentration camps or in combat), or who were potentially exposed to trauma (i.e., by living in Europe or serving in a war zone). Others, in contrast, focus on parents who meet formal criteria for PTSD.

In addition, while some studies focus on offspring with no specific exposure to trauma, others focus on those who have been exposed to trauma (whether from their parents' behavior or from nonfamily sources), and a third group has focused on those children who have been exposed to trauma *and* have been diagnosed with PTSD or other psychological problems. Overall, studies that focus on trauma survivors and their nontraumatized offspring have shown weak intergenerational affects (Schwartz *et al.*, 1994). In contrast, studies of children of parents with diagnosed PTSD have shown far stronger intergenerational affects (Kulka *et al.*, 1990a), as have studies of the children of traumatized parents who themselves were traumatized and/or who also manifest PTSD (Fontana & Rosenheck, 1993; Solomon *et al.*, 1988) We feel these differences between samples in the degree of trauma exposure and symptomatology may play a central role in determining the strength of the observed intergenerational effects of trauma. These issues have not received adequate attention. Table 1 illustrates the six possible combinations of parental and second-generation status with respect to trauma and PTSD, and summarizes the proportion of empirical studies in each category showing significant intergenerational affects. In this summary, *all* of the nonconfirming studies have involved nontraumatized offspring.

In this chapter, we seek to enlarge our empirical understanding of intergenerational aspects of the genesis of Vietnam-related PTSD by exploring the impact of having a combat veteran father on (1) childhood family relationships, (2) current psychopathology, and (3) social adjustment and alienation from authority. Toward this end, we present findings from two studies in which we compare Vietnam veterans whose fathers served in combat with those whose fathers did not—one involving 400 Vietnam veterans seeking treatment for PTSD from VA's PTSD Clinical Teams program (Fontana & Rosenheck, 1993), and the second involving over 1,400 male veterans in the national community sample surveyed in the NVVRS (Kulka *et al.*, 1990a). In the course of our investigation, we examine the differential effects of parental combat exposure on offspring who (1) were exposed to little or no war-zone trauma, (2) were exposed to high levels of war-zone trauma, and (3) evidenced symptoms of PTSD.

Table 1. Proportion of Empirical Studies Demonstrating Intergenerational Psychological Effects of Trauma

	Parental exposure	
Offspring exposure	Trauma	PTSD
None	3/12 (25%)[a]	2/3 (67%)[b-d]
Trauma	NA	NA
PTSD	2/2 (100%)[e,f]	NA

Note: Studies are classified by the nature of parent and offspring exposure to trauma and PTSD.
[a]Schwartz, Dohrenwend, & Levav (1994)
[b]Kulka *et al.* (1990a)
[c]Harkness (1994)
[d]Davidson, Smith, & Kudler (1989)
[e]Solomon, Kotler, & Mikulincer (1988)
[f]Fontana & Rosenheck (1994a)
NA = No studies available.

STUDY 1: TREATMENT-SEEKING VIETNAM VETERANS' METHODS

Sample

Data for this study were gathered as baseline assessments in the national evaluation of the Department of Veterans Affairs (VA) PTSD Clinical Team (PCT) Program. Six teams, located in Boston, Massachusetts, Jackson, Mississippi, Kansas City, Missouri, New Orleans, Louisiana, Providence, Rhode Island, and San Francisco, California, were invited to participate in an intensive outcome monitoring study. During 1990–1991, 439 male veterans who served in the Vietnam theater of war completed baseline assessments. Each veteran was asked if his father was a veteran ($n = 256$, 58.3%) and if he had been involved in combat ($n = 155$, 39.5%). This study focuses on a comparison of two groups: those whose fathers were exposed to combat ($n = 155$, 39.5%) and those who were not ($n = 241$, 61%). The father's combat exposure did not differ significantly among the six sites.

Measures

Veterans in these two groups were compared on measures in four principal domains: (1) demographic characteristics, (2) premilitary family environment and personal adjustment, (3) conditions of military entry and war-zone experiences, and (4) current symptomatology and social adjustment.

Demographic Characteristics. Data on age (mean = 42.9 years; $SD = 3.13$) and race ($n = 283$, 72.2% white; $n = 94$, 23.9% black; $n = 4$, 0.9% Hispanic; and $n = 12$, 3.0% other) were recorded for each veteran.

Premilitary Family Environment. A negative family environment was assessed by two measures. One was the Family Stability Scale (Kadushin, Boulanger & Martin, 1981) which is coded in the direction of family instability (mean = 3.0, $SD = 2.15$). This scale is composed of 11 dichotomous items covering experiences before the age of 18, such as parental separation, divorce, or death; father being out of wok; or family income less than $5,000 per year.

The second measure is composed of two questions concerning whether either parent had been hospitalized for a psychiatric or substance-abuse problem during the veteran's childhood ($n = 43$, 9.9%), or whether either parent seemed to the veteran to have a problem with alcohol or drug abuse ($n = 141$, 32.6%). They were combined to identify families in which there was evidence of parental psychological problems ($n = 161$, 37.2%).

A positive family environment was identified by questions concerning whether the veteran felt emotionally close to his or her family ($n = 307$, 70,9%) and whether he or she was free of physical or sexual abuse by either parent ($n = 389$, 88.5%). We combined these two items to identify close, nonabusive families ($n = 291$, 67.1%).

Premilitary Personal Adjustment. Conduct disorder in childhood was measured by an index composed of behaviors such as being in trouble with the law or school officials, playing hookey, being suspended or expelled, or doing poorly academically (Helzer 1981) (mean = 1.54, $SD = 2.08$).

Positive adjustment prior to entry into the military was measured by an Adolescent Social Adjustment Index (ASAI) that we constructed as the sum of three aspects of the veteran's interaction with his or her peers: (1) having close friends, (2) dating, and (3) being actively involved in extracurricular activities (mean = 6.1, SD = 1.97, alpha = 0.67).

Military Entry and Experience.   Age at entry into the military was recorded (mean = 18.93, SD = 1.84), as was the issue of whether the veteran entered the military willingly (n = 278, 64.7%) or reluctantly (n = 152, 35.3%). Specific war-zone experiences were assessed by three variables. Exposure to combat was measured by the Revised Combat Scale (mean = 10.72, SD = 2.74). Laufer, Yager, Frey-Wouters, & Donnellan, 1981). Witnessing and participating in abusive violence were assessed, following the convention advocated by Laufer and his colleagues (Laufer, Brett, & Gallops, 1985), as two mutually exclusive categories: witnessing abusive violence perpetrated by others only (n = 173, 39.4%), and participating in abusive violence oneself (n = 138, 31.4%).

Current Symptomatology.   PTSD symptoms were measured with the Mississippi Scale for Combat-Related PTSD (mean = 126.02, SD = 20.7) (Keane, Caddell, & Taylor, 1989), and general psychiatric symptoms with the Global Severity Index of the Brief Symptom Inventory (BSI-GSI) (mean = 2.18, SD = 0.79). (McLellan *et al.,* 1985). A Suicidal Behavior Index (0 = never made a suicide attempt, 1 = made one or more attempts but never required medical hospitalization, 2 = made at least one attempt that required medical hospitalization) was constructed as an indicator of severe psychiatric problems (mean = 0.49 SD = 0.76). Guilt was measured by the Guilt Inventory (Laufer & Frey-Wouters, 1988) (mean = 2.75, SD = 0.98), an instrument specifically designed to assess issues of war-related guilt. Change in religious faith during Vietnam service was also assessed, using a 5-point scale, with scores below 3 representing loss of faith, and scores above 3 representing strengthened faith (mean = 2.69, SD = 1.04). Eight items concerning violent behavior (each rated on a 5-point scale) were used to create a violence index (mean = 10.18, SD = 6.56, alpha = 0.77). The Addiction Severity Index (ASI; McLellan *et al.,* 1985) was used to measure alcohol problems (mean = 0.12, SD = 0.20) and drug abuse problems (mean = 0.04, SD = 0.11).

Social Adjustment

Several aspects of postwar social adaptation were assessed: (1) educational attainment (mean = 13.09 years, SD = 2.39), (2) marital status (n = 208 married, 47.4%), (3) current full-time employment (n = 134, 30.5%), (4) total monthly income (mean = \$1,187, SD = \$1,134), (5) the number of people with whom the veteran felt close (mean = 10.37, SD = 7.47), and (6) the number of people from whom the veteran felt he could currently receive advice, material assistance, or psychological support (mean = 8.49, SD = 5.14, alpha 0.78). Current (7) recreational and social activity was measured using the Katz and Lyerly (1963) index (mean = 11.09, SD = 5.33). Antisocial adjustment since leaving the military was also measured, by (8) the number of arrests for different categories of felonies (mean = 1.0, SD 1.49) and (9) misdemeanors (mean = 0.89, SD = 0.97).

Analyses

The significance of differences in all measures between the two groups was tested using t tests for continuous variables and chi-square tests for categorical variables. One-way analysis of covariance (ANCOVA) was then used to determine whether significant differences in symptoms and social adjustment between father–combat groups in the bivariate comparisons could be accounted for by premilitary or wartime experiences that also differed significantly between the groups.

Results from Study 1

Bivariate Analyses.   Table 2 shows that Vietnam veterans whose fathers also served in combat were currently younger than other veterans, but they were not significantly different in race or on any measure of premilitary family environment or childhood behavior. Veterans

Table 2. Comparison of Vietnam Veterans in VA's PCT program According to Whether Their Father Ever Served in Combat

	Father not in combat N = 284 (60.5%)	Father in combat N = 155 (39.5%)	T	Chi-Square	N
Demographics					
Age	43.3	42.3	3.37		0.00
Race				5.44	NS
White	70.5%	79.6%			
Black	25.7%	15.9%			
Hispanic	1.3%	0.8%			
Other	3.2%	2.9%			
Premilitary behavior and family environment					
Family Stability Index	3.06	2.87	0.89		NS
Close, nonabusive family	63.9%	68.9%		1.07	NS
Parent mentally ill	35.4%	41.9%		1.67	NS
Childhood Problem Index	1.45	1.66	0.98		NS
Adolescent Social Adjustment	6.02	6.16	0.67		NS
Military service					
Age at entry to military	19.14	18.57	3.23		0.00
Reluctant service entry	37.3%	32.3%		1.04	NS
Combat scale	10.58	10.73	0.50		NS
Witnessed abusive violence	43.2%	38.2%		0.96	NS
Participated in abusive violence	27.4%	37.6%		4.56	0.03
Current symptoms					
Mississippi PTSD Scale	122.8	129.7	3.30		0.00
BSI-GSI	2.07	2.29	2.67		0.01
Suicidal Behavior Index	0.38	0.63	3.17		0.00
Laufer–Parson Guilt Inventory	2.61	2.98	3.78		0.00
Change in religious faith	2.80	2.50	2.76		0.01
Violence Index	10.02	10.61	0.87		NS
Alcohol Index (ASI)	0.11	0.13	1.01		NS
Drug Index (ASI)	0.03	0.04	0.99		NS
Current social adjustment					
Highest education	13.09	13.21	0.51		NS
Never married	48.6%	45.9%		0.28	NS
Currently working	39.0%	32.5%		3.68	NS
Income (past month)	$1,206	$1,189		0.15	NS
Social activities (Katz, 1963)	11.4	10.5	1.64		NS
People feel close to	10.83	9.45	1.82		0.06
Social support	8.6	8.44	0.30		NS
Major crimes	0.92	1.12	1.33		NS
Misdemeanors	0.90	0.88	0.17		NS

whose fathers saw combat were also younger when they entered the military, and they participated more frequently in abusive violence, although there were no differences in the frequency
of witnessing abusive violence, or in combat exposure. Significant differences were found on
four symptom measures: the Mississippi PTSD Scale, the BSI-GSI, the Suicidal Behavior Index, and the Guilt Inventory. There was also a significantly greater loss of religious faith
among those whose fathers saw combat (Table 2). There were no significant differences in current social adjustment.

One-Way Analyses of Covariance.   After controlling for current age, age at entry into
the military, and participation in abusive violence, a significant relationship persisted between
father's combat experience and all five measures that had shown a significant difference in the
bivariate analyses: the Mississippi PTSD Scale ($F = 4.17$; $df = 1, 435$; $p < .05$), the BSI-GSI ($F
= 3.90$; $df = 1, 435$; $p < .05$), the Suicidal Behavior Index ($F = 8.44$; $df = 1, 435$; $p < .01$), the
Guilt Inventory ($F = 7.03$; $df = 1, 435$; $p < .01$), and the loss of religious faith ($F = 4.30$; $df =
1, 435$; $p < .05$). Thus, after controlling for other potentially explanatory variables, veterans
whose fathers saw combat still had more severe and pervasive psychological symptoms than
other veterans. It is notable that these differences emerge in the absence of any measured differences in childhood experience that might explain them.

STUDY 2: A COMMUNITY SAMPLE—THE NATIONAL VIETNAM VETERANS READJUSTMENT SURVEY (NVVRS) METHODS

Sample

The NVVRS was conducted on a national sample of veterans who served in the U.S.
Armed Forces during the Vietnam era. The sampling frame was a national screening sample of
military personnel records and is described in detail in the original publications on the survey
(Kulka *et al.,* 1990a, 1990b). Blacks and Hispanics were oversampled.

Measures

As in the previous study, the full sample of Vietnam theater veterans were classified as
those who reported that their fathers had served in combat ($n = 278$, 26.8%) and those who
reported that their fathers had not served in combat ($n = 761$, 73.2%). Unfortunately, no data
were available on whether their fathers had suffered psychological or other sequelae of their
wartime service.

Characteristics of these veterans that are of relevance to assessing the impact of their father's combat service were grouped into five sets of variables. Only males were included in this
study.

Demographic Characteristics.   Data on age (mean = 41.9 years, $SD = 5.6$) and race ($n =
519$, 50% white; $n = 283$, 27% black; $n = 237$, 27% Hispanic) were obtained on all subjects.

Premilitary Family Environment.   Family instability was measured, as in the VA study,
by (1) the Family Stability Scale (Kadushin *et al.,* 1981) (mean = 2.88, $SD = 1.91$). Other measures of premilitary experience included (2) indicators of exposure to physical violence or
abuse in the family before the age of 18 ($n = 223$, 21.5%); (3) having a parent who suffered

from substance abuse or mental illness ($n = 227$, 21.8%); (4) positive qualities in the veteran's relationship to his or her father (the average of five items that assessed affection, sharing of interests, confiding, closeness, and helpfulness on a series of 5-point scales) (mean = 3.27, SD = 1.08, Cronbach's alpha = 0.89); (5) positive qualities in his or her relationship to his or her mother using the same items (mean = 4.04, SD = 0.86, Cronbach's alpha = 0.88); (6) how much the veteran wanted to be like his or her father (mean = 3.13, SD = 1.44); and (7) the veteran's history of conduct disorder, measured, as in the VA study, by reports of behaviors occurring before the age of 15 (Helzer, 1981) (mean = 1.78, SD = 1.89).

Period of Military Service. The veteran's initial experience of the military was documented by (1) age at entry to the military (mean = 20.00, SD = 2.22), and (2) whether the veteran had been reluctant to enter the military (i.e., was drafted or volunteered under pressure) ($n = 281$, 27.12%). War-zone traumatic experience was assessed (3) by the same scale of exposure to combat used in the VA study (Laufer *et al.*, 1981) (mean = 7.64, SD = 4.37), and by (4) dichotomous determinations of participation in abusive violence (i.e., atrocities) ($n = 344$, 33.08%) and witnessing abusive violence committed by others ($n = 195$, 18.7%). Several measures of war-zone exposure was combined to identify veterans exposed to high levels of war-zone stress (Kulka *et al.*, 1990a) ($n = 445$, 42.8%).

First Year of Postmilitary Readjustment. Three measures assessed immediate postmilitary social experiences. The first is a scale based on questions that addressed the availability of people with whom the veterans could talk about personal matters during the first year after discharge (mean = 24.15, SD = 2.30, alpha = 0.60). The second measure was based on questions concerning the availability of material and emotional support during the year after discharge (mean = 7.46, SD = 1.06, alpha = 0.78). The third is a measure of the degree to which the veteran felt welcomed home or appreciated by the nation he or she had served (mean = 20.21, SD = 5.32, alpha = 0.79).

Subsequent Postmilitary Period. Several features of postmilitary psychiatric adjustment were examined. PTSD was assessed using the Mississippi Scale for Combat-Related PTSD (mean = 72.08, SD = 22.28) (Keane *et al.*, 1988) and demoralization with the Demoralization subscale of the Psychiatric Epidemiological Research Instrument (PERI) (Dohrenwend, Shrout, Egri, & Mendelsohn, 1980) (mean = 76.08, SD = 22.28). Veterans with a Mississippi scale score of 89 or greater were considered to be PTSD cases, as determined by an extensive validation procedure ($n = 262$, 25.2%) (Kulka *et al.*, 1990b). Survivor guilt was assessed with a single, 3-level severity assessment (mean = 0.07, SD = .35) and past suicidal behavior with a 3-level scale (0 = no attempt or gesture, 1 = gesture, 2 = serious attempt) (mean = 0.05, SD = 0.29). Lifetime psychiatric diagnoses other than substance abuse ($n = 212$, 20.36%) and a diagnosis of substance abuse ($n = 451$, 43.36%), based on a diagnoses of either alcohol abuse or dependence ($n = 425$, 40.9%) or drug abuse or dependence ($n = 70$, 6.7%) were assessed by the Diagnostic Interview Schedule (DIS) (Robins, Helzer, Croughan, & Ratcliff, 1981).

Postmilitary education (mean = 13.38 years, SD = 2.37), marital status ($n = 741$ married, 71.28%), personal income (mean = $2,179, SD = $1,017), social support (measured by 10 questions concerning access to assistance of various types) (mean = 19.02, SD = 2.00, Cronbach's alpha = 0.96), and criminal activity (major crimes: mean = 0.14, SD = 0.76; and misdemeanors: mean = 0.04, SD = 0.22) were also evaluated. A 7-item scale was used to assess violent behavior (mean = 7.71, SD = 4.33, Cronbach's alpha = 0.63). Finally, a measure of social alienation assessed the degree to which the veteran felt victimized by societal forces and by powers that exploited or took advantage of him or her (mean = 25.11, *SD* = 6.06, Cronbach's alpha = 0.74).

Analyses.   Potential areas of intergenerational influence were assessed first by comparing veterans whose fathers served in combat with veterans whose fathers did not on all measures using *t* tests for continuous variables and chi-square tests for categorical variables.

In view of our literature review and especially Solomon *et al.*'s (1988) finding of significant differences in severity in the response of second-generation Holocaust survivors who suffered from combat stress reactions, we classified veterans into three trauma/PTSD categories according to their levels of war-zone stress and PTSD (*n* = 594 with low war-zone stress, 57.17%; *n* = 175 with high war-zone stress but not meeting the symptom cutoff for PTSD, 16.84%; and *n* = 270 with PTSD, 25.99%). We then conducted a two-way ANOVA in which we evaluated the interaction of having a father who served in combat within each level of the trauma/PTSD classification. Where the ANOVA showed significant differences, *t* tests were used to compare veterans whose fathers served in combat and those whose fathers did not, within each level of the trauma/PTSD classification.

Two-way ANCOVA, in which premilitary variables, and the pre- and postmilitary variables were included as covariates, was used to determine whether significant differences in symptoms and social adjustment between father–combat groups in the first set of ANOVAs could be accounted for by either premilitary family experiences alone or by the addition of postmilitary homecoming experiences.

Finally, in view of our findings from the VA clinical sample, we repeated the comparison of veterans whose fathers served in combat with those whose fathers did not on the subgroup of NVVRS respondents who reported any past use of VA mental health services.

Results from Study 2

Table 3 shows that in the entire national sample, there were few significant differences between veterans whose fathers served in combat and those who did not. As in the VA treatment sample, those whose fathers served in combat were younger and had entered the military at a younger age than other veterans. The only other significant difference, that they were less likely to be black, is most likely due to the smaller number of blacks who served in combat World War II, as compared to Vietnam (4.9% vs. 9.1%)) (Rosenheck & Fontana, 1994). A significant difference was also noted for one postmilitary variable, lifetime alcohol abuse. Because of these differences, age and black ethnicity were included as covariates in subsequent analyses.

Significant interactions (Table 4) showed that among veterans whose symptoms exceeded the cutoff for PTSD, those whose fathers served in combat had poorer relationships with their mothers when they were children, less help at the time of their homecoming, higher Mississippi PTSD Scale scores, more survivor guilt, greater lifetime prevalence of drug abuse, and lower levels of current social support. In contrast, there were no significant differences between veterans whose fathers served in combat and other veterans who had either high or low exposure to war-zone trauma without PTSD.

ANCOVA showed that adjusting for the effect of premilitary family variables (family instability, relationship with mother and father, wanting to be like father, ever were hit in the family, having a parent with psychiatric or substance-abuse problems) had no effect on the results. Significant differences were still observed, among those with PTSD, between veterans whose fathers were in combat and those whose fathers were not, in PTSD symptoms (*F* = 3.43;

Table 3. Comparison of Male Vietnam Theater Veterans Whose Fathers Served in Combat versus All Others: NVVRS

	Father no combat N = 772 74.3%	Father saw combat N = 283 27.2%	T	Chi-Square	P
Premilitary					
Age	42.62	40.74	5.88		0.000
Race				12.53	0.000
White	47.9%	58.5%			
Black	27.5%	18.1%			
Hispanic	23.4%	21.6%			
Other	1.3%	1.8%			
Family instability	2.65	2.54	0.91		NS
Ever hit in family?	21.5%	20.6%		0.11	NS
Parent had mental illness or substance abuse	21.0%	21.8%		1.12	NS
Relationship with father	3.30	3.20	1.24		NS
Relationship with mother	4.04	3.96	1.45		NS
Wanted to be like father?	3.10	3.24	1.43		NS
Conduct disorder	1.69	1.86	1.27		NS
Military service					
Age at entry to the military	20.09	19.85	1.36		NS
Reluctant to enter service	73.3%	71.4%		0.36	NS
Combat exposure	7.53	7.84	0.99		NS
Participated in atrocities	31.7%	34.8%		0.91	NS
Witnessed atrocities	18.2%	19.5%		0.24	NS
Homecoming					
People to talk with at homecoming	24.24	24.17	0.46		NS
People offered help at homecoming	7.52	7.43	1.18		NS
Felt welcomed and appreciated	20.42	19.96	1.23		NS
Current psychiatric status					
PTSD (Mississippi scale)	75.16	75.83	0.42		NS
Survivor guilt	0.06	0.10	1.45		NS
Demoralization (PERI)	54.81	53.83	0.75		NS
Suicide Attempt Scale	0.04	0.06	0.78		NS
Violence	7.56	7.71	0.54		NS
Any non-PTSD psychiatric diagnosis	19.8%	18.7%		0.16	NS
Depression	6.0%	5.0%		0.38	NS
Manic	0.8%	1.8%		1.97	NS
Dysthymia	6.0%	3.6%		2.38	NS
General anxiety disorder	16.2%	16.7%		0.03	NS
OCD	2.2%	2.5%		0.07	NS
Panic disorder	1.8%	4.3%		5.12	0.024
Substance abuse (lifetime)	41.5%	47.7%		3.17	NS
Alcohol abuse	39.2%	46.3%		4.28	0.039
Drug abuse	6.1%	8.2%		1.44	NS
Current social adjustment					
Married	72.4%	75.6%		1.09	NS
People feels close to	10.86	10.32	1.00		NS
Social support	19.16	18.93	1.60		NS
Major crimes	0.13	0.11	0.36		NS
Misdemeanors	0.04	0.03	1.15		NS
Alienation	25.07	24.87	0.47		NS
Education	13.38	13.53	0.97		NS
Income (monthly)	$2,174	$2,317	1.86		NS

Table 4. Comparison of Male Veterans Whose Fathers Served in Combat versus All Others by War-Zone Stress and PTSD Status (ANCOVA)[a,b]

| | | Served in VN | | War-zone Stress | | | | ANCOVA Interaction Term | |
| | | No Warzone Stress | | No PTSD | | PTSD | | Father in combat | Trauma |
	N	No Father in combat	Father in combat	No Father in combat	Father in combat	No Father in combat	Father in combat	F	P
		N = 438	N = 156	N = 127	N = 48	N = 196	N = 74		
		42.2%	15.0%	12.2%	46.%	18.9%	7.1%F		
Premilitary									
Family instability	1,039	2.41	2.19	2.39	2.29	3.36	3.45	0.50	NS
Ever hit in family?	1,037	0.16	0.16	0.22	0.17	0.33	0.28	0.32	NS
Parent had mental illness or substance abuse	1,035	0.19	0.21	0.19	0.19	0.28	0.36	0.90	NS
Relationship with father	1,039	3.30	3.33	3.42	3.29	3.22	2.94	2.53	NS
Relationship with mother	1,033	4.07	4.09	4.18	4.01	3.91	3.64a	3.25	0.0391
Wanted to be like father?	1,014	3.06	3.25	3.23	3.36	3.25	3.20	0.17	NS
Conduct disorder	1,039	1.46	1.56	1.51	1.79	2.32	2.61	0.46	NS
Military service									
Age at entry to the military	1,039	20.21	20.20	20.07	19.77	19.89	19.22	2.15	NS
Reluctant to enter service	999	0.73	0.68	0.71	0.75	0.76	0.76	0.31	NS
Combat exposure	1,039	5.34	55.8	11.36	11.81	10.06	10.04	0.18	NS
Participated in atrocities	1,038	0.12	0.13	0.56	0.65	0.59	0.61	0.52	NS
Witnessed atrocities	1,037	0.14	0.19	0.32	0.25	0.19	0.18	1.47	NS
Homecoming									
People to talk with at homecoming	1,039	24.70	24.81	24.42	24.45	23.14	22.71	1.47	NS
People offered help at homecoming	1,039	7.74	7.84	7.63	7.65	7.01	6.43b	10.45	0.0001
Felt welcomed and appreciated by nation	1,039	21.95	21.90	20.38	20.05	17.08	15.97	0.77	NS

Current psychiatric status

PTSD (Mississippi scale)	1,039	63.59	62.35	70.60	69.52	104.06	108.54a	4.49	0.0114
Survivor guilt	1,031	0.02	0.01	0.01	0.00	0.20	0.35b	5.71	0.0034
Demoralization (PERI)	1,039	47.78	46.55	49.30	48.16	74.30	73.40	0.04	NS
Suicide Attempt Scale	1,033	0.01	0.04	0.03	0.04	0.13	0.12	0.23	NS
Violence	1,039	6.38	6.75	7.02	6.90	10.48	10.35	0.24	NS
Any non-PTSD psychiatric diagnosis	1,039	0.09	0.11	0.18	0.06	0.46	0.43	1.95	NS
Depression	1,039	0.01	0.00	0.01	0.00	0.20	0.19	0.01	NS
Manic	1,039	0.00	0.00	0.00	0.00	0.03	0.07	2.66	NS
Dysthymia	1,039	0.01	0.01	0.02	0.00	0.19	0.12	1.48	NS
General anxiety disorder	1,039	0.08	0.10	0.16	0.06	0.35	0.36	1.55	NS
OCD	1,039	0.00	0.00	0.01	0.00	0.08	0.09	0.32	NS
Panic disorder	1,039	0.01	0.01	0.01	0.00	0.04	0.15b	11.15	0.0001
Substance abuse (lifetime)	1,034	0.36	0.39	0.36	0.38	0.58	0.72	1.22	NS
Alcohol abuse	1,037	0.35	0.38	0.33	0.38	0.54	0.69	1.36	NS
Drug abuse	1,033	0.03	0.03	0.06	0.00	0.14	0.25b	5.51	0.0042
Current social adjustment									
Married	1,039	0.77	0.81	0.75	0.83	0.61	0.61	0.26	NS
People feels close to	1,038	11.86	11.64	12.10	11.83	7.83	6.85	0.35	NS
Social support	1,038	19.50	19.53	19.52	19.47	18.14	17.32b	4.03	0.0181
Major crimes	1,021	0.02	0.02	0.16	0.09	0.34	0.32	0.08	NS
Misdemeanors	1,021	0.03	0.01	0.02	0.01	0.10	0.07	0.33	NS
Alienation	1,038	23.91	23.25	24.19	23.63	28.16	19.17	1.67	NS
Education	1,038	13.66	13.74	13.20	13.67	12.92	12.93	0.37	NS
Income (monthly)	1,011	$2,395	$2,535	$2,319	$2,575	$1,581	$1,672	0.18	NS

a Age and race (black vs. other) are included as covariates in all analyses.

b Key: $a = p < .01$; $b = p < .0001$

$df = 13, 990; p < .03$), survivor guilt ($F = 7.45, df = 2, 982; p < .0006$), help at the time of homecoming ($F = 8.93; df = 2, 990; p < .0001$), lifetime panic disorder ($F = 7.28; df = 2, 990; p < .0007$), lifetime drug abuse ($F = 6.00; df = 2, 984; p < .0026$), and current social support ($F = 3.42; df = 2, 989; p < .04$).

ANCOVA showed that adjusting additionally for the effect of homecoming variables (someone to talk with after the war, help adjusting after the war, and feeling welcomed home) eliminated the significant differences in PTSD symptoms and current social support, but not in lifetime panic disorder ($F = 6.21; df = 16, 987; p < .02$), survivor guilt ($F = 6.96; df = 16, 979; p < .002$), or drug abuse ($F = 4.96; df = 16, 981; p < .008$). These analyses suggest that the lack of support at the time of homecoming is significantly related to the greater level of PTSD symptoms and current social support, but not to survivor guilt, panic disorder, or drug abuse, which appear to be related to other, unmeasured factors.

Finally, in a replication of the VA study presented (Study 1), using NVVRS data, we found a significant difference between veteran subgroups who had used VA mental health services: Veterans whose fathers had served in combat had higher scores on the Mississippi PTSD Scale than others ($t = 2.47; df = 42; p < .02$).

Discussion

The data presented here largely confirm findings of previous studies of the multigenerational impact of trauma. In addition, they help to integrate what previously appeared to be conflicting and contradictory findings. Before reviewing the findings, it is important to emphasize that we focused exclusively on the intergenerational effect of trauma rather than on the effect of PTSD, since no data were available on PTSD among the fathers of the veterans in either of our samples. In this respect, our study parallels previous studies of children of survivors of the Holocaust. This, we contend, is the appropriate focus of intergenerational studies. In studies that focus on the effect of PTSD on children, the effect of trauma is confounded by the many other factors that contribute to the genesis of PTSD (Fontana & Rosenheck, 1993; Fontana & Rosenheck, 1994a).

Our examination of the community sample of Vietnam theater veterans surveyed in the NVVRS, consistent with the majority of community studies of the children of Holocaust survivors, found very limited evidence of greater psychopathology, demoralization, or maladjustment among veterans whose fathers served in combat. The only differences were in age, race, and lifetime alcohol abuse.

Unlike some studies of second-generation Holocaust survivors, however, we failed to find evidence of differences in childhood family relationships or in alienation from authorities. This may reflect the fact that most of the combat veteran fathers of Vietnam veterans served in World War II. Although many of these fathers experienced severe trauma, they fought for a popular cause that succeeded in its objectives and were publicly praised and honored when they returned home. Their children, although aware of the honor of their fathers' service, typically had little idea of the horror of war (Kovic, 1977; Puller, 1993; Rosenheck, 1986). For Holocaust survivors, in contrast, there were no victories, and no proud celebrations—only survival and continued endurance of unspeakable grief and loss (Danieli, 1981, 1988).

The picture changed substantially when we considered specific subgroups of veterans. Most striking is the observation that among veterans who met the diagnostic threshold for PTSD, veterans whose fathers served in combat had more severe PTSD symptoms, more survivor guilt, less current social support, and were more likely to meet criteria for lifetime panic disorder and drug abuse. Curiously, these clinical differences are associated with only limited evidence of more severe problems with parental relationships in childhood or with family instability. Rather, they were associated with reports of less help from family and friends at the time of homecoming. Furthermore, when the effect of the homecoming experience was controlled through multivariate techniques, the differences between groups in PTSD symptoms and social support were no longer significant, suggesting that the observed differences in symptom levels may have been partially attributable to differences in homecoming experience.

The more negative homecoming experience among Vietnam veterans with combat veteran fathers is not hard to understand. Vietnam veterans with severe, disabling PTSD (Rosenheck, 1985a, 1985b), as well as others such as Ron Kovic (1977) and Lewis Puller (1993), report serious conflicts or misunderstanding with their World War II veteran fathers after the war. There were vast differences between military service in these two eras: in the nature of the fighting (Rosenheck & Fontana, 1994; Fontana & Rosenheck, 1994b); in the outcome of the fighting; and in public attitudes toward the war. Never in our history have warrior fathers and warrior sons had such diametrically opposed experiences of service to their country. We have suggested previously (Fontana & Rosenheck, 1994a) that the lack of a supportive reception after the Vietnam War may have impeded the resolution of PTSD symptoms for many veterans. This seems to have been an especially important factor for those who served in Vietnam and found themselves contending, on their return, with fathers whose wartime experience was in "The Good War."

Our findings on this subgroup of veterans with PTSD are also consistent with those of Solomon *et al.* (1988) among veterans of the Lebanon War. Our findings, in particular, suggest that the greater severity of PTSD symptoms among second-generation trauma survivors may also have less to do with pretrauma vulnerability for PTSD, and more with greater difficulties with coping and recovery at the time of homecoming.

The central finding in our sample of VA patients with PTSD (that those whose fathers served in combat had more severe PTSD symptoms than other veterans) was replicated in our examination of the subgroup of veterans in the NVVRS community sample who had used VA mental health services. To determine whether this finding was specific to users of VA mental health services, or whether it applied equally to those who had sought mental health treatment from non-VA providers, we repeated these comparisons on the subgroup of veterans who had used non-VA mental health services. In this subgroup, there were no significant differences between veterans whose fathers had served in combat and veterans whose fathers did not. We have shown elsewhere that Vietnam veterans with PTSD are more likely to use VA than non-VA mental health services (Rosenheck & Fontana, 1995), and we believe that observed VA-related effects are due to the greater proportion of veterans with PTSD in those samples. The more dramatic results in the VA clinical sample, as compared to the NVVRS subgroup, most likely reflect the fact that all of these veterans were seeking services for PTSD. The NVVRS sample of VA mental health service users had sought help for diverse emotional or family problems, not just for PTSD.

Our interpretation that intergenerational effects are strongest among those who are exposed to trauma and suffer resulting ill effects may also help to account for the diverse conclusions of studies of the second generation of Holocaust survivors. Several commentators have suggested that differences between children of Holocaust survivors and comparison groups are most robust in studies that rely on small samples drawn from religious or other groups with a special interest in the Holocaust, whose subjects have strong identities as children of survivors, or in studies biased by poor response rates (Schwartz *et al.*, 1994; Sigal & Weinfeld, 1989). These samples are likely to include greater proportions of help-seeking offspring with emotional problems or secondary posttraumatic conditions (Rosenheck & Nathan,

1985) and those with strong identifications with their parents (Epstein, 1979). Our examination of data from several veteran subgroups, therefore, suggests that it is among the most troubled segments of the population that second-generation effects are strongest.

The good news of intergenerational studies of trauma is that, in most cases, the horrors of the parents are not visited on the children, at least as long as there is not further exposure to trauma. This does not mean, of course, that these children are indifferent to or uninterested in the suffering of their parents. As Erikson (1968, p. 29) put it almost 50 years ago, the core issue for all people, "identity . . . is a generational issue." But although the children of Holocaust survivors and war veterans may be interested, concerned, or even preoccupied with the experiences of their parents, they are not generally made ill by them.

It does appear, however, that some members of the next generation, should they be exposed to their own traumatic experiences and suffer from PTSD, may have a more difficult time recovering from those experiences than those whose parents did not experience trauma. This may be either because they cannot easily obtain needed support directly from their families of origin during the recovery period, or because they did not fully develop internalized self-healing capacities when they were young, perhaps because, as suggested by Krystal (1988), the healing capacities of their parents were so thoroughly overwhelmed.

ACKNOWLEDGMENTS: We would like to thank Yael Danieli and Paul Errera for their suggestions and assistance in the preparation of this chapter.

REFERENCES

Barocas, H. A., & Barocas, C. B. (1973). Manifestations of concentration camp effects on the second generation. *American Journal of Psychiatry, 130,* 820–821.

Bergmann, M. S., & Jucovy, M. E. (Eds.). (1982). *Generations of the Holocaust.* New York: Basic Books.

Danieli, Y. (1981). Families of survivors of the Nazi Holocaust: Some short- and long-term effects. In C. D. Spielberger, I. G. Sarason, & N. Milgram (Eds.), *Stress and anxiety* (Vol. 8) New York: McGraw-Hill/Hemisphere.

Danieli, Y. (1985). Treatment and prevention of long-term effects and intergenerational transmission of victimization: A lesson from Holocaust survivors and their children. In C. R. Figley (Ed.), *Trauma and its wake: Vol. I. The study and treatment of post-traumatic stress disorder* (pp. 295–313). New York: Brunner/Mazel.

Danieli, Y. (1988). Mourning in survivors and children of survivors of the Nazi Holocaust: The role of group and community modalities. In D. R. Deitrich & P. C. Shabod (Eds.), *Problems of loss and mourning: Psychoanalytic perspectives* (pp. 427–460). Madison, CT: International Universities Press.

Danieli, Y. (1993). Diagnostic and therapeutic use of the multigenerational family trees in working with survivors and children of survivors of the Nazi Holocaust. In J. P. Wilson & B. Raphael (Eds.), *International handbook of traumatic stress syndromes* (pp. 889–898). New York: Plenum Press.

Davidson, J., Smith, R., & Kudler, H. (1989). Familial psychiatric illness in chronic posttraumatic stress disorder. *Comprehensive Psychiatry, 30,* 339–345.

Davidson, S. (1980). The clinical effects of massive psychic trauma in families of Holocaust survivors. *Journal of Marriage and Family Therapy, 6,* 11–21.

Dohrenwend, B. P., Shrout, P. E., Egri, G., & Mendelsohn, F. (1980). Measures of nonspecific psychological distress and other dimensions of psychopathology in the general population. *Archives of General Psychiatry, 37,* 1229–1236.

Egeland, B., Jacobvitz, D., & Papatola, M. (1987). Intergenerational continuity of abuse. In R. Gelles & J. Lancaster (Eds.), *Child abuse and neglect: Biosocial dimensions* (pp. 255–276). New York: Aldine Gruyter.

Epstein, H. (1979). *Children of the Holocaust: Conversation with sons and daughters of survivors.* New York: Putnam.

Erikson, E. H. (1968). Identity: Youth and crisis. New York: Norton.

Felsen, I., & Erlich, H. S. (1990). Identification patterns of offspring of Holocaust survivors with their parents. *American Journal of Orthopsychiatry, 60*(4), 506–520.

Fontana, A. F., & Rosenheck, R. A. (1993). A causal model of the etiology of war-related PTSD. *Journal of Traumatic Stress Studies, 6,* 475–500.

Fontana, A. F., & Rosenheck, R. A. (1994a). PTSD among Vietnam theater veterans: A causal model of the etiology in a community sample. *Journal of Nervous and Mental Disease, 182,* 677–684.

Fontana, A. E., & Rosenheck, R. A. (1994b). Traumatic war stressors and psychiatric symptoms among World War II, Korean, and Vietnam veterans. *Psychology and Aging, 9,* 27–33.

Fryberg, J. T. (1980). Difficulties in separation–individuation as experienced by children of Nazi Holocaust survivors. *American Journal of Orthopsychiatry, 50,* 87–95.

Harkness, L. (1994). Intergenerational transmission of combat related trauma. In J. P. Wilson, & B. Raphae (Eds.), *The international handbook of traumatic stress syndromes* (pp. 635–643). New York: Plenum Press.

Helzer, J. E. (1981). Methodological issues in the interpretations of the consequences of extreme situations. In B. S. Dohrenwend & B. P. Dohrenwend (Eds.), *Stressful life events and their contexts* (pp. 108–129). New York: Prodist.

Hunter, R., Kilstrom, N., & Kraybill, E. (1978). Antecedents of child abuse and neglect in premature infants: A prospective study in a newborn intensive care unit. *Pediatrics, 61,* 629–635.

Jordan, B. K., Marmar, C., Fairbank, J. A., Schlenger, W. E., Kulka, R. A., Houogh, R. L., & Weiss, D. S. (1992). Problems in families of male Vietnam veterans with posttraumatic stress disorder. *Journal of Consulting and Clinical Psychology, 60,* 916–926.

Kadushin, C., Boulanger, G., & Martin, J. (1981). *Long-term stress reactions: Some causes, consequences, and naturally occurring support systems. Legacies of Vietnam: Comparative adjustment of veterans and their peers* (Vol. 4). Washington, DC: House Committee Print No. 4, U.S. Government Printing Office.

Katz, M. M., & Lyerly, S. B. (1963). Methods for measuring adjustment and social behavior in the community: I. Rationale, description, discriminative validity and scale development. *Psychological Reports, 13,* 503–535.

Keane, T. M., Caddell, J. M., & Taylor, K. L. (1989). Mississippi Scale for Combat-Related Post-Traumatic Stress Disorder: Three studies in reliability and validity. *Journal of Consulting Clinical Psychology, 56,* 85–90.

Kestenberg, J. S. (1982). Survivors parents and their children. In M. S. Bergmann & M. E. Jucovy (Eds.), *Generations of the Holocaust* (pp. 83–102). New York: Basic Books.

Kovic, R. (1977). *Born on the fourth of July.* New York: McGraw-Hill.

Krystal, H. (1988). *Integration and self-healing.* Hillsdale, NJ: Analytic Press.

Krystal, H., & Niederland, W. G. (1968). Clinical observations on the survivor syndrome. In H. Krystal (Ed.), *Massive psychic trauma* (pp. 327–348). New York: International Universities Press.

Kulka, R. A., Schlenger, W. E., Fairbank, J. A., Hough, R. L., Jordan, B. K., Marmar, C. R., & Weiss, D. A. (1990a). *Trauma and the Vietnam War generation: Report of findings from the National Vietnam Veterans Readjustment Study.* New York: Brunner/Mazel.

Kulka, R. A., Schlenger, W. E., Fairbank, J. A., Hough, R. L., Jordan, B. K., Marmar, C. R., & Weiss, D. A. (1990b). *The National Vietnam Veterans Readjustment Study: Tables of findings and technical appendices.* New York: Brunner/Mazel.

Last, V., & Klein, H. (1981). Impaet de l'Holocaust: Transmission aux enfants der vecu des parents. *Evolution Psychiatrique, 41,* 735–388.

Laufer, R. S., Brett, E., & Gallops, M. S. (1985). Dimensions of posttraumatic stress disorder among Vietnam veterans. *Journal of Nervous and Mental Diseases, 173,* 538–545.

Laufer, R. S., & Frey-Wouters, E. (1988, October 22–26). *War trauma and the role of guilt in post-war adaptation.* Paper presented at the annual meetings of the Society for Traumatic Stress Studies, Dallas, TX.

Laufer, R. S., Gallops, M. S., & Frey-Wouters, E. (1984). War stress and trauma: The Vietnam veteran experience. *Journal of Health and Social Behavior, 25,* 65–85.

Laufer, R. S., Yager, T., Frey-Wouters, E., & Donnellan, J. (1981). *Legacies of Vietnam. Vol. III. Post-war trauma: Social and psychological problems of Vietnam veterans and their peers.* Washington, DC: House Committee Print No. 14, U.S. Government Printing Office.

Leon, G. R., Butcher, J. N., Kleinman, M., Goldberg, A., & Almagor, M. (1981). Survivors of the Holocaust and their children: Current status and adjustment. *Journal of Personality and Social Psychology, 41,* 503–516.

Matsakis, A. (1988). *Vietnam wives.* Kensington, MD: Woodbine House.

McLellan, A. T., Luborsky, L., Cacciola, J., Griffith, J., Evans, F., Barr, H. L., & O'Brien, C. P. (1985). New data from the Addiction Severity Index: Reliability and validity in three centers. *Journal of Nervous and Mental Diseases, 173,* 412–423.

Nadler, A., Kav-Vanaki, S., & Gleitman, B. (1985). Transgenerational effects of the Holocaust: Internalization of aggression in second-generation Holocaust survivors. *Journal of Consulting and Clinical Psychology, 53,* 365–369.

Niederland, G. (1968). Clinical observations on the "Survivor Syndrome." *International Journal of Psychoanalysis, 49,* 313–315.

Puller, L. B. (1993). *Fortunate son: The autobiography of Lewis B. Puller, Jr.* New York: Bantam.

Rakoff, V., Sigal, J. J., & Epstein, N. B. (1966). Children and families of concentration camp survivors. *Canada's Mental Health, 14,* 24–26.

Robins, L. N., Helzer, J. E., Croughan, J., & Ratcliff, K. S. (1981). National Institute of Mental Health Diagnostic Interview Schedule: Its history, characteristics, and validity. *Archives of General Psychiatry, 38,* 381–389.

Rosenheck, R. (1985a). Malignant post-Vietnam stress syndrome. *American Journal of Orthopsychiatry, 36,* 538–539.

Rosenheck, R. (1985b). Father–son relationships in malignant post-Vietnam stress syndrome. *American Journal of Social Psychiatry, 5,* 19–23.

Rosenheck, R. (1986). Impact of posttraumatic stress disorder of World War II on the next generation. *Journal of Nervous and Mental Diseases, 174,* 319–327.

Rosenheck, R. A., & Fontana, A. F. (1994). Long-term sequelae of combat in World War II, Korea and Vietnam: A comparative study. In R. Ursano, B. McCaughey, & C. Fullerton (Eds.) *Individual and community responses to trauma and disaster: The structure of human chaos.* New York: Cambridge University Press.

Rosenheck, R. A., & Fontana, A. F. (1995). Do Vietnam era veterans who suffer from posttraumatic stress disorder avoid VA mental health services: *Military Medicine, 160,* 136–142.

Rosenheck, R., & Nathan, P. (1985). Secondary traumatization in children of Vietnam veterans. *Hospital and Community Psychiatry, 36,* 538–539.

Schwartz, S., Dohrenwend, B. P., & Levavy, I. (1994). Nongenetic familial transmission of psychiatric disorders? Evidence from children of Holocaust survivors. *Journal of Health and Social Behavior, 35,* 385–402.

Sigal, J. J. (1971). Second generation effects of massive psychic trauma. In H. Krystal & W. G. Neiderland (Eds.), *Psychic traumatization: Aftereffects in individuals and communities* (pp. 55–66). Boston: Little, Brown.

Sigal, J. J., & Weinfeld, M. (1989). *Trauma and rebirth: Intergenerational effects of the Holocaust.* New York: Praeger.

Solomon, Z., Kotler, M., & Mikulincer, M. (1988). Combat-related posttraumatic stress disorder among second-generation holocaust survivors: Preliminary findings. *American Journal of Psychiatry, 145,* 865–868.

Trossman, B. (1968). Adolescent children of concentration camp survivors. *Canadian Psychiatric Association Journal, 13,* 121–123.

Weiss, E., O'Connell, A. N., & Siiter, R. (1986). Comparison of second generation Holocaust survivors, immigrants and non-immigrants on measures of mental health. *Journal of Personality and Social Psychology, 4,* 828–831.

Youngblade, L. M., & Belsky, J. (1990). Social and emotional consequences of child maltreatment. In R. T. Ammerman & M. Hersen (Eds.), *Children at risk: An evaluation of factors contributing to child abuse and neglect* (pp. 109–146). New York: Plenum Press.

15

Children of Military Personnel Missing in Action in Southeast Asia

EDNA J. HUNTER-KING

... women and children—rebuilding their lives and perhaps building houses of cards with the hands they've been dealt ...

DAVE SMITH, *The Los Angeles Times*, 1976

INTRODUCTION

Children of wartime prisoners of war (POWs) and those missing in action (MIAs) experience a *prolonged, ambiguous stressor* that may have long-term effects on their later personal psychosocial adjustment and health—either positively or negatively. What are those effects? Several studies of children of World War II concentration camp survivors suggest there are deleterious second-generational, perhaps even third-generational, residuals of extreme parental trauma (Bergman & Jucovy, 1982; Danieli, 1985, 1988a, 1988b; Rakoff, 1966; Segal, Hunter, & Segal, 1976; Sigal, 1971). To date, no definitive study has been carried out on the long-term effects on Vietnam-era MIA children, although several preliminary efforts have been made to determine what these effects might be (Benson, McCubbin, Dahl, & Hunter, 1974; Boss, 1980, 1988, 1990; Hunter, 1980, 1982, 1983a, 1983b, 1986a, 1986b, 1988). Comparing the Vietnam War MIA situation and the Holocaust tragedy, the reader may also wonder how those two experiences differ in their future effects on surviving family members.

In reviewing the literature on the long-term effects on children caused by wartime parental loss, it quickly becomes apparent that the task is more complex than it appears. First, the impact of loss varies, depending upon whether one looks at children whose fathers were killed and whose bodies were not recovered (BNR), taken POW, or who continue in the MIA status. When the POW father returned, one must also consider whether the family remained

EDNA J. HUNTER-KING • Advisory Committee on Former Prisoners of War, Department of Veterans Affairs, Washington, DC 20420.

International Handbook of Multigenerational Legacies of Trauma, edited by Yael Danieli. Plenum Press, New York, 1998.

together after the war ended. Among MIA families, the focus of this chapter, one must consider whether the mother, eventually able to accept the possibility that the MIA husband was indeed dead, perhaps then remarried or became career oriented and began a new life, or whether she and her children continued to wait and hope that the husband or father is still alive and held against his will.

Indeed, some family members whose sons, husbands, or fathers were declared missing during the Vietnam era maintain hope that the men will be found alive, even 25 years after they disappeared into the jungles of Southeast Asia. Families that continue in this state of ambiguous, unresolved grief are figuratively "stuck in time" and unable to go forward. A collage of quotes from the 1988 interviews with the adult children of these men (Hunter-King, 1993) can perhaps best illustrate their inability to resolve the grieving process, their continuing feelings of frustration and helplessness, and the perception of a gap in their lives even today:

> One of the most difficult aspects that I've had to deal with is the feeling of frustration and depression of not knowing where my Dad is or if he is alive, and the inability to do anything about it. It's very difficult to have your life revolve around someone who may not even be alive.

> The years of pain [have been the most difficult] . . . of not knowing . . . missing a loved one and never being able to put them to rest in death . . . the wondering and the periodic mourning. It's an issue that you don't want to die, but wish it would.

> It would be better if my father's body were returned. At least there would be an end. . . . My family is very close (my mother, brother, and myself) but I do miss my father. . . . Around holidays I get very sentimental and am often thinking of my Dad. . . . Every major event growing up included a poignant moment wishing my father could be there. . . . I have difficulty putting it behind me since it's an open issue.

This chapter specifically looks at what we know about the long-term effects on the now "adult" children of American military personnel declared MIA during the Vietnam era. Much of the information is derived from my small pilot survey, carried out in 1988, over 15 years after the Vietnam conflict ended (see Hunter-King, 1993, for a fuller report of that study). For a better understanding of the impact on children of a missing father, it is first necessary to review (1) some background information on the Vietnam War (1964–1973); (2) the tireless efforts, since 1969, of the National League of Families of American Prisoners and Missing in Southeast Asia; and (3) the research program of the San Diego Center for Prisoner of War Studies (CPWS) from 1971 through 1978.

THE UNITED STATES WAR IN VIETNAM (1964–1973):
AN UNPOPULAR WAR

Unlike World War I, World War II, and the recent Gulf War in the Middle East, the war in Southeast Asia, like the war in Korea, was very unpopular with the American public in general. There was much antiwar sentiment, especially among high school and college-age students. Many posed the question: "Why are we there?" Military personnel were sometimes scorned, even spat upon in public. They were called "war criminals" and "baby-killers" by antiwar activists. Until 1969, the government insisted that U.S. military personnel were there merely as "advisors," not as combatants. Most American civilians were unaware of the thousands of military personnel serving in Southeast Asia in the early years.

The first men were missing or captured in 1964; at that time, the government instructed the families not to mention that their sons, husbands, or fathers were missing or imprisoned.

The government insisted that it was not at war and did not share with these families the fact that many others were experiencing similar losses. Fearful that it would hurt their loved ones if they told anyone of their situations, the families obediently kept quiet. They coped alone; there was no support from the government and little from friends, who knew nothing of their loss. Some mothers did not even share with their own children the fact that their fathers were missing or imprisoned in a foreign land. Imagine how difficult it must have been for these children, growing up during such an unpopular war. Some did not share with their peers the knowledge that their fathers were missing, but it was not for being "obedient" as their mothers may have been. Over the years, the war itself and the entire POW/MIA issue had become thoroughly "politicized."

These children were very proud of their fathers, yet some felt an underlying, inexplicable shame that they themselves did not understand. Some, who did share their plight with peers, were told, "Your father should not have been fighting a criminal war. He deserved to be captured!" Older children, especially, were puzzled by ambivalent feelings that they were unable to verbalize at the time. One college-aged daughter of an MIA expressed her feelings in a video as follows:

> The real conflict for me on campus came when my friends were actively marching and actively participating in the antiwar movement. . . . something I wanted to do, but yet I couldn't perceive the war in simple "black and white" terms that my friends were talking about at that time. . . . I don't think I ever resolved that conflict. . . . It's easy to say I was intimidated by the telegram that threatened if I said anything publicly, something would happen to my father . . . but I don't think it's that simple. . . . I think it has to do with my still clinging onto that blind faith you have in your father. You say to yourself, "Well, there's a reason he's there; there's a reason he chose to do that; he just didn't have time to tell me." (Smith, 1978).

It was only recently—almost 30 years later—that the young woman just quoted was able to bring closure to her loss. In 1995, she returned to Vietnam, located her father's crash site, and was finally able to say "Good-bye" to him (R. Smith, June 4, 1995, personal communication). Other children of MIAs have yet to bring closure to their grieving.

THE NATIONAL LEAGUE OF FAMILIES OF AMERICAN PRISONERS AND MISSING IN SOUTHEAST ASIA

The Vietnam-era POW/MIA families continued their grieving alone and in silence from 1964 until 1969, the year when North Vietnam threatened to execute the POWs they held as "war criminals." It was then that the families themselves became activists. They banded together, and the National League of Families of American Prisoners and Missing in Southeast Asia was created. The nucleus of the League was informally organized in late 1966 in San Diego, California, by two wives of missing men, who tracked down 33 other families in their same circumstance. The League was officially incorporated in the District of Columbia on May 28, 1970. It is composed of the wives, children, parents, and other close relatives of American POWs, MIAs, BNRs, and former Vietnam-era POWs. Its current membership numbers over 3,800, the majority of whom are Air Force families. (It is noteworthy that more Air Force men were held captive than Army and Navy personnel; also, Air Force families were the *only* service families not included in the follow-up research of the Center for POW Studies.) The League is a nonprofit, nonpolitical, tax-exempt organization, financed by contributions from concerned citizens and the families themselves. The organization's objectives are to obtain the release of all POWs and achieve the fullest possible accounting for the MIAs, including the return of the remains of these Americans who died serving their country during the Vietnam War.

Had it not been for the persistence of the League over the past two decades, the issue of full resolution of the POWs/MIAs would probably have faded from national attention in 1973, when 566 POWs held in Hanoi were released, or in 1975, when the war in Southeast Asia finally came to an end and South Vietnam collapsed in defeat. Despite numerous "live sightings," the White House steadfastfully maintained for many years that there were no more men held in Southeast Asia until Ronald Reagan took office as President of the United States. For the first time since 1973, a President suggested that a *possibility* existed that there could still be live American POWs held in Southeast Asia.

It should be noted that after the French defeat by Vietnam in 1954 at Dien Bien Phu, 13 live, French POWs were returned unexpectedly over 16 years after the war ended. Since 1954, French authorities and citizens have been literally "buying back" the remains of their dead. Reportedly $50,000 was paid for one set of bones as late as March 1981 (Hunter, 1982). (We hear little about the French experience in Vietnam because their humiliation was so great that the French government prohibited any publications on the matter for fifty years!)

All these MIA children remember the unexpected release by Hanoi of United States Marine PFC Robert Garwood in 1979, after 14 years in captivity (for an account of Garwood's controversial return, see Hunter, 1983a). They may also remember the return, after 19 years, of Richard Fecteau, when he was unexpectedly released by the Chinese Communists. He had been shot down with Gary Powers in the infamous U-2 incident, and no one back home suspected that he had survived. Finally, there is the more recent escape from North Korea of a South Korean prisoner after 43 long years! *History shows that no Communist nation has ever released all known living POWs at the end of hostilities.* This knowledge gives hope to Vietnam-era MIA and BNR families that perhaps a *few* American men may yet return after these many years.

After years of denial, when the admission was finally made by top U.S. government officials that some men might indeed be still held captive in Southeast Asia, the hopes and frustrations of MIA family members immediately increased, especially for the children and brothers and sisters, who were now ready to "take the flag" from their mothers and grandparents, and carry the issue toward full resolution.

Many of these MIA "children" had been included in a 7-year longitudinal study of POW/MIA families carried out at the Center for Prisoner of War Studies from 1971 to 1978. At the time of the project's inception, it was not known which of the fathers were actually prisoners and which were missing, since Hanoi had furnished no lists of men held, and some men had not written letters home. Thus, *all* Army, Navy, and Marine Corps POW/MIA families were included in the prehomecoming personal interviews conducted by the Center's professional staff.

THE CENTER FOR PRISONER OF WAR STUDIES

By 1970, it appeared that the war in Vietnam was winding down. Prior to the release, the number of men held captive was thought to be in excess of 600. Over 2,500 were listed as MIA, since there was no evidence that they had been taken captive. Homecoming plans began, and the Naval Health Research Center, San Diego (the Navy's primary research organization studying stressful environments), was provided funding to set up a Center for Prisoner of War Studies (CPWS; Hunter, 1986b).

Research under the Umbrella of Preventive Medicine

The research studies at the Center for Prisoner of War Studies were set up under the umbrella of preventive medicine. The logic was that if the families were doing well during captivity, and if the men were given good medical attention at the time of Operation Homecoming and counseling was provided for both the men and their families subsequent to that period, perhaps there would be fewer long-term problems for this group of ex-POWs than had been found for former POWs after World War II and Korea. Those former captives had received minimal assistance (Beebe, 1975; Schein, 1957). At the time the Center was set up, it was not known whether the POWs would be released in 2 months, 6 months, a year, or ever. However, subsequent to homecoming, the research plan called for monitoring the physical, psychological, social, and family adjustments of Army, Navy, and Marine Corps returnees for a 5-year period after their return, whenever that event might occur. The MIA families were no longer followed by CPWS after the return of the men in the early spring of 1973; families of returned POWs were followed until 1978.

The Center was disestablished in 1978, although the medical follow-up of the returned Navy POWs has continued at the Navy Aerospace Medical Institute in Pensacola, Florida, since that time. The Center was jointly funded by the Navy Bureau of Medicine and Surgery and the Office of the Army Surgeon General, and included all Army, Navy, and Marine Corps POWs/MIAs. Although the Air Force also examined its returned POWs medically at the time of homecoming, participation was voluntary in subsequent years, and the decision made by Air Force operational planners prior to the men's release was *not* to include families in their research planning.

Planning for Homecoming

Why did the Center include families as part of its planning? The families were viewed as both potential *stress producers* and *stress alleviators* for the returning POWs. The rationale was that if the families were functioning well at the time of release, they were more likely to be stress alleviators, rather than stress producers. In 1972, professional CPWS staff traveled throughout the United States, to Hawaii, Puerto Rico, and Europe with the goal of interviewing *all* parents of POW/MIAs who were dependent financially upon their missing/captured sons, the men's wives, and their children. The goal was to discover the extent of family adjustments that might be necessary when homecoming arrived. Over half the families of all married Army, Navy, and Marine Corps POW/MIAs had been interviewed when word came in January 1973, that release was imminent. At that point in time, all interviewing ceased until after the men came home.

As mentioned earlier, at the time of the initial interviews, many families did not know whether their sons–husbands–fathers were dead or held captive. At homecoming, over 2,500 men did not return, and many of those families have yet to resolve their state of prolonged, ambiguous grieving. Today, 2,205 Americans are still missing and unaccounted for from the Vietnam War. Their parents (those few who are still alive), their brothers and sisters, their children, and now their grandchildren (whom they have never seen) still seek resolution. *Resolution* has been defined by the National League of Families as the return of all live prisoners, the fullest possible accounting for those still missing, and repatriation of all recoverable remains (National League of Families, 1995).

RESEARCH ON CHILDREN OF THE MISSING

From a research perspective, the Vietnam War provided a unique opportunity to study the effects of prolonged wartime parental absence upon children, one that could never have been duplicated in a laboratory setting (Hunter, 1986a, 1988; Hunter-King, 1993). Initial studies of the CPWS examined POW/MIA children together as one group. Data collected during the fathers' absence indicated that the impact of wartime father absence on children was determined to a large extent by three major factors, all relating to the mothers' adjustments: (1) the mothers' attitudes toward the separation; (2) the mothers' satisfaction with their marriages prior to the separation; and (3) the mothers' abilities to cope satisfactorily with the separation period (Hunter & Nice, 1978; McCubbin, Hunter, & Metres, 1974). Thus, the mother's role appeared very important in predicting how children would cope at that point in time.

The Center's follow-up data, obtained 5 years after the release (Nice, McDonald, & McMillian, 1981), dealt only with children of returned POWs. Although the study by Nice and colleagues may shed light on what type of military family is best able to cope with *any highly stressful situation,* their conclusions are perhaps misleading if one attempts to use them to delineate long-term effects of MIA parental absence, which has been not only prolonged but also highly ambiguous (Hunter-King, 1993).

LATER ADJUSTMENT OF CHILDREN OF VIETNAM-ERA MIAs

In 1988, the 1988 Survey of Vietnam-Era MIA Children (Hunter-King, 1993) was mailed to all children of MIAs/BNRs who were currently members of the National League of Families. The survey was designed to examine various areas of functioning, such as emotional/psychological adjustment, occupational adjustment, friendships, family relationships, and members' relationships with their own children. Participants in the study were also asked to provide comments on (1) the most difficult aspects of their MIA experience, (2) whether there had been any specific advantages because of their MIA status, (3) what current problems/issues they were dealing with that might be directly related to being the child of an MIA father, and (4) what advice they might give to children who suddenly found themselves in a similar situation. Not all Vietnam-era MIA children are members of the National League. Therefore, results from the survey may not precisely reflect attitudes of the total population of MIA children. Nonetheless, information obtained from the 1988 study provided a better understanding of how these children had coped with the situation than was available heretofore.

MIA Children in 1988

A review of the findings from the 1988 study showed that of those, now adult, children who completed the survey, over half (50.6%) were daughters and half (49.4%) were sons. Almost two-thirds of the participants were married, and over 40% now had children of their own. Almost three-fourths were children of Air Force personnel whose fathers, in most cases, first became listed as missing between the years 1964–1967. At the time of the fathers' casualties, their children ranged in age from less than 1 year to 20 years of age. By 1988, slightly over half (51.2%) the mothers of these children had not remarried. Data also indicated that those children whose mothers had not remarried were less likely themselves to have married.

Although the majority of the mothers had been active in the National League of Families since its founding in 1969, most of the children had only recently become active. Also, if mothers had *never* been active in League activities, their children were *more* likely to rate relationships with their own children as having been more affected by the MIA experience. As for the various areas of personal functioning that these young adults believed were affected by having been children of MIAs, they rated emotional/psychological adjustment as most affected, followed by family relationships, occupational adjustment, and marital relationships. According to their ratings, friendships had been affected least (Hunter-King, 1993). Unfortunately, from the manner in which the questions on the survey were asked, it was impossible to determine whether these effects were in a positive or negative direction.

Long-Term Effects on MIA Children

From the 1988 study, there appeared to be long-term effects on children whose fathers became missing during the war in Southeast Asia. Some effects were perceived as having had a negative impact on their lives, whereas others were viewed as having had a positive influence.

Negative Effects.   By far, the most difficult problem, and one with which all participants still struggled, was the prolonged and ambiguous nature of the loss and their inability over many years to achieve any enduring sense of resolution. Examples of the children's feelings were expressed as follows:

> My father never came home! I'm always waiting for Daddy. . . . I resent him for leaving me—yet I'm so proud of him. I've gone on with my life, but every day I wonder about him. Every success, every accomplishment makes me realize how much I miss his not being here. No matter how much we know that Dad is gone, we're still waiting for him to come home. (Daughter of an MIA, 1988)

> [The most difficult aspect] is the unrequited grief. From time to time I have to overcome feelings of isolation and loneliness. [One must] recognize the inevitable roller coaster between despair and frustration and hope. There will always be hope. I wish my Dad could see his grandchildren. (Son of an MIA, 1988).

Several children believed having an MIA father resulted in long-term effects on their own attitudes toward close relationships, including marriage, especially for daughters. It was as if they hesitated to make deep emotional commitments for fear that they would again experience loss or abandonment. Some of these young women reported that they had developed a fierce sense of independence over the years to ward off any possibility of becoming dependent upon a husband who might suddenly disappear. A selection of comments illustrates how these young adults believed the MIA experience had produced long-term effects on close relationships:

> I've developed an overfatalistic attitude toward life and sometimes have trouble becoming close to people, perhaps for fear they will disappear and not return.

> Each in our own way (my brothers, sisters, and I) have had difficulties in romantic relationships.

> I have an irrational fear of my spouse dying at an early age—a fear of ending up a single mother.

> I put off having children for 11 years because I wanted to make sure I had a career, should anything happen to my own husband.

> [My mother and other relatives] put [my Dad] on a pedestal. By the time you're grown, no mate (or you) can ever compare to the "God" they've become!

> Each one of us [four children] had different reactions and have suffered in various ways. My only brother, who was 3 years old at the time my father was shot down, is still struggling with who his father was, what was he like, etc. (MIA daughters' comments, 1988)

Sons of the missing have reported effects that often differed from those reported by daughters. Eldest sons, especially, found the responsibilities heaped upon them when their fathers disappeared overwhelming at times. Lacking a father to whom they could go for advice and counsel, and look to as a role model of husband and father, was particularly problematic. Matriarchal families were also viewed as a very difficult issue for those sons who lacked an extended family that included uncles and grandfathers. Perhaps a few comments from these grown sons can better illustrate their particular concerns:

> The most difficult problem was the self-imposed responsibility of being the "man of the family."

> There are hardly any males on either side of my family. I'm the only son. The hardest part for me was the lack of older male companionship. Neighbors were always promising fishing trips, hunting trips, ballgames, etc., which never seemed to materialize. Being at the door with fishing pole in hand ready to go and not having them show up really hurt.

> I have been raised in a fourth-generation female-run household. I was constantly surrounded by women—sisters, mother, her friends, my sisters' girlfriends, etc.

> I have had some problems dealing with the role of father. I think I have idealized my own father to the extent that it has been hard to live up to that image. (MIA sons' comments, 1988).

For a small segment (probably less than 10%) of these adult children of MIAs, over the years, there was a growing mistrust of the government (A. M. Griffiths, April 25, 1995, personal communication). A few reported viewing the Vietnam War as a "farce" and said they are still bitter toward the fathers who "deserted them and never returned." According to some of their comments made in 1988, they were certain that the North Vietnamese lied, their own Government had lied, and they did not even trust the National League of Families, as they believe "its leadership is in bed with the government." As one embittered daughter strongly advised,

> Identify these officials who want to kill your father (through indifference). Remember who the real enemy is. In Vietnam, President Carter and Henry Kissinger were as responsible for the deaths of unreturned POW/MIAs as any Vietnamese. Don't trust anyone! (Daughter of MIA, 1988)

Positive Effects.   Were there any benefits or advantages perceived by these young adults specifically derived from being children of missing fathers? Many of these young adults reported that there indeed were. The most frequently mentioned advantage was that their MIA family status had afforded them the financial means to obtain a college education. Most added the caveat, however, that such financial aid in no way compensated for the loss of their fathers during their formative years.

A second advantage mentioned by the majority of the adult children surveyed in 1988 was the development of closer relationships with their mothers and siblings than might otherwise have been the case. Also, they felt they had stronger appreciation of the value of life and had developed a more mature outlook on life in general than others who had not been in their situation. Two examples reflect on this family closeness and the mature "worldview" that evolved for many of these children from the MIA experience:

An experience like this really brings a family together. An inseparable bond is formed. [We] learned to depend on each other for strengths—support in ways I have not experienced in other families. Today we are still as close. (Daughter of an MIA, 1988)

[When in this situation] you must try not to feel guilty if you are happy or joyful. . . . Such guilt is inevitable, yet it must be channeled into positive action, not self-inflicted punishment. [Being the child of an MIA] you will develop a sense of eternal hopefulness in all things [and] you will be burdened with a sense of loss at all acts of thoughtlessness and hatred. You will eventually see the joy in living and the meaning of how much freedom costs. . . . Others will look to you for direction and understanding. . . . I have learned from this ordeal that, while I still feel [there is] a certain romance in war and combat, any type of conflict (war, terrorism, etc.) is brutal and unmerciful. (Son of an MIA, 1988)

In other words, the positive results of having coped with the missing father were the greater maturity and greater personal strengths that these children believed they had attained over the years, compared with their peers. Many reported that the experience made them emotionally stronger individuals. They believed they had reached a higher level of maturity earlier in life. Coping with the loss had also resulted in their being more realistic, determined in their actions, and highly independent. They had learned to face problems head-on with the attitude "If I could cope with Dad's loss, I should be able to handle other difficult situations in life." Philosophically, one MIA adult "child" commented,

It is ironic that the most painful event in my life has also brought about the most changes of a positive nature. I have learned to value and appreciate relationships and life itself, for it can be so very short. I have pondered the existential questions of life at any early age, and in so doing, it has enriched me with wisdom to help me through life's ups and downs. I have learned the importance of being honest with myself and others, for my life may be short and I may not have a second chance to make things right. [Nonetheless] it is difficult at times to live with unanswered questions. Some questions may never be answered. (Adult daughter of an MIA serviceman, 1988)

Recognition of the Need for Support Systems

Over the years, these children experienced varying degrees of difficulty as they sought answers that could perhaps bring final resolution to a situation that seemed to have no end. When interviewed in 1988, many of these young adults talked about how important seeking support from others had been. Some found help within their own families or extended families. Others went outside to teachers, friends, or therapists. Many found the strengths they needed to cope with their loss through working with POW/MIA organizations in their attempts to bring public attention to the issue and prompt more effective governmental actions to determine the fate of the missing men. When asked what advice could be given to other children who might find themselves in a similar situation, these young adults offered a variety of suggestions, many of which advocated requesting assistance:

Tell *somebody*—a teacher, a relative, a friend. . . . Don't "shut down" your emotions to cope with the loss. Get it out or you'll spend the rest of your life fighting to share feelings, instinctively "swallowing" your feelings. . . . Admit your anger or you'll never be able to forgive. Don't withdraw. . . . Stay involved, or you'll always feel like you're on the outside looking in.

I feel very strongly that the entire family should get into counseling as soon as possible to be taught how to deal with what sometimes seems like an unbearable, unending situation. If your family won't do this as a whole, visit a therapist yourself.

Make sure the surviving parent gets counseling of some sort. We were emotionally abused by our mother because she could not cope with the enormity of the situation. She eventually sought help after we all left home.

Don't give up your own childhood to take care of the surviving parent!

The Importance of Mothers in Children's Coping

Throughout the 25 years I have worked with children of MIAs, the role of the mother in the children's coping with the loss of their fathers has appeared to be the most critical factor in determining effective coping. Her importance was evident when POW/MIA families were first interviewed by the staff of CPWS in 1972, prior to the release of POWs (Hunter & Nice, 1978; McCubbin, Dahl, & Hunter 1976; McCubbin *et al.,* 1974), and it was even more apparent in later, follow-up studies (Hunter, 1983b, 1988; Hunter-King, 1993).

While preparing this chapter, I discussed the critical role mothers had played in their children's ability to cope with prolonged and ambiguous grieving with the Executive Director of the National League of Families (she is also the sister of an MIA serviceman), an individual who has probably been more closely involved with the MIA issue than any other person (A. M. Griffiths, April 25, 1995, personal communication). Many of her comments corroborated my own opinions, which are based upon 25 years of research, and added depth to some of those findings. In our discussions, an attempt was made to clarify why a small group of these "children" have grown extremely distrustful over the years—almost to the point of irrationality— in dealing with any attempt to resolve the MIA issue. The majority of the grown children of the missing, although still harboring unanswered questions and repeated frustrations, have become mature, caring adults, who surprisingly perceive that a variety of actual benefits have accrued from their tragedy. One must ask, what makes the difference? Again, it appears to be the mothers whose attitudes and behaviors have set the stage for adequate functioning. Mothers made the difference.

> [Of] those mothers who were open and talked with their children about their missing fathers and let them know who their fathers were, [it is their children who] are the more rational ones today. [Of the] mothers who ignored the situation, or asked quickly for a presumptive finding of death (but the kids always thought the father was dead or found out later the father had been declared dead without additional information obtained by the government), their children are those who now have a more unrealistic or less objective approach. (Griffiths, April 25, 1995, personal communication)

In other words, those children with whom their mothers did not share information from the very beginning, children who never knew the father because they were very young, whose mothers themselves perhaps told the child, "Your father should never have been in Vietnam in the first place," those are the young adults who today have adopted an extreme antigovernment stance. In commenting on the importance of mothers in the coping process, one mature MIA son recently stated that he believed that those mothers who were "typical" military wives were more likely to have reared well-adjusted children, since those mothers were more involved and experienced within the military culture, and were affiliated with other military families who understood their problems. He also believed that MIA families "who immediately retreated back into the civilian world had a more difficult time" (M. L. Stephensen, May 30, 1995, personal communication).

Grandparents have also been very important in the coping equation for MIA children. If mothers stayed in touch with the paternal grandparents over the years, the children appeared to have been raised in a much warmer, more supportive situation (A. M. Griffiths, April 25, 1995, personal communication).

INTERGENERATIONAL TRANSMISSION OF TRAUMA IN MIA CHILDREN

As is apparent from the previous discussion, parents, wives, and children of American servicemen declared missing in Southeast Asia experienced personal traumata that have been both prolonged and ambiguous. That war was the longest conflict in U.S. history, extending from 1964 until 1973, when American troops hastily pulled out in defeat. During that 9-year period, wives of MIAs did not know whether they were wives or widows; MIA wives continued to wonder after the war ended. Shortly after the release of the POWs in 1973, one MIA wife related a dream she had. She was going about her job as usual, but in the backseat of her station wagon was the body of her missing husband. She went about her tasks as if there were absolutely nothing unusual about having her husband's body in there, remarking, "That's precisely the way it is. I'm *sure* my husband is dead, and yet I can't bury him. He's always with me wherever I go" (Hunter, 1982). MIA mothers and their children have ridden an emotional roller coaster month after month, year after year, for almost three decades; their husbands and fathers still ride in the backseats.

Transmission of Trauma from Mothers to Children

Because of the U.S. government's secrecy surrounding the war in Vietnam in the early years (prior to 1969), some mothers did not share with their in-laws or their own children the fact that their husbands were missing. After 3 or 4 years in "limbo," some wives did not want to deal any longer with an issue they felt powerless to resolve. They could no longer "mark time in place." Some of the wives formed new relationships and went forward with their lives, despite the fact there was no legal way to file for divorce from a "missing" husband. Some children did not learn until they were older that the man they thought was their father was not. In-laws sometimes found that they could not forgive women who "abandoned their sons" and/or chose not to participate in efforts to resolve the fate of their sons because they could not handle the situation emotionally. Thus, some children lost not only their fathers, but also access to paternal grandparents.

Many children were too young when their fathers became missing to retain any memories of them. In recent years, these children have persistently sought information about the fathers they never knew. Some became active in the National League of Families only recently, adopting the attitude: "I cannot abandon my father as my mother and the government have done." On the other hand, for some children, their mothers were so totally immersed in POW/MIA activities outside the home that it was almost as if they had lost *both* parents. Older children who knew their fathers, but whose mothers did not include them in their efforts to get answers from the government about their fathers' status, also tended to feel abandoned. A similar situation existed for brothers and sisters of MIAs, whose mothers spent every waking moment dealing with issues and activities concerning their missing sons, resulting in perceived neglect by some of these siblings. A teenage son, the brother of an MIA, once emotionally commented during a group session: "I guess I'll have to commit suicide before my mother will pay some attention to me, instead of thinking about my missing brother all the time!"

MIA Children and Children of Holocaust Survivors

It is exceedingly difficult to compare such two very different experiences as the children of World War II Holocaust survivors and the children of military men still missing in action following the Vietnam War. Unlike the Holocaust, mothers of MIA children were not suddenly uprooted from their homes and deprived of their possessions, countries, and cultures. They did not lose parents, siblings, and husbands to programmed incineration. They were not subjected to incarceration, underfed, and abused, as were Holocaust victims. Of course, we do not know what tortures the missing fathers faced, and we may never know.

On the other hand, most children of Holocaust survivors have not waited for over a quarter of a century in a state of ambiguous grieving, wondering whether their parent is dead or alive, as children of MIAs have done. Both groups, however, have perceived the *conspiracy of silence* between survivors and society, and between survivors and their children, categorized by Danieli (1988a, 1988b) as the most pervasive consequence of the Holocaust experience. For children of MIAs, this conspiracy of silence was between the U.S. government and the families in the early war years, and between mothers and children in instances in which the mothers "closed out" the missing men's role within the family in order to cope with their absence.

In 1973, at the time of homecoming of the POWs released by Hanoi, MIA families were eager to speak with them to see what they knew of the fate of their missing men. Here, again, MIA family members were sometimes met with "silence." Although some returnees felt they "owed a debt" to these MIA families and tried to help them, others avoided them and were reluctant to talk with them. Analogous to individuals who dealt with Holocaust survivors, for some returned Vietnam-era POWs, there was a degree of *survivor guilt.* They felt that those men who did not return were the real heroes, not them. In more recent times, pressure for silence from these MIA families has come from some individuals, both within government and in the civilian community, who want to put Vietnam behind them and/or to open up full diplomatic recognition of the former "enemy" for economic gain. The continuing politicizing of the MIA issue augments and prolongs the plight of these families.

Is There a "Child-of-Survivor Syndrome"?

For both groups (children of MIAs and children of Holocaust survivors), no single "child-of-survivor syndrome" has been delineated. For Vietnam-era MIA children, research has shown that much was determined by whether children remembered their fathers, their ages at the time of casualty, their sex, whether support was available from an extended family, and, most importantly, by their mothers' openness with them. I agree with Yael Danieli, who pointed to the *heterogeneity* of responses to the Holocaust legacy, and who suggested that there was a "need to match appropriate intervention to particular forms of reaction if optimal therapeutic or preventive benefits are to be obtained" (Danieli, 1988a, p. 236). As one adult child of a missing Vietnam-era father stated in a 1988 interview,

> [I think you will find that] children of MIAs haven't coped much differently than other children with one deceased parent. They just go on with their lives. They cry over their loss, they feel proud of their dads. They feel bitter about the lies and about the abandonment of the dads. But they go on and live normal lives. The one difference you will find is that no matter how much we know that Dad is gone, we're still waiting for him to come home.

CONCLUSION

It becomes readily apparent in talking with the children of servicemen who have been missing in Southeast Asia for over a quarter of a century, that, for most of these MIA adult children, *unless they are convinced that the fullest possible accounting has been made,* and/or *unless the fathers' remains are located, adequately identified, and returned to the family,* their prolonged, ambiguous grieving will continue indefinitely. For some "children," there will never be a final resolution of their loss, and this lack of resolution could result in intergenerational effects on the grandchildren of the missing men. For some families of MIAs, closer marital and family relationships developed, because nuclear relationships became more valued after the loss of the fathers. For other families, there was diminished closeness because the families, immediately after the loss, turned their emotions inward to insulate themselves against further loss and pain.

Research has shown that the response of the wives of the missing men appeared to be the key variable in predicting the degree and direction of intergenerational effects in their children. Research also suggests that immediate support from friends, extended family, and governmental agencies played a critical role in the wives' abilities to cope with the MIA experience. Thus, we must recognize that *adequate support for these families, immediately subsequent to their loss, could play a preventive role in the intergenerational transmission of the effects of prolonged, ambiguous trauma.*

REFERENCES

Beebe, G. W. (1975). Follow-up studies of World War II and Korean War prisoners: II. Mortality, disability, and maladjustments. *American Journal of Epidemiology, 101,* 400–422.

Benson, D., McCubbin, H., Dahl, B., & Hunter, E. (1974). Waiting: The dilemma of the MIA wife. In H. McCubbin, B. Dahl, P. Metres, Jr., E. Hunter, & J. Plag (Eds.), *Family separation and reunion* (pp. 157–167). Washington, DC: Government Printing Office (Cat. No. D-206.21:74-70)

Bergman, M. S., & Jucovy, M. E. (Eds.). (1982). *Generations of the Holocaust.* New York: Basic Books.

Boss, P. (1980). The relationship of psychological father presence, wife's personal qualities and wife/family dysfunction in families of missing fathers. *Journal of Marriage and the Family, 42,* 541–549.

Boss, P. (1988). *Family stress management.* Newbury Park, CA: Sage.

Boss, P. (1990). Family therapy and family research: Intertwined parts of the whole. In F. Kaslow (Ed.), *Voices in family psychology* (Vol. 2, pp. 17–32). Newbury Park, CA: Sage.

Danieli, Y. (1985). The treatment and prevention of long-term effects and intergenerational transmission of victimization: A lesson from Holocaust survivors and their children. In C. R. Figley (Ed.), *Trauma and its wake* (pp. 295–313). New York: Brunner/Mazel.

Danieli, Y. (1988a). Confronting the unimaginable: Psychotherapists' reactions to victims of the Nazi Holocaust. In J. Wilson, Z. Harel, & B. Kahan (Eds.), *Human adaptation to extreme stress* (pp. 219–238). New York: Plenum Press.

Danieli, Y. (1988b). Treating survivors and children of survivors of the Nazi Holocaust. In F. Ochberg (Ed.), *Post-traumatic therapy and victims of violence* (pp. 278–294). New York: Brunner/Mazel.

Hunter, E. J. (1980, January). Combat casualties who remain at home. *Military Review,* pp. 28–36.

Hunter, E. J. (1982, July). Marriage in limbo. *U.S. Naval Institute Proceedings,* pp. 27–32.

Hunter, E. J. (1983a). Coercive persuasion: The myth of free will? *Air University Review, 34*(2), 100–111.

Hunter, E. J. (1983b, August). Let no war put asunder: Families are holding together 10 years after Vietnam. *LADYCOM,* pp. 34–36, 60.

Hunter, E. J. (1986a). Families of prisoners of war held in Vietnam: A seven-year study. *Evaluation and Program Planning, 9,* 243–251.

Hunter, E. J. (1986b). Missing in action. In T. Rando (Ed.), *Parental loss of a child* (pp. 277–239). Champaign, IL: Research Press.

Hunter, E. J. (1988). Long-term effects of parental wartime captivity on children: Children of POWs and MIA servicemen. *Journal of Contemporary Psychotherapy, 18*(4), 312–328.

Hunter-King, E. J. (1993). Long-term effects on children of a parent missing in wartime. In F. Kaslow (Ed.), *The military family in peace and war* (pp. 48–65). New York: Springer.

Hunter, E. J., & Nice, D. S. (Eds.). (1978). *Children of military families: A part and yet apart.* Washington, DC: U.S. Government Printing Office. (Cat. No. 008-040-00181-4)

McCubbin, H., Dahl, B., & Hunter, E. (1976). Research on the military family: A review. In H. McCubbin, B. Dahl, & E. Hunter (Eds.), *Families in the military system* (pp. 291–319). Beverly Hills, CA: Sage.

McCubbin, H., Dahl, B., Lester, G., & Ross, B. (1975). The returned prisoner of war: Factors in family reintegration. *Journal of Marriage and the Family, 37,* 471–478.

McCubbin, H., Hunter, E. J., & Metres, P., Jr. (1974). Children in limbo. In H. McCubbin, B. Dahl, P. Metres, Jr., E. Hunter, & J. Plag (Eds.), *Family separation and reunion: Families of prisoners of war and servicemen missing in action* (pp. 65–76). Washington, DC: U.S. Government Printing Office. (Cat. No. D-21:74-70)

National League of Families of American Prisoners and Servicemen Missing in Southeast Asia. (1995, April 27). News bulletin, Washington, DC.

Nice, S. D., McDonald, B., & McMillian, T. (1981). The families of U.S. Navy prisoners of war five years after reunions. *Journal of Marriage and the Family, 43,* 431–437.

Rakoff, V. A. (1966). A long-term effect of the concentration camp experience. *Viewpoints, 1,* 17–22.

Schein, E. H. (1957). Reaction patterns to severe chronic stress in American Army prisoners of war of the Chinese. *Journal of Social Issues, 13,* 21–30.

Segal, J., Hunter, E. J., & Segal, Z. (1976). Universal consequences of captivity: Stress reactions among divergent populations of prisoners of war and their families. *International Social Sciences Journal, 28,* 593–609.

Sigal, J. (1971). Second generation effects of massive psychiatric trauma. *International Psychiatry Clinics, 8,* 55–65.

Smith, D. (1976, September 3). Vietnam POWs rebuild their lives. *Los Angeles Times.*

Smith, R. (1978). *He's only missing* [video, producer: Robin Smith]. Boston: Boston University.

16

The Legacy of Combat Trauma

Clinical Implications of Intergenerational Transmission

MICHELLE R. ANCHAROFF, JAMES F. MUNROE, and LISA M. FISHER

INTRODUCTION

Posttrauma symptoms can have a profound effect on the manner in which a trauma survivor relates to others, including, perhaps most significantly, family members. Survivors are markedly changed by their experiences. The psychological impact of trauma is well established in a variety of survivor populations (e.g., Burgess & Holmstrom, 1974; Davis & Friedman, 1985; Figley, 1978; Foa, Rothbaum, Riggs, & Murdock, 1992; Kilpatrick, Veronen, & Best, 1985; Koopman, Classen, & Spiegel, 1994; Laufer, Frey-Wouters, & Gallops, 1985; Titchner, Kapp, & Winget, 1976). These posttrauma symptoms include (1) experiencing the trauma through flashbacks, nightmares, and persistent thoughts; (2) cognitive and phobic avoidance of trauma-related stimuli; (3) hyperarousal symptoms of irritability, startle response, and sleep disturbance (American Psychiatric Association, 1994). It is easy to understand how survivors' numbing of responsiveness, social withdrawal, and irritability, with episodic outbursts of rage, can make it difficult for them to maintain interpersonal relationships. In turn, children of traumatized patients may be affected directly or indirectly by their parents' posttrauma symptoms. For example, Rosenheck and Nathan (1985) described a child of a combat veteran with posttraumatic stress disorder (PTSD) as having insomnia; headaches; tearfulness; feelings of helplessness; fears of being kidnapped, shot, or killed; attention problems at school; and fantasies similar to his father's flashbacks. These authors coined the term *secondary traumatization* to describe this phenomenon. Others have referred to this as transgenerational transmission of trauma (Harkness, 1993). Although the terminologies differ, common to these descriptions is the notion that children are affected by their parents' posttrauma sequelae. Despite a plethora of descriptive information, intergenerational transmission of trauma is a poorly defined empirical construct, and one that is not well understood within the professional community. We do not know the extent to which parental trauma affects the next generation or how many generations may be influenced. One of the best predictors for PTSD is the intensity and duration

MICHELLE R. ANCHAROFF, JAMES F. MUNROE, and LISA M. FISHER • Department of Veterans Affairs Outpatient Clinic, National Center for Posttraumatic Stress Disorder, Boston, Massachusetts 02114.

International Handbook of Multigenerational Legacies of Trauma, edited by Yael Danieli. Plenum Press, New York, 1998.

of exposure to traumatic events (Gleser, Green, & Winget, 1981; van der Kolk, 1988). We can speculate that one of the best predictors for secondary trauma in children may be the intensity and duration of trauma exposure of their parents. Combat veterans are a group that has been exposed to extensive trauma and, therefore, represent a population in which intergenerational transmission is likely. The objectives of this chapter are to describe the legacy of combat trauma on the children of Vietnam veterans and identify the mechanisms through which these cognitive, affective, and behavioral patterns are handed down. In addition, this chapter explores issues of how to determine if, when, and how to intervene.

BACKGROUND

Anecdotal Literature

Holocaust Survivors. Intergenerational transmission of trauma was first described among the children of Holocaust survivors (e.g., Freyberg, 1980; Krystal & Niederland, 1968; Rakoff, Sigal, & Epstein, 1966; Sigal & Rakoff, 1971). Some authors noted pathological symptoms in children and families of Holocaust survivors (Rakoff, 1966; Trossman, 1968). In contrast, other authors observed no specific behavioral disturbances in this population (Klein, 1971), except a tendency to avoid separations from parents, overt expressions of anger, and the desire to protect their parents from emotional pain. In addition, these children manifested a low tolerance toward hearing parental trauma memories (Klein, 1971; Prince, 1985). Other authors noted that children of survivors were apathetic and uncertain about career goals (Krystal & Niederland, 1971), manifested neurotic and psychotic symptoms similar to or symbolic of their parents' trauma (Kestenberg, 1983; Krell, 1982; Link, Victor, & Binder, 1985; Rodin & Rodin, 1982), and experienced what appears very similar to dissociation and emotional numbing (Epstein, 1979). Similarly, Epstein (1979) reported episodes of daydreaming the content of which bore a striking resemblance to the traumatic experiences of the parents. Finally, Danieli (1985) and Wardi (1992) suggested that children of Holocaust survivors seemed to have special significance for their parents. Danieli described a constant psychological presence of the Holocaust in the homes of survivors and their children and how this presence was absorbed through "osmosis" (Danieli, 1985, p. 299). Neither Epstein nor Danieli found these children to be a pathological population. Rather, these children seemed to struggle silently with war-derived messages from their parents, including belief that the world is not a secure place, the future is uncertain, evil exists in the world, and their parents were fragile, despite outward appearances (Epstein, 1979). The anecdotal descriptions suggest that these children demonstrate a range of emotions and behaviors that may be associated with their parents' traumatic experiences.

Internees. Descriptions of children whose parents were interned in Japanese Civil Internment Camps in the Dutch East Indies during World War II (Doreleijers & Donovan, 1990) document survivor parents' massive denial of trauma, the communication of trauma-related messages to children, and the subtle encouragement of children's aggression. These authors postulated that the traumatized parents equipped their children with the same defenses that were useful to them during their internment. Similarly, internment of Japanese Americans in the United States has been found to impact survivors and their children (Nagata, 1991). Nagata described inhibited communication about the trauma in these families that heightened a sense of foreboding and awareness of parental trauma in the children. Also, these children experienced a greater sense of vulnerability than those whose parents were not interned, and in psychotherapy they manifested rootlessness, emotional constriction in the family, feeling burdened by the silence in the family, low self-esteem, vocational concerns, problems with assertiveness, and identity issues.

Vietnam Veterans.   Intergenerational transmission of trauma has also come to the attention of clinicians working with combat veterans. Figley (1985) referred to this as a chiasmal effect (p. 410) whereby traumatic symptoms are transferred to supporters. In a case report, Rosenheck and Nathan (1985) documented symptoms of a young boy that mimicked those of his combat-veteran father. They hypothesized that PTSD can disrupt the psychosocial and academic functioning of children through direct exposure to parents' traumatic material, and through parental repetitions of the trauma. Many latency-age children of Vietnam veterans were observed to manifest significant levels of psychopathology during the course of group therapy (Jacobsen, Sweeney, & Racusin, 1993), particularly in the areas of affect modulation, coping with stress, and the ability to elicit help from adults. Harkness (1991) also reported that children of veterans manifested difficulties in academic performance, peer relations, and affective coping. Similar to some descriptions of children of Holocaust survivors, she did not report extremely severe symptoms in children of Vietnam veterans but, rather, described general deficits in psychosocial functioning. Vietnam veterans are often observed, according to Harkness, to maintain an extremely close, overprotective, and overcontrolling relationship with their children. Jurich (1983) observed that families of Vietnam veterans have enmeshed parent–child ties between the veteran and his children. Adolescence appears to be a time of great difficulty for both the veteran and his children in terms of identity development in the child and the resurrection of identity foreclosure (p. 356) in the parent. The risk of intergenerational transmission is high at this time.

Although the literature is compelling in its rich and comprehensive description of intergenerational phenomena, most observations are made by clinicians working with families with identified psychopathology that may not accurately reflect the true heterogeneity of the population. There is no consensus among authors about the specific symptoms experienced by the children of survivors, and adequate empirical support for conclusions has not been provided. Until the 1980s, the literature on children of Holocaust survivors presumed existence of psychopathology, and the prognosis was considered poor. Later accounts focused more on the meaning of the parental trauma to the child and the role this played in the development of adaptational styles, vocational choices, and relationships (Danieli, 1981).

Empirical Literature

Holocaust Survivors.   A recent review of the literature found a very mixed picture of children of survivors (Ancharoff, 1994). Clinical observations of psychopathology of children of Holocaust survivors have not been substantiated by research results (Baron, Reznikoff, & Glenwick, 1993; Keinan, Mikulincer, & Rybricki, 1988; Leon, Butcher, Kleinman, Goldburg, & Almagor, 1981; Rose & Garske, 1987), although they may be vulnerable to stress responses subsequent to trauma in adulthood (Solomon, Kotler, & Mikulciner, 1988). Unique styles of defensive functioning have been reported, most likely related to the meaning of the expression of certain types of affect (i.e., aggression, anger, anxiety; Lichtman, 1984; Nadler, Kav-Venaki, & Gleitman, 1985). No specific style of family interaction or structure has been found to be linked directly to parents' survivorship status; however, children of survivors do appear to struggle more with independence and autonomy than children of nonsurvivors (Rose &

Garske, 1987). There exists a high degree of affective avoidance and feelings of parental responsibility in children of Holocaust survivors (Nadler *et al.,* 1985; Rose & Garske, 1987; Zwerling *et al.,* 1984); however, parental communication was found to be significantly related to personality variables rather than survivorship status (Lichtman, 1984). Cultural variables and immigrant status may also influence emotional expressiveness in families (Rose & Garske, 1987). Child-rearing practices do not appear significantly different in families of Holocaust and non-Holocaust survivors (Halik, Rosenthal, & Pattison, 1990; Weiss, O'Connell, & Siites, 1986).

Many of the empirical studies suffer from methodological weaknesses that may have resulted in their failure to detect true differences between groups of Holocaust survivors and nonsurvivors, and their children. For example, studies examining child-rearing practices did not consistently use comparison groups to control for the effects of parental trauma on child rearing. Conclusions about the impact of parental trauma on child rearing in families of Holocaust survivors, are, therefore, difficult to reach. Examination of children of Holocaust survivors was based on the retrospective accounts of these adult children, and in many studies, objective indices of psychological status and functioning of the children were not obtained. Parental diagnoses were also not obtained, so the relationship between the psychological states of these parents and their children is unclear. There is insufficient evidence to conclude that psychopathology is common in the children of Holocaust survivors, and the population appears to be more heterogeneous than people originally thought (Danieli, 1985).

Vietnam Veterans.   Although symptoms have been described in children of Vietnam veterans that appear to be directly related to their fathers' war experiences, few controlled studies have been conducted to test these observations. Harkness (1993) examined the effect of fathers' combat-related PTSD and violent behaviors on their children. Results revealed that parents viewed their children as depressed, anxious, somatized, schizoid, uncommunicative, hyperactive, aggressive, and delinquent. Boys were viewed by parents as being more disturbed than girls. Additionally, lower levels of family functioning, paternal combat experience, and paternal violence were significantly associated with child behavior problems, academic difficulties, and poor social competence. Harkness's study, however, evaluated outcome based on the presence or absence of violence in fathers with PTSD. Harkness suggests that violence in the family may be more influential in the development of child psychopathology than either the fathers' PTSD or the level of family functioning, but she did not include a non-PTSD comparison group. Since outbursts of anger, however, can be considered a PTSD Criterion D symptom of increased arousal, and violence may be incorporated into traumatic reexperiencing (particularly in Vietnam veterans), the study can still be considered to lend support for the hypothesis of intergenerational transmission of trauma. Parsons, Kehle, and Owen (1990) also found that combat-veteran fathers perceived their children to manifest dysfunctional behavior, including aggression, hyperactivity, delinquency, and social difficulty.

Davidson, Smith, and Kudler (1989) evaluated family histories of psychiatric illness in Vietnam, Korean, and World War II veterans with PTSD, nonpsychiatric controls, depressed patients, and alcohol-abusing individuals. Their results revealed that more children of PTSD patients received psychiatric treatment than did those of nonpsychiatric controls and manifested significant psychiatric and developmental problems such as attention deficit disorders, anxiety, behavioral and academic difficulties, and anorexia nervosa. A study of 1,200 Vietnam veterans (out of 3,016 veterans who had engaged in interviews as part of the National Survey of the Vietnam Generation, a component of the NVVRS study (Kulka *et al.,* 1990), found that veterans with PTSD were more likely to report martial, parental, and family adjustment problems (in terms of adaptability and cohesion, and family violence) than veterans without PTSD (Jordan, Marmar, Fairbank, & Schlenger, 1992). Overall, the results of empirical studies of Vietnam combat veterans and their children are consistent with clinical observations of this population. There is some evidence to suggest that psychopathological responses may be transmitted to children by their fathers.

Wives of combat veterans also incur secondary trauma in the relationship with their husbands. Verbosky and Ryan (1988) found increased levels of stress, feelings of worthlessness, poor self-esteem, and ineffective coping in wives of veterans with PTSD. Many have also been battered in their relationships with these combat veterans (Maloney, 1988; Matsakis, 1988; Williams, 1980) and have been found to show psychiatric symptoms (Solomon, 1988, 1990). Factors that have been found to contribute to wives' mental health include the degree of expressiveness in the marital relationship (Solomon, Waysman, Avitzur, & Enoch, 1991). De-Fazio and Pascucci (1984) observed common interpersonal patterns between Vietnam veterans and their wives which appeared to influence the marital relationship and, one can speculate, the potential for transmission of trauma.

Traumatic events impact survivors along a continuum of psychological functioning. Not every child of a trauma survivor will become a dysfunctional adult. Conversely, a parent does not necessarily have to meet criteria for PTSD to communicate traumatic beliefs and assumptions about the world. Children receive trauma-related communications about beliefs and assumptions that may result in emotional and behavioral problems, or more subtle disruptions in psychosocial functioning and adjustment.

DEFINITIONS AND CONSTRUCTS

The information-processing theories of Janoff-Bulman (1992) and McCann and Pearlman (1990a) provide a theoretical framework for understanding the traumatic beliefs and assumptions that survivors communicate to their children. Janoff-Bulman (1992) uses the concept of schemata to explain how trauma influences the development of these beliefs and assumptions about the world. A schema is a mental structure that represents organized knowledge about a given concept or type of stimulus. Based upon early interactions with caregivers, individuals develop a set of beliefs, assumptions, or internal representations of the self and others that guide subsequent interactions with others. According to Janoff-Bulman, fundamental assumptions are generally the grandest schemata, the most abstract, generalized knowledge structures. Individuals tend to perceive and understand the world in schema-consistent ways. Once basic assumptions develop, they are usually resistant to change except when trauma is experienced.

The psychological sequelae of trauma stem from the shattering of three fundamental assumptions about the world and the self: (1) the world is benevolent, (2) the world is meaningful, and, (3) the self is worthy. Differential responses to trauma arise, in part, from the nature of the traumatic event and the basic assumption most threatened by it. The world is no longer considered safe and secure; thus, a new worldview is constructed. According to Janoff-Bulman (1992), the breakdown of any one assumption is sufficient to disrupt a victim's feeling of personal safety and security in the world.

In constructivist self-development theory, McCann and Pearlman (1990a) also utilize these concepts to explain the impact of trauma on the survivor. They postulate the self as the basis for an individual's identity and inner life that develops as a result of (1) reflection, (2) interactions with others, and (3) reflection upon these interactions. The self is composed of four elements: (1) basic capacities to maintain inner identity and self-esteem, (2) ego resources that regulate interactions with the world, (3) psychological needs that motivate behavior, and (4) cognitive schemata, which are beliefs, assumptions, and expectations through which an individual interprets his or her experience. These components of the self are affected by trauma interdependently, and the individual's dominant needs determine his or her psychological response to events. Early experience with others creates particular patterns of salient needs within each individual. The needs hypothesized to be most affected by traumatic experience include (1) frame of reference, (2) safety, (3) trust and dependency, (4) esteem, (5) independence, (6) power, and (7) intimacy. Trauma disrupts the individual's salient needs; schemata are the cognitive manifestations of these needs.

It is these disrupted schemata of the traumatized parent that are transmitted to the children, influencing their basic assumptions, worldviews, and beliefs. Transmission of trauma has been observed in other populations as well, including therapists who work with trauma survivors (Chrestman, 1994; Danieli, 1988a; McCann & Pearlman, 1990b; Munroe, 1991; Schauben & Frazier, 1995). Intergenerational transmission of trauma may occur in children whose parents are survivors of trauma. It refers to thoughts, feelings, and behaviors that parallel those of the trauma survivors, are generated from the survivors' experiences, and are transmitted to them from the survivors (Munroe, Shay, Fisher, Zimering, & Ancharoff, 1993).

The distinction between primary and secondary trauma is not necessarily clear. A child who is the victim of violence is being primarily traumatized. A child who learns the parent's traumatized worldview in the context of the relationship might more accurately be described as being secondarily traumatized. Both can occur simultaneously, and the distinction between the two is more academic than real. They may be difficult to separate or label in practice.

Children who have been primarily traumatized, as well as those who have been secondarily traumatized, may manifest intrusions of traumatic material in the form of daydreams and fantasies. Both groups may also manifest behavioral change in response to environmental and/or ideational stimuli symbolic of the trauma. Directly traumatized children may encode the trauma in visual memory, subsequently replaying the image in their minds. Similarly, children of traumatized parents may experience recurrent visual images of parental trauma that they have constructed from fantasy and information acquired from parents or other sources. In response to intrusions, both directly traumatized children and those who have experienced secondary trauma may remain in a state of anxious arousal or hypervigilance. Finally, both groups of children, without words sufficient to describe or process the traumatic material, may act it out through play or develop trauma-related fears.

Conceptual models to understand secondary traumatization or intergenerational transmission are less clear than the theories on the impact and effects of primary trauma. We hypothesize the following as variables influential in the transmission of traumatic beliefs: the severity of parental trauma; the degree to which beliefs and assumptions have been disrupted, the degree to which a parent has integrated the traumatic event and restored meaning to life, and the number and frequency of stimuli that may trigger traumatic recollections and reexperiencing.

It is important for clinicians to remain aware of the functional utility of the messages that are transmitted from traumatized parents to their children. Not all messages, beliefs, or assumptions are necessarily pathological in the context of the imperfect society in which we live. Aspects of a traumatized parent's worldview may, at times, be helpful. Although a combat veteran, for example, remained vigilant for any sign of ambush even after Vietnam, it may not be maladaptive for his child to be moderately cautious while walking along city streets. The most malignant component of the transmission is the raw, unintegrated affect that has never been processed in the parents and, consequently, becomes internalized in the children in another place and time. The goal of treatment is not necessarily to restore a "Pollyannaish" worldview in children and families of survivors, but to help them integrate the traumatic experiences of the parent's past and create a worldview that incorporates realistic considerations and maintains an overall feeling of safety, meaning, and value in the present.

Perhaps adaptive or maladaptive consequences of transmission are not the central issue. What is more important is the nature of the transmission and the degree of choice regarding behavior. Transmission of trauma implies that trauma, in some way, narrows the choices one has with regard to behavior, based upon beliefs and assumptions that have been shattered. When children of survivors feel compelled to reenact parental traumatic experiences, their choices are, by definition, narrowed. Choice is based upon messages communicated by parents about the world in which the child never lived, except, perhaps, vicariously.

MECHANISMS OF TRANSMISSION

The mechanisms of transmission (secondary, as opposed to primary) described herein should be regarded as simplified working models. They are not mutually exclusive and, in practice, show considerable overlap. They are neither good nor bad. They can transmit healthy or maladaptive messages. These mechanisms are silence, overdisclosure, identification, and reenactment.

Silence

Silence can often communicate traumatic messages as powerfully as words. Danieli (1984) wrote about a "conspiracy of silence" in society, in general, and in therapists working with Holocaust survivors, in particular, that she found maintained and exacerbated the effects of trauma. From a systemic perspective, silence communicates rules, myths, and metamessages to which the family may unquestioningly adhere. Silences in the family may develop in one of two ways. First, family members may be empathically attuned to the survivor parent's emotional distress. To avoid arousing further distress, they may work hard to shun issues they believe may trigger discomfort and further symptomatology in the parent. This is especially relevant for children of survivors, who sense that something terrible must have happened to their parent and that he or she is fragile as a result. Second, the parent's behavior may inhibit discussion about sensitive issues. For example, a combat veteran may react to issues that trigger recollections of combat trauma with extreme anxiety, outbursts of rage, or a flashback. Children learn quickly to avoid discussion of events, situations, thoughts, or emotions they believe may provoke such behavior. Families collude to maintain these silences to protect themselves and the survivor from posttrauma reactions. The breach of silence may precipitate the use of diversionary tactics or crises in the family to maintain distance from the traumatic material. These may include simply changing the subject, scapegoating a child, or a marital argument. As a result, the focus of the family interaction changes from the father's trauma to relatively more benign issues. Subsequent anxiety in the children may be related to the anticipation of their parent's symptoms and to fantasies about the uncommunicated material.

A variant of silence is underdisclosure. When only partial details of the parents' trauma are known, children may struggle to complete the story and gain closure. In an effort to know and feel closer to their parents, children may fantasize or imagine the trauma their parents experienced, which can be as horrifying, or more horrifying than accurate information.

Overdisclosure

Bearing witness to traumatic experience can challenge even the most firmly held beliefs that the world is a safe place, that there is a meaning to what happens to us, and that we are worthy. Sharing the process with another person has therapeutic value in terms of alleviating the intense isolation of a trauma survivor. It is problematic if the other is not equipped to share the intensity of the experience in its raw form.

Children of trauma survivors vary with respect to awareness and knowledge about their parents' traumatic experiences. Frequently, trauma survivors want to protect family members from the emotional pain of their memories. However, direct disclosure does occur and may traumatize the children. Traumatic information relating to parents' experiences must be conveyed to children in age-appropriate ways and in doses that permit children to listen to the experiences and receive appropriate parental support. The ability of parents to confide appropriately about their trauma, however, is a function of the degree to which they can cope with their symptoms, and perhaps the extent to which their assumptions have been altered. Trauma survivors who have not sufficiently integrated their experiences often have difficulty choosing how much to disclose and modulating associated affect. It is difficult to hear and empathize with the emotional pain of those we care about. It is also distressing to hear traumatic details without concomitant affect. The impact of such direct disclosure on children may be horror, particularly when delivered in a flat, nonchalant way. This has also been noted in psychotherapists working with trauma survivors (Danieli, 1988a). Graphic disclosures of trauma-related information may be made by parents with urgency to prepare their children to survive in a world in which they believe there is no trust and danger is omnipresent.

Identification

Children who live with a traumatized parent may be continually exposed to posttrauma reactions, which can be unpredictable and frightening. Children tend to feel responsible for their parents' distress and feel that if they could just be good enough, their parents would not be so sad or angry. Thus, the child makes extreme efforts not to disturb them further. Children of trauma survivors are similar to the frequently parentified children of depressed or alcoholic mothers (Gizynski, 1983; Greenfield, Swartz, Landerman, & George, 1993; Harkness, 1993). These roles may arouse significant anxiety in children who are not prepared to handle the functions and demands of adulthood. This anxiety may parallel, for example, the inexperienced combat veteran suddenly placed in the middle of a firefight.

Children seek out their parents' acceptance and recognition. Children of combat veterans identify with their father's experience to know him better and attempt to feel what he feels, possibly leading to the development of parallel symptomatology (Harkness, 1993). Additionally, PTSD intrusion and avoidance cycles may be particularly confusing and disruptive for children. Survivors may be unpredictable and explosive during intrusions, unable or unwilling to explain what is happening to them. Subsequently, they may feel guilty for having put the family through this experience, and may isolate themselves and feel emotionally numb and unable to connect with their children. The child may manifest the same feelings and behaviors.

The survivor's propensity for hypervigilance may be conveyed to children through observation and modeling as well. A child of a Vietnam combat veteran may observe the father angrily insisting on sitting in the far corner of a restaurant to have a full view of the room, so no one can surprise or ambush him. The child may learn to manifest similar hypervigilance on the playground, believing there are dangers in the world against which he or she must be perpetually on guard. Emulating parental behavior is also a way to gain acceptance from a parent who has difficulty with intimacy because of trauma.

Survivor guilt has been an associated with PTSD (American Psychiatric Association, 1987), perhaps reflecting the need of trauma survivors to maintain a view of the world as meaningful (Janoff-Bulman, 1992) and reverse the helplessness associated with their traumatic experience, while maintaining loyalty to the dead (Danieli, 1985). Children of trauma survivors may also experience a type of survivor guilt. They may ruminate about their behavior to make sense of what appear to be arbitrary, random parental reactions to common events. This behavior may also facilitate the child's ability to maintain a connection with the traumatized parent. Without this connection, severely traumatized parents may be absorbed in their own traumatized world and be unreachable in many ways to their children.

Reenactment

Trauma survivors tend to reenact their trauma. Traumatic experiences, however, may not be reenacted alone. Others may be engaged or induced to participate in relationships based on this worldview and to act out various roles that vary in accordance with the specific dynamics of the original trauma (Munroe et al., 1995). Affect is aroused in others that parallels the survivors' original trauma experience by their participation in the reenactment. These interactions repeatedly test the validity of the traumatized worldview in a way that tends to confirm it. People close to trauma survivors can find themselves thinking, feeling, and behaving as if they, too, had been traumatized or were perpetrators. Although the content of the interaction may vary, the themes and the affect it generates in others remain the same. Essentially, what is created is an isomorph of the survivor's experience in another person, a relationship that generates a pattern or structure parallel to the survivor's trauma experience and produces feelings, thoughts, and behaviors common to that experience.

Behavioral isomorphs engage children directly in the traumatized world of their parents. Engagement in scenarios that are thematically reminiscent of the parent's trauma forcefully transmit the parent's worldview. For example,

> A Vietnam veteran who had experienced severe combat exposure, disillusionment with his superiors in Vietnam, and with the government upon his return, took his 3-year-old son to the playground. His son wanted to ride down the slide but was afraid and repeatedly asked his father to catch him at the bottom of the slide. The father agreed. However, when the child reached the bottom of the slide, the father broke his promise and deliberately did not catch him. When asked why, the father said his child needed to learn to distrust what people told him. (J. F. Munroe, personal communication, November 18, 1993)

This message of distrust is exactly what the father learned in Vietnam. Superiors often made lethal decisions, stating they had the best interest of their men at heart, decisions that cost the lives of friends and innocent civilians. In the aforementioned interaction with his father, the little boy experienced a betrayal parallel to the one his father experienced in his unit. In essence, this man was teaching his son how to survive in an unsafe world. The father did not need words or reference to Vietnam to teach this lesson, yet the content of the message was powerfully transmitted, as Danieli (1985) has noted in children of Holocaust survivors.

Reenactments transmit trauma by setting up participatory isomorphs that produce in others parallel but perhaps less intense trauma experiences of the survivor. These may be produced intentionally, but often involve unconscious acting out of the trauma worldview. When participants experience this, they are being secondarily traumatized. The affective experience of this participation is described by others as projective identification (Catherall, 1992b) or countertransference (Wilson & Lindy, 1994). The isomorphic reenactment produces parallel thoughts and behaviors, as well as feelings.

> An intoxicated, suicidal Vietnam veteran was found in the basement of his home by his adolescent son, who had just come home from school at the regular hour. The father, reliving a combat experience in a fit of rage, was crying, and holding a revolver to his head. Having seen his father's rages before, the son experienced each one to be as anxiety provoking as the first. He felt responsible for his father's life, both powerful and helpless, as well as angry. (J. F. Munroe, personal communication, February 25, 1994)

This situation paralleled the overwhelming helplessness the veteran felt in the middle of a firefight and the intense feeling of power that often accompanies the combat experience. The child's anger may have also paralleled the veteran's rage at having been forced into a situation with which he was ill-equipped to cope.

As described earlier, all of these mechanisms may overlap. For example, while watching television with his 8-year-old son, something he saw triggered a memory of the war for a combat veteran, who began to talk about his experiences, which soon led to describing atrocities. As if attacked by his own horror, the father made up some excuse and left the house quickly in an attempt to contain his feelings. The son had been exposed to the horror of wartime atrocities (overdisclosure). His father's abrupt departure left him without closure and with having to speculate on what else happened, and what it meant (silence). With no one to talk to, he went outside and played basketball to try to force the information out of his mind (identification). He was left with the parallel feelings of knowing about the horrors of war but not being allowed to speak about them, and perhaps thinking that nobody would believe him anyway (isomorphic reenactment). A portion of the father's combat experience had been transmitted to the son to be incorporated into his worldview.

CASE EXAMPLES

The following are some examples of the messages Vietnam veterans can pass on to their children. They illustrate a range of negative and positive behaviors that might occur, but do not imply that all or most children of Vietnam veterans will experience such problems.

Case 1

Laura was 16 when she attempted suicide by an overdose of street drugs and medications prescribed for her mother. Prior to her suicide attempt, her grades had slipped from a B average to failing all her courses. Her steady boyfriend also used drugs, and she hung out with an older group of friends.

Her parents had separated $2^1/_2$ years earlier, but they still maintained intermittent contact. Laura, her old brother, and younger sister lived with their mother but had contact with their father. Laura was described as her father's favorite. He would often take her for walks when she was little, and she was the one who could coax him out of his "moods." She remembered her father saying to a family therapist that he had been in the woods with a loaded gun to his head, but he could not pull the trigger because he saw Laura's face.

Laura's father, Mike, served as a field medic in Vietnam. Following his return, he reported constantly seeing the faces and bodies of soldiers he could not save. Although he had been a promising student and athlete before Vietnam, Mike was not able to "get it together" when he got back. While his three brothers went on to successful professional careers, Mike had a long history of alcohol and heroin addiction. He would be able to maintain sobriety for 6 months to 2-year periods. During these clean-and-sober periods, he would become very involved with work. As sleep, negative images, and relationships at work worsened, he would gradually go back to using substances. After his last relapse, he and Laura's mother separated.

Gail, Laura's mother, said, "Laura is always the one who seems to take things most seriously."

Laura was a quiet, sweet child. She was often the family peacekeeper and the one who tried to make everyone happy. She would prepare dinner for the family when Gail worked late and make little cards and gifts for Mike to cheer him up. Mike and Gail said that this made it even more confusing when she started running around with an older crowd and getting into trouble.

Laura was, at first, extremely reticent to talk in sessions. She alternated between anger and silence. Shortly after her suicide attempt, she told the emergency-room physician, "I made a mess out of everything, and now I just want to die!"

Case 2

Kevin, a 12-year-old boy, was brought in by his father, Jake, to his Veterans Affairs therapist for evaluation after a motorcycle accident from which Kevin still suffered nightmares. Jake was being seen at Veterans Affairs because his PTSD symptoms from Vietnam combat interfered with his job advancement and social functioning. Kevin was a soft-spoken, pleasant young man who often looked to his father for direction, and he stated a preference that his father remain with him during the first session.

Jake was a 46-year-old Vietnam combat veteran. He completed 2 years of community college before being drafted and sent to Vietnam. Because of his intelligence, greater maturity, and physical abilities, he soon became a squad leader. Although he performed admirably and received medals and commendations, many of the men in his squad were killed in an ambush that he felt he should have been able to prevent. After coming home, Jake took a job with the telephone company but persistently turned down promotions and had difficulty getting along with his bosses.

Kevin and Jake described the accident in which an older man and his wife turned out of a driveway in front of the motorcycle Kevin and his father were on. Kevin said that his father tried to swerve away from the car, but the car kept coming, and they hit it anyway. Kevin's leg was badly scraped and bleeding. He remembered how angry his father was, threatening to kill the driver. They kept shouting at each other. Finally, the police arrived, and Kevin was taken to the hospital and released the same day.

Jake was worried that the accident had traumatized Kevin. He was surprised when he heard the content of Kevin's dream. In his dream, the accident was about to happen and Kevin could not warn his father. Jake got so angry over his son's injury that he pulled out a gun and shot the man in the car, and the police took Jake away. Kevin was then able to tell his father that he was more afraid of his father's anger (and his being the cause of it) than he was bothered by the accident or the injury.

Kevin said that he often felt he caused his father's upsets. With some prompting, Jake was able to tell his son that, as a squad leader, he had felt very responsible for his men and sometimes still reacts today the way he did then. At the therapist's urging, he gave a few examples of how this happened at work as well. He reassured his son that he was not the cause of his anger.

IDENTIFICATION OF INTERGENERATIONAL TRANSMISSION OF TRAUMA IN CLINICAL PRACTICE

There is no single answer to the question of what we should look for in the child of the survivor of combat trauma. The legacy of trauma is complex. It depends on the initial trauma, the ways in which it is handed down, the mediators in the child's environment, and his or her makeup. Sometimes the symptoms may mirror those of the parent's PTSD, but the legacy may manifest itself in other forms. Green (1993) described the category of trauma, individual factors, and the recovery environment as the three factors relevant to the presentation of a traumatized person. These factors are also relevant for the child of a traumatized combatant. It is important to remember that the effects are not always only negative. Since these children are often still living in an environment influenced by the traumatized parents, assessment is neither static nor easily standardized. Asking the right questions does not mean drawing standardized conclusions for a child.

The degree to which transmission of traumatic beliefs will affect children cannot be presently predicted, because no tools exist to measure adequately the construct and the differential impact of primary and secondary trauma. But risk factors, based on historical and interpersonal data, can be identified. A comprehensive assessment should include a thorough evaluation of the child's cognitive, affective, and psychosocial functioning. The assessment extends to an evaluation of the parents' psychosocial and marital functioning (as traumatic reenactments occur within the entire family). To uncover the family's worldview, the clinicians must be alert to family myths, common themes and assumptions, beliefs, as well as patterns of engagement.

The child who is having problems may be identified through the school, the parents, or a treatment or social service agency, as in the case examples. Harkness (1993) pointed out that the child may not behave or be perceived the same way in all situations. A child who appears to pose few problems at home or school may come to the attention of a treatment or social service agency because of the parents' behaviors. There are many ways to assess a child's behavior (e.g., child behavior checklists filled out by parents, teachers, or observers; educational core evaluations; parent interviews; direct observations).[1] The place in which the child is identified often determines how the child is assessed. Some of the symptoms found in children of Vietnam veterans include impaired self-esteem, poor reality testing, trouble following rules, hyperactivity and aggressive behavior, difficulty coping with feelings, intrusive thoughts, and nightmares (Harkness, 1993; Rosenheck & Nathan, 1985). Because these are also found in many other disorders, knowledge of the parent's primary trauma and the interaction patterns in the family are important in determining if secondary trauma is a factor. Understanding the behavioral context is equally important in terms of identifying ways in which trauma may be reenacted and ascertaining the degree to which the reenactment is impinging upon daily functioning. Examining behavior patterns seen in other children of combatants with PTSD [e.g., Harkness's (1993) descriptions of the vicariously traumatized child, the nurturant rescuer, and the emotionally isolated child] may also be helpful in determining the existence of secondary trauma. Psychoeducation and trust building, discussed in the interventions section below, may need to precede data gathering in many instances.

Beyond the nature of the parent's trauma, how it has been communicated to the child (overtly, covertly, or by reenactment), its behavioral manifestations in the father and its parallel in the child, exploring the family dynamics is extremely important. Mason (1990) poig-

---

[1]Krinsley and Weathers (1995) reviewed assessment measures for trauma and emphasize that the definition of trauma, the dimensions of trauma (subjective and objective), and the examination of a broad range of stressful events are important. Some of the measures they reviewed include the Familial Experiences Inventory (Ogata *et al.,* 1990) and the Retrospective Assessment of Traumatic Experiences (Gallagher, Flye, Hurt, Stone, & Hull, 1992). Similarly, McNally (1996) reviews assessment tools for evaluating PTSD in children. Pynoos *et al.*'s (1993) description of age-related behaviors in traumatized children, and developmental models of childhood traumatic stress (Pynoos, Steinberg, & Wraith, 1995) might also apply to children of traumatized parents as a result of either primary or secondary traumatization. Pynoos and Eth's (1988) interview for traumatized children might also be adapted to those suffering the legacy of trauma. In these cases, it would be assumed that the child's behavior is parallel with, or reactive to, the traumatized parents' behaviors.

nantly described the role that wives often take in families of traumatized veterans: selfless, enabling, pacifying, and, usually, depressed and angry. Wives may experience primary as well as secondary traumatization in their leadership with their husbands and may transmit aspects of both within the context of their relationship with the children. Figley (1989) suggested exploring issues related to functioning in families in which one or more members has PTSD, such as their understanding of how the stress affects them, their inclination to conceptualize their difficulty as a family problem versus identification of the traumatized parent as the damaged member, flexibility of family roles, and the level of intrafamily violence. Ben-David and Lavee (1992) described and categorized family reactions to outside stressors as being secure, indifferent, cautious, or anxious. Measures such as the Family Environment Scale (Moos & Moos, 1986) assess various dimensions of family relating. Danieli (1985) identified specific categories of adaptational styles in families of Holocaust survivors. She described victim families, fighter families, numb families, and families of "those who made it." These patterns may also emerge in families of Vietnam veterans as clinicians and researchers continue to study Vietnam veterans with regard to the specific nature of the combat experience, as well as the homecoming they received. For example, the child of a combat veteran, who was taught that life was expendable and its value low, might show the aforementioned symptoms of low self-worth. Children of veterans who saw authority as incompetent and had negative homecomings are not likely to see the world as benevolent and may have a very difficult time following rules that society has set. A rigid pattern may affect behavior and self-esteem over time. A traumatic family pattern that may work moderately well when children are small (e.g., allies and enemies) may fall apart in their adolescent and young adult years, when the child desires a degree of independence and autonomy. A father who had been uninvolved in a child's early years may identify and become more engaged with his or her adolescent rebellion.

The social context is also very important in assessing the legacy of trauma. When the environment is dangerous (e.g., war zone, certain inner-city neighborhoods), teaching survival behaviors may be quite adaptive. The cultural context must be evaluated as well. The child may come from a group of people that has been persecuted or traumatized in addition to the war experiences of the combatant parent. The family may be one that has experienced generations of trauma and sees this as the norm. Contextualizing the story in an integrated fashion is crucial. Messages communicated within a family can relate a history or a legacy such that important aspects of their past are not forgotten. Within this communication, however, there must be a context or a place within which the affect may be held, so that it does not overwhelm the family as a whole, or any of its members. There is usually an element of truth in the anxiety communicated within the family of a trauma survivor. Evaluative skills must be taught to help families ascertain the probability of the traumatic event occurring in the present. Families of trauma survivors, and children more specifically, have difficulty accurately assessing the risk of the past repeating itself.

Mediating variables are also extremely important. Sources of support outside the immediate family can often provide an alternative worldview. Unique strengths the child may have should be assessed and utilized appropriately. Socioeconomic factors may also be involved.

INTERVENTION

Combat-veteran status, alone, does not automatically imply the necessity for clinical intervention. Neither are the problems that children may manifest automatically attributable to the father's combat experience. Combat experience may, instead, serve as a framework for intervention if it is warranted. It is important to identify the behavior of the child, the context in which it occurs, and whether it is related to the father's combat trauma. A child who has difficulty reading and does not get along with teachers may have a learning disability and subsequent problems with teachers, or may be acting out the father's difficulty with authority in a subsequent lack of attention to reading. Interventions on both levels may be appropriate.

When the child's behavior does seem clearly related to secondary trauma, it is important to avoid blaming the father. He may already be suffering a great deal of guilt; moreover, he may be worried that he is harming his child. Blaming the victim of the combat trauma is unlikely to increase the possibility for effective intervention with either the father or the family. Involving the father as part of the solution is more likely to produce results that will benefit both generations. Engaging the mother is equally important. The wife, a recipient of secondary trauma, may also need help, but the parental team is, by far, the most powerful influence on addressing transmissions. There is no clear guideline on when to intervene. In general, intervention should be considered when the worldview transmitted by the trauma generates thoughts, feelings, and behaviors that may be inappropriate for the current environment.

Interventions are either preventive or reactive. Preventive responses are appropriate when awareness of the father's traumatic experience exists and he and his family can be informed of the possible impact of intergenerational transmission. Reactive responses are called for when problems in the children of veterans become apparent. The relationship between these difficulties and paternal combat trauma should be explored. If the child's problems surface in school, the staff may not know whether the father is a veteran and if he has been traumatized by combat. Since transmission is not limited to combat trauma, it would be wise to take a full trauma history from both parents.

Intervention strategies can be either informative or interactive. Similar to the mechanisms of transmission that they address, these strategies overlap considerably and the differences may be more conceptual than actual. Informative strategies are essentially psychoeducational and include pamphlets, books, video- or audiotapes, lectures, and presentations. Many veterans who suffer from PTSD do not know what it is. They often assume that they are crazy or inadequate, and that nobody else experiences the world the way they do. And even those who are aware of the influence that trauma can have on individuals may be totally unaware of the process of such transmission. Framing PTSD as a normal response to abnormal experiences can relieve a great deal of pressure on both the veteran and his or her family. The explanation should include effects on loved ones and families of those traumatized. Transmission does not require a diagnosis of PTSD. Once some of the effects of trauma are identified and explained, family members can begin to consider some control over their behaviors. These are fairly passive activities for the clinician, in that the family determines what actions are to be taken. Material may be presented on the formal definitions and symptoms of PTSD, as well as on the less formal effects (e.g., where the veteran will sit in a restaurant, the avoidance of family social gatherings such as weddings and holidays). The mechanisms of transmission described earlier, of how those who are close to the combat veteran can begin to think, feel, and behave as if they were in combat, may also be explained. Strategies might include a family information meeting that is followed by questions and answers, a spousal support group, or a workshop that included both parents and children. Family members can learn how trauma influences their own lives. Recommendations for further information should be provided. The specific content and style of such an intervention will vary according to the needs of the participants the clinicians assess throughout the meeting.

Interactive strategies consist of the active involvement by mental health professionals, directed at the mechanisms of transmission, in the process of therapy. They help identify the messages, the specific means of transmission, and alternative communication patterns. To succeed, therapeutic interventions must rely on first having established and maintained trust. Trauma involves the betrayal of basic trust. Moreover, in combat veterans, the loss of trust in authority is crucial (Munroe *et al.,* 1995). This mistrust may be an integral part of what is transmitted to other family members, including children. Therapists who rely on the role of "professional authority" may be quickly rejected. A successful interactive strategy requires attention to the ongoing tests of trust that the traumatized veteran and his or her family may pose.

The mechanisms of transmission are problematic when they cannot be identified or discussed. Transmitted messages, once elucidated, can be evaluated for their current appropriateness. Silence and overdisclosure do not allow opportunity for discussion. Identification and reenactments are essentially nonverbal exchanges. It may be very hard to decipher the messages on a conscious level. In the example in which the father allowed his son to fall off the slide, the messages and worldview were not open to discussion or analysis. The girl whose father did not shoot himself because he saw her face could neither articulate her sense of being thrust into the impossible responsibility for life and death, nor know how it may have paralleled her father's experience of being thrust into combat. Therapy focuses on the mechanisms in order to verbalize the resultant transmitted messages.

Ideally, it would be most efficient if the entire family were available and interested in therapy, but this is quite frequently not the case. Also, since trauma disrupts the ability to trust or negotiate relationships, a broad definition of what constitutes a "family" may be necessary. Interventions can be targeted to the parents, partners, children, relatives, friends, or other therapists. The trauma survivor may be the person least receptive to outside influence as a result of the deep violation of his or her sense of trust. The veteran who is in treatment may resist involving the family out of the wish to protect them. Veterans are frequently concerned that therapy will result in overdisclosure that may harm the family or cause them to reject him or her. It is crucial to allow the family to have some degree of control over the process. It is also important to tailor the therapy to the needs of the recipients to prevent further traumatization. For example, the amount and nature of information about war should differ when disclosed to a school-age child and to a grown child who is considering enlisting in the military.

Recovery from trauma is enhanced when trauma is viewed as a family problem rather than an individual problem (Catherall, 1992a; Danieli, 1988b, 1993; Figley, 1988). The objective of interventions directed at intergenerational transmission is to help family members examine the appropriateness of the various components of their current worldview in light of past traumatic events. Once the problems with silence or overdisclosure are identified, families can begin to talk about what questions need to be asked and how detailed the answers need to be. Once family members are aware of identifications or isomorphic reenactments, they can begin to distinguish between reactions to the past and responses to the present. A worldview that is dominated by trauma restricts the ability to respond to changing world conditions. The objective of any intervention is an expanded worldview that allows all family members a greater range of responses.

CLINICAL IMPLICATIONS

There is little doubt that combat trauma can have devastating and long-lasting effects on those directly exposed to it. It is important to recall, however, that prior to 1980, the diagnosis of PTSD did not exist, and the view held by the clinical community was that people should recover from combat exposure within 6 months. Those who did not recover were presumed to

have a premorbid condition. The field has developed and revised the criteria for PTSD to evaluate the impact of primary trauma, but secondary effects are not well understood. Similarly,
there may be a tendency to deny the legacies of combat trauma on successive generations.

The extent of the damage that transmitted trauma can incur is yet unclear. The number of
generations affected remains ambiguous, as is the specific nature of the transmissions and the differential vulnerability of family members. There is some evidence that children's symptoms may
parallel those of the combat-veteran father, but additional consequences are unknown. Children
of combat veterans may be more likely to exhibit parallel symptoms of PTSD, but they may also
be more likely to exhibit symptoms of other disorders of childhood. Combat veterans received a
wide variety of inappropriate diagnoses prior to 1980, and it is possible that many of the diagnoses given to their children have been similarly inaccurate. There is clearly much research to be
done, but clinical experience demonstrates the need to address secondary effects. Clinicians must
address it or become part of the "conspiracy of silence" (Danieli, 1981, 1984, 1988a).

Bloom (1995) has proposed a germ theory of trauma. Following Pasteur, she suggests
that, just as bacterial agents external to an individual cause infection, traumatic experience
external to the survivor cause PTSD symptoms. Similarly, one can speculate that such an infection may be contagious to successive generations. Pasteur's discoveries led to direct interventions on causal agents and the mechanisms of infectious transmissions. With respect to the
legacies of combat trauma, the causal agent is known. Techniques for addressing it in those directly exposed are continually being refined. If trauma has an infectious aspect, we should not
treat just the traumatized individual.

As stated earlier, silence does not prevent the transmission of trauma but, on the contrary,
acts as a mechanism of its transmission. Many combat veterans, their spouses, as well as their
therapists, are understandably reluctant to expose children to the horrors of war. Age and developmental level of children are crucial in determining the nature of what and how much they can
process. The messages, however, are transmitted even if the content of the trauma is not. A portion of the raw affect of the original trauma may be transmitted without processing its meaning.
Any effort to prevent the potential damage of transmission necessitates a careful analysis of just
how much of the traumatic detail is disclosed and when. Full disclosure is not an objective of
treatment. Allowing the family greater control over disclosure and transmitted messages is a more
appropriate goal. Understanding the mechanisms of transmission allows therapist and family
members to examine the messages conveyed, with or without disclosure of details of the trauma.

The implications of transmission should be an immediate concern for clinicians working
with combat veterans. Therapists working with children should be sensitive to the possibility
that the behavior observed may be related to the symptoms of a combat veteran father. A thorough assessment should include a trauma history, and should not be limited to combat trauma.
A family history of exposure to traumatic events should be taken to identify potential "conta-
gions," as extrapolated from the germ theory. Interventions should focus on the family whenever possible. The mechanisms provide clinicians with expanded choices about how to address
intergenerational transmission.

REFERENCES

American Psychiatric Association. (1987). *Diagnostic and statistical manual of mental disorders* (3rd edition, rev).
    Washington, DC: Author.
American Psychiatric Association. (1994). *Diagnostic and statistical manual of mental disorders* (4th edition). Wash-
    ington, DC: Author.

Ancharoff, M. R. (1994). *Intergenerational transmission of trauma: Mechanisms and messages.* Unpublished doctoral thesis, Graduate School of Professional Psychology, University of Denver.

Baron, L., Reznikoff, M., & Glenwick, D. S. (1993). Narcissism, interpersonal adjustment, and coping in children of Holocaust survivors. *Journal of Psychology, 127*(3), 257–269.

Ben-David, A., & Lavee, Y. (1992). Families in the sealed room: Interaction patterns of Israeli families during SCUD missile attacks. *Family Process, 31,* 35–44.

Bloom, S. (1995). The germ theory of trauma: The impossibility of ethical neutrality. In B. Stamm (Ed.), *Secondary traumatic stress: Self-care issues for clinicians, researchers, and educators* (pp. 257–276). Lutherville, MD: Sidran.

Burgess, A. W., & Holmstrom, L. L. (1974). Rape trauma syndrome. *American Journal of Psychiatry, 131,* 981–986.

Catherall, D. R. (1992a). *Back from the brink: A family guide to overcoming traumatic stress.* New York, Bantam.

Catherall, D. R. (1992b). Working with projective identification in couples. *Family Process, 31,* 355–367.

Chrestman, K. R. (1994). *Secondary traumatization in therapists working with survivors of trauma.* Unpublished doctoral dissertation, Nova University, Fort Lauderdale, Florida.

Danieli, Y. (1981). Therapists' difficulties in treating survivors of the Nazi Holocaust and their children. *Dissertation Abstracts International, 42,* 4947-B.

Danieli, Y. (1984). Psychotherapists' participation in the conspiracy of silence about the Holocaust. *Psychoanalytic Psychology, 1*(1), 23–42.

Danieli, Y. (1985). The treatment and prevention of long-term effects and intergenerational transmission of victimization: A lesson from Holocaust survivors and their children. In C. R. Figley (Ed.), *Trauma and its wake: The study and treatment of post-traumatic stress disorder* (pp. 295–313). New York: Brunner/Mazel.

Danieli, Y. (1988a). Confronting the unimaginable: Psychotherapists' reactions to victims of the Nazi Holocaust. In J. P. Wilson, Z. Harel, & B. Kahana (Eds.), *Human adaptation to extreme stress: From the Holocaust to Vietnam* (pp. 219–238). New York: Plenum Press.

Danieli, Y. (1988b). Treating survivors and children of survivors of the Nazi Holocaust. In F. Ochberg (Ed.), *Post-traumatic therapy and victims of violence* (pp. 278–294). New York: Brunner/Mazel.

Danieli, Y. (1993). Diagnostic and therapeutic use of the multigenerational family tree in working with survivors and children of survivors of the Nazi Holocaust. In J. P. Wilson & B. Raphael (Eds.), *International handbook of traumatic stress syndromes* (pp. 889–898). New York: Plenum Press.

Davidson, J., Smith, R., & Kudler, H. (1989). Familial psychiatric illness in chronic post-traumatic stress disorder. *Comprehensive Psychiatry, 30*(4), 339–345.

Davis, R. C., & Friedman, L. N. (1985). The emotional aftermath of crime and violence. In C. R. Figley (Ed.), *Trauma and its wake: The study and treatment of post-traumatic stress disorder* (pp. 90–112). New York: Brunner/Mazel.

DeFazio, V. J., & Pascucci, N. J. (1984). Return to Ithaca: A perspective on marriage and love in posttraumatic stress disorder. *Journal of Contemporary Psychotherapy, 14*(1), 76–89.

Doreleijers, T. A. H., and Donovan, D. (1990). Transgenerational traumatization in children of parents interned in Japanese civil internment camps in the Dutch East Indies during World War II. *Journal of Psychohistory, 17*(4), 435–447.

Epstein, H. (1979). *Children of the Holocaust: Conversations with sons and daughters of survivors.* New York: Penguin Books.

Eth, S., & Pynoos, R. S. (Eds.). (1985). *Post-traumatic stress disorder in children.* Washington, DC: American Psychiatric Association Press.

Figley, C. R. (Ed.) (1978). *Stress disorders among Vietnam veterans: Theory, research, and treatment.* New York: Brunner/Mazel.

Figley, C. R. (1985). From victim to survivor: Social responsibility in the wake of catastrophe. In C. R. Figley (Ed.), *Trauma and it's wake: the study and treatment of post-traumatic stress disorder* (pp. 398–415). New York: Brunner/Mazel.

Figley, C. R. (1988). A five-phase treatment of post-traumatic stress disorder in families. *Journal of Traumatic Stress, 1*(1), 127–141.

Figley, C. R. (1989). *Helping traumatized families.* San Francisco: Jossey-Bass.

Foa, E. B., Rothbaum, B. O., Riggs, D. S., & Murdock, T. (1992). A prospective examination of post-traumatic stress disorder in rape victims. *Journal of Traumatic Stress, 5*(3), 455–475.

Freyberg, J. T. (1980). Difficulties in separation–individuation as experienced by offspring of Nazi Holocaust survivors. *American Journal of Orthopsychiatry, 50*(1), 87–95.

Gallagher, R. E., Flye, B. L., Hurt, S. W., Stone, M. H., & Hull, J. W. (1992). Retrospective assessment of traumatic experiences (RATE). *Journal of Personality Disorders, 6,* 99–108.

Gizynski, M. N. (1983). The effects of maternal depression on children. *Clinical Social Work, 11,* 339–350.

Gleser, G. C., Green, B. L., & Winget, C. (1981). *Prolonged psychological effects of disaster: A study of Buffalo Creek.* New York: Academic Press.

Goodwin, J. (1988). Post-traumatic symptoms in abused children. *Journal of Traumatic Stress, 1*(4), 475–488.

Green, B. L. (1993). Identifying survivors at risk: Trauma and stressors across events. In J. P. Wilson & B. Raphael (Eds.), *International handbook of traumatic stress syndromes* (pp. 135–144). New York: Plenum Press.

Greenfield, S. F., Swartz, M. S., Landerman, L. R., & George, L. K. (1993). Long-term psychosocial effects of childhood exposure to parental problem drinking. *American Journal of Psychiatry, 150*(4), 608–613.

Halik, V., Rosenthal, D. A., & Pattison, P. E. (1990). Intergenerational effects of the Holocaust: Patterns of engagement in the mother–daughter relationship. *Family Process, 29,* 325–339.

Harkness, L. (1991). The effect of combat-related PTSD on children. *National Center for Post-Traumatic Stress Disorder Clinical Newsletter, 2*(1), 12–13.

Harkness, L. (1993). Transgenerational transmission of war-related trauma. In J. P. Wilson & B. Raphael (Eds.), *International handbook of traumatic stress syndromes* (pp. 635–643). New York: Plenum Press.

Holaday, M., Armsworth, M. W., Swank, P. R., & Vincent, K. R. (1992). Rorschach responding in traumatized children and adolescents. *Journal of Traumatic Stress, 5*(1), 119–129.

Jacobsen, L. K., Sweeney, C. G., & Racusin, G. R. (1993). Group psychotherapy for children of fathers with PTSD: Evidence of psychopathology emerging in the group process. *Journal of Child and Adolescent Group Therapy, 3*(2), 103–120.

Janoff-Bulman, R. (1992). *Shattered assumptions: Towards a new psychology.* New York: Macmillan.

Jordan, B. K., Maarmar, C. R., Fairbank, J. A., & Schlenger, W. E. (1992). Problems in families of male Vietnam veterans with post-traumatic stress disorder. *Journal of Consulting and Clinical Psychology, 60*(6), 916–926.

Jurich, A. P. (1983). The Saigon of the family's mind: Family therapy with families of Vietnam veterans. *Journal of Marital and Family Therapy, 9*(4), 355–363.

Keinan, G., Mikulincer, M., & Rybricki, A. (1988). Perception of self and parents by second generation Holocaust survivors. *Behavioral Medicine, 14,* 6–12.

Kestenberg, J. S. (1983). Psychoanalyses of children of survivors from the Holocaust: Case presentation and assessment. *Journal of the American Psychoanalytic Association, 28,* 775–804.

Kilpatrick, D. G., Veronen, L. J., & Best, C. L. (1985). Factors predicting psychological distress among rape victims. In C. R. Figley (Ed.), *Trauma and its wake: The study and treatment of post-traumatic stress disorder* (pp. 113–141). New York: Brunner/Mazel.

Klein, H. (1971). Families of Holocaust survivors in the kibbutz: Psychological studies. *International Psychiatry Clinics, 8,* 67–92.

Koopman, C., Classen, C., & Spiegel, D. (1994). Predictors of post-traumatic stress symptoms among survivors of the Oakland/Berkeley, California, firestorm. *American Journal of Psychiatry, 151*(6), 888–894.

Krell, R. (1982). Family therapy with children of concentration camp survivors. *American Journal of Psychotherapy, 36*(4), 513–522.

Krinsley, K. E., & Weathers, F. W. (1995). The assessment of trauma in adults. *PTSD Research Quarterly, 6,* 1–6.

Krystal, H., & Niederland, W. G. (1968). Clinical observations on the survivor syndrome. In H. Krystal (Ed.), *Massive psychic trauma* (pp. 327–348). New York: International Universities Press.

Krystal, H., & Niederland, W. G. (Eds.). (1971). *Psychic traumatization: Aftereffects in individuals and communities.* New York: Little, Brown.

Kulka, R. A., Schlenger, W. E., Fairbank, J. A., Hough, R. L., Jordan, B. K., Marmar, C. R., & Weiss, D. S. (1990). *The National Vietnam Veterans Readjustment Study: Tables of findings and technical appendices.* New York: Brunner/Mazel.

Laufer, R., Frey-Wouters, E., & Gallops, M. S. (1985). Traumatic stressors in the Vietnam war and post-traumatic stress disorder. In C. R. Figley (Ed.), *Trauma and it's wake: The study and treatment of post-traumatic stress disorder* (pp. 73–89). New York: Brunner/Mazel.

Leon, G., Butcher, J., Kleinman, M., Goldburg, A., & Almagor, M. (1981). Survivors of the Holocaust and their children: Current status and adjustment. *Journal of Personality and Social Psychology, 4,* 503–516.

Lichtman, J. (1984). Parental communication of Holocaust experiences and personality characteristics among second-generation survivors. *Journal of Clinical Psychology, 40,* 914–924.

Link, N., Victor, B., & Binder, R. L. (1985). Psychosis in children of Holocaust survivors: Influence of the Holocaust in the choice of themes in their psychoses. *Journal of Nervous and Mental Disease, 173*(2), 115–117.

Maloney, L. J. (1988). Posttraumatic stresses on women partners of Vietnam veterans. *Smith College Studies School of Social Work, 58*(2), 122–143.

Mason, P. (1990). *Recovering from the war.* New York: Viking Penguin.

Matsakis, A. (1988). *Vietnam wives.* Kensington, MD: Woodbine House.

McCann, I. L., & Pearlman, L. A. (1990a). *Psychological trauma and the adult survivor: Theory, therapy, and transformation.* New York: Brunner/Mazel.

McCann, I. L., & Pearlman, L. A. (1990b). Vicarious traumatization: A framework for understanding the psychological effects of working with victims. *Journal of Traumatic Stress, 3*(1), 131–149.

McLeer, S. V., Deblinger, E., Atkins, M. S., Foa, E. B., & Ralphe, D. L. (1988). Post-traumatic stress disorder in sexually abused children. *Journal of the American Academy of Child and Adolescent Psychiatry, 27*(5), 650–654.

McNally, R. S. (1996). Assessment of post-traumatic stress disorder in children and adolescents. *Journal of School Psychology, 0,* 000–000.

Moos, R. H., & Moos, B. S. (1986). *Family environment manual scale.* Palo Alto, CA: Consulting Psychologists Press.

Munroe, J. F. (1991). Therapist traumatization from exposure to clients with combat related post-traumatic stress disorder: Implications for administration and supervision. *Dissertation Abstracts International, 52*-03B, 1731.

Munroe J., Shay, J., Fisher, L., Makary, C., Rapperport, K., & Zimering, R. (1995). Preventing compassion fatigue: A team treatment model. In C. R. Figley (Ed.), *Compassion fatigue: Coping with secondary traumatic stress disorder in those who treat the traumatized* (pp. 209–231). New York: Brunner/Mazel.

Munroe, J., Shay, J., Fisher, L., Zimering, R., & Ancharoff, M. (1993). *Preventing traumatized therapists: Coping with survivor engagement patterns.* Workshop conducted at the 9th Annual Meeting of the International Society for Traumatic Stress Studies, San Antonio, TX.

Nadler, A., Kav-Vanaki, S., & Gleaitman, B. (1985). Transgenerational effects of the Holocaust: Externalization of aggression in second generation of Holocaust survivors. *Journal of Consulting and Clinical Psychology, 53*(3), 365–369.

Nagata, D. K. (1991). Transgenerational impact of the Japanese-American internment: Clinical issues in working with children of former internees. *Psychotherapy, 28*(1), 121–128.

Ogata, S. N., Silk, K. R., Goodrich, S., Lohr, N. E., Westen, D., & Hill, E. M. (1990). Childhood sexual and physical abuse in adult patients with borderline personality disorder. *American Journal of Psychiatry, 147,* 1008–1013.

Parsons, J., Kehle, T. J., & Owen, S. V. (1990). Incidence of behavior problems among children of Vietnam war veterans. *School Psychology International, 11*(4), 253–259.

Prince, R. M. (1985). Second generation effects of historical trauma. *Psychoanalytic Review, 72*(1), 9–29.

Pynoos, R. S., & Eth, S. (1988). Witness to violence: The child interview. In S. Chess, A. Thomas, & M. Hertzig (Eds.). *Annual progress in child psychiatry and child development, 1987* (pp. 299–326). New York: Brunner/Mazel.

Pynoos, R. S., Nader, K., Black, D., Kaplan, T., Hendriks, J. H., Gordon, R., Wraith, R., Green, A., & Herman, J. L. (1993). The impact of trauma on children and adolescents. In J. P. Wilson & B. Raphael (Eds.), *International handbook of traumatic stress syndromes* (pp. 535–657). New York: Plenum Press.

Pynoos, R. S., Steinberg, A. M., & Wriath, R. (1995). A developmental model of childhood traumatic stress. In D. Cicchetti & D. J. Cohen (Eds.), *Developmental psychopathology: Vol 2. Risk, disorder, and adaptation* (pp. 72–95). New York: Wiley.

Rakoff, V. (1966). A long-term effect of the concentration camp experience. *Viewpoints, 1,* 17–22.

Rakoff, V., Sigal, J., & Epstein, N. (1966). Children and families of concentration camp survivors. *Canada's Mental Health, 14,* 24–26.

Rodin, R. G., & Rodin, M. M. (1982). Children of Holocaust survivors. *Adolescent Psychiatry, 10,* 66–72.

Rose, S., & Garske, J. (1987). Family environment, adjustment, and coping among children of Holocaust survivors: A comparative investigation. *American Journal of Orthopsychiatry, 57,* 332–344.

Rosenheck, R., & Nathan, P. (1985). Secondary traumatization in children of Vietnam veterans. *Hospital and Community Psychiatry, 36*(5), 538–539.

Schauben, L. J., & Frazier, P. A. (1995). Vicarious trauma: The effects on female counselors of working with sexual violence survivors. *Psychology of Women Quarterly, 19,* 49–54.

Sigal, J., & Rakoff, V. (1971). Concentration camp survival: A pilot study of effects on the second generation. *Canadian Psychiatric Association Journal, 16,* 393–397.

Solomon, Z. (1988). The effect of combat-related posttraumatic stress disorder on the family. *Psychiatry, 51*(3), 323–329.

Solomon, Z. (1990). *From front line to home front: Wives of PTSD veterans.* Paper presented at the 6th Annual Meeting of the Society for Traumatic Stress Studies, New Orleans, LA.

Solomon, Z., Kotler, M., & Mikulincer, M. (1988). Combat-related post-traumatic stress disorder among second-generation Holocaust survivors: Preliminary findings. *American Journal of Psychiatry, 145*(7), 865–868.

Solomon, Z., Waysman, M., Avitzur, E., & Enoch, D. (1991). Psychiatric symptomatology among wives of soldiers following combat stress reaction: The role of the social network and marital relations. *Anxiety Research, 4*(3), 213–223.

Terr, L. C. (1979). Children of Chowchilla: A study of psychc trauma. *Psychoanalytic Study of the Child, 34,* 552–623.

Terr, L. C. (1983). Chowchilla revisited: The effects of psychic trauma four years after a school-bus kidnapping. *American Journal of Psychiatry, 140,* 1543–1550.

Terr, L. C. (1985). Children traumatized in small groups. In S. Eth & R. S. Pynoos (Eds.), *Post-traumatic stress disorder in children* (pp. 45–70). Washington, DC: American Psychiatric Association Press.

Terr, L. C. (1990). *Too scared to cry: Psychic trauma in childhood.* Grand Rapids, MI: Harper & Row.

Terr, L. C. (1991). Childhood traumas: An outline and overview. *American Journal of Psychiatry, 148*(1), 10–20.

Titchener, J. L., Kapp, F. T., & Winget, C. (1976). The Buffalo Creek syndrome: Symptoms and character change after a major disaster. In H. J. Parad, H. L. P. Resnick, & L. G. Parad (Eds.), *Emergency and disaster management* (pp. 283–294). Bowie, MD: Charles Press.

Trossman, B. (1968). Adolescent children of concentration camp survivors. *Journal of the Canadian Psychiatric Association, 13,* 121–123.

Verbosky, S. J., & Ryan, D. A. (1988). Female partner of Vietnam veterans: Stress by proximity. *Issues in Mental Health Nursing, 9*(1), 95–104.

Wardi, D. (1992). *Memorial candles: Children of the Holocaust.* London: Tavistock/Routledge.

van der Kolk, B. A. (1988). The trauma spectrum: The interaction of biological and social events in the genesis of the trauma response. *Journal of Traumatic Stress, 1*(3), 273–290.

Weiss, E., O'Connell, A. N., & Siites, R. (1986). Comparisons of second generation Holocaust survivors, immigrants, and non-immigrants on measures of mental health. *Journal of Personality and Social Psychology, 50,* 828–831.

Williams, C. (1980). The veteran system with a focus on women partners: Theoretical considerations, problems and treatment strategies. In T. Williams (Ed.), *Post-traumatic stress disorders of the Vietnam veteran* (pp. 169–192). Cincinnati, OH: Disabled American Veterans.

Wilson, J. P., & Lindy, J. D. (Eds.). (1994). *Countertransference in the treatment of PTSD.* New York: Guilford.

Zerling, I., Podietz, K., Belmont, H., Shapiro, M., Ficher, I., Eisenstein, T., & Levick, M. (1984). Engagement in families of Holocaust survivors. *Journal of Marital and Family Therapy, 10*(1), 43–51.

V

Intergenerational Effects Revealed after the Fall of Communism

17

Intergenerational Aspects of the Conflict in the Former Yugoslavia

EDUARD KLAIN

INTRODUCTION

The war on the territory of the former Yugoslavia surprised almost the whole world. It began with the 4-day "war operetta" in Slovenia in the summer of 1990, then extended into a heavy war in Croatia, and reached its climax in Bosnia and Herzegovina. We often ask ourselves whether we could have foreseen such development. It is not easy to answer that question. Serbs, who had prepared for that war, did foresee it. Among victims, only Herzegovinians (part of the Croatian population in Bosnia and Herzegovina) anticipated a war and began preparing for it. Historical memory in western Herzegovina probably helped people to expect the worst. So we have come to the possibility of understanding the intergenerational transmission of emotion that might warn us that something awful might happen. In this chapter, I try to consider the remote historical events in these regions and their influence on transmission of emotions from generation to generation, which, at a certain moment, produces an explosion (i.e., a terrible conflict). The interpretations I offer can only be in accordance with my work and education, so they will necessarily be psychoanalytical and group analytical.

The collective psychosis that seized people in the former Yugoslavia was in fact a generalization of paranoid projections onto another nation and religion, with no chance for critical judgment and rational consideration of the facts. Destructive slogans could be heard, such as "Only a dead Chetnik" (pejorative name for Serbs) or "a dead Ustasha" (pejorative name for Croats) "is a good Chetnik or a good Ustasha" or "All Serbs are the same; there are no loyal Serbs," and so on. Collective paranoia overcame all social strata. Thus, for instance, each member of the "enemy" nation was a suspect with whom it became dangerous to associate or work. Such collective projection has also very real repercussions for people who lose apartments, jobs, and so on. The old prejudices were aroused, and new ones were created, or, as Di Maria (1995), writes,

> Nations break down, barriers fall, everybody can freely move from one place to another. We
> mingle together, change position, "confuse" roles. However, prejudices still rule the world,

EDUARD KLAIN • Clinic for Psychological Medicine, Kišpatićeva 12, HR–10000, Zagreb, Croatia.

International Handbook of Multigenerational Legacies of Trauma, edited by Yael Danieli. Plenum Press, New York, 1998.

often latent, but ready to violently explode in moments of crisis. So, when we talk about barbarians, foreigners, people's moves from one country to another, we are entering the field of prejudice and the crossbridge to racism is an easy one. It is the hatred versus any difference. It is ethnocentrism, and the use of diversities to gain advantages against the others, as it is in any colonization (pp. 2–3).

The whole history of humanity is in fact the history of waging war. Most often, wars were being waged against somebody or something like a neighbor, someone richer, or people of another faith, another ideology. Rare were the wars for improvement of living conditions, for freedom, for justice, and so on. One such imperialistic war in which racism was one of predominant driving forces was World War II, which had an enormous impact on the relations among people in the former Yugoslavia, and which was, I dare say, the strongest link in the chain of intergenerational transmission of emotions. I wrote about this in the book *Psychology and Psychiatry of a War* (Klain, 1992a):

> The Second World War was an ideal occasion to realize all the destructive aggressions in Yugoslavia suppressed from the moment that the new state was born. Paranoid projections prevailed with the help of external groups, i.e., the warring European states. The destructive–cannibalistic needs of different ethnic groups dressed up as projections (revenge) were realized during the war. What happened in that war was something that is latent in us at all times and that, under normal conditions, only psychotic patients realize: as Freud warned us, the very thin layer of human culture and civilization broke and groups clashed like primal hordes. The group superego manifested itself only within the framework of its aggressive and destructive component. The libidinous component of the loving superego was deeply suppressed. In Bion's theory, only the fighting situation of the group was realized. The end result of such group developments was the destruction of human life and of family groups. The most important consequence is the memory of scenes of separation in the minds of the surviving members of these groups: the killing of their parents before their eyes, forced separation of mothers and their children in concentration camps, etc. Such frustrations influence the group memory of the aggression perpetrated by members of the other nation. The transmission of wartime memories also takes place in groups, leading to a transgenerational remembrance of injury, murder and destruction laid at the door of the enemy nation. All this is crucially important for an understanding of the current ethnic and other confrontations among the different groups in Yugoslavia (pp. 77–78).

HISTORICAL ASPECTS

In his book *The Evil of the Great Spleen: History and Non-History of Croats, Montenegrins, Muslims, and Serbs* (1996), Ivan Rendić-Miočević, a professor of history at the Faculty of Philosophy in Zadar, who had studied the distant history of the peoples of Illyricum, connects the remote past of the peoples who lived in these region with present-day events. One of his fundamental theses is that the patriarchal society developed in these regions has not changed throughout their history. Rendić-Miočević writes, "If we can say that this society, usually called patriarchal, has not changed for centuries, or has changed very little, then we must conclude that, in fact, it has no history" (p. 53). V. Dvorniković (1939) emphasized this problem long ago:

> Yugoslavs, like other Slavs, were non-historical people of space for a long time, and on entering the history—when they came to the present-day south—historical fate and nature of their new habitation made them turn back into non-historical people of the space. We could even say that the life destiny of Yugoslavs as a whole consisted in permanent struggle for that transformation from people of space into people of time. And this struggle is still go-

ing on. The Yugoslavs are still struggling with the space, the geographic dominant of their lives. They have not surmounted this dominant, although they have reached the crucial point towards political synthesis and against geographical spacial forces which have not favoured this synthesis (p. 114).

Rendić-Miočević (1996) includes within the traditional patriarchal territory Montenegro, mountain regions of Serbia and Bosnia, Herzegovina, Dalmatian hinterland, Lika, and Macedonia. This is very important, since in these regions live Serbs, mostly Bosnian and Croatian Serbs, Croats, and, in smaller part, Muslims. These tribes that lead patriarchal lives are called Dinaric by Dvorniković. According to him, a patriarchal man hates work, for work is the death of heroism. This will remind the reader of the Serbian President Milošević's saying, at the beginning of the present-day Serbian aggression: "We don't know how to work, but we know how to fight" (speech given at the meeting of the Serbian Assembly in 1990). Dvorniković also emphasizes morality and sanctity of revenge: "A patriarchal man can not forgive because he equates forgiveness with self-defeat. In this ethical dilemma, he always remains a fighter, a Balkan, and not a Christian soul. The ethos of fighting and solidarity of a patriarchal person has two poles: On one side, undoubted virtues developed through ages of family life, but on the other side, brutality and robbery in their worst forms" (p. 798). However, not everything is so bleak, as can be seen in the following citation of Ivan Rendić-Miočević (1996): "Besides tribal society, there are other models like the Mediterranean one and the cooperative one in Croatian Zagorje. In the Serbs, besides the "Dinaric" model, there is also a "Moravic" one, tending to compromise and rationalization" (p. 125).

Dubrovnik is an example of an ambivalent relationship between the hinterland and the coastland. Historical sources mention the attacks from eastern Herzegovina (Serbian territory) in the second half of the 15th century and the first half of the 16th century, when people in Konavle and Dubrovnik were robbed and killed. In 1896, when Dubrovnik was under French control, Russians attacked the French. The Russians were supported by Montenegrins who robbed, killed, and set fires. They impaled the head of the French commander and showed it to the French soldiers. The French ambassador in Dubrovnik, the commander of the Russian army, and the writer Vojnović described these atrocities, wondering how such a thing could happen in civilized Europe. The year 1991 witnessed very similar pictures when Konavle and Dubrovnik were attacked barbariously by these same Montenegrins and Serbs from eastern Herzegovina, and when there were also appeals to the world. The reaction was the same as in 1806: none. According to my own experiences from World War II and the present-day war against Croatia and Bosnia, and Herzegovina, a more primitive population exhibits more hatred and envy than better-educated and often richer populations. After World War II, the communist rulers, most of whom were uneducated and came from poor regions, confiscated the property of rich people in towns and arrested them. Unfortunately, there are similar examples today. One can see constant conflicts and confrontations among people from certain regions (e.g., Dalmatia, Zagorje, Herzegovina, continental Croatia, etc.). This is an important element that influences the aggressive and destructive behavior of individual persons and groups, and is transmitted transgenerationally.

BIRTH AND DEATH OF YUGOSLAVIA

Yugoslavia has been unfortunate since its beginning. It was set up after World War I, under the terms of the Treaty of Versailles, and after World War II by agreement of the Allied powers, created to meet the needs of foreign parties (i.e., the great European powers) rather than in response to the needs of its peoples and the nations into which they had divided. From the outset, it was made up of very heterogeneous peoples who were forced to live together. In a sociopolitical context, one way to make very heterogeneous people live together in a state is through the use of authoritarian repression carried out under the aegis of an idealized or demonized supreme leader who relies on a small ruling group to execute his orders. This was the formula according to which a large group of 20 million people, still called Yugoslavia, functioned (Klain, 1992b, 1995).

From 1918 to 1941, the supreme authority in Yugoslavia was the Serbian king, which meant that repression was carried out by the police, and power was vested in the majority people (the Serbs). The remaining two large nations in the state (Croats and Slovenes) played a subordinate role, while other nations and ethnic minorities were denied their identities as groups. The mutual rivalry of the three main groups (Serbs, Slovenes, and Croats) caused them to act out from time to time, while the repression established a false cohesion behind which destructive aggression, accompanied by projection of the archaic instinctual needs, was hidden.

Yugoslavia as a monarchy disintegrated in 1941, only a week after its leadership, the king and everybody around him, fled the country. World War II provided an ideal opportunity to release the destructive aggressions suppressed in the Yugoslav subgroups since the formation of the union.

Perhaps most important at present is that the surviving members of these groups, as mentioned earlier, carry memories of awful scenes of separation derived from World War II. The Nazis occupied all of Yugoslavia. Both Croatia and Serbia were created as puppet states with quisling regimes. Minority extremist groups in Croatia (Ustashas) and in Serbia (Chetniks) sided with the Nazis and carried out atrocities against the peoples of other nations. Such traumatic scenes also influenced group memories about aggression perpetrated by the "members of the *other* nation." The transmission of feelings engendered by war experiences was carried by particular national groups as their history, leading to transgenerational memories of insults and destruction, the blame for which was laid upon the "enemy people" as a whole. The consequences of this transmission of affects and memories are of utmost importance for understanding present-day confrontations among the various ethnic groups in Yugoslavia.

The second Yugoslavia was formed in 1945. The repressive authority of the tyrannical leader relied on two groups: members of the leading, and only, party (somewhat less than 10% of the population) directly, and the dominant Serbian nation indirectly, through the group that called itself the federal administration (1–1.5% of the population). The number of competing national groups increased in the new state, because new nations and ethnic minorities were accepted, thus further reducing the country's overall cohesion and increasing the intragroup tensions. The number of "enemy groups" as potential targets for negative and destructive projections also increased. The functioning of the contesting subgroups could only be achieved by the organization of repressive forces in the two hierarchically dominant groups—the police and the army—that were actually unified, since they were conducted from one and the same center. A difference in the later organization and administration of the police and army resulted in the different behavior of these groups in the war to come.

We are considering the prevailing influence of groups of people whose common characteristic is their nationality. In all crisis situations in Yugoslavia, groups form around the symbols of "nation" and "religion," two cohesive attractors that are so highly correlated in the Balkans as to be often (but not always) functionally synonymous.

The Serbs have been in the majority, and have ruled the country directly in the first Yugoslavia and indirectly (through the Communist Party and the federal state administration) in the second. They have a warlike tradition, transmitted from generation to generation: Elders tell children about Serbian heroes of the past. A cult of warriors and military leaders has been cherished. Group cohesion is formed around a leader-warrior: a king, a duke, or a Marshal Tito, rather than around the church and religion, although the Serbian Orthodox Church is authochthonous. (The Orthodox churches are not only national but also independent; that is, they are autocephalous.) In summary, the church is a cohesive factor, but more as an aspect of Serbian national identity and less as a religious symbol.

The Serbs as a group have long considered themselves the leading nation in Yugoslavia because they are the strongest, and because they founded Yugoslavia. As a people, they have idealized certain external groups, in particular the former U.S.S.R. and France (the latter was the cultural cradle of the Russian czars). In relation to the national groups in the western part of the country, however, the Serbs may be described as harboring feelings of inferiority because they perceive their own culture as being at a "lower" level. They try to rid themselves of these feelings by means of various defense mechanisms, such as negation, projection, denial, and ambivalence, but the destructive element remains. The heightened Serbian militancy suggests a defensive group tendency to view the world from a "schizoid–paranoid" position (Klein, 1946) in which whatever is "good" is felt to come from within and whatever is "bad" to come from the outside. This seems especially so when the Serbs are compared to the Croats who, as discussed next, are more prone to Klein's "depressive" position.

The Croatian nation is the Serbs' greatest rival. Due to very different external and internal influences upon the development of this group, they have built their own cohesiveness based on labor, dialogue, obedience, and an expectation of understanding and justice. Their religious idealizations are more pronounced than those of the Serbs. As a result, they have more readily accepted authorities from outside their national group and developed dependency on them. Compared to the Serbs, the Croats as a group may be said to express the "depressive position" described by Klein (1946). This position is characteristic of personalities that are more prone to feelings of guilt about their self-perceived destructiveness than fear of anger vis-à-vis hostile or threatening assaults from the "outside world." These feelings of guilt, no matter how irrational they may be, are expressed by, among other things, the notably stronger Croatian tendency to rely on prayer to resolve conflict and bring about relief from pressing problems.

The Slovenes, the third nation-building component in the first Yugoslavia, have, as a group, always been a little outside the interactions of the main groups. Very homogeneous as a national group, they benefited over the years from the continuous confrontations between the Serbs and Croats, and were able to develop as a group relatively undisturbed. They succeeded in reaching a more mature capacity for political interaction and developing political communications without any great need for authoritarian leaders (as will be elaborated later in the analysis of the war in Slovenia). They succeeded in integrating the Catholic Church into their group concept at a more mature level. For instance, if we compare the Slovenes and the Croats during the recent years, we can see a difference in their need for religious and national symbols accompanied by national euphoria. As distinguished from the Croats, the Slovenes had no need for coats of arms and flags, or frequent cardinal masses and processions, in order to create their group identity, thus proving that regressive processes are less marked in their group. Having a more mature group identity, the Slovenes also have no need of charismatic group leaders. They are able to use, in a more mature way, their group self to realize the needs of the whole group, and not the needs of a charismatic leader.

The Macedonians were recognized as a nation in the second Yugoslavia. As a group, they are ambivalently linked with the Bulgarians, Greeks, and Albanians. In the interaction with these neighboring peoples, they try to prove their identity as a nation, which these same neighboring peoples have denied. As the Macedonians consist of ethnically heterogeneous people, their group cohesion is rather loose. On the other hand, like any newly formed group, they have a need to idealize their group identity.

While the Montenegrins were given their minirepublic in the second Yugoslavia, they had already existed as a nation for centuries. Historically, they felt connected with Russia, a nation into which they project the libidinal (desirable) parts of their group self. They are split into two subgroups: one which values their separate identity from Serbs more than their kinship ("greens"), and one which does not ("whites"). They have an extremely heroic–militant tradition. They possess a libidinal (loving) and rigid (harsh, punitive) superego, which manifests itself as pride and honesty. Their economy is rather backward and has had a limiting effect on their societal and cultural development in spite of their long history.

The Bosnians live in the Republic of Bosnia and Herzegovina, together with Serbs and Croats. They are essentially a Slavic people who, after occupation by the Turks, converted to Islam. They have no intrinsic relationship, tribal, or blood ties with other Islamic nations. As a nation, they were recognized only in the second Yugoslavia. They refer to themselves as *Bosniacs,* a term that bears an ethnic rather than only a religious connotation. This subgroup comprises the majority of the population of Bosnia and it differs socioculturally from the Croatian and Serbian subgroups. They are very traditional and conservative, with the father's authority being sacrosanct. They live in large families in which sexual differentiation is marked by the absolute predominance of the male.

The Albanians form the majority in the former Kosovo Autonomous Province, "annexed" by the Republic of Serbia in 1989. As mentioned earlier, a large group of Albanians live in Macedonia. Most of them are Muslims, and the majority of the population is engaged in agricultural work and has not assimilated Western technology and culture to the same extent as other Yugoslav regions. At present, Albanians are exposed to destructive, genocidal acts by the communist Serbian government. Using their usual formula of announcing that they were endangered as a national minority, Serbs began to kill, arrest, and expel people from their homes. The same scenario was seen in Croatia, and now in Bosnia and Herzegovina. In Kosovo, they have abolished Albanian autonomy.

There are many other ethnic minorities in Yugoslavia, but those mentioned here provide an insight into the group map of Yugoslavia, which consists of numerous national and religious groups, all intermingled and opposed to each other. These are groups of different and mutually alien cultures and influences (not only from the Islamic countries, Turkey, Greece, Bulgaria, Albania, but also from Hungary, Austria, Germany, Italy, France, Great Britain, the United States, and the former U.S.S.R.).

This conglomerate of heterogeneous groups, formed on the basis of a variety of external and internal influences, has few homogenizing factors but much that is confrontational and destructive in its structure. Thus, it was inevitable that Yugoslavia would disintegrate, given the presence of destabilizing conditions.

Most of the members of these large national groups were not aware of very serious economic and political realities. They were protected by idealization and projection, dynamics that are often observed in large groups (Kreeger, 1975). This balance was disrupted in 1980 by the death of the great leader. His cult continued through numerous rituals, beginning with a great show at his funeral, followed by pilgrimages to his tomb and the establishment of a (still another) museum. A large number of people needed all this for the mourning process, which lasted for years. However, the space for idealization narrowed with time. The illusion of a good, giving breast began to collapse. Economic difficulties arose, and variously organized groups began to split apart. The weakest link (i.e., the Communist Party of Yugoslavia) was the first to break down. This process was supported by the dissolution of the Soviet Union. The rigid rules that governed the Communist Party hierarchy deteriorated, the group lost its clear boundaries, and subgroups formed, confronting one another. At the same time that the split within the Communist Party took place, the large group, the state, split into subgroups as well. This process was slower and resulted in the war launched by representatives of one political idea against the other.

From June 27 to July 2, 1990, the Yugoslav army waged war against Slovenia. The Yugoslav army initiated this war to demonstrate its strength, but for various reasons it gave up Slovenia. Unrest in Croatia began in the summer of the same year. It is interesting that Serbs rebelled first in Knin and its vicinity, a very undeveloped region, where people were poor and marginalized. In 1992, the most bloody part of the war began: the occupation of Bosnia by Bosnian Serbs and Serbia, which caused the greatest number of victims. During that war, a conflict between Bosnian Muslims and Bosnian Croats also took place.

MEDIATORS OF "INHERITED" EMOTIONS

The Patriarchal Family

A product of a patriarchally organized society, the patriarchal family is most important for transmission of emotions from one generation to the next. As mentioned already, in the territory of the former Yugoslavia, such a family appeared mostly in mountainous and poor regions. It represented a source of petrified rules that would not allow any development or progress, but, on the contrary, imposed severe sanctions on everyone who violated the rules. Former Yugoslavia was not the only place with patriarchal families, where rigid rules and numerous prejudices were transmitted from generation to generation. In his study on the Mafia, Lo Verso (1995) presents his thesis that the patriarchal family is present in the "south." Referring to the south anthropologically rather than geographically, in addition to southern Italy, he includes in it Northern Africa and Latin America, among others, and states that all of them have underdevelopment and poverty as common characteristic. In a patriarchal family, the mother plays the dominant role in transmitting various emotions and rules. Lo Verso writes, "From the psychodynamic point of view, transmission of values, culture, models of object relations, symbolism and emotionality goes through mother. From this point of view women have an important role in the Mafia" (pp. 117–118). In patriarchal families, transmission of emotions and other rules, both preoedipal and oedipal, has also been mostly through the mother. The relations between father and child, which also means father and son, are less frequent and appear in a later phase of upbringing. Also, we should not neglect the intergenerational transmission of oedipal envy of the son in relation to his father which, ever since the primal horde, leads to killing the father and possessing the mother. Through generations, Laius's revenge pervades, which in the modern form means sending the sons to war to be killed, wounded, and physically and psychically mutilated. It is especially important to point out the meaning of psychic mutilation. Young people have been reeducated for killing, and their oedipal fascination with arms and power has brought about psychological disturbances and inability to adapt to civilian life afterwards. Destructive as well as identification needs have extended from the patriarchal family to the tribe, then to the nation, which, in fantasy, has taken on the meaning of the group, which is linked by blood ties to the primitive patriarchal family. There are examples in the former Yugoslavia, when Tito tried, through his behavior, dress, and pompousness to become an important identification object. In the beginning of this war Rašković, a psychiatrist, the leader of Serbian rebellion in Croatia, wore a long beard and played the role of the good Father of his nation. The Croatian leader, Tudjman, behaves in a similar way.

Superego

In his work, *The Ego and the Id,* Freud (1923) presents his thesis that many habits, cultural manifestations, ideals, ethical principles, and the like are inherited through the superego. In his opinion, a child's superego is formed not according to its parent's ego but according to its parent's superego, and all precipitates of general principles that are in the superego are thus transmitted to future generations. When we try to understand the behavior of people in war, this thesis is very important, because we know that in certain subcultures, there are rules and regulations that do not fit into European and North American civilization and culture. We can mention here superego of a *haiduk* in former Yugoslavia, superego of a pirate, superego of a hired killer, and so on. The similarity is with the superego of a mafioso described by Lo Verso (1995). A primitive patriarchal family will often develop through identification a similar superego in children, who are marginalized, exposed to their father's rage, beaten and abused, and, in fact, marginalized in their own families. Such a superego will help to choose people for special tasks in a war, such as liquidating civilians. It would be wrong to think that these persons do not experience conflicts within their personality after committing acts they were ordered to do. Along with destructive and aggressive elements, guilt feelings also exist in their superego. In a group, their most frequent reaction is projection, which is being shifted from the enemy to the government. Such aggressive manifestations are associated with paranoid projections that they will be liquidated because they know too much. Freud's idea expressed in his letter *Why War* (1933) can be applied to them: "The death instinct changes into destructive instinct when it is turned to the outside, to the object. In this way one keeps his own life by destroying another person's life" (p. 203). In a group of war veterans, a patient stated that his only problem was aggression. This veteran had attacked a man who entered his shop only because he was blond; his jailor, who beat him, was blond. He slapped two Albanians because they spoke Albanian, a language he could not understand. Later, he became aware that his behavior is aggressive, but he could not prevent it. His death instinct and his unconscious guilt feeling are so intense that he is not able to stop these aggressive behaviors.

Folk Songs and Literature

Folk songs and literature have remained, unfortunately, generators of transmission of interethnic hatred, especially in Serbs and Montenegrins. For example, the epic *Death of Smail aga Čengić,* which has been included in all textbooks for schoolchildren, is presented as a historical truth and has for generations produced hatred toward Muslims. In that epic, a Turkish aga tortures people and takes away all their crops, then kills them. Grmek, Gjidara, and Šimac (1993) mention *Gorski Vijenac,* a well-known Montenegrin epic, a breviary of interethnic hatred and generator of its transgenerational transmission. In Serbian and Montenegrin epics and legends, the greatest hatred is directed toward Turks (i.e., Muslims). It is therefore not surprising that in this war too, the Serbs manifested their hatred toward Croats and Muslims in decasyllables. The following verse was thus created after the fall of Vukovar in November 1991: "Slobodane (Milošević) šalji nam salate, bit će mesa klat ćemo Hrvate" [Slobodan (Milošević) send us salad, there will be meat, we shall butcher the Croats]. (The song was sung by Serbian military groups in Vukovar on November 19, 1991.) In 1992, Serbian soldiers sang:

> Pored doma na selo kidišu Dušanovi rafali ih zbrišu. Medo kaže povlači se brate ko će po-
> bit tolike Hrvate. Dule reče čeka još ovoga da osvetim djeda voljenoga, jer za svakog našeg
> Srbina treba ubit bar dvadeset psina.

> After the house they attack the village, Dušan's bursts of fire destroy them. Medo says, with-
> draw, my brother, who can kill so many Croats. Dule says, wait, just one more, to avenge my
> beloved grandfather, because for each of our Serbs, at least twenty dogs should be killed.

Such poems seem strange in Europe at the end of the 20th century, but if we know the *haiduk* tradition, according to which slaughter, robbery, and abduction were no offenses, we can understand these "popular poems." Cvijić (1922) explains the function of folk songs for the Dinaric Serbs in the following way:

> To kill many Turks means for a Dinaric man not only to avenge his ancestors, but also to re-
> lieve their pains of which he, too, suffers. It is significant that all Dinaric Serbs—from those
> in the northern Croatia along the border with Kranjska, to those living at Skadar—know the
> main events of Serbian history, which have been conveyed through folk-songs and narra-
> tives from one generation to the other. National morality and national idea are heritage of a
> long history (p. 83).

Thus, we can conclude that the motifs of folk songs live in Serbian people and can easily inspire instrumentalized aggression stimulated by Serbian rulers.

Church and Religion

In the former Yugoslavia, there have been three main religions: Catholic, Orthodox, and Muslim. In Communist Yugoslavia, religions were suppressed by the government. The people of the nations of the former Yugoslavia felt, as members of these religions, although relatively few were true believers adhering to religious principles, that the Communist regime persecuted primarily the Catholic Church because it was the best organized and a part of the Vatican. The Orthodox church, and especially the Muslim Church, were less active and therefore minor threats to the Communist regime. Thus, for example, celebration of Catholic holidays was forbidden, while customs connected with the Orthodox Church and Muslim faith were tacitly allowed. In the current war, accusations have been revived against the Catholic Church, which, allegedly, baptized Serbs during World War II. The fact is that many people, in order to save their lives, converted to the religion that was welcomed in their territory. The aggressivness of the Orthodox Church was manifest during this war through abandoning its own people by the priests, accusing the entire Croatian population of genocide, and through advocating myths and stirring up revenge toward Croats and Muslims. The Orthodox Church has never apologized for the crimes committed by its believers. On the other hand, the Catholic Church pleaded for peace, apologized for the crimes committed by its believers, and has never accused the whole Serbian nation of genocide. If we follow the events in Yugoslavia between the two world wars, we can see that the traditional attitude of the Serbian Orthodox Church was closely connected with the state, along with incitement and direct calls for hatred. Along these lines, S. Pribičević (1990) accuses directly Serbian orthodoxy:

> For the whole period since 1918 up to the present day, there has never been heard a patriarch's
> sermon about religion and church, relationship of man towards God, about love for one's
> neighbor, about the needs of soul, about morality and goals in life, but always about questions
> of national and political meaning in the sense of imperialism and megalomania (p. 87).

The autonomy of the Orthodox Church makes it more closely connected to the nation and state, while the Catholic Church, because of its internationalism, seems to be at some distance from the nation and state. The lives of the Orthodox priests and their families are intimately ingrained in the lives of their communities. Their educational level is also not much higher than their people's. All these elements influence their reactions to difficult war situations.

Myths

Throughout their history, the Serbs cherished two myths: one about their heroism and courage, the other of committing genocide of the surrounding nations.

It is known that the Turks defeated the Serbs in 1389, in the Battle of Kosovo. The saying goes (not a historical fact) that the Turks, after their victory over the Serbs, killed all male children and raped all young Serb women so that they would give birth to Turks. In the Eastern religion, the father determines the child's religious identity. He is the seed, while the mother represents only the earth into which the seed is placed. This myth about Turkish behavior after the Battle of Kosovo has remained vivid in Serbian people up to the present day, and in this war, it has been the generator of revenge against the Muslims because of the events that had happened 600 years ago. During the last 10 years, the Serbs have been celebrating the Battle of Kosovo as if it were their victory, not defeat. In the nationalistic euphoria that seized both the Croatian and Serbian ruling classes, the Serbs have turned back to the czar, Lazar, who was defeated at Kosovo, and carried his bones triumphantly around Serbia. Their myths about heroism have been transmitted also through popular songs. The most characteristic hero is Prince Marko, who is described in a series of poems as an extremely courageous man who always conquered the Turks, especially his rival Musa Kesedžija. But the truth was quite the opposite. Marko was a Turkish vassal who served them obediently. From 1945 to the present, the Serbs have been spreading propaganda throughout Yugoslavia and all around the world about the Croats as genocidal, equating them with Hitler's minority of 50,000 Ustashas. These people, who originated from the patriarchal regions of Croatia (Herzegovina, Dalmatian hinterland, and Lika) were extremely brutal and destructive. They killed and tortured members of other nations, primarily Jews, as did also the Serbs (Chetniks) and the Communists. The Ustashas had a concentration camp in Jasenovac, in which, according to the historians, about 50,000–70,000 Serbs, Jews, Gypsies, and Croats were killed. But in Serbian propaganda, Jasenovac was the grave of 700,000 Serbs.

WHAT IS BEING TRANSMITTED FROM GENERATION TO GENERATION?

Hate and Rage

Unfortunately, the most frequent emotions that have been transmitted in the ways described are deep hatred and rage, accompanied by aggression and destruction. So, for instance, the methods of torture and killing have not changed since the Roman and Turkish times. It is difficult to believe that at the end of the 20th century in Europe, people get crucified, impaled, barbecued, skinned alive, their ears and noses cut off, and so on. Only if we remember that the patriarchal tribes have no history, and that in their destructiveness, nothing has changed, can we try to understand such reactions. The wave of hatred and rage overflowed the churches, cultural monuments, cemeteries, and homes. As mentioned several times already, one of the main reservoirs of hatred and rage, but also of revenge, was World War II, when the Croats and the Serbs committed the greatest crimes first, followed by the Communists belonging to different nations. Significantly, some of the future generals of the Yugoslav national army were children of people killed by the Ustasha's knives or torn away from arms of their mothers, who were taken to prison camps. It is not easy to find out why, of all the nations in the former Yugoslavia, hatred and rage were most manifest in the relationships between the Serbs and Croats. True, they were two dominant nations, their languages are almost identical, and they are very alike. Diatkine (1993) applied Freud's concept of narcissism of small differences to the relationships between these two nations: as brotherly rivals as to which is better, stronger, more cultured, or more prominent internationally.

Revenge

Revenge includes many emotions such as hatred, rage, and guilt. Its character is projective, and it is primitive and archaic in its manifestations. Both the Serbs and the Croats emphasize their need for revenge, but the Serbs aim it toward the Muslims as well as Croats. The Serbs lament that they have always been endangered, that, particularly in the period before the Serbian attack and uprising in Croatia, they have always lost at the negotiating table, even though they conquered on the battlefield. They also felt they were losers during the Communist regime, despite having ruled in almost all the republics of the state. The Croatian feeling of neglect and injustice was manifest between the two wars, when the Ustasha movement was founded. The maxim of revenge, of "revolution by blood and arms" was emphasized from the very beginning, in 1932. In each issue of the journal *Ustašah,* one could read, "Knife, gun and bomb are idols that have to give the peasant back the fruits of his land, to worker his bread, and to Croatia freedom" (printed on the first page of each issue of the journal *Ustašah*). These who drink blood of Croatian people should be slaughtered, so that no such evil appears ever again in Croatian territory (see Jelić-Butić, 1978; Kavran, 1944). After World War II, Croats felt endangered, and the militant among them emigrated and prepared for revenge.

The ever-present need for revenge in the national groups resulted in the heavy crimes in this war. First, Serbian rebels and the Serbian army imprisoned not only a large number of soldiers but also civilians. They not only tortured soldiers and policemen, but also children and old people. For example, it is known that four old men were beaten to death in the prison camp "Manjača." They also killed an 80-year-old woman, whose only crime was that she had given birth to, as they said, an Ustashah. The Serbs exhibited special cruelty toward Muslims. Raping women and sexual abuse of men were only one kind of torture and humiliation. Earlier, I mentioned the myth of the Battle of Kosovo and the alleged Turkish rape of Serbian women. In this war, the Serbs performed mass rape of Muslim women, along with other kinds of torture. They then kept many of the pregnant women in prison through the eighth month of their pregnancy, so that the women had to bear these children. The following describes our first field experience with a rape case:

M. is a 21-year-old Muslim from a village near the Bosnian town of Ključ. When the Serb forces occupied her village, they began by physically and psychically maltreating the local people. They took their crops and cattle, restricted their movements, and finally took them to the Manjača detention camp. M.'s father, as well as all male members of her extended family, including adolescents, was also taken. Some were killed. As the oldest child in the family (M. has two younger sisters and two younger brothers), her mother sent her to pay some obligatory taxes at the local Serb-held community offices. Upon her arrival, two soldiers grabbed her and called another soldier. All three of them raped her on the premises and then let her go. She did not dare to tell her mother anything. When she realized that she was pregnant, she attempted to conceal it by wearing large clothes. She could not eat or sleep and lost 15 kgs. She became depressed and had suicidal thoughts. She felt guilty and was too ashamed to tell anyone about her troubles. After the whole family was expelled from the village, they came to a refugee settlement near Zagreb. They were soon joined by their father, who was exchanged as a prisoner of war with another member of their extended family. As her term was coming, she felt worse and progressively more suicidal, and confided in an old aunt, who was a dominant person in the extended family. The aunt helped her to get professional medical help, and she gave birth to a child in one of the Zagreb hospitals, where one of our psychiatrists talked to her. M. did not want to see the child. Her major concern was how to get back to her family, who considered her pregnancy a sin.

The psychiatrist realized that M.'s parents had to be prepared for her return and went with a colleague to talk to them. Despite long-term psychiatric experience and work in psychiatric institutions, they were anxious. M.'s parents and her extended family greeted them warmly and talked in detail about their traumatic experiences. Each individual described his or her experiences, but nobody said anything about M. After several visits to the settlement, the family accepted M.'s return, but her trauma was never discussed in front of them. M. had 15 regular sessions. She married a young man from the settlement after 1 year.

The negation of rape was a basic finding in all clients in the beginning. In cases where the women delivered a child after rape-induced pregnancy, the child was usually abandoned and left for adoption (Arcel *et al.,* 1995).

The revenge of the victim is seldom spoken about. The tortures and killings by Serbs have brought about similar reactions by Croats and Muslims. The victim's revenge is, in fact, one of the hardest blows to the victim by his or her persecutor and tormentor, because in this way the victim becomes like him or her.

Guilt and Shame

Our knowledge about intergenerational transmission of guilt comes from analyses of Holocaust victims and from the therapies of the members of the second generation. While we cannot speak yet of transmission of guilt feelings from this war, we can imagine which people and which traumas will bring about transmission of guilt feelings. One such victims group is of the wives and mothers of men missing in the war. They could neither elaborate their losses, nor go through the usual mourning process, because they still do not know the fate of their missing loved ones.

The very rigid and punitive superego of some groups of war victims makes rather difficult any therapeutic approach and elaboration of psychic trauma. First are the raped women and sexually abused men. They developed strong, unconscious guilt feelings because of what had happened to them and suffer especially from narcissistic injury, shame, and loss of self-respect. The suicides in this group, in my opinion, are a consequence of a "deserved" punishment by the superego, because the ego could not endure the heavy reproaches from the superego. We know that rapes in this war were a planned action to humiliate the victims and an effective method to force them to cleanse themselves ethnically (i.e., to leave their homes). Knowing each other's subculture, the torturers knew that by raping a woman they, in fact, degraded her husband and, in a symbolic way, killed him. Therefore, these women often refuse to speak of such experiences, which results in psychosomatic reactions, depression, and suicide. In a study comprising 55 men who were sexually abused, the researches found out that all of these men developed depression, and most of them manifested symptoms of psychic impotence and had much difficulty in socialization. The predominant emotions in these sexually abused men were guilt and shame because they experienced their suffering as degradation to the female level. It is interesting and characteristic that they very seldom seek or accept therapy for their disturbances.

Transmission of Authority

Transmission of the father's authority in a patriarchal family from one generation to another is important for understanding certain events in the countries of the former Yugoslavia over the last 5–6 years. In a patriarchal family, the father's power is an untouchable authority that is transmitted from generation to generation. Family members are afraid to move out of its group, because everything strange is dangerous and hostile. Arrival in town from the country is an enormous change, and in these families, young people who come to town look for their fellow tribesmen and often call them "cousin" and "countryman," which reflects belonging to the same group.

Authoritarian education encourages the development of numerous projections onto the enemy and idealizations as well as identifications with authoritarian figures. These mechanisms spread onto the large group, which may be the neighborhood, the town, or the state. Persons thus brought up need an inviolable authority and are lost without it. Examples in the countries of the former Yugoslavia are Ante Pavelić in the Ustasha state, Tito in Communist Yugoslavia, and Tudjman and Milošević in the present. For example, Tomšić (1942) wrote,

> Leaders, authority and sovereignty of the Independent State of Croatia are embodied in the person of Dr. Ante Pavelić, whose official title was *Poglavnik* (Chieftain). He was the source of all the power and his was the last word. The Ustasha state was conceived as a widened family of patriarchal type in which all the authority was in the hands of its superior. Most of the leaders and ideologists of the Ustasha state come from the country in the Dinaric part of Croatia, where peasants are still living in large families of the strictly patriarchal type (p. 341).

The present situation in Croatia and Serbia is very important for both the future generations and the development of democracy. The authoritarian behavior by Croatian leaders, compared with that of Serbian leaders, is less explicit. Autocratic and repressive tendencies are attenuated in Croatia by freer and louder opposition groups in Croatia, and by the media, who were themselves partly responsible for having removed governmental controls on democratic processes in the first place. Also, the parliamentary elections in Croatia did help the people realize a considerable amount of freedom.

Both Serbian and Croatian leading groups demonstrate a penchant for supporting charismatic leaders. Dr. Franjo Tudjman of Croatia, while proclaiming democracy, manifests a similar authoritarian style and shares traditional family origins similar to those of Josip Broz Tito. They both come from peasant families in Hrvatsko Zagorje. The small group around the Croatian ruler is entirely dependent on his direction, having little opportunity to mature as autonomous political individuals. It seems as if the electoral victory brought about an oceanic feeling of bliss in this small group (marked by carelessness and self-satisfaction), but it did not last long, because they were soon faced with enemy groups from within their environment. As if awakened from a pleasant dream, they reacted aggressively and regressively, not allowing anyone to oppose them, thus increasing resistance and hostility in other groups, especially in the Serbs in Croatia, who actually had for years been persistently indoctrinated through propaganda directed from Belgrade.

MITIGATING THE CONSEQUENCES OF CONFLICT
IN THE FORMER YUGOSLAVIA

Current Situation

In various parts of Yugoslavia, especially those striken by the war, which means Croatia and Bosnia and Herzegovina, the victims are still full of hatred and wish for revenge. Hatred exists also on the other side. It has stimulated this war, and today, when, according to the Dayton agreements, they must surrender some territory, that hatred is even more obvious. Once again, the Serbs seem to have lost at the negotiating table what they had won on the battlefield. In many people's minds, there still echo the last words of their fellow soldiers when they died under torture or were killed by destructive shells: "Avenge me," which left a permanent impression on the survivors. Particularly vulnerable is the group of families of the missing and persons taken away by force. In order to further torture psychologically their families, the Serbs refuse to give any information about them. Hatred in families of the killed prevails, as well as wish to avenge. The war victims themselves, like the disabled, released prisoners of war, refugees, and displaced persons, also suffer serious scars and wish for revenge. As far as we could observe, the atmosphere in the groups of war victims is less aggressive and revengeful today than it was 2 or 3 years ago, due perhaps to the conciliatory attitude of the Catholic Church, which lectures on forgiveness. But there is still rather frequent and dangerous inducement of children by their parents, primarily mothers, to avenge their killed or missing parents. This reminds us of the mother, wife of a killed Mafia chief, who used to wake up her son every morning with the words: "Go and kill the murderers of your father."

Distrust in the "enemy" is the most widely spread reaction both in the war victims and in those persons all over the former Yugoslavia who did not suffer as much. A good illustration comes from the refugee camp in The Netherlands. Children of Bosnian, Croatian, and Serbian refugees played together. When they quarreled, they would insult each other, calling each other by pejorative names: "Ustasha," "Chetnik," and "balija" (for Muslim). Similarly, the relationships in the group of adults in the same camp depended on the situation on the battlefield. Distrust and separation of nations were constantly present. An example of much distrust between Croats and Bosnian Muslims is the current situation in divided Mostar. Inability to come to an agreement about fixing administrative boundaries is, in fact, an inability to agree on making the city unique, so its citizens can live in the same groups as they were living with before the war. A poignant example of distrust, due to the irrational fear that they will all be killed, is the emigration of Serbs from those parts of Sarajevo that belonged to the Bosnian–Croatian federation. It is difficult to gauge the extent to which this fear is the result of unconscious guilt feelings because of what they had done in Sarajevo during the war. Their digging up their dead, putting them into coffins, and taking them away was especially archaic.

Another dangerous situation that will generate intergenerational transmission of hatred is the tendency to generalize responsibility and guilt. Serbs will neither confess their crimes nor ask for pardon. When they talk about the causes of this war, they neglect the fact that they themselves attacked Croatia and Bosnia and Herzegovina, but use the maxim: "All are equal." It would be more correct to say that "all have become equal."

Equally dangerous for future generations is the opinion of Croats when they say: "All Serbs are criminals, there are no loyal Serbs." One has yet to see how much the International Criminal Tribunal for the Former Yugoslavia in the Hague can do to help reduce the destructive projections and contribute to the feeling that justice has been satisfied.

What we can observe today in the countries of the former Yugoslavia are idealization and demonization of the government occurring at the same time. The refugees and the displaced persons regressively expect to return to their villages and towns. They hope that not everything has been destroyed, that something has been left. They expect the state to give them back everything they lost and to enable them to have a normal life in the future in the places where they had lived before the war. Return of the displaced and the refugees is psychologically a most complex operation, and one cannot avoid being afraid that it will provoke aggressive and destructive impulses that will be transmitted to children and future generations. The best example is the town Mostar, where Muslim Bosniacs and Croats expect all their problems to be solved by the European Union-appointed administrator, Hans Koschnik, performing magic. Here, of course, each side has in mind the solution desired and suggested by itself.

The actual situation in this war brought about new "victims." So, for instance, in Croatia, members of Serbian nationality, besides being "suspicious" citizens, are exposed to being thrown out of their homes, losing their jobs, and the like. The situation in 1945, when families of the Ustasha officers and soldiers were brutally thrown out to the street without any means for living, is repeated. Many of the innocent Ustasha and *Domobran* officers were sentenced to long imprisonments, and their families were left without any means of subsistence.

How to Help?

To help the situation in the long run, we will have "to break the chain of intergenerational transmission of hatred, rage, revenge and guilt." I am already aware of the utopian nature of this sentence. I would like only positive emotions of love to be selectively transmitted. This sentence reminds me of the experience of a female colleague who lives and works in one of the countries of the former Yugoslavia not directly exposed to the war's destruction. She has been engaged in helping child refugees from Bosnia. She explained to me that an important motivational factor of her activity was the fact that she, herself, as a Jewish child, was hiding during World War II and well treated by the peasants of that country.

What would breaking the chain of intergenerational transmission of "negative" emotions mean? In our case, this would mean that a patriarchal family transforms into a modern family, that people outgrow their need for an absolute authority, and that there are no more uncritical nationalisms connected with xenophobia. It would mean, in fact, creating a dynamic group matrix characterized by cohesion and coherence, as in a good analytic group. This may be an illusion that might never come true. As is the case in some countries, perhaps it will be possible to create a democracy in ethnically mixed groups. But we are aware that these democracies, too, are not free of much that has been written in this chapter. Therefore, a change of identification objects is necessary. Only when the group and its goals replace the authority as identification objects can a real change of identity and ideals in these groups occur. Then, for example, it will be possible to isolate an individual criminal from his or her group, or in our case, from his or her nation.

A refugee psychiatrist talked with a child complaining of some psychological disturbances. The child and his mother were expelled from their home and maltreated by Serbian soldiers. The doctor, a refugee himself, said angrily, "Serbian mothers will also cry." The eight-year-old boy replied, with tears in his eyes, "No, don't let Serbian mothers cry." Recently I met a female doctor, a refugee from Bosnia, who has participated in a team offering psychosocial help to displaced persons. She told me: "Earlier I used to say that all I have gone through should never happen to anybody again, but now I tell everybody, let all this happen to everyone." I responded to her: "This is not good for you, because it makes you full of bitterness and hatred, which destroy you."

There are experiences around the world in which different people or ethnic groups are brought together to talk, such as groups of black and white persons (Ferron, 1992), Germans and French (Heenen-Wolff & Knauss, 1991), and Germans and Jews (Heenen-Wolff, 1992; see also Chapter 5 in this volume). Most of these groups have the very important common characteristic of having been formed many years after the actual conflict between the nations or races ceased. Notably different are the groups for Israelis and Arabs. In the territory of the former Yugoslavia, the situation is still very fresh, which makes it extremely difficult to establish a dialogue. Recent attempts to gather a group of members of different nations failed. Nevertheless, we will continue in this direction, because I think that it is very important.

I believe that adequate work with children war victims could best mitigate the intergenerational transmission of pathogenic emotions. Their parents should also be included in that work. Thus, the priority of psychological work in the countries of former Yugoslavia should be psychotherapeutic work with children who could then speak, express, and integrate their feelings and suffering connected with this war. I am sure that this would help to relieve the emotions that are transmitted.

REFERENCES

Cvijić, J. (1922). *Balkansko poluostrvo i južnoslavenske zemlje: Osnove antropogeografije, Knjiga I* [Balkan peninsula and southslavic countries: The bases of antropogeography, Book I], p. 115. Zagreb: Hrvatski štamparski zavod.

Cvijić, J., quoted by Rendić Miočević, I. (1996). *The evil of the great spleen: The history and non-history of Croats, Montenegrins, Muslims, and Serbs*, p. 87. Split: Književni krug.

Di Maria, F. (1995). *Planet, society, and group.* Paper presented at the 12th International Congress of Group Psychotherapy "Groups at the Doorstep of the New Century." Buenos Aires, Argentina.

Diatkine, G. (1993). La cravate croate: narcissisme des petites differences et processus de civilisation. *Revue française de Psychanalise, 4,* 1058–1071.

Dvorniković, V. (1939). *Karakterologija Jugoslavena* [Characterology of the Yugoslavs], pp. 81–95. Beograd: Geca Kon.

Ferron, E.G. (1992). The black and white group. *Group Analysis, 24,* 201–211.

Freud, S. (1923). Ego and id. *SE,* Vol. XIX, pp. 28–40. London: Hogarth Press.

Freud, S. (1933). Why war. *SE,* Vol. XXII, pp. 203. London: Hogarth Press.

Grmek, M., Gjidara, M., Šimac, N. (1993). *Le nettoyage etnique: Documents historiques sur une ideologie serbe,* pp. 53–75. Paris: Fayard.

Heenen-Wolff, S., & Knauss, W. (1991). Analyse de groupe autour de conflits dits "interculturels." *Connexions, 58,* 31–40.

Jelić-Butić, F. (1978). *Ustaše i Nezavisna država* Hrvatska [Ustashas and the independent state of Croatia], *II izdanje,* pp. 53–67. Zagreb: Sveučilišta naklada Liber, Školska knjiga.

Kavran, B. (1944). Ustaški pokret i Nezavisna Država Hrvatska. In *Hrvatska na novom putu* [Ustashas and the independent state of Croatia, in Croatia on the new path), pp. 100–138. Zagreb: Nakladna knjižara Velebit.

Kirigin, I. (1942, May). Hvalospjev četničkim zločinima [Praising of Chetniks'atrocities]. Rijeka: Novi list (newspaper).

Klain, E. (1992a). *Psychology and psychiatry of a war.* Zagreb: Faculty of Medicine, University of Zagreb, p. 77.

Klain, E. (1992b). Yugoslavia as a group, I. *Croatian Medical Journal, 33,* 3–13.

Klain, E. (1995). Yugoslavia as a group, II. In M. F. Ettin, J.W. Fidler, B. D. Cohen (Eds.), *Group process and political dynamics* (p. 166). Madison, NJ: International Universities Press.

Klein, M. (1946). Notes on some schizoid mechanisms. *International Journal of Psycho-Analysis, 27,* 99–110.

Kreeger, L. (1975). *The large group.* London: Constable, pp. 57–58, 145–159.

Lo Verso, G. (1995). Mafia e follia: Il caso Vitale. Uno studio psicodinamico e psicopatologico [Mob and insanity: Vitale case. Psychodynamic and psychopathology study]. *Psycoterapia e scienze umane, 3,* 99–121.

Mažuranić, I. (1965). Smrt Smail-age Čengića, u: Pet stoljeća hrvatske književnosti, knjiga 32 [Death of Smail-aga Čengić]. In *Five centuries of Croatian literature,* Book 32. Zagreb: Zora, Matica Hrvatska, pp. 43–77.

Pribičević, S. (1990). *Diktatura kralja Aleksandra* [Dictatorship of King Alexander]. Zagreb: Globus, p. 87.

Rendić-Miočević, I. (1996). *Zlo velike jetre: povijest i nepovijest Crnogoraca, Hrvata, Muslimana i Srba* [The evil of the great spleen: History and non-history of Croats, Montenegrins, Muslims, and Serbs]. Split: Književni krug, pp. 139–272, 315–343.

Rippa, B. (1992). *One year after: Groups in Israel during the Gulf War.* Paper presented at the 11th Congress of Group Psychotherapy, Montreal, Canada.

Tata Arcel, L., Folnegović-Šmalc, V., Kozarić-Kovačić, D., Marušić, A. (1995). *Psycho-social help to victims of war: Women refugees and their families from Bosnia and Herzegovina and Croatia.* Copenhagen: International Rehabilitation Council for Torture Victims (IRCT) and Rehabilitation Center for Torture Victims (RCT), p. 69.

Tomašić, D. (1942). *Croatia in European politics.* Quoted in I. Rendić-Miočević (1996). *The evil of the great spleen: History and non-history of Croats, Montenegrins, Muslims, and Serbs.* Split: Književni krug, p. 341.

18

Three Generations in Jewish and Non-Jewish German Families after the Unification of Germany

GABRIELE ROSENTHAL and BETTINA VÖLTER

INTRODUCTION

How do three generations of families live today with the family and the collective past during the Nazi period? What influences do this past of the first generation, and its own ways of dealing with it, have upon the lives of its offspring and on the ways in which the latter come to terms with their family history? These are the general empirical questions put forward by our current research (Rosenthal, 1998).[1] The specific focus of our study lies in comparing different family constellations based on whether the first generation can be categorized as victims, perpetrators, or Nazi followers during the Nazi period. Particularly from a sociological perspective, we also investigate how biographically different family histories after 1945—in Israel, in West Germany (FRG), and in the former East Germany (GDR)—affect the process of transmission from one generation to the next. In three generations of Jewish and non-Jewish German and Israeli families, we examine the process by which the family history is passed down through the generations. The aim is to reconstruct constellations in life stories that may facilitate the psychological and social integration of people burdened with a threatening collective and family past.

We have been conducting narrative–biographical interviews[2] of at least one member per generation in each family. Following the individual interviews, we conducted family interviews

---

[1]This study is carried out by a project run by the Deutsche Forschungsgemeinschaft, under the aegis of Fritz Schütze (Magdeburg University) and Regine Gildemeister (Kassel University) in cooperation with Dan Bar-On (Ben Gurion University of the Negev, Israel). Our coworkers in Israel are Noga Gilad and Yael Moore. Revital Ludewig-Kedmi participated in recording the interviews with the Basler family presented here.

[2]This interview technique (Rosenthal, 1995a, Schütze, 1976) works by means of an initial opening question in order to elicit and maintain a longer narration. This narration—the so-called main narration—is not interrupted by further questions but is encouraged by means of nonverbal and paralinguistic expressions of interest and attention. In the second part of the interview—the period of questioning—the interviewer initiated, with narrative questions, more

---

GABRIELE ROSENTHAL and BETTINA VÖLTER • University of Kassel, Faculty of Social Work, 34109 Kassel, Germany.

International Handbook of Multigenerational Legacies of Trauma, edited by Yael Danieli. Plenum Press, New York, 1998.

in order to examine the dynamics within family dialogue. At this stage, we have completed interviews of members of 20 Israeli and 19 German families. At the beginning of the individual interview,[3] we asked the biographer[4]: "Please tell me (us) your family story and your personal life story. I (we) am (are) interested in your whole life." The biographers were not interrupted by the interviewers as they narrated; only after they had finished did we start to put forward questions regarding details about parts of their lives and events that interested us.

The interviews are done in a research rather than a clinical setting. None of our interviewees had ever been hospitalized for psychological reasons. But it should be noted that we understand our interviews as a social–therapeutic intervention facilitating communication. Our experiences made obvious the effect of the interviews on opening the family dialogue, which can be considered as the start of familial restructuring.

The method used in analyzing the narrated family and life stories is one of hermeneutical case reconstruction.[5] The general questions posed for analysis can be formulated this way: In what way is the collective and the family past integrated into the presentation of the individual life story? What meaning is given to it in the biographical construction of the biographer? What biographical repair strategies are used in order to heal the effects of a threatening past?

An empirical comparison of families from the FRG, the GDR, and Israel clearly demonstrates that the structural differences inherent in familial dialogue with regard to National Socialism result less from differing socialization processes after 1945 and more from differences before 1945; that is, these pasts constitute the deep structure of the biographer to a far great extent than the family histories after 1945, be it in Israel, in the FRG, or under socialism in the GDR. Of crucial importance for the life stories of the subsequent generations, as well as for dialogue within the individual family, are whether and in what way were the great-grandparents, grandparents, or parents persecuted in Europe, and how they survived such persecution. Or, on the other hand, to what extent were they involved in Nazi crimes?

Based on these empirical findings, we would first like to discuss the similarities and dissimilarities between families of the persecuted and those of perpetrators or Nazi followers. Second, we will illustrate the differences among Israel, the GDR and the FRG. In order better to understand the mechanisms with which the family's past is handed down through generations, we introduce a detailed case study of a family from the ex-GDR. The Basler family[6] consists of both Jewish and non-Jewish members. This case study illustrates, on the one hand, the ways in which one deals with the persecuted past of the Jewish family members in the GDR, and, on the other, what kinds of repair strategies one employs to normalize the Nazi past of the non-Jewish family members. This case study further serves to clarify the extent to which the collapse of socialist society and the unification changed these individual life stories, as well as the interactively produced family story.[7]

elaborate narrations on topics and biographical events already mentioned, and locked-out issues were addressed. The method is based on the assumption that the narration of an experience comes closest to the experience itself. Narration of biographical events gives the social scientist the chance to glimpse some of the motives and interpretations guiding the actions of his subject.

[3]Some interviews were carried out by two interviewers.

[4]We prefer to use the term *biographer* instead of the term *autobiographer* in this context. In our opinion, the latter term does not place adequate emphasis on the social construction of life stories.

[5]For elaboration of the procedure of hermeneutical case reconstruction, see Rosenthal (1993, 1995a). Essential principles in this method are reconstruction and sequentiality. The texts are not subsumed under specific categories, but the meaning is analysed in the context of the entire text (= interview). The sequential compilation of the text of the life story, as well as the chronology of the biographical experiences in the life history, play an essential role.

[6]All names and some biographical data have been changed to protect their identity.

[7]By life story, we mean the narrated personal life as related in conversation or written in the present time; by life history, we mean the lived-through life. By family story, we mean the shared construction of one family history in the family dialogue.

SIMILAR AND DISSIMILAR WAYS OF DEALING WITH THE PAST IN FAMILIES OF SURVIVORS AND PERPETRATORS

At first glance, one can observe similarities when comparing ways of dealing with the traumatic past during National Socialism within Jewish families in which the grandparents either survived the Shoah or managed to flee Germany in time, with the same in families in which the grandparents were either perpetrators or active National Socialists. At the level of the individual life stories of the following generations,[8] these similarities manifest themselves in many ways: blocking out information about the family past, acting out the past through fantasies and psychosomatic reactions, fear of extermination, guilt feelings, and disturbed autonomy processes. Additionally, one may also observe similar mechanisms within families of the persecuted and the persecutors with regard to inner family dynamics. The silence about the past that has institutionalized itself within perpetrator families extends itself to families of the persecuted as well (Danieli, 1982). Moreover, in both kinds of families, one finds an enormous effect of family secrets (Karpel, 1980), a mutual obstructing of one another with regard to any thematizing of the past, accusations that render family dialogue impossible, the institutionalization of family myths (Ferreira, 1963) in order to circumvent familial conflict, and a bounded family system (Stierlin, 1981) resulting from the problematic past.

Behind these manifest similarities at the superficial level, however, lies the level of the latent, deep structure, which is constituted differently in each case by the experience of the family past. In other words, no matter how strong the superficial similarities, their function within the family system, and, more specifically, their psychological effect on individual family members continue to be divergent, based on the differences in the family pasts.

An aura of secrecy and shame hangs over survivor families when crucial information and experiences are not handed down to the subsequent generations. "The children develop fearful and embarrassed attitudes to the 'family secret' and often weave horrifying fantasies about what was done to their parents and how they survived" (Davidson, 1980, p. 19). In their fantasies, they fill in the gaps in their knowledge by imagining their relatives as active agents rather than as passive sufferers. In contrast, in perpetrator families, this is substituted by justification strategies and myth building that attests to the victim status of the family during National Socialism.

In survivor families, the silence of the grandparents regarding their experiences is connected to totally different problems and motives from the silence of those grandparents who actively participated in Nazi crimes. Similarly, different reasons motivate the frequently encountered reactions of children or grandchildren of survivors from those of the offspring of perpetrators. Examples include when they withdraw from the horror depicted in survivors' narrations of persecution and killing, when they fail to grasp the full meaning of certain details of the experience, or when they even repeatedly forget the communicated information. These gestures of self-protection are aimed at warding off very different pressures from those of the children or grandchildren in perpetrator families, even when the latter employ similar, self-protective methods. Grandparents, who were active Nazis, had enveloped themselves in a cocoon of silence and denial for fear of accusations and loss of familial affection. Their children and their grandchildren protect themselves from having to be aware of the gruesome activities of their near and dear. They also try to ward off feelings of guilt, as well as the fear that they themselves will be judged by the grandparents or parents as unfit to live (Rosenthal & Bar-On, 1992). One grandmother, who survived the ghetto

---

[8]In contrast, there are significant differences in the ways in which members of the first generation—victims, perpetrators, and Nazi followers—deal with the past (Rosenthal, 1991).

and extermination camp, does not deny her persecuted past, as is the case with perpetrators or Nazi followers. However, if she, too, does not articulate this past, it is because, among other things, she tries to protect her children and grandchildren from the daydreams and nightmares that haunt her. Survivors very often use their silence to spare their children the pressures they themselves are exposed to, and to avoid burdening others with their painful experiences (Danieli, 1982).

Our case analyses clearly show that silence and family secrets, as well as family myths, constitute some of the most effective mechanisms ensuring a continued impact of problematic family past. This is true in families of survivors, perpetrators, and Nazi followers. Generally formulated, this reads: The more closed or guarded the familial dialogue, or the greater the attempt to make a secret of, or to whitewash, the past, the more sustained will be the impact of the family past on the second or third generation (Bar-On, 1995; Danieli, 1993; Sigal, Silver, Rakoff, & Ellin, 1973). Our biographical case reconstructions show that these subsequent generations often unconsciously suffer from extremely detailed fantasies concerning undisclosed family history or family secrets.

The respective family secrets differ both in content and function within the families of survivors and perpetrators and of Nazi followers. Furthermore, the fantasies built around these secrets by subsequent generations are correspondingly different in content. These either revolve around the powerlessness and suffering experienced by a survivor, or around the criminal actions of a perpetrator. Moreover, their psychological dynamics also differ. Examples from the Sonntag and the Steinberg families offer preliminary insight into these differences. Both in the former, in which the grandfather was most likely a participant in Nazi crimes, and in the latter, in which the grandmother survived the Shoah, the children and grandchildren have access only to partial information and fill in the gaps with their fantasies. Fantasy building demonstrates, how, in spite of narrative silence, a latent handing down of the experiences and actions of the grandparents takes place.

In the Sonntag family[9] the grandfather, who, as archival research shows, was possibly involved in constructing death ovens in concentration camps, continues to ponder how so many corpses could still be left over after 1945. After all, he argues, one did try to burn all the bodies. His whereabouts during the war, and the crimes he was actively involved in, continue to be a secret within his family. His son, however, continues to pose "burning" questions with regard to his own life story, preoccupied as he is with whether he could bring himself to shoot people or even burn to death women and children locked inside a church building. He subsequently concludes that if he were required to carry out such orders, he would not risk "burnt fingers" by refusing to do so. He primarily excuses the perpetrators guilty of such crimes by allocating responsibility and guilt to the victims. One of his main arguments puts forward the view that it was the victims' support of the partisans that led to the liquidation of entire populations by the Nazis in some places. On the other hand, in the Steinberg family,[10] the interview with the mother, who was subjected to torture as a political prisoner, as well as incarceration in several concentration camps, is riddled with unspecified allusions to repeated sexual abuse and rape. In her own narrative, the daughter, who is extremely close to the mother, makes cloaked allegations against her. She is unconsciously haunted by the fantasy that her mother prostituted herself to the Nazis.

These scenarios reveal a son of a possible perpetrator, who tortures himself with his own potential to become one, thereby excusing the real perpetrators and, instead, turning the ac-

---

[9]A detailed discussion of this perpetrator family can be found in Rosenthal (1998).
[10]For a detailed discussion of this family, see Zilberman and Rosenthal (1994).

cusation onto the victims. In contrast, the daughter of a survivor struggles with suppressed accusations against her mother and with related guilt feelings. This scenario clearly signifies the handing down of a pattern already present in the first generation. While the real perpetrators attempt to deflect responsibility from themselves by accusing the victims (Rosenthal, 1992), survivors continue to be plagued by guilt for having survived, repeatedly calling into question their desertion of their parents, their failure to help others in certain situations, and why, during the "selection," they only thought of themselves rather than of those who were sent to be gassed.

A comparison of survivor and perpetrator families also illustrates structural differences with regard to the content of family myths. Within survivor families, the construction of and identification with such myths are focused on the themes of "strength" and "resistance" (e.g., the fantasy that the grandfather had boxed an SS officer in the ear). In families with a Nazi past, this takes on the form of stressing the victimhood of the family members (e.g., the grandfather as a victim of the war and subsequently of imprisonment, an image that concretizes itself in the process of fantasy building). A noticeable feature in Jewish families is the fact that children and grandchildren of grandparents, both of whom survived concentration or extermination camps, take a particular interest finding "fighting" parts in their family history. For instance, the Goldstern family, whom we interviewed in Israel, strongly identify with the grandmother's brother who was killed in action during the War of Independence in Israel. The enlargement of his photograph is put up very visibly in the grandparents' living room, whereas the unenlarged photographs of the murdered great-grandparents lie stored away in the grandparents' sleeping room. The analysis of this family dialogue made clear that identification with this great-uncle served as a repair strategy, in an attempt to heal the intense feelings of powerlessness. This is especially true of the grandmother who witnessed the murder of babies and of her best girlfriend in the ghetto of Lodz.[11] Although on a superficial level this phenomenon might be explained as an expression of collective patterns of interpretation institutionalized in Israel, we also find it in the families of Jewish survivors living in Germany.

In non-Jewish German families, one increasingly comes across the myth of the "clean" soldier, who, in the midst of injustice, succeeded in helping enemy civilians or even in treating prisoners of war with respect and a sense of justice. This belief corresponds to the long-standing social myth of the "clean" Wehrmacht, whose members, unlike those of the SS, supposedly did not participate in dishonorable criminal activities.[12]

DIFFERENCES IN SOCIAL AND FAMILIAL DIALOGUE IN ISRAEL, WEST GERMANY, AND THE FORMER EAST GERMANY

The phenomenon of collective silence can be found in each of these three societies despite the emergence of a more open social dialogue about the Holocaust in recent years.

In Israel, the opening up of such dialogue has undergone several stages. Until the Eichmann trial, which began in 1961, the Holocaust was more or less a taboo topic in public discussion. Only with the public radio broadcast of the trial, which contained the accounts and testimonies of the persecution and sufferings of the victims, could it come to the forefront of

[11]For a detailed discussion of this family and a comparison with the myths in a family of a perpetrator, see Rosenthal (1998).

[12]This myth has partly been called into question in Germany by, among others, exhibitions and publications of the Hamburger Institut für Sozialforschung, under the heading "war of extermination" (Heer & Naumann, 1995). The exhibition was taken to several cities in Germany and gave rise to innumerable controversies.

public attention (Danieli, 1980; Segev, 1993). The Yom Kippur war in 1973 was the first time that Israel, caught by surprise, started to be more identified with the helplessless of the victims of the Holocaust. However, until the early 1980s, one could still observe an effective, socially imposed tendency to focus on the "heroic" in Israel, with issues of powerlessness remaining unvoiced. This conspiracy of silence "was accompanied by harsh value judgments, which blamed the survivors who went, it was said, like sheep to the slaughter" (Bar-On, 1995, p. 19). During the last 10–15 years, survivors are being denounced less and less for having exhibited any weakness during the persecution, and an increasing number of them have begun to speak about their past. In fact, the end of the 1980s marks the beginnings of a public discussion—both in films and in literature—on the tribulations not only of the survivors but also of their descendants.

In West Germany, widespread silence had institutionalized itself on the topic of Nazi crimes, and what prevailed was the myth of the innocent populace that unsuspectingly followed Nazism. This enabled perpetrators responsible for the crimes of Nazism to be freed of charges, and the collective majority of Germans could mutually reassure themselves that they had seen or heard nothing concerning the persecution of Jews and other persecuted people until 1945. Empirical analyses of life stories of nonpersecuted Germans (Rosenthal, 1990, 1991) illustrate the multiple ways in which members of all generations attempt to extricate accounts of their lives from any possible complicity with the Nazi regime. Although for several years the mass media have attempted to thematize Nazi crimes in a general way, this has hardly ever taken the form of the lived reality of people at the time. This silence on questions or perpetrators and of the lived experience of Nazi atrocities led in the course of time to certain established rules that, in turn, effectively obstructed any intergenerational as well as intragenerational dialogue. Even the enormous energy that members of the so-called (19)68 generation brought to the discussion on antifascism in West Germany could not prevent them from unconsciously submitting to the same rules, in spite of their effort to seriously examine fascism, criticize the continuities between the "Third Reich" and postwar society, and squarely face their parents' generation with its complicity with the Nazis. Our interviews with the 68 generation show how little they know about their own family histories. The act of accusing their parents or grandparents of being Nazis often works as an enormous defense mechanism against any concrete knowledge of their actual pasts as perpetrators of Nazi followers (Rosenthal, 1995b). The genocide of the Jews has, however, become a topic of public discussion, leading to greater social dialogue following the initial broadcasting of the American television series *Holocaust* in 1979. This increased discussion of the persecution and the fate of the persecuted in the media,[13] in schools, and even within families does not, however, rule out the hesitation, or even resistance, in directly addressing the question of perpetrators in either public discourse or within the family.

While in West Germany all discussion centered around the Holocaust more or less ignored the political resistance, in the case of the former East Germany, exactly the opposite held true. There was an overemphasis on communist resistance to Nazism and a corresponding underplaying of the Shoah. Jewish resistance fighters were routinely exalted as antifascists, whereby their Jewish antecedents were bracketed out. Our interviews illustrate how this lack

---

[13]The stir caused by Daniel Jonah Goldhagen's Ph.D. thesis, recently published in both the United States and in Germany, reveals more about the American and German discourse in public on topics concerning Nazi Germany and the Holocaust than about internal scientific discussion. Goldhagen's findings are not new. The myth of an unwitting and uninvolved majority of Germans, with only a small number of persecutors, has long been dispelled in academic and also in public discourse in Germany, and has been further discredited by the exhibitions and publications of the Hamburger Institut für Sozialforschung (see footnote 10).

of a public discourse on racial persecution led to even less discussion in GDR families on the Holocaust and Jews than in FRG families. In the GDR, bourgeoise resistance groups gradually became included in public discourse, and since the mid-1980s, there was even an official attempt to rebuild structures to commemorate the Jews, such as reconstructing the New Synagogue in Berlin. However, it was only with the unification in 1989 that an unambiguous reinterpretation of the Nazi past was ushered in. Sites of public commemoration, such as the memorials where the concentration camps of Sachsenhausen and Buchenwald once stood, could now be given a new emphasis. The Holocaust exhibits were rearranged to allocate more space to the genocide, and the magnitude of the exhibition devoted to political resistance was reduced.

In general, it is necessary to emphasize that the silence about the Nazi past stems from similar motives in both East and West Germany, whereas in Israel, these motives are altogether different. Examining the different ways in which Jewish families in the FRG, in the former GDR, and in Israel deal with the past should shed further light on the differences in social dialogue on the Holocaust in the three countries.

In the former GDR, until well into the 1980s, one could find a strong tendency to remain silent about Jewish antecedents and about the persecution, or even about anti-Semitism experienced after 1945. Instead, the antifascist elements and the history of political resistance in the family would usually be stressed. This was part of an uncritical identification with the antifascist myth propagated by the East German state and the obligatory loyalty to the system. In other words, this way of dealing with the family history was symptomatic as well as reflective of the general social treatment of the Nazi past. Moreover, the state laid little importance on the development of Jewish self-awareness. According to the official definition, only someone who was registered as a member of one of the eight religious communities was considered Jewish (Runge, 1990). Secular Jews were considered "GDR citizens of Jewish origin" at best (Schoeps, 1991, p. 374). In addition, many Jewish functionaries and intellectuals consciously did not profess their Jewishness (Ostow, 1988). These defense mechanisms, functioning partly as mechanisms of denial, contributed to a refusal to acknowledge anti-Semitism as prevalent in East Germany. Somewhat before the wall came down in 1989, however, these mechanisms were already losing their effectiveness. The more the belief in the socialist state crumbled, the stronger became the need for some people to reflect on their Jewish origins. Others began to stress the difference between Jews and non-Jews, once based, of necessity, on their different experiences, and to take an interest in their family history. For instance, around the mid-1980s in Berlin, a group came together to build a circle of people with Jewish origins who were interested in questions of culture rather than religion.

In contrast, the self-definition of Jews living in West Germany was based more strongly on their Jewishness. However, until well into the 1980s, even here, many of them kept this relatively inconspicuous and learned a form of self-presentation by which they could avoid being necessarily identified as Jewish within non-Jewish circles. Moreover, they, too, did not raise within the realm of public discourse questions on the topic of Nazi crimes. Finally, however, some children of families with Jewish background began to voice their thoughts in an openly political way.

While Jews in the former GDR identified with the East German state, those in West Germany suffered from a negative identification with their country of domicile. When comparing Jewish families in the two countries, it should also be taken into account that the life histories of their grandparents had considerably different trajectories prior to 1945. In the west, the grandparents mainly consisted of survivors of the camps who were of Eastern European origin, and who immediately after the liberation lived in displaced-person camps (Richarz, 1988). In the east, on the other hand, they were either part of the resistance or among those who had emigrated out of Germany before 1939 and, as members of the Communist party, decided to live in a socialist state after the war.

This group that was forced to emigrate and subsequently returned to the GDR shows interesting similarities to the group that left Germany before 1939 with the Youth-Aliyah for Israel. In Israel, both the first and the second generation of these families mostly live in the Kibbutz, and often hold to a strong, decidedly Zionistic persuasion. Analysis of interviews with them shows that such identification serves, among other things, to alleviate the guilt that torments the first generation (Rosenthal, Völter, & Gilad, 1998): the self-accusation that they had left their relatives to die in Europe, while they themselves could build a new life in Israel. Both the Zionist identification in Israel and the identification with the socialist state in the former GDR are, therefore, accompanied by an underplaying of the negative aspects of their respective systems.

A FAMILY WITH JEWISH AND NON-JEWISH MEMBERS IN EAST GERMANY: ANTIFASCISM AS A SUBSTITUTE MOURNING?

The Baslers[15] are typical of a family of Jewish origin in the former GDR, both with regard to the trajectory of their family history and their way of dealing with the history of persecution. We conducted five interviews with them: with the grandmother Gertrud Kersten, with her son, Gerhard, with his non-Jewish wife, Silvia, and with the grandsons, Ralf and Roland. Both Gertrud and her son, Gerhard, refused to participate in a family interview.

Let us now look at the life story of each member individually.

The First Generation

Gertrud, the grandmother, was born in 1919 near Heidelberg. Her family lived strictly according to Jewish rules. Her father was a tailor, and her mother owned a fabric shop. Gertrud had seven siblings. In 1933, at the age of 14, she began to work as a maid in several Jewish households. One by one, these families began to emigrate out of Germany. By 1939, four of her older siblings had also emigrated, with the help of her father's relatives, to Australia. In May 1939, Gertrud herself emigrated to Sweden on her own steam. In her interview, she only hinted at her feelings of rivalry toward her older siblings.

Shortly after her arrival in Sweden, she was initiated into the KPD (Communist Party of Germany) by her new circle of friends. There, she met her future husband, Manfred, who was non-Jewish and had fled Germany as well. When the Nazis came to power in 1933, Manfred and his brother, Paul, a well-known philosopher, were active as communists in the resistance against National Socialism. While Manfred managed to escape to Sweden, his brother was captured by the Nazis and died in a Gestapo prison.

Gertrud and Manfred married in 1940, and, in 1944, their son was born. In 1946, the Baslers returned to Germany and lived in the west, until 1949, when they went over to the GDR. Not too many years later, Gertrud and her husband separated.

---

[15]The following discussion of this case study is result-oriented (i.e., the process of interpretation cannot be reconstructed here). Therefore, we would like to make the reader aware of the fact that the analytical method applied here (Rosenthal, 1993, 1995a) implies that both the construction and the examination of hypotheses takes place in each concrete case.

Since her return to Germany, Gertrud has repeatedly tried to look for information on her family that stayed behind. In 1947, she had received archival information that her younger sister was transported to an extermination camp and died there. One of her brothers was murdered along with his family. She also found out that her paternal grandparents had been killed in Holland. Some years after the war, she was able to determine that her parents had been taken to the concentration camp in Theresienstadt. It was only after 1989 that Gertrud turned to the archive at the Theresienstadt memorial and found out that her mother and father were transported from Theresienstadt to different camps at different points in time. In spite of this knowledge, she tried to alleviate her grief for losing parents by imagining that they died together in the gas chambers. She insists that her mother, 11 years younger than her father, voluntarily accompanied him to his death: "It was typical of my mother to say that she wouldn't let my father go alone. I'm convinced that this is how it happened. And she must definitely have fought so they could go together." Gertrud finds it easier to live with this fantasy than with the possibility that her father might have died alone. The thought that her mother fought against the passivity of her situation is equally relieving. Alone with her grief and her thoughts, she hardly ever has the opportunity to talk about her parents' deaths or to share her pain with others. "Not a day goes by when I don't think about these things. . . . I was the only one who went away to Sweden. . . . I always lived without my family." How little of this is spoken of within the family becomes clear, especially in the interviews with her grandsons.

Exactly how threatening these memories of her family can be for Gertrud also becomes clear from the text structure of her biographical self-presentation. Despite repeated attempts on the part of the interviewer to motivate her into talking about her family, her childhood, and growing up, she answers purely with descriptions of everyday routine in a religious household, refusing to relate any stories about her parents or her siblings. Although she begins her interview by recounting relevant dates in her family prior to her emigration, her presentation focuses to a much greater extent on her own experiences of persecution after she left home at the age of 14. Rather than speak about her family, she concentrates her narrative from 1933 to 1939 (i.e., up to the point of her departure), mainly on her life outside the family. We interpret this text structure as being influenced by her guilt at having survived. Like many of her generation, Gertrud was in a situation of despair. Her parents and younger sister had written to her for help, even for money, so they could pay for visas in order to emigrate, but she was in no position to help.[16] Especially in the months before the war broke out, her days were entirely taken up with the "problem, how to get the parents out of there." The last set of letters Gertrud exchanged with her parents and her sister, providing further insight into this inner-family conflict, was in 1941. After a long silence, she writes to tell them about her marriage. Her parents and sister write back, complaining about her long silence, adding that they regretted that she had married a non-Jew. The mother writes: "However, since it is already the case, then let it be so. As a mother, I wish you and your husband every happiness and send my blessings. I pray to God that your marriage may be a happy one." Gertrud did not reply to this letter. Nor did she exchange any more letters with her siblings in Australia.

Her political ideas and her related lifestyle, as well as her marriage to a non-Jewish academic, drew her further and further away from her background. She had moved away not only from her family but also from her life as a Jew and had found instead a new home for herself in an atheist, communist world. Her marriage and her new circle of like-minded people were definitely a great help during her adjustment to a foreign country. When she moved to the

[16]The feeling that one could integrate into a life outside Germany, while one's family was persecuted and killed by the Nazis, is a constellation in the children's life stories that leads to tremendous guilt at having survived (Rosenthal *et al.*, 1998).

GDR, she was asked by the communist party to make a clear decision as to whether she identified as a practicing Jew or not. The party line did not allow one to be a member of the Jewish congregation and of the SED at the same time. In the early 1950s, Gertrud therefore renounced her Jewish identity. We surmise that this is a further reason for her feeling guilty, especially after the wall came down in 1989.

Her efforts to construct a memorial, together with her family, to her non-Jewish brother-in-law, Paul Basler, in his hometown, provide further insight into her difficulties in dealing with her family history. Every year, the family conducts a memorial service there. As the interviews with Gertrud's son and her grandsons also show, this non-Jewish member of the resistance, whom she personally knew, is the only victim of National Socialism who is openly commemorated by the entire family. In psychoanalytic terms, this could be a displacement of the grief surrounding the killings of her Jewish family members onto a process of grieving for a political resistance fighter from the non-Jewish side of the family. In this context, it is possible to use the term *substitute mourning*. This displacement is also influenced by the social discourse in the former GDR, where members of the communist resistance earned far greater respect and acceptance in public memory than did religious Jews.

Biographical case reconstruction shows that Gertrud Basler had replaced her Jewish self-understanding with her communist identity. While exacerbating her guilt regarding her parental family, this, at the same time, helps her to block these feelings and provides her with means to occupy herself with the politicized, non-Jewish side of her family. However, in contrast to other Jewish families interviewed, Gertrud feels deeply connected to the time in her life she spent growing up in a Jewish milieu. As opposed to many other Jewish communists, she was still a member of the Jewish congregation during the initial years in the GDR. She says, "Everyone who knows me, knows that I'm Jewish. It has always been that way." However, she still sees herself as a communist and continues to be a member of the Partie des democratischen Socialismus (PDS), the party that came out of the former SED. If she were to question this identification, her distance from her parental family would become an even greater problem for her.

The Second Generation

Gerhard Basler, born in 1944, is the only son of Gertrud and Manfred Basler. He works as a historian and was an active member of the SED.

Asked to narrate his family history and his life story, he begins with his biographical self-presentation: "I was born in Sweden, on (. . .), in 1944, as the son of an emigrant family." After this introductory statement, which we may read as an identity tag, Gerhard narrates his family history under the rubric "emigration." His life is shaped specifically by the fact that his parents could escape persecution, and that after he was born, the family moved from a West European country to the GDR. Concretely, however, he knows little about his family history prior to 1945. Although he can talk at length about the latter part of his life story, when it comes to the topic "family history," he suffers from a total block, able only to hint at certain things, and he often breaks off his report or lapses into silence. While, to his relief, he can recount a few "facts" about his maternal family, his knowledge about his paternal family is totally fragmentary. But from his implications and the gaps in his knowledge, we may surmise that there were some Nazis in this branch of the family. At least one of his father's brothers was a member of the Nationalsozialistische deutsche Arbeiterpartei (NSDAP) and therefore a potential threat to Manfred and his communist brother, Paul. However, this aspect of their past was never discussed openly in the Basler family. This tendency to remain silent about, or even make a secret of, the unpleasant parts of family history comes up in other contexts as well. For instance, only after many pointed questions did Gerhard admit that his father died while under psychiatric treatment, in Gerhard's words "surrounded in mental darkness."

In his interview, Gerhard, moreover, displays a noticeable need for harmony with regard to the relationships in his family. For example, he refuses to distinguish between people he feels close to and those he does not. He can only partly meet the request of the interviewer to illustrate this with the help of a family sculpture,[17] when he is asked to attach dots in distances to signify his emotional relationship with different members of his family. After he has stuck the dots representing his wife, his sons, his mother, and her partner on top of each other, to signify that he is equally close to each of them, he refuses to position his uncles and aunts. He likens the request to demonstrate emotional closeness and distance through graphic representation with Nazi practice, which divided people into categories that read "fit or unfit to live." He says, "I refuse to hierarchize human beings. I cannot do it. Even apart from the Holocaust, when one has two children one compares them and asks of oneself, which of the two do you love more. This question cannot be answered and I refuse to evaluate in this way. I don't consider it human."

In the conversations that followed regarding his vehemence on the matter, it became clear how strongly he fears the question of which of his sons he feels closer to, a question he often finds himself asking. He feels a tremendous pressure that it is wrong to differentiate within the realm of his family. In this context, Gerhard begins to talk about his mother having survived the persecution, as opposed to her sister and her brother. When asked whether he thinks that his mother experiences guilt, he responds strongly: "I think it's possible. But I would never discuss it with my mother. It's too personal, I wouldn't want to trespass. I would only hurt her with a question like that and I don't want to dig around in the past in that way."

Like numerous members of the second generation of emigrants who returned to the GDR, Gerhard had identified with socialism for as long as he can remember, and had worked to fulfill its goals. After the wall came down in 1989, bringing with it a crisis in his work life as well, he began to question his own behavior during GDR times. The revival of Nazism, rascism, and anti-Semitism in Germany deepened his insecurity and lent greater importance to his Jewish origins. While earlier he would identify more strongly with the communist tradition within his family and definitely knows more about it even today, his connection to his Jewish family history grew in importance in the newly unified Germany. What remains important for him, however, is the difference between the family history of his father, who was part of the communist resistance, and that of his mother, whose family members, according to him, "went to their death unresistingly." Gerhard would like, above all, to resolve this difference. This becomes clear not only through his actions—he, too, displaces his grief onto the non-Jewish resistance fighter Paul—but also in his dreams. When asked what kinds of dreams he had as a child about his grandparents' fate, he describes persistent dreams in which he saw himself on the way to the gas chamber: "Pretty realistic dreams, where someone says, 'Let's see if you all are brave enough and if you can march in there,' and I knew what it meant."

Gerhard interprets this situation of ultimate powerlessness (i.e., the journey to the gas chamber) as a courageous act in his dreams, thereby dissolving the difference in the family histories of his father and his mother into one shared picture. Moreover, in this way, he continues with his mother's fantasy in which she imagines her own mother fighting to be allowed to accompany her husband to the gas chamber.

[17]After the interview, we asked our interviewees to build a family sculpture, to associate to it, and to explore its meanings further in a manner following the one used in family therapy (Jefferson, 1978, Papp, Silverstein, & Carter, 1973, Simon, 1972).

In 1973, Gerhard married Silvia Scholz, a daughter of non-Jewish parents. Silvia was born in 1949. She, too, is a trained historian and was an active member of the SED.

Silvia's grandfather worked for the Reichsbahn (railways) and was transferred in an important capacity to Posen, in the annexed part of Poland, when the war broke out. The Reichsbahn administration in Posen was responsible for loading Jews onto trains from Wartheland for transportation to the extermination camps (Hilberg, 1990), and it seems highly probable that he was involved in the process. Silvia never got to know this grandfather. In her family, he is considered missing, presumed dead as of 1945. Her statements about her grandfather's potential involvement in Nazi persecution are fairly unreflective, and she blocks out the emotional underpinnings entirely. When asked by the interviewer whether her grandfather had anything to do with the transportation of Jews, she answers succinctly: "I think that in Posen he [the grandfather] did, because it was a railway junction, and trains to Ausschwitz and Treblinka had to pass through it."

Silvia herself was born out of wedlock. Her father was a commanding officer in the Red Army and was stationed in the Soviet-occupied zone. He lived together with her mother and her until she was a year old and then returned to the Soviet Union. Since then, she has lost all contact with him, and he is never mentioned in the family: "That was always something that strained relations between my mother and me, because we never really talked about it." In 1954, her mother married again. Although Silvia always knew she had a different father, her mother kept his identity from her until she was 18. The secrecy around his real identity was sometimes the topic of gossip outside the family. When she was a child, Silvia was once told by a friend, "'My mother said your father is a Russian.' I said, 'No, that can't be, that's not true.' And I said it with total confidence." Today, she herself makes a secret of her father's existence within the family. In her interview, she emphasizes that her sons should not learn about him. For them, her stepfather is her actual father. The decision to keep the existence of their real grandfather from them has far-reaching consequences for the family. Boszormeny-Nagy (1975) writes in a similar context: "One such decision makes every subsequent effort at honesty and openness among family members concerning important matters in life impossible" (p. 296). Silvia's husband is also forced into the role of the accomplice. The grandfather becomes part of internal family secrets (Karpel, 1980) with which the parents keep parts of the family history from the children. Silvia therefore puts her children in a situation similar to the one she was in as a child, and one day, they too could be confronted with statements such as "Your grandfather is a Russian."

The thematic field in which Silvia's life story is embedded is her political trajectory as a socialist. Silvia and her husband's common political orientation helps them ignore unpleasant parts of their respective family histories. Her marriage to a Jew, who identifies himself as a communist first and foremost, enables her to distance herself from the Nazi elements in her family background and at the same time identify with the victims without having to deal with her grandfather's involvement in their persecution. Their common political ideas also take care of any potential conflict within the family that could otherwise result from the difference in their sensibilities and perspectives owing to different family histories.

The Third Generation

The grandsons, Ralf and Roland, were born in 1975 and 1978, respectively, and are still in school. Their presentation of their family history also begins with the topic of "grandmother's emigration," and they know nothing of their family history prior to this point.

The younger brother, Roland, when asked to recount his life story as well as his family history, begins: "Well, I know that my grandmother (3-second pause) went over to Sweden with her entire family during the Nazi era." It is clear from the first sentence that Roland has never found out or felt the need to repress the threatening part of his family history, for instance, that his great-great-grandparents, his great-grandparents, and his grandmother's siblings were killed, and that the grandmother was alone in Sweden. He continues: "And there she (2-second pause) gave birth to my father (5-second pause, takes a deep breath) and then her brother and other relatives remained in Sweden or moved to Australia."

At this point, Roland introduces his granduncle, Paul Basler, the communist resistance fighter, into the narrative, along with the information that he died of an illness in a concentration camp. Then, he goes on to speak about himself: "Well, that I have Jewish roots (2-second pause) and I don't really know in which, phf, well, I think my father's family is Jewish and my mother's is not. My mother comes from M. and (2-second pause) um . . . (3-second pause) well, I don't know anything about that (5-second pause). . . ."

Roland is not sure who was or is Jewish in his family. His confusion about who is related to whom, in which way, is so great that he thinks Paul Basler is his grandmother's brother and therefore a Jew. The numerous pauses in his recounting of his mother's family point to his own confusion, and, above all, the darkness her family history is cloaked in. However, at the very least, Roland has some vague feeling that there were Nazis in this branch of his family:

> ROLAND: Grandmother also said they had all cheered Hitler at the time, he gave them work. . . . Obviously, it was a dictatorship, and anyone who didn't go along was done away with, and so they preferred to go along. . . . More than anything he (Hitler) enticed them. Everyone could get a job, and the Jew is to blame, and once the Jews have been removed, your situation will improve.

> INTERVIEWER: Can you imagine that your grandmother also thought this way?

> ROLAND: Well, I would rather not imagine that. . . . I don't know.

As a result of family traditions and his socialist education, Roland identifies strongly with the communist resistance. Faced with the question of what meaning he attributes to whether someone was persecuted as a Jew or as a communist, his initial response is based on a scene from the television series *Holocaust* in which "thousands of Jewish families were transported away, and there were only about 20 guards. And the Russians made a run for it because they recognized they were numerically stronger and the Jews didn't try to defend themselves."

In his imagination, Jews, as opposed to communists, are passive. Since, however, he makes his granduncle, Paul Basler, out to be a Jew, this causes great confusion. When asked, "And on which side do you see your uncle?" he answers, "If he was in the resistance, he must have been a communist, but he was (3-second pause) a Jew" (15-second pause).

> I: Are these mutually exclusive?

> R: (*3-second pause*) Well, I can't say now how I place him, as a Jew or as a communist (*15-second pause*).

> I: what would you rather see him as?

> R: As a communist (*4-second pause*) but (*16-second pause*) I don't know (*6-second pause*).

> I: What's going through your head at this moment?

> R: I don't mean that I'm ashamed that he was a Jew (*3-second pause*). That was stupid of me (*5-second pause*). I'm a Jew myself.

I: Have you ever thought about how you would have behaved?

R: As a communist or uh, or how. If I wasn't alone, I would put up a fight. If one does that alone and not in a group, it makes little sense. One always has to be part of a larger mass (*7-second pause*).

I: How do you imagine Paul Basler in the camp, alone or in a group?

R: Well, as an outsider, because those in the camps were mostly either Jews or communists and he was both.

For Roland, Jews and communists do not belong in the same schema. Jews who are communists at the same time do not belong to any group. This crucial statement in the interview corresponds equally to how Roland feels about his life postunification. As the son of communist parents, he falls under the most attacked minority in Germany today. As a "leftist" and a Jew he fears the neo-Nazis and "Right Radicals" who are now active in his school. However, he tells the interviewer that he is even friends with them. They are "sportsmen," and therefore unpolitical and not so radical. Obviously, he fears the role of the outsider and the thought of having no one to stand by him. As a result, he harmonizes his relationship with his potential persecutors, despite having been attacked by neo-Nazis in the subway once. By arranging the past and the present of both persecuted and persecutor into a harmonious picture, Roland tries to do away with the threat such a reality would otherwise present. This shows how behavior patterns present in the earlier generations of his family—the refusal to disturb or deal with certain family connections to National Socialism—are handed down.

This confusion around the process of mourning and the handing down of family history produces a sense of diffusion in the members of the third generation that defines their entire identity. Even if one interprets this in the case of 15-year-old Roland as lack of orientation during middle adolescence, in the case of his 18-year-old brother Ralf, it becomes increasingly clear that this confusion results equally from their specific family dynamics. In Ralf's case, both his confusion regarding his relatives and the lack of a concrete sense of identity that results from this are more pronounced. Although at the time of the interview he was 18 years old, he could barely narrate either his family history or his own life story.

His markedly brief response when asked to recount his family history and life story can be broken down into four headings: emigration, lack of knowledge about when his paternal grandfather actually died, Jewishness in the family, and his granduncle Paul: "Well, I know nothing of what happened before World War II. I only know that they escaped to Sweden, America, and Australia, and got to know many of their present friends at the time. My father's father died there. I don't know if that was in the war or before. . . . Well, they are very interested and involved in Jewish culture, museums, and so forth, and they built a memorial or some such thing to my uncle. He was some kind of a philosopher and, well, (6-second pause) I guess that's it for starters."

In his fantasies, Ralf lets his grandfather die before his return to Germany. This is probably because no one in the family ever mentions that the grandfather died while in psychiatric treatment. Ralf's interview also illustrates that he substitutes the dethematization of his Jewish family members with thematizing his non-Jewish granduncle Paul. When asked what he had been told by his grandmother about her past, he replied, "Well, actually, we only spoke about the philosopher all the time, not much about the rest of the family." Ralf's confusion around his family history is especially striking with regard to his mother's family: "I don't know whether they (the grandparents) were Jews or not." He also wonders if they emigrated out of Germany during National Socialism. However, he clearly considers his mother

Jewish: "As far as I know, she's Jewish. She's very into Jewish culture." In his understanding, Jewishness is obviously defined by Jewish culture. He defines himself as a Jew but also fears being identified as one and tries to keep his Jewish family background as inconspicuous as possible in his school. He is especially fearful of the neo-Nazis in his class, "although we get along very well." Asked to narrate his own life story, he says, "Hm, well, hm, so I was born at some point, and what really impressed me, well (3-second pause), hm (2-second pause), difficult to say (2-second pause), because the last thing I know is the radical change, the turning point here in the GDR, that's really impressive. . . . The last 2 years, now, also left their mark on me, because neo-Nazism and hatred toward foreigners and such like keep growing in Germany (2-second pause). That's also a little confusing (5-second pause) hm, (6-second pause) . . ."

For Ralf, as for his younger brother Roland, the fall of the wall brought about a sense of insecurity in their self-understanding, a simultaneous strengthening of the awareness of their Jewish origins and a growing fear of the neo-Nazis.

CONCLUDING REMARKS

The Baslers represent the type of family in which the focus on the emigration within the family story allows a denial and warding off of the unpleasant and threatening parts of their family history. This repair strategy helps achieve two things. First, the mourning around the murdered Jewish members of the family is split off. Second, the actions of the non-Jewish members from 1933 to 1945 are bracketed out of the family history. In other Jewish families, in which the grandparents were also forced to leave Germany, we observed the same repair strategy. Both in families in the GDR and in Israel, the family histories and life stories are narrated under the latent heading "Shoah" and the manifest ones of "emigration" and "living in the new society." In the ex-GDR families, the heading "emigration" could and still can be embedded in the socialist self-understanding of all three generations, because, for the grandparents, the "antifascist" trajectory began or could continue with such emigration.

What is GDR-specific in the Basler family is that they commemorate the victims of National Socialism in a peculiarly indirect way, through strategies of mourning directed supposedly at a non-Jewish resistance fighter. This corresponds to its public variant in the former GDR, reduced as it was to mourning the murdered communists exclusively. Antifascism therefore fulfills the function of a substitute mourning in such families.

As in other Jewish families, with the Baslers, the fact of the Nazi past of some members remains undisclosed. Instead, the family's common identification with communism is emphasized, and, in this way, the divergent family pasts are harmonized. The specific family dynamics that arise from such harmonization correspond to the larger social dynamics in the GDR. In this context, it is necessary to note that in order to present itself as the new, antifascist Germany, the GDR state rejected all continuity or connection with the Nazi past. Only that which bound everyone was stressed after 1945 (i.e., the building of a socialist society), and the difference in family histories resulting from different backgrounds could not be thematized. Even when both persecuted and persecutor could be found in one's family history, this social reality strengthened, indeed demanded, the individual need for harmony and denial. This mechanism, institutionalized over years, was seriously called into question after the wall came down in 1989. However, although this crisis widely affects such family histories, it may not be wrong to assume that as a first reaction, it will usher in even stronger defense mechanisms rather than an immediate opening up of familial dialogue.

For the Baslers, the denial of divergent family pasts spawned family secrets and the myth of the communist resistance fighter. These can only be revised with the help of far-reaching biographical processes of reinterpretation in the future. In the case of the grandsons, the existence of these secrets and myths has led to extreme confusion regarding both their own life stories and the general family history. This insecurity is strengthened by the fall of the wall, bringing, as it did, the possibility of new forms of self-definition and religious identification for ex-GDR citizens in general (Völter, 1994, 1998). Today, this transformation is not only a possibility but also a demand they are socially required to meet. Social transformations require reorientation of biographies, so hitherto unquestioned family and individual pasts have to be looked at anew. This process of looking back into the past may bring up more difficulties than one is equipped to deal with, and this, in turn, may lead to renewed blocking or excuses for certain sections of one's past.

REFERENCES

Bar-On, D. (1995). *Fear and hope: Three generations of the Holocaust.* Cambridge, MA: Harvard University Press.
Boszormeny-Nagy, I. (1975). Dialektische Betrachtung der Intergenerationen-Familientherapie. *Mariage - Ehe. Zentralblatt für Ehe- und Familienkunde.* Tübingen: Katzmann Verlag, 12, 117–131.
Danieli, Y. (1980). Countertransference in the treatment and study of Nazi Holocaust survivors and their children. *Victimology, 5*(2–4), 355–367.
Danieli, Y. (1982). Families of survivors of the Nazi Holocaust: Some short- and long-term effects. In C. Spiegelberger & I. Srasason (Eds.), *Stress and Anxiety Series in Clinical and Community Psychology,* (vol. 8, pp. 405–421). New York: Hemisphere.
Danieli, Y. (1993). Diagnostic and therapeutic use of the multigenerational family tree in working with survivors and children of survivors of the Nazi Holocaust. In J. P. Wilson & B. Raphael (Eds.), *International handbook of traumatic stress syndromes* (pp. 889–898). New York: Plenum Press.
Davidson, S. (1980). The clinical effects of massive psychic trauma in families of Holocaust survivors. *Journal of Marital and Family Therapy, 6*(1), 11–21.
Ferreira, A. J. (1963). Family myth and homeostasis. *Archives of General Psychiatry, 9,* 457–462.
Goldhagen, D. (1996). *Hitler's willing executioners.* New York: Knopf.
Heer, H., & Naumann, K. (Eds.). (1995). *Vernichtungskrieg: Verbrechen der Wehrmacht 1941–1944.* Hamburg: Hamburger Edition.
Hilberg, R. (1990). *Die Vernichtung der europäischen Juden.* Frankfurt a.M.: Fischer.
Jefferson, C. (1978). Some notes on the use of family sculpture in therapy. *Family Process, 17,* 68–76.
Karpel, M. A. (1980). Family secrets. *Family Process, 19,* 295–306.
Ostow, R. (1988). *Jüdisches Leben in der DDR.* Frankfurt a.M.: Athenäum.
Papp, P. Silverstein, O., & Carter, E. (1973). Family sculpting in preventive work with "well families." *Family Process, 12,* 197–212.
Richarz, M. (1988). Juden in der Bundesrepublik Deutschland und in der Deutschen Demokratischen Republik. In M. Brumlik, D. Kiesel, C. Kugelman, & J. Schoeps (Eds.), *Jüdisches Leben in Deutschland seit 1945* (13–30). Frankfurt a.M.: Athenäum.
Rosenthal, G. (Ed.). (1990). *"Als der Kreig kam, hatte ich mit Hitler nichts mehr zu tun." Zur Gegenwärtigkeit des "Dritten Reiches" in erzählten Lebensgeschichten.* Opladen: Leske & Budrich.
Rosenthal, G. (1991). German war memories: Narrability and the biographical and social functions of remembering. *Oral History, 19*(2), 34–41.
Rosenthal, G. (1992). Antisemitismus im lebensgeschichtlichen Kontext. Soziale Prozesse der Dehumanisierung und Schuldzuweisung. *ÖZG, Österreichische Zeitschrift für Geschichtswissenschaften, 3*(4), 449–479.
Rosenthal, G. (1993). Reconstruction of life stories: Principles of selection in generating stories for narrative biographical interviews. *Narrative Study of Lives, 1*(1), 59–91. Newbury Park, CA: Sage.
Rosenthal, G. (1994). Zur Konstitution von Generationen in familienbiographischen Prozessen. Krieg, Nationalsozialismus und Genozid in Familiengeschichte und Biographie. *ÖZG, Österreichische Zeitschrift für Geschichtswissenschaften, 5*(4), 489–516.
Rosenthal, G. (1995a). *Erlebte und erzählte Lebensgeschichte.* Frankfurt a.M.: Campus.

Rosenthal, G. (1995b). Familienbiographien: Nationalsozialismus und Antisemitismus im intergenerationellen Dia-
log. In I. Attia, N. Bosque, U. Kornfeld, G. Lyivanga, B. Rommelsbacher, P. Teimori, S. Vogelmann, & H.
Wachendorfer (Eds.), *Multikulturelle Gesellschaft und monukulturelle Psychologie? Antisemitismus und Rassis-
mus in der psychosozialen Arbeit* (pp. 30–51). Tübingen: Dgvt-Verlag.
Rosenthal, G. (Ed.). (1998). *The Holocaust in three-generations: Families of victims and perpetrators of the Nazi
regime.* London: Cassell.
Rosenthal, G., & Bar-On, D. (1992). A biographical case study of a victimizer's daughter. *Journal of Narrative and
Life History, 2*(2), 105–127.
Rosenthal, G., Völter, B. & Gilad, N. (1998): Israeli families of Forced Emigrants from Germany. In G. Rosenthal
(Ed.), *The Holocaust in three generations* (pp. 144–153). London: Cassel.
Runge, I. (1990). Grauzone des Wartens. *Blätter für deutsche und internationale Politik, 8,* 942–951.
Segev, T. (1993). *The seventh million: The Israelis and the Holocaust.* New York: Hill & Wang.
Schoeps, J. H. (1991). Jüdisches Leben in Nachkriegsdeutschland. In A. Nachama, J. Shoeps, & E. van Voolen (Eds.).
Jüdische Lebenswelten (pp. 352–281). Frankfurt a.M.: Jüdischer Verlag bei Suhrkamp.
Schütze, F. (1976). Zur Hervorlockung und Analyse von Erzählungen thematisch relevanter Geschichten im Rahmen
soziologischer Feldforschung. In Arbeitsgruppe Bielefelder Soziologen (ABS) (Eds.), *Kommunikative Sozial-
forschung* (pp. 159–260). Munich: Fink.
Sigal, J., Silver, D., Rakoff, V., & B. Ellin. (1973). Some second generation effects of survival of the Nazi persecu-
tion. *American Journal of Orthopsychiatry, 43*(3), 320–327.
Simon, F. (1972). Sculpting the family. *Family Process, 11,* 49–57.
Stierlin, H. (1981). The parent's Nazi past and the dialogue between the generations. *Family Process, 20*(4), 379–390.
Völter, B. (1994). "Ich bin diesen Feind noch nicht losgeworden." Verschärfter Identitätsdruck für ostdeutsche junge
Erwachsene. *ÖZG, Österreichische Zeitschrift für Geschichtswissenschaften, 5*(4), 547–566.
Völter, B. (1998). East German families of forced emigrants. In G. Rosenthal (Ed.), *The Holocaust in three genera-
tions* (pp. 198–239). London: Cassell.
Zilberman, T., & Rosenthal, G. (1994). The effects of the untold stories: The Steinberg/Noifeld family. In G. Rosen-
thal, N. Gilad, B. Völter, & T. Zilberman-Paz (Eds.), *Der Holocaust im Leben von drei Generationen.* Arbeits-
bericht für die Deutsche Forschungsgemeinschaft (pp. 124–150). Kassel/Berlin/Tel-Aviv.

19

Intergenerational Responses to Social and Political Changes
Transformation of Jewish Identity in Hungary

FERENC ERŐS, JÚLIA VAJDA, and ÉVA KOVÁCS

Jewish identity in the diaspora has always had its problematic sides, particularly in the last 100 years. As a consequence of factors such as secularization, the erosion or dissolution of traditional communities, and rapid assimilation processes, Jewish identity became more problematic, and its borders and definitions more vague, doubtful, or flexible. Definitions of "being a Jew" were relativized; they became various points on a scale that may range from belonging to a ritual community, to a distinct ethnic, religious and/or linguistic group, through belonging to more or less well-defined subcultures and/or traditions, to the point where no Jewish identity exists at all.

Nevertheless, before the rise of totalitarian regimes, it was, at least theoretically, the decision of the individual person where he or she wanted to belong or what form of Jewish identity among the existing choices he or she would prefer to maintain, cultivate, and pass on to the next generations. The assimilation process of Hungarian Jewry, however rapid and massive it was from the second half of the nineteenth century on, did leave open some room for individual choice. One could have been perfectly "assimilated" according to most of the sociological parameters (including choice of name, education, or even marriage and religion); this fact, however, did not necessarily prevent the individual from maintaining spiritual, social, or solidarity ties with other people perceived as Jewish. (On the assimilation process of Hungarian Jewry see, e.g., Hanák, 1984; Kovács, 1984; McKagg, 1989; Vágó, 1981). Moreover, Jews could belong to more than one community at the same time: They could be members of the Jewish community and, simultaneously, be full-fledged members of the political nation of which they were citizens.

It was the political anti-Semitism of the thirties and forties, raised to the level of official state policy, that first deprived them of their Hungarian identity and then imposed on them an externally and forcefully defined Jewish identity, based on race and blood. The Holocaust, the

FERENC ERŐS • Institute of Psychology, Hungarian Academy of Sciences, Teréz Krts. 13, H–1067 Budapest, Hungary.   JÚLIA VAJDA • Institute of Sociology, ELTE University, Budapest, Hungary.   ÉVA KOVÁCS • Institute for East European Studies, Budapest, Hungary.

International Handbook of Multigenerational Legacies of Trauma, edited by Yael Danieli. Plenum Press, New York, 1998.

annihilation of the Jews, was, in this sense, the logical consequence of a policy that denies and forcefully determines identity as an act of state. The Holocaust was the final deprivation of human identity and, for the majority, of life.

For the survivors of the Holocaust and their offspring, communism, the new totalitarian system emerging after 1945, promised a new society where no discrimination, whether racial, ethnic, or national, would exist. The universalistic claims of communist ideology were particularly appealing for a significant portion of Jews, because this ideology and this form of social organization were perceived as a guarantee that at least one category of identity—human identity as such—could not be denied to Jews or to other groups. In addition, the new regime offered special benefits for Jews as being practically the only major group in the country that was in no way affected or infected by the right-wing or fascist movements and ideologies of the recent past. The price for all this was, however, very high: Those who decided to find their place in the new regime had to give up the remnants of their Jewish identity, at least in all areas in public view. Jewish identity was marginalized again, and this marginalization was concomitant with the repression of the memory of the Holocaust. (On this topic, see more details in Karády, 1984, 1992, 1993.)

The crucial question is: What happened to Jewish identity in the intersection of repression and marginalization? How was it further distorted under the superimposing effects of the Holocaust and communism?

Forty years after the Holocaust, in the early 1980s, András Kovács, Katalin Lévai, and Ferenc Erős started a research project on Hungarian Jewish identity (see the following reports on this research: Erős, Kovács, & Lévai, 1985, 1988; Erős & Kovács, 1988; Erős, 1996). The project was basically a collection of detailed life histories of people belonging to the "second generation," whose parents survived the Holocaust. Most of our respondents were born in the period between 1945 and 1960. We found the signs of identity crisis and the search for identity in both what the respondents told us and what they did not talk about; the speech and the silence, the urge to talk as well as the fears and anxieties associated with raising these issues, all of this reminding us of our own ambivalent feelings. For many of us, the interview situation was the first step in a communicative experience; the interviews convinced both interviewer and interviewee that they were not quite alone in their ambivalences, in their dubious, vague feelings and knowledge about being Jewish—that there must be, however latently and marginally, a community or a group to which they could relate their own personal feelings.

From the scientific point of view, we were interested primarily in the specific features of identity formation, socialization, and personality development among the "second generation" in postwar Hungary. In the course of this research, we collected about 150 in-depth interviews, which are still only partly worked up. However, due to the sudden and, in many ways, unexpected political and social changes in the late eighties and early nineties, our interview materials became, in a way, "obsolete"; they belong now, so to speak, to the historical past. As is well known, in the past few years, the public representation of Jewish identity changed dramatically in Hungary. Nowadays, Jewish identity, or at least various elements of a Jewish identity, can be openly expressed. There are now different organizations, cultural and educational facilities, and there is a revival of, or at least a growing interest in, religious and cultural traditions and values. On the other hand, as is also well known, there is a growing, or at least more visible, tendency towards anti-Semitism in the country. (On anti-Semitism after 1989, see Erős & Fábiá, 1995; Postma, 1996.) The large-scale political, social, and economic transformation process has created new types of conflicts for Jews as well as non-Jews in Hungary.

When we conducted our interviews in the eighties, the hegemony of the communist party state was still, at least seemingly, unbroken. To be sure, the questions were the same as today;

for example, who is a Jew, what is a Jew, what does it mean to be Jewish in Hungary, what are the basic factual and ideological elements of a Jewish identity? However, these questions were pronounced only in the privacy of the interview situation. Let us now examine in some details the construction of Jewish identity as seen through these interviews.

THE HOLOCAUST AND JEWISH IDENTITY

Our research project originated, historically, as a sociopsychological study of the post-Holocaust generation. It was no coincidence that the Holocaust was central in our questions. First, we felt that it was precisely the issue that was forcefully (and also voluntarily) excluded from public discussion; second, we learned, at that time, of the clinical, psychological, and psychoanalytical studies dealing with the traumatizing effects of the Holocaust and the (unconscious) transmission of the trauma to the next generation. These studies had been done in Western countries and in Israel, but similar work was started also in Hungary in the early eighties, almost parallel to our interviews, by Teréz Virág (1984, 1988, 1994; see also other relevant Hungarian psychoanalytic studies: Cserne, Pető, Szilágyi, & Szőke, 1992; Mészáros, 1990, 1992; Pető, 1992; Szilágyi, 1994; Vánai, 1994; Virág & Vikár, 1985; Vikár, 1994). Virág's work and the subsequent works of other therapists and researchers also revealed the so-called "Survivor's Syndrome" and the "Second-Generation Syndrome," which are so well known in the psychoanalytic literature on the Holocaust (e.g., Bergman & Jucovy, 1982; Daneli, 1982; Kestenberg, 1982; Krystal, 1968; Wardi, 1992).

Our interviews were, of course, not psychoanalytic, though we endeavored to utilize some principles and methods of analytic interview technique. When talking about their parents, many respondents described them as completely depressed, emotionally emptied persons who were, or still are, unable to talk about or cope with the memory of the extreme situations they survived, including the deaths of their close kin. When talking about themselves, our interviewees related their fears, anxieties, persecution dreams, and daydreams that haunt this generation. It was clear from our interviews that the memory of persecution was psychologically transmitted to the subsequent generation, which, in turn, made the Holocaust to appear as a primary constituent of identity. This process and its outcomes well agreed with the psychoanalytic finding that trauma would destroy the most primal, earliest attachments of the person, the very core of any healthy identity. Extreme traumatization may lead to silence and incapacity to communicate, and the traumatic experience becomes inaccessible, encapsulated in the psyche. Unconsciously transmitted to the second generation, this aspect of the trauma created the "Second-Generation Syndrome," a secondary, though somewhat fainter blueprint of the original "Survivor Syndrome." Our interview subjects more or less displayed the signs of this syndrome—albeit not so dramatically or consistently as what was reported in the clinical papers on the related population. The most striking feature of our interviewees was what is termed "object relational problems" in psychoanalytic literature: disturbed, ambivalent relations, or sometimes a complete inability to communicate with relevant "objects" of the external world—with parents, partners or peers, and so on.

These ambivalences and disturbed object relations were characteristic for many respondents in their relationship to Judaism itself. For most of them, Jewish identity essentially meant belonging to a persecuted group, being "children of the Holocaust." One of our respondents expressed it in the following way: "Among surviving Jews, there is a kind of . . . disunited or unconscious sympathy toward the person who—if not himself, then his parents—suffered through the same thing. You cannot ignore it, if, when you are speaking with someone, his shirtsleeve slides up and discloses a number tattooed on his arm. Among a person's close and distant acquaintances, there is certain to be someone who fell victim . . . but even if everyone in the entire family survived the catastrophe, that, too, will have caused terrible damage. Of course, this . . . is a kind of unifying force."

We can conclude that at the depth of Hungarian Jewish identity in the eighties, the trauma of the Holocaust was still a major determining factor. The reduction of Jewish identity to the common experience of being victimized or being a child of victims signifies the fact that in the decades after the war, there was practically no possibility for Jews in Hungary to work through the past; the public taboo contributed to the prolongation of private sufferings. This reduction was, on the other hand, part of another tendency: assimilation.

In our interviews, we attempted to explore sociological and historical dimensions, too, by asking our respondents to narrate the life histories of their family members going back three generations. These life histories reveal typical assimilation strategies. Identity formulations, themselves based on the Holocaust and on the awareness of common sufferings, worked, in many cases, as a special assimilation strategy. We mean here that someone can be perfectly un-aware of the elements of Jewish religion, tradition, or culture; someone might have no essential relationship to Judaism at all, but, at the same time, the person can assume that there is no need to rediscover such ties, because being a child of survivors is sufficient by itself to make him or her belong to the Jewish group, in such a way and to such an extent as the person might wish it. In principle, then, someone can be a good Hungarian, a good Christian, a good Communist, and so on; being Jewish has nothing to do with the person's actual group affiliations. In other words, for most of our respondents, being Jewish meant belonging to some kind of secondary or vir-tual community, based not so much on common interactions as on allusive identifications.

THE STRATEGY OF SILENCE

In the second layer of Hungarian Jewish identity, we found what we called the "strategy of silence." Whereas secondary traumatization means unconscious transmission of the trauma suffered by the parents, the "strategy of silence" means a more or less conscious effort on the part of the parents to conceal the fact of their belonging to the once-persecuted group. Chil-dren growing up in these families experienced an inconceivable family secret and were social-ized in an environment where tradition had been more or less eliminated and the generational continuity of the family history broken. Analysis of the interview material within the context of the question, "How did you come to realize that you are Jewish?", revealed that, for many respondents, even learning that they were Jewish proved to be an extremely conflictual emo-tional experience. Often, they had been "enlightened" by strangers, and, even when the "en-lightenment" took place in the family, it was typically a reaction to a painful situation experienced by the child or adolescent outside the family (see more details in Erős *et al.,* 1985, 1988). A respondent told us: "At the age of 13, I didn't know what it meant to be Jewish. I didn't even know the word. This may sound strange, but at that time, when I first heard the word, it was not from them [the parents], but from a friend 4 years older than myself. He told me that we were Jews and all about what happened to the Jews. It was then that I learned for the first time what happened to us, and I became very frightened, and ever since then, I haven't been able to accept these facts. The truth of the matter is that I have never been particularly willing or able to deal with it, believing, as a matter of principle, that if I close my eyes, they cannot see me. In short, if I don't deal with the problem, then there won't be any, just there won't be any anti-Semitism."

JEWS AND COMMUNISTS

The previous quotation speaks for itself. If you don't speak about the problems, they don't exist, and what is more important, if you close your eyes, they cannot see you. The strategy of silence and "closed eyes" was, first of all, characteristic of those families where communism was the dominant ideology. "We were communists, not Jewish." "Our family had nothing to do with Jews. It was only an accident that we were Jewish; we were communists, and it was much more important. . . . We belonged to a larger family, and in relation to this, our being Jewish had no significance." These and similar statements show the efforts of the parents to get rid of their Jewishness by accepting and enforcing the "universalistic" values of communism. One of our respondents found—in her later years—the cadre file of his father. In the cadre file, she read the curricula vitae (CVs) her father was forced to write in the early fifties. Each year, the father wrote: "I have a 4- [or 5-, 6- . . .] year-old daughter. My greatest wish is to raise her so that she becomes a valuable member of our socialist society." As these children were growing up, they were told, "If people ask you what your religion is, you should tell them that you have no religious affiliation." For children growing up in the fifties, this itself sometimes became the basis of discrimination. For example, in contrast to the majority of their classmates, they celebrated not Christmas but the birthday of Comrade Stalin (December 21). It would be easy to argue that these parents refused to be Jewish because they strongly believed in communist ideology. We think, however, that there were deeper and more complex motives. These motives are clearly stated in a sentence quoted by one of our respondents from his father, who was a high-ranking functionary: "There is no God after Auschwitz. After all those things happened to us, there is, there must, be no God." If there is no God, there are no traditions; one has to break with everything that, even distantly, has associations with God. In this respect, communism was a radical negation of religion, because it absolutely excludes the existence of God. Communism is a revenge against the God who allowed all this to happen. The same respondent told us: "When I was a little child, I needed a circumcision for simple health reasons. The doctor said, 'He must be circumcised!' But my parents did not consent to the operation. My father somehow procured some penicillin (it was very difficult in the fifties), and I was cured."

He related then the following story. An uncle smuggled food to the ghetto in a Hungarian Nazi (arrow-cross) uniform. He was caught, made to pull down his trousers, and beaten almost to death. This narrative explains clearly the deeper, nonrational motive of affiliating with communism. It was depression, the emptiness of the self. "My father," our respondent told us, "did not exist inside. . . . After Auschwitz there was no inside, as there is no Jewish life. This is our tragedy, and this will be the tragedy of our children: the inhibition of the internal family life. In a certain sense, this made the family dead . . . because we were in the selection process. If there had been any family life, any inside solidarity, it should have been Jewish. But who wanted it?"

BREAKING THE SILENCE

Is this the end of the story? In a certain way, it was only the beginning. The next layer is what we would call the "breaking the silence." For many respondents, these interviews were the first occasion at which they could speak about this topic in a more or less systematic way. We asked them to tell as many family legends, stories, childhood memories (even the most insignificant ones) as they could remember. "Just tell everything that occurs to your mind in relation to this topic!" We were then able to observe the narrative construction of Jewish identity, the process by which identity was created through telling "stories." These stories were full of pictures of a lost world, secondhand memories, and incomprehensible words that were, for the first time, put together into a systematic narrative. In this way, the process of reconstruction of the continuity of the family history may have begun.

To be sure, most of the identity-relevant statements were formulations of a marginal identity. To be Jewish means a vague feeling of being different, but the terms in which these differences are measured are not always clear. The majority of our respondents stated that most of their friends, as well as their partners, were Jewish, without their having consciously sought out only Jewish contacts. In any case, however, the discovery of whether another person is Jewish or not is basically a metacommunicative experience, as it is very difficult to formulate the criteria verbally by which a person's affiliation can be ascertained.

This is the ideological side of identity, the ideological elaboration of group differences: what it means to be Jewish. It is the elaboration of group differences, that is, the way of finding out in what way Jews and non-Jews differ from each other. Most of our respondents worked out highly personalized criteria for this. They often described Jews as being more emotional, more family loving, more intelligent, possessing a greater sense of self-irony and humor, and drinking less alcohol. We also encountered highly intellectualized ideologies concerning the role of Jews played in Hungarian or European history and culture.

Beyond the ideological formulations, there is another aspect of identity that we may call "interactional identity." It is an identity model according to which the person manifests his or her self in actual social situations that can be sometimes conflictual and tense. According to our experience, "being Jewish" in concrete situations is a "borderline" problem. This means that Jewish identity may come up only as a reaction to an extreme situation, for example, if one becomes target of anti-Semitic statements or attacks. "Basically, I am not Jewish, but if I meet an anti-Semite, I become Jewish" is the typical formulation of a reactive, marginal, "borderline" Jewish identity manifested in concrete interactions.

BEYOND IDENTITY CRISIS

In our interviews, however, we discovered the beginnings of another kind of Jewish identity: a positive relation to Judaism, the recognition that "being Jewish" means not just humiliation, suffering, psychological disturbance, and discrimination. The development of a positive identity comes after "breaking the silence." This creates a new situation. When "being Jewish" appears primarily as an intrapsychic, emotional problem, there are no open conflicts. After "breaking the silence," however, one has to choose and reveal one's identity in public situations, too. The previous regime, the Kádár era, when our interviews were done, was the world of "private deals" between citizens and the state. The problem of "being Jewish" was, in a way, an "underground" problem; Jewish identity existed as a marginal identity. The open, public manifestation of identify was blocked out by a series of political and social obstacles. One of the basic experiences of post-Holocaust second-generation Jews was that the topic of Jewry was silenced and treated as a taboo; it was considered a kind of hidden secret in both public and informal channels of social communication. Discussion of the topic between generations and peers could only take place in a restricted family–friend environment. Such an experience—depicted in interviews, case studies, and other reports—determined and accompanied early and late (adolescence, youth) socialization and identity development of the second generation.

However, at the end of the seventies and early eighties, in an era of changing social, ideological, and political conditions, a series of historical, sociological literary works and films cracked the wall of silence by giving access to the topic of the history of the Hungarian Jewry, anti-Semitism, and certain other topics related to the Holocaust. The fact that a problem that remained hidden for long decades has now surfaced proves that silencing has been replaced by processes involving remembering and working through. A condition for initiating such processes was realized by establishing communication and collective reflection related to the topic of Jewry. István Bibó's study (1984) on the Jewish question in Hungary, originally published in 1948, became accessible to the larger public in this era, a basic study, to date, concerning political and historical discussion of the subject. The basic traits of the history of Hungarian Jewry—especially its modern, 20th-century history—commenced to be defined in works published in the seventies and eighties. Publications presented themes involving the role of Jewry in the establishment of a modern Hungary and Hungarian bourgeois culture, the contradictory process of assimilation and its tragic dilemmas, development of modern anti-Semitism and its process of radicalization, detailed research of the history of the Hungarian Holocaust, and, last but not least, the place of the Jewry as a social group in the Rákosi and Kádár regimes—sociological and social psychological aspects of the relationship between Jews and non-Jews (see, e.g., Bibó, 1984; Braham, 1990; Ember, 1994; Hanák, 1984; Kovács, 1984; Várdy, 1984).

Historical, sociological, and artistic debates in the late seventies and early eighties played a major role in open public discussion and intellectual awareness of problems related to Jewry, and served as a basis for establishing a Jewish identity for second-generation Jews. For this generation, it became more and more important to search for "roots," to discover the repressed and forgotten past and Jewish culture, to become acquainted with Jewish history and tradition, and to establish group experiences that would create a solid ground for Jewish identity (Jewish cultural groups, discussion groups meeting in private apartments, introduction and performance of religious rituals and customs, and self-organization within the framework of politically determined limits). Therefore, some of our interviewees started to reflect on the question: Which of the existing models of Jewish identity should they accept? Religious, traditional, cultural, ethnic, and national models and their combinations had already emerged as possible models of Jewish identity.

In our day, the problem of Jewish identity seem to be acquiring new aspects. On the one hand, new and public appearances of anti-Semitism or "neo-anti-Semitism" awaken the feeling of being Jewish even in some of those people who, until now, tried to avoid the problem by applying the "strategy of silence." On the other hand, the new, sometimes rather harsh anti-Semitic propaganda evokes new fears and anxieties. In general, however, it is hoped that the emerging new, autonomous civil society will give the full possibility for renewal of Jewish identity and commitment to this identity without any external and internal constraint. It is difficult to predict what models and forms of Jewish identity will be dominant, or even if any of these will be dominant. It seems to us that it is not possible to prescribe any uniquely valid identity model. The plurality of identity models can really be developed only after "breaking the silence," that is, only in a process in the course of which the elements of social and individual pathology gradually lose their significance. This development also presupposes that there are no social and political situations in which certain categories of identity are forcefully exiled to the margin. In this respect, the question of Jewish identity is a question of democracy—as are all questions of minority identity throughout the world.

In the newly started Jewish ethnic renaissance, we see three major tendencies. One is the religious one, strengthening of religious identity, which is not limited to either the more intensive approach to religion by families who had been religious even earlier, or to stricter observance of religious rules, though the latter was supported by newly emerging possibilities (kosher food shops, Jewish schools, and so on). However, individual conversions, returning to the Jewish religion, can be observed in Hungary in increasing numbers. The American Foundation School is, for example, a creation of this religious renaissance. The second trend is modern Zionism, forming Jewish identity as a national one. The symbolic system of this identity is well elaborated and through the intervention of Israeli and American Zionist organizations, it has already appeared in Hungary. Still, it seems to us that Zionism is not an attractive force at this time. The third, most intensive trend is the creation and strengthening of a group identity defined by liberal Jewish Hungarian traditions. Specific elements of this identity are liberal political attitudes, preserving Jewish Hungarian cultural traditions, the lifestyle of large-city (Budapest) intellectuals, secularism, and stressing only the cultural and historical elements of the religion. Javne Lauder Community School "targets" the demands of this liberal Jewish intellectual subculture.

In the fall of 1989, two independent twelfth-grade Jewish schools were founded in Budapest: the American Foundation School and the Javne Lauder Community School. These schools have not only played an important role in the identity transformations of the adult generation, but also created new possibilities for the younger generation. The Jewish character of these schools is, of course, important for the parents, though to various degrees. For some of them, the Jewish nature itself is the most important, but there are many parents who appreciate the tolerant or even liberal mentality of the schools, or just the mere fact that twelfth-grade schools may save their children from high school enrollment on a strong, competitive basis. Nevertheless, the Jewishness of the school is always a decisive element of choice. Parents who take their children to these schools allow the world to identify them through the school as Jews, and as "liberals," too. In this context, choosing a school means choosing an identity as well (see the extensive sociological and social psychological research on the Jewish schools in Budapest done by É. Kovács and Vajda, 1994).

The life of the third generation is not thoroughly determined by the communist period. They were born in the era of "consumer socialism," and they are thus children of a more pragmatic, up-to-date, technocratic world. By the time a genuine sensitivity to social problems developed in them, the old political regime was over. For them, the polyphony of the world is much more natural than for the earlier generation. They are not even surprised by the fact that a Jewish school can be created from one day to the next. Of course, we know from psychotherapeutic case studies that this generation may also carry the trauma of the Holocaust. Nevertheless, they are the ones—especially those who go to Jewish schools or actively participate in Jewish organizations—who fulfill a kind of a mediating role between Jewish culture and tradition, and the older generations. They are the ones who "take home" Jewish culture, and they are the ones who make their parents and grandparents encounter and face their Jewish origin. (On the "third generation," see also Gur, 1992.)

These are the main trends that determine the identity of three Jewish generations after 1945. Individual family histories, life stories, and personal experiences may greatly vary within them. As to the changes in relation to Jewish identity, the situation of members of the second generation is the hardest, since they, even if born Jewish, had been growing up as if this fact had not played a role in their identity. For many of them, it was truly traumatic in adolescence or in young adulthood to face the fact and weight of their origin. This was then followed by a quiet period in the seventies, when the problem of Jewish origin was pushed into the background, only to emerge again in the eighties. Among the many taboos touched upon during the change of the political regime, claims to conceptualize Jewish identity came into the forefront again. Jewish institutions have been mushrooming. Now, this euphoria seems to have disappeared, as if Jewish identity and related discussions are not so important any longer. To reveal the causes of this phenomenon is a task of further research. Members of this generation reflect social changes in a rather sophisticated way, since their relation to their own identity is closely connected to these problems. This phenomenon is interesting even in itself, since this generation fluctuates between choosing or pushing into the background ethnic or cultural identity. If so, then we face a typical Central European "identity," which other ethnic groups in the region share, because traumas caused by permanent changes of political systems and state boundaries in the last century, and also ethnic polyphony, might have made other ethnic groups uncertain as to their identity as well.

REFERENCES

Bibó, I. (1984). Zsidókérdés Magyarországon 1944 után [The Jewish Question in Hungary after 1984]. In P. Hanák (Ed.), 135–294. In German: *Zur Judenfrage. Am Beispiel Ungarns nach 1944*. Frankfurt am Main, 1990.

Bergman, M. S., & Jucovy, E. H. (Eds.). (1982). *Generations of the Holocaust*. New York: Basic Books.

Braham, R. L. (1990). *A magyar Holocaust*. Budapest: Gondolat. (Originally published as *The politics of genocide: The Holocaust in Hungary*, New York: Columbia University Press, 1981.)

Cserne, I., Petõ, K., Szilágyi, J., & Szõke, G. (1992). Az elsõ és a második generáció [The first and second generation]. *Psychiatria Hungarica, 7*(2), 117–131.

Danieli, Y. (1982). Families of survivors of the Nazi Holocaust: Some short- and long-term effects. In N. Milgram (Ed.), *Psychological stress and adjustment in time of war and peace* (pp. 405–421). Washington, DC: Hemisphere.

Eitinger, L., & Major, E. F. (1993). Stress of the Holocaust. In L. Goldberger and S. Breznitz (Eds.), *Handbook of Stress. Theoretical and Clinical Aspects*. 2d ed (pp. 617–640). New York: Free Press.

Ember, M. (1994). A Holocaust a magyar prózairodalomban. [The Holocaust in the Hungarian prose] Kabdebó, L., and Schmidt, E. (Eds.), *A Holocaust a mûvészetekben*. Pécs: Janus Pannonius Egyetemi Kiadó. 155–159.

Erõs, F. (1988). Megtörni a hallgatást [Breaking the silence]. In *Múlt és Jövõ: Zsidó kulturális antológia* (pp. 19–27). Budapest: Szimultán.

Erõs, F. (1996). The construction of Jewish identity in the 1980s. In Y. Kashti, F. Erõs, D. Schers, & D. Zisenswine (Eds.), *A quest for identity: Post-War Jewish identities. Studies in Jewish culture, identity and community* (pp. 51–70). Tel Aviv: School of Education, Tel Aviv University.

Erõs, F., & Fábián, Z. (1995). Antisemitism in Hungary 1990–1994. In W. Benz (Ed.), *Jahrbuch für Antisemitismusforschung 4* (pp. 342–356). Frankfurt and New York: Campus Verlag.

Erõs, F., & Kovács, A. (1988). The biographical method in the study of Jewish identity. In T. Hofer & P. Niedermüller (Eds.), *Life history as cultural construction/performance* (pp. 345–356). Budapest: Institute of Ethnography of the Hungarian Academy of Sciences.

Erõs, F., Kovács, A., & Lévai, K. (1985). Comment j'en suis arrivé à apprendre que j'étais juif? *Actes de la Recherche en Sciences Sociales, 56,* 63–68.

Erõs, F., Kovács, A., & Lévai, K. (1988). Wie ich schliesslich gemerkt habe, dass ich Jude bin: Interviews mit ungarischen Juden aus der Nachkriegeneration. *Babylon. Beiträge zur jüdishen Gegenwart.* Heft 3, 65–79.

Gur, N. (1992). A kortárscsoport szerepe a magyarországi zsidó fiatalok identitásának kialakulásában [The role of the peer group in the development of identity of young Hungarian Jews]. In M. M. Kovács, Y. Kashti, & F. Erõs (Eds.), *Zsidóság, identitás, történelem* (pp. 141–155). Budapest: T-Twins.

Hanák, P. (Ed.). (1984). *Zsidókérdés, asszimiláció, antiszemitizmus* [Jewish question, assimilation, anti-Semitism]. Budapest: Gondolat.

Karády, V. (1984). Szociológiai kísérlet a magyar zsidóság 1945 és 1956 közötti helyzetének elemzésére [A sociological attempt to analyze the situation of the Hungarian Jewry between 1945 and 1956]. In P. Kende (Ed.), *Zsidóság az 1945 utáni Magyarországon* (pp. 37–180). Paris: Magyar Füzetek.

Karády, V. (1992). A Shoah, a rendszerváltás és a zsidóság azonosságtudata Magyarországon [The Shoah, the change of the political system, and the identity of the Jews in Hungary]. In M. M. Kovács, Y. Kashti, & F. Erõs (Eds.), *Zsidóság, identitás, történelem* (p. 23–48). Budapest: T-Twins.

Karády, V. (1993). Beyond assimilation: Dilemmas of Jewish identity in contemporary Hungary. *Discussion Papers,* No. 2. Budapest: Collegium Budapest.

Kestenberg, J. (1982). Survivor-parents and their children. In M. S. Bergman & E. H. Jucovy (Eds.) *Generations of the Holocaust* (pp. 83–102). New York: Basic Books.

Kovács, A. (1984). A zsidókérdés a mai magyar társadalomban [The Jewish question in the contemporary Hungarian society]. In P. Kende (Ed.), *Zsidóság az 1945 utáni Magyarországon* (pp. 1–35). Paris: Magyar Füzetek.

Kovács, A. (1988). Az asszimilációs dilemma [The dilemma of assimilation] *Világosság, 8–9,* 605–613.

Kovács, E., & Vajda, J. (1994). *"I have a certificate of not being an anti-Semite." Identity of a "Social Jew": Its roots in life history.* Paper presented at the 13th World Congress of Sociology, Bielefeld, Germany.

Kovács, E., & Vajda, J. (1995). *Blacks are not usually labelled Jews: Why does a mulatto boy got to a Jewish school?* Paper presented at the conference of the European Sociological Association, Budapest, Hungary.

Kovács, E., & Vajda, J. (1996). *Three versions of a story: A menorah in a non-Jewish family.* Paper presented at the Conference on the Linguistic Construction of Social and Personal Identity, Évora, Portugal.

Kovács, M. M., Kashti, Y., & Erős, F. (Eds.). (1992). *Zsidóság, identitás, történelem* [Jewry, identity, history]. Budapest: T-Twins.

Krystal, H. (Ed.). (1968). *Massive psychic trauma.* New York: International Universities Press.

McCagg, W. O. (1989). *A history of Habsurg Jews, 1670–1918.* Bloomington: Indiana University Press.

Mészáros, J. (1990). A társadalmi elfojtások megjelenése a pszichoanalízisben [The appearence of social repressions in psychoanalysis]. *Thalassa, 1*(1), 131–138.

Mészáros, J. (1992). Az elfojtott visszatér [The return of the repressed]. In M. M. Kovács, Y. Kashti, F. Erős (Eds.), *Zsidóság, identitás, történelem* (pp. 114–172). Budapest: T-Twins.

Pető, K. (1992). Engem za antiszemitizmus sodort a zsidók közé [Anti-Semitism pushed me among the Jews]. In M. M. Kovács, Y. Kashti, F. Erős (Eds.), *Zsidóság, identitás, történelem* (pp. 128–140). Budapest: T-Twins.

Postma, K. (1996). *Changing prejudice in Hungary. A study on the collapse of state socialism and its impact on prejudice against Gypsies and Jews.* Groningen: Rijksuniversiteit Groningen.

Szilágyi, J. (1994). Egy zsidó származású páciens analízise [Analysis of a patient of Jewish origin]. *Thalassa, 5*(1–2), 160–168.

Vágó, B. (1981). *Jewish assimilation in modern times.* Boulder, CO: Westview.

Várdy, P. (1984.) A magyarországi zsidóüldözések a hazai történetírásban. [The persecution of the Jews in the Hungarian historiography]. In P. Kende (Ed.), *Zsidóság az 1945 utáni Magyarországon* (pp. 181–219). Paris: Magyar Füzetek.

Várnai, G. (1994). A Holocaust késői pszichoszomatikus és pszichoszociális hatásai [Late psychosomatic and social effects of the Holocaust]. *Thalassa, 5*(1–2), 147–159.

Vikár, G. (1994). Zsidó sors(ok) az analitikus rendelés tükrében [Jewish fate[s] in the mirror of analytic therapy]. *Thalassa, 5*(1–2), 139–146.

Vikár, G., & Virág, T. (1985). Pszichotrauma elaborációja a gyermekpszichoterápiában [The elaboration of psychological trauma in child psychotherapy]. *Magyar Pszichológiai Szemle, 2,* 129–139.

Virág, T. (1984). Children of the Holocaust and their children's children: Working through current trauma in the psychotherapeutic process. *Dynamic Psychotherapy, 2*(1), 47–60.

Virág, T. (1988). A Holocaust-szindróma feldolgozása már folyamatban lévő pszichoterápiában [The elaboration of the Holocaust syndrome in the course of psychotherapy]. In *Klinikai Gyermekpszichológiai Tanulmányok* (pp. 72–82). Budapest: Akadémiai Kiadó.

Virág, T. (1994). A Holocaust-szindróma megjelenése a pszichoterápiás gyakorlatban [The appearance of the Holocaust syndrome in the practice of psychotherapy]. *Thalassa, 5*(1–2), 129–138.

Wardi, D. (1992). *Memorial candles: The children of the Holocaust.* London-New York: Tavistock-Routledge. (1995 Hungarian translation, Budapest: Ex Libris)

VI

Indigenous Peoples

20

Intergenerational Aspects of Trauma for Australian Aboriginal People

BEVERLEY RAPHAEL, PATRICIA SWAN, and NADA MARTINEK

Australian Aboriginal peoples constitute a multitude of tribal and cultural groups. Their presence on the Australian continental land mass can be established as going back as far as 60,000 years, and they represent the oldest continuous, identified culture of people in the world today. They were generally a nomadic people, although with different communities and family occupying relatively defined areas of land, their tribal lands. These lands were identified through knowledge passed down in oral traditions. Particular understandings and "Law" were held by tribal elders, but the rich cultural heritage was for the most part understood and valued by all peoples. There were over 600 languages and groups.

In 1788, the first white settlement was established formally in Australia, the Colony of New South Wales, at Sydney. The Australian continent had been claimed by Captain James Cook for the British in 1770, although there had been other non-Aboriginal explorers, including Dutch and Portuguese. A core understanding that must be incorporated into any consideration of intergenerational aspects of trauma is that in claiming this land for the British and in colonizing it, it was seen as "Terra Nullius" (i.e., a land of no peoples). This meant that from the very beginning, there was a denial by the white colonizers of the reality of Aboriginal peoples as human beings, and of their rights to the land they had inhabited for millennia. This loss of land is a potent background to understanding trauma and its intergenerational effects for Aboriginal people, for it impacted on their well-being and has continued to do so in many ways.

This was the more so because of the close relationships between the tribal groups and their land, their own places of being, in terms of spiritual meanings as well as physical survival. Indeed, Aboriginal peoples' understanding and management of the ecology of their land was

BEVERLEY RAPHAEL • Director, Centre for Mental Health, NSW Health Department, North Sydney, NSW 2059 Australia.   **PATRICIA SWAN** • Aboriginal Health Resource Cooperative, Box 1565, Strawberry Hills, NSW 2012 Australia.   **NADA MARTINEK** • Department of Psychiatry, The University of Queensland, Brisbane, Australia.

International Handbook of Multigenerational Legacies of Trauma, edited by Yael Danieli. Plenum Press, New York, 1998.

complex and sophisticated. Similarly, their interpersonal relationships, kinship, and communities were complex and governed by requirements for behavior, relating, and understandings that were sophisticated and balanced, and showed among other things, gender equity.

In considering Aboriginal people as of little consequences, the white invaders set the pattern for the next 200 years. Aboriginal people were not given the right to vote until 1967, and it was only in June 1992 that the High Court in the Mabo decision acknowledged the land rights of Aboriginal peoples.

Thus, the first pervasive and ongoing level of trauma experienced by Aboriginal peoples in Australia was dispossession and denial of their rights. O'Shane (1995), speaking of the psychological impact of white colonization on Aboriginal people, emphasises how pervasive this impact was and is. "Dispossession, defined in terms of land, is however, too narrow a view of the experience of dispossession that has been ours. In the process of expropriation of the land the colonisers also destroyed our communities" (p. 150). She goes on to recount how families were driven or taken from their homelands, and how this continued until the most recent times.

A second component of this pervasive and ongoing traumatization related to a complete denial of the human rights of Aboriginal people, who were seen by the early colonists as "sub-human." This was associated also with a failure to recognize the family and kinship structure of Aboriginal life. Not surprisingly, there is also a history of repeated attempts to "wipe out" Aboriginal groups with massacres, poisoning of food and water supplies, and virtual annihilation in some states, such as Tasmania. Subjugation of surviving Aboriginal peoples and enforcement of non-Aboriginal language and culture led to a breakdown of traditional family life, which was essential to the passing on of Aboriginal ways of life, language, and cultural practice. Thus, active discrimination, denigration, the breaking down of culture, racism, and denial of the most basic rights added a second level of ongoing traumatic experience to the background of distress impacting on Aboriginal peoples. As O'Shane states, "The psychological impact of these experiences of dispossession, racism, exclusion, extermination, denigration and degradation are beyond description" (p. 157) and "they strike at the very core of our sense of being and identity" (p. 151).

Many specific policies introduced by the colonizers, allegedly for their good and protection, also had traumatic effects. One such group of policies focusing on Aboriginal children and families demands particular attention (Kendall, 1994). Describing the history of removal of Aboriginal children in Australia Kendall stated that this had been a constant theme from the time of colonization, later formalized in specific legislation and regulation. The six states and the Commonwealth Government had each introduced "policies which contributed to large numbers of Aboriginal children being removed from their families, communities and culture" (p. 18). Such policies arose, she suggests, to blend Aboriginal people with the white population, to assimilate and civilize them, and to train them for the "lower orders of white society." These specific aims were formally spelled out in many of the policies; for instance, "dissociating the children from camp life must eventually solve the Aboriginal problem." Particular emphasis was placed on children who were "half-caste" or had other levels of Aboriginal/white mix. It was expected that the race would gradually fade out, as the circumstances of living of those left behind would lead to their extermination, and their offspring, reared among the whites, would gradually become more "white." It is not surprising that Aboriginal people interpreted this as genocide. Every aspect of the lives of Aboriginal peoples was controlled, including where they could go and who they could marry throughout much of this period, unless they lived in such remote places as not to have interacted with the colonizing groups, whose influence spread rapidly through pastoral holdings and later mining. Those children taken away were reared for domestic work (girls) or farm labor (boys), or for adoption by white families.

The traumatic ways in which these separations took place, and their impact on both parents and children, are conveyed in the following examples taken from the recent report "Learning from the Past" (1994).

One of the most common memories is of a government car driving up the road to the mission: "They just took them. . . . Parents were never asked for consent. . . . That's why when a car came with officials the children would run away and hide" (Edwards, 1982). One man interviewed for this report said he would have "defied anyone to find me and my sister in the little hideout mum and dad made in the bush for us," and remembered how he hid in a cave. "As soon as the police used to come up the hill, mum used to scream, and we used to run and hide, even too frightened to breathe. . . . If we heard mum outside we wouldn't even speak until mum came and got us." A woman again reports: "After we were stolen . . . mum had another child, a boy, and he was also taken. How could they do that? How could they pick on us? No one to this day has told us why we were taken away and why we were told that our mother was dead. How horrible it has been; why do they do these things?"

Justification for taking children in these ways often came from the appalling conditions in which Aborigines and their families were living. But poor conditions arose because of the ways in which Aboriginal people had been treated. Their rich cultural and community life, which placed such a strong emphasis on kinship, family, and the care of children, was denied, and the physical circumstances of their existence in fringe camps or on white properties invalidated their competence and capacities.

Children were also taken as infants and when very young, and frequently were reared as "white," so that many grew up knowing nothing of their Aboriginal heritage. In some instances, brothers and sisters were kept together; in others, they were separated and could not comfort, or did not know the fate of one another. One woman, taken with other Aboriginal girls, remembers "screaming like mad because I wanted to go back to my mother." She and her sisters, when in the Half-Caste Home "used to try to run away," but couldn't escape, "so we just cried all the time to go back to our country."

These and innumerable other accounts attest to the intense, traumatic, and painful separation and loss experienced by Aboriginal children and families in these horrific circumstances. While policies eventually changed, after Aboriginal people attained equity in terms of citizenship (1967), they persisted to a degree beyond that time. And formal policies, no longer politically correct, were replaced by more subtle and institutionalized forms of separation that continue to the present. Kendall (1994) reports from the point of view of her organization, Link-Up, which was developed to help Aboriginal people find their families: "we who were being removed until very recently and in some areas are still being removed from our families." "The oldest client in our organisation is 107 years old and the youngest is still being born" (Kendall, 1994, p. 18). The current basis of such separations resides in welfare and community service actions, and in the high levels of incarceration of Aboriginal young people in welfare and juvenile justice institutions. Many sources document the ongoing extent of separations. For instance, Aboriginal youth in 1990 were overrepresented in detention in juvenile justice systems by a factor of 12 in Queensland, 16 in New South Wales, and 62 in Western Australia (Hunter, 1994). Hunter suggests that this reflects a social construction of Aboriginal children as problems.

The children who experienced these systematic processes of separation from family and homeland became known as the "Stolen Generations" (Read, 1981). In examining the stressors they experienced, and their impact, a number of different elements can be identified. These then provide a framework from which to examine trans- or intergenerational effects. But such effects must, of course, be seen in the context of other ongoing stressor experiences for Aboriginal people, including separation, loss, and trauma. Overall, it is estimated that over 100,000 people have been so affected, with direct effects for, at the very least, 1 in 10 families.

Stressors experienced by these children included intense separation distress; searching behaviors; multiple grief, which was chronic and often unresolvable; emotional and behavioral disturbances in childhood, which arose naturally upon their distress; dislocation stressors from loss of home and place; denial and stigmatization of their Aboriginality and cultural heritage; and loss of identity. Swan (1988) vividly describes the impact of these experiences in her report, "200 Years of Unfinished Business."

> The devastating experiences of Aboriginal parents and families brought on by the removal of their children, the loss of control over their lives, powerlessness, prejudice, and hopelessness, have left many problems for us to deal with today. The theft of Aboriginal children . . . has produced the background for many years of horrific memories, distress, and mental health problems that still need to be addressed.

In addition to these direct effects and consequences of separation and removal, other problems arose. Many Aboriginal children were emotionally, physically, and sexually abused in the institutions or foster homes in which they were placed. Hunter (1994) suggests that the pain caused by all those experiences is "enduring and unquantifiable." He reports that in one area he worked, in an urban Aboriginal population, one-half of his patients had been separated as children, and, among the women, about a half of the population had been sexually abused in a foster home.

IMPACT OF THESE STRESSOR EXPERIENCES

In studies of non-Aboriginal communities, the extent of such traumatic separation, loss, abuse, dislocation, and dehumanization can only be found in populations subjected to systematic torture, genocide, concentration camps, or urban or family violence. Data from such populations provide a basis for considering how these experiences may have impacted on Aboriginal people themselves, and also how such effects may influence subsequent generations. Comparisons of this kind are necessary, as there is as yet only the most rudimentary information from which inferences may be drawn.

Such studies have described the impact on a shortened life span, with illnesses occurring in the survivors lives (Eitinger & Strom, 1973). Although more recent studies, such as that of Tennant, Goulston, and Dent (1993), suggest that mortality rates are no different. Eitinger and Strom (1973) found from their own work and in reviewing other studies that death rates from tuberculosis and infectious diseases, lung cancer, coronary heart disease, chronic bronchitis, diseases of the liver, and violent death were all higher, especially in the first decade after these experiences.

Suicide and accidents were high throughout. These results were seen to be general rather than specific. Similarly, clinical symptoms of depression and anxiety are prevalent in populations surviving prisoner-of-war camps (Tennant *et al.,* 1993).

Posttraumatic stress syndromes, particularly posttraumatic stress disorder (PTSD), are the most prevalent and specific forms of morbidity likely to follow such experience, both with effects in childhood and subsequent adult life. Judith Herman (1992) described complex PTSD, a syndrome that reflected the outcome of such chronic experiences of traumatization. These symptom constellations include a wide range of general psychological and somatic symptoms (and somatization patterns), impact on personality and identity, and vulnerability to self-harm, suicide, revictimization, and further abuse. Substance abuse is also prevalent.

Unfortunately, no broad systematic data are available on relationships between such trauma and health, but examination of health data available currently from Aboriginal populations shows patterns that are not dissimilar.

TRANSGENERATIONAL ASPECTS

Harkness (1993) has reviewed intergenerational aspects of transmission of PTSD, particularly war-related trauma. As she indicates, psychological reverberations of traumatic events can affect other family members, particularly the next generation, the children. Effects may be direct, linked to genetic vulnerability, experienced by both parent and child, or the result of psychological or social factors associated with the traumatic morbidity, for instance, family breakdown, impaired parenting and relating skills, violence, or antisocial behaviors. Danieli (1985, 1989) has described the intergenerational effects for children of Holocaust survivors and shown how burdens of guilt, reactions to overprotectiveness, unspeakable family secrets, and many other factors can be transmitted to the next generation. McFarlane, Blumbergs, Policansky, and Irwin (1985) demonstrated that ongoing parental PTSD contributed to a significant level of disaster-related morbidity in their children. Another aspect may be vicarious traumatization of the child who identifies closely with the traumatized parent and may reflect similar symptoms or traumatic patterns. Of concern may also be those circumstances in which intergenerational effects lead the child to become the nurturer, not only of the impaired parent, but perhaps pathologically so of others. This is what Bowlby (1979) described as care of the vicarious object, where, through the mechanism of projective identification, the individual cares for the wounds of others as he or she would wish to be cared for. Harkness's (1993) own study of the behavioral problems of children of Vietnam veterans found that lower levels of family functioning, the father's past combat experience, and the father's current violent behavior were the strongest predictors of problems in children. Girls with violent fathers were more withdrawn and delinquent, and demonstrated both externalizing aggressive and internalizing anxious/depressive patterns. Boys who were younger showed high externalizing scores, and those in the adolescent age group revealed violent and aggressive patterns resembling those of their fathers. These effects were seen as arising from many sources, ranging from intergenerational transmission of violence, to trauma in the family and social factors.

TRANSGENERATIONAL IMPACTS AFFECTING ABORIGINAL CHILDREN AND ADULTS

Studies carried out with Aboriginal people are limited and, in the past, were often poorly informed, or took little account of Aboriginal perceptions and views. The earlier workers who contributed an understanding of mental health problems in Aboriginal communities usually did so using either ethnographic models or applying Western models of psychiatric diagnosis. Few took into account the extent of trauma, loss, and separation experienced by Aboriginal people, or used conceptualization that would provide understanding of intergenerational effects. Some have been identified in the most recent work in the mental health field (e.g., Brady, 1995; Hunter, 1994; McKendrick, 1993; McKendrick & Thorpe, 1992, 1994), or through inquiries related to attempts to identify the source of particular problems (e.g., Royal Commission into Aboriginal Deaths in Custody, 1991). More potently, however, the extent, nature, and severity of effects have been presented by Aboriginal people themselves in reports, discussions, and a range of other responses. It must be emphasized here, however, as earlier, that it may often be difficult to distinguish particular intergenerational transmission when considerable vulnerability must be related to the extensive and pervasive ongoing effects of dislocation, dispossession, deprivation, and discrimination.

History of childhood separation from parents is strongly correlated with a wide range of problems found in many of the studies reported earlier. This may have had a direct effect in leading to morbidity, or indirect effects in that problems of the parental generation, or experienced by them, impacted on the child. Kamien's study (1978) in Bourke found that among the 320 adults interviewed, one-third had been separated for more than 5 years between the ages of 5 and 14. Separation in the family history was found to be very frequent in populations in McKendrick's study and correlated with the very high levels of depression found in these Aboriginal people seeking primary health services.

Hunter (1994) comments particularly on effects on males, where these histories are powerfully influenced by the loss of fathers, both through such separations and through the criminal justice system, and where the models for and initiation into mature malehood are often sorely lacking. He sees this in contrast to women's ongoing primacy in domestic and child-rearing settings, and their greater financial security with welfare payments. He also shows how this occurs, particularly in remote communities, where "paternal roles are further compromised in the confusion of changes which included dislocation, entry into the cash economy, unemployment and the consequences of heavy drinking which became widespread after the repeal of prohibition" (the prohibition in Australia applied only to Aboriginal people) (p. 17). Hunter goes on to point out that "early mortality and excess morbidity from alcohol-related causes, enormous rates of arrest and detention, absence from communities and families in pursuit of alcohol, and the dysfunctionality of intoxication, all disproportionately impact the availability of males as parents" (p. 17).

Clayer (1991) assessed 530 Aboriginal people in South Australia. This group explored suicidal ideation and behaviors, and mental health and behavioral problems. A high proportion of those assessed (31%) had been separated from parents before age 14. Absence of the father, and absence of traditional Aboriginal teachings, were found to correlate significantly with attempted suicide and mental disorder (likelihood of having a disorder, as indicated by score on a screening measure, the General Health Questionnaire 12). Suicidal behavior was not infrequent, with 16% of males and 15% of females having attempted suicide in their lifetime. Demoralization, or anomie, as measured by an eight-question factor from the BSI (Brief Symptom Inventory) also related very significantly to attempted suicide and alcohol and drug use. While suicidal behaviors were at a much higher level than in non-Aboriginal populations, mental ill health was at much the same level, at least in this study. Anomie may thus contribute in an important way to this suicidal behavior, and may reflect the effects of intergenerational transmission of the types of stressors described here.

Brady (1995), considering vulnerability to drug and alcohol abuse among Aboriginal people, describes the negative way in which state welfare authorities are viewed because of the traumatic and powerful memories that they evoke by their actions in the past. Particular problems relate to failure to understand the nature of Aboriginal family life and seeing it as pathological, for instance, shifting households and raising of children by other Aboriginal people. Similar to others reporting on trauma and separation, she comments on the high level of parental separation experienced by Aboriginal people who died in police custody (43 of 99) and who had been separated as children from their natural families "by intervention by the state, mission organisations or other institutions" (p. 11). She also quotes figures from the Australian Bureau of Statistics (1995), which indicate that 10% of Aboriginal people over age 25 years had been taken away from their natural parents. While Brady acknowledges that it is impossible to define exact connections to alcohol- and drug-use problems, there is much to suggest that this is highly likely to contribute to vulnerability.

Swan (1988) suggests that the major impact of these traumata and losses on the next generations occurs through the effects on child-rearing practices, the passing on of culture, and the lack of role models. The transmission of culture, normally from parents to children, is particularly disrupted. Where culture is not transmitted because of such separations, it is likely that a sense of uncertainty and strain will be engendered. Aboriginal people so separated may seek their origins consciously and be assisted through organizations such as Link-Up or reunions. This is a painful and uncertain process, as they may not know from whence they have come, or their names, in a culture where identity is defined by name and place of origin. Many who were reared in non-Aboriginal families and not told of their origins may only discover this in later life, by accident or foster parents telling them subsequently, and may then have the struggle to accept their status as well as coping with their need to search for their roots. Tragic stories abound of people who found all their family members to be deceased, or whose families had been told they were dead or had been shown a false certificate of death, or who found a parent or sibling, only to lose that person shortly after. Thus, the search is for both family and identity. Swan describes how the loss of vital attachments may prevent these children from achieving their full potential, attaining cultural identity, developing a conscience, becoming self-reliant, coping with stress and frustration, and knowing the importance of family and relationships. All these factors may adversely impact on their mental health and well-being.

Aboriginal people, in their National Mental Health Conference (1993), identified important areas of need. It was recommended that "family links should be encouraged, especially with the extended family by: breaking the cycles of kids being placed in care from mothers who were in homes" and that "putting people back in touch with their families is a priority in achieving Aboriginal well-being and mental health" and that "the importance of grieving the loss of family caused by forced removal of children be acknowledged" (p. 29).

Kendall (1994) comments on the special problems of identity that may result for Aboriginal people who have experienced these traumata, and also the stresses involved in moving into Aboriginal society when reared as non-Aboriginal. This may be the more so for those who are fair-skinned and had "passed as white." She sees education, support, and counseling as necessary to provide "a positive pathway for our children."

O'Shane, a magistrate and University Chancellor (President), speaks compellingly of the consequences of the forced assimilation practices described earlier. While acknowledging that there has not been a full description or analysis of these effects, she states:

> From what we know of the effects generally of dislocation, dispossession and breakdown of social structures, we may infer that these assimilation practices . . . have had further [than high levels of mental illness], far-reaching ramifications on the behaviors of the individual family members, compounding the generational effects of the original dispossession of land, culture and children; and including not only the mental health and general health problems, but also child behavior problems, and violence. It is no exaggeration to say that many Aboriginal families and communities spend their entire lives in crisis (p. 197).

She concludes that there is a great need for specific programs and therapies to address these issues. Later, she describes her own experience in childhood and adult life with the brutality of the practices of dispossession, assimilation, and removal of children. She states that the psychological impact of these "strike at the very core of our sense of being and identity" (p. 151). "I recognised the thing that happened to the thousands of other Aboriginal families like our family and I marvelled that we weren't all stark, raving mad" (p. 153). O'Shane herself had suffered such psychological impact and had been treated by psychiatric systems that had recommended that she have a lobotomy. Fortunately, she did not do so, but her grief and distress are still issues for her in terms of her own and her people's losses.

Lorraine Peters (1995) vividly describes the way in which she came to terms with her experience of being removed from her family and the loss of that family and her Aboriginal heritage for many years. She states: "I was only 4 years old when I was removed from my family and placed in a home for Aboriginal children." She remembers little of the removal but does remember some of her subsequent experiences. "I was told I was there because my family didn't want me and that they didn't care for or love me, and that all Aboriginal men (they called them dirty blacks) were dangerous. They also said that my culture was not important and that we had to forget about it and never talk about it" (p. 154). She goes on to speak of her life later, with all the girls being turned out of this home at 15 to find work and lives of their own. Deeply ingrained in her mind was the word *welfare*. She married, but states that progressively all she focused on was her children and trying to make sure "no one was going to take my children away." She did not tell her husband or anyone of these fears, but kept the children and house clean all the time in case "they would come." This same fearfulness and protectiveness extended to her grandchildren. While attending a reunion of her "stolen generation," she became able to face some of her grief and encompass her family of origin and work through these issues. Such experiences inevitably affected her sense of identity, her anxieties, and her parenting skills. She concludes: "I will not be free of pain, of my lost years, of a lost childhood they took from me. But at least my children and grandchildren will be free of having their lives and minds screwed up" (p. 157).

TRANSMISSION OF VIOLENCE AND ABUSE

There is considerable evidence that being abused as a child is associated with greater risk of becoming an abusive adult (i.e., transmitting the pattern of abuse to the next generation). Oliver (1993) has reviewed many of the studies addressing these issues, and has also carried out his own research. He found that approximately one-third of child victims of abuse grow up to have significant difficulties parenting, or they become abusive of their own children. One-third do not have these outcomes, but the other one-third remained vulnerable, and, in the face of social stress, there was an increased likelihood of their becoming abusive. The capacity of the child to grow up with the ability to face the reality of past and present relationships, to develop a strong personality and other supportive relationships, particularly a supportive adult partner, could protect against these negative outcomes.

There have been no studies to document these issues as they affect Aboriginal people, but it seems very likely that such patterns will contribute, particularly in view of the systematic abuse suffered by Aboriginal people in their own childhood, as outlined earlier. High levels of child abuse are reported by Aboriginal people as central to their concerns, as being related to breakdown of parenting skills, alcohol abuse, and violence (Swan & Raphael, 1995). Current Australian statistics show the rates of abuse and neglect for Aboriginal and Torres Strait Islander children (15.2 per 1,000 children ages 0–16 years) were much higher than for all children (5.7). Aboriginal and Torres Strait Islander children ages 0–4 years had the highest rate of abuse and neglect in the population, with a rate of 16.3 per 1,000 children (Angus & Woodward, 1995).

Hunter describes how the impact of profound social change on parents may be transmitted to the next generation, leading to social problems and other negative outcomes for these offspring. He reports that in the remote Kimberley region in the 1980s, there has appeared "a spectrum of self-harmful behaviors in which alcohol plays a part, with the most serious (completed suicide) primarily involving males" (Hunter, 1990, p. 192). These increases in set behavior and violence in this region were also reflected in rising rates of convictions for murder and rape among Aboriginal males in this state. He believes that, until the previous generation, this region had to some degree been insulated against change, but changes did occur in the 1960s, with the "dramatic social transformations" that occurred during that time. These changes included the cash economy, changes in structure of Aboriginal communities and lives, and, most particularly, the sudden ready availability of alcohol. This led to many social changes and adverse impact on health, for instance, increases in deaths from external causes. Those who were young adults during this period of destabilization are the antecedents of the current group among whom the recent increases in self-harming behaviors is occurring. These changes are mixed with many of the other factors noted earlier. Furthermore, the separations experienced by the earlier generation (15–27% among those ages 30 and older who were children prior to the 1970s) continued but appeared to be related to heavy parental drinking. These effects may also be reinforced by the related antisocial spectrum of behaviors affecting the earlier generation and leading to incarceration and absence of parental figures, especially fathers. There is, Hunter suggests, transmission to the next generation of the violence and abusive and antisocial outcomes. This may be through lack of positive factors, so that the negative identifications and stressor effects predominate both at family level and in broader social groups. Hunter (1993, 1994) believes males are particularly vulnerable, with females perhaps protected to a degree by the relative power of their female role models in economic and family domains.

PARENTING AND THE IMPACT OF EARLIER LOSS AND TRAUMATIZATION

Aboriginal people themselves have identified the pattern of loss of parenting skills for the "stolen generations" (Swan & Raphael, 1995). As described earlier, children were taken from parents at many different ages, but mostly in younger childhood. The vast majority were then raised in institutional settings with few primary, caring parental figures. Both the traumatic effects of such separations and loss, and the loss of role models of parenting are likely to have had profound psychological effects, disrupting attachment and creating vulnerabilities to anxiety and depression. Most communities suggest the need for special programs to support young Aboriginal people and to redevelop parenting skills both in terms of child rearing generally and traditional practices. The inability of many women experiencing childhood separation to care for their own children has led to these children being passed on to other family members or institutions, with a cycle that continues to further generations if satisfactory parenting is not achieved.

Grandmothers, aunts, and women in traditional roles of support for childbirth and child rearing are frequently left to provide care. This has led in many instances to what is known as the "stressed-out granny," a grandmother caring for many grandchildren when her own children have been unable to respond through outcomes of illness, loss of parenting skills, alcohol abuse, or other problems. As pregnancies occur at a younger age than in the non-Aboriginal population, the giving status of womanhood, and fertility rates are higher, this is a substantial problem. Support may, however, be very effective in assisting these young women, especially with extended kinship groups. Young women in urban settings may be more vulnerable as they lack access to some degree to such networks, or face greater stresses and vulnerabilities with violence and alcohol abuse.

The whole impact of the processes of colonization, dispossession, discrimination, deprivation, and removal of children has affected indigenous family life in multiple ways and thus impacted broadly as well on successive generations. Dodson (1994) has outlined how the extended family or kinship system had traditionally managed most areas of social, economic and cultural life, and governed relationships between people such as marriage and responsibility for children. The family, and child rearing, were the frameworks for transmission of knowledge, language and culture. Dodson contends that Aboriginal people have a right not to be prevented from transmitting their culture and, indeed, should be encouraged to do so. Many of the processes mentioned, as well as "direct intervention, but more indirect effects of the social environment and the dominant non-indigenous culture have severely interfered with the ability of indigenous cultures to transmit our cultures" (p. 36). He goes on to point out that the "dismantlement" of indigenous families has had profound effects for Aboriginal children. He sees these factors as contributing in ongoing ways to the disproportional levels of problems among these children, including the high levels of social problems, addictions such as petrol-sniffing, and extraordinarily disproportionate rates of incarceration. There is a need for "culturally relevant national legislation relating to Aboriginal and Islander child development" (Secretariat of National Aboriginal and Islander Child Care, 1992).

HEALTH CONSEQUENCES TRANSGENERATIONALLY

Aboriginal people have great inequities in health, as indicated by excess morbidity and mortality. For instance, there are high death rates among the young, particularly from external causes. Maternal and infant mortality rates are higher than those of the general population. Infant mortality is 2 to 3 times higher, and general Aboriginal mortality is 2 to 8 times higher than the nonindigenous population. The life span for an Aboriginal woman is 20 years less, and for an Aboriginal man, 18 years less than for whites. There are more frequent hospital admissions and disproportionate incidences of certain diseases including diabetes, circulatory disorders, respiratory illness, renal disease, ear and eye disorders, and infectious diseases including hepatitis B and other sexually transmitted diseases. In national surveys, more than one-third of Aboriginal people rate their health as poor or fair. Mental health problems are pervasive. Although it is likely that rates of major psychosis and related disorders are at much the same level as the general population, depression, anxiety, and trauma-related morbidity are likely to be much higher, though systematic studies are not currently available. McKendrick and colleagues (1992, 1994), whose work attempts to address these issues, found high rates of depression, and that separation histories were a significant risk factor for it.

Sibthorpe (1988) outlines how these premature deaths and illnesses also impact on family structure and children. She quotes Gray (1987), who stated that "parental death and preceding parental illness is a constant accompaniment to the process of growing up Aboriginal" (p. 16). Aboriginal children who lost their fathers were also much more likely to have lost their mothers. Thus, there is an immersion in death, dying, and loss. Sibthorpe's own work leads her to conclude that the psychosocial stressors experienced in this way by Aboriginal people have a *direct* effect on their health. It might be hypothesised that the stressors described here impact on parental generations in many ways, and that these effects are likely to contribute to their physical health problems and vulnerabilities through psychoimmune, neuroendocrine, and other mechanisms. Then, the illnesses and problems of those parents, and their premature deaths, are likely to set a further substrate for health problems for subsequent generations.

NARRATIVES AND OUTCOMES CONCERNING THE INTERGENERATIONAL TRANSMISSION OF TRAUMA AND LOSS

A great many Aboriginal people tell individual stories that are compelling examples of the impact of ongoing factors of dispossession and discrimination, with superimposed patterns related to trauma, separation, and loss. The painful search for lost families, the joys and grief of reunion, are increasingly apparent as both social and political processes begin to recognize the extent and nature of the past and its ongoing effects for present generations. Many Aboriginal people have given testimony to these experiences in moving ways (e.g., Peters, 1995; O'Shane, 1995). A report on Aboriginal Mental Health in New South Wales identified the centrality of these issues for mental health and well-being. The Human Rights Commission Inquiry into Mental Health in Australia (Burdekin, 1993) also described the importance of these issues, as has every other major investigation concerning Aboriginal people's health and well-being.

A recent National Consultancy to develop a strategic plan for Aboriginal mental health (Swan & Raphael, 1995) found that Aboriginal people and communities across the country reported these problems as critical to their future. Particular emphasis was placed on the effects on children and young people, a much larger proportion of the indigenous population, in which 40% of the population is below 15 years of age. It is well recognized in communities that these children are profoundly impacted upon by transgenerational effects, and that these children are the future. Various counseling, prevention, and support programs are seen as essential and many have been developed through centers for Aboriginal health. A model of Narrative Family Therapy (Howson, Graham, Hall, & Jenkins, 1994) has been seen as particularly appropriate to address the needs of parents and children, and in light of the oral tradition and role of kinship in the Aboriginal culture. Other models such as holistic counseling frameworks, building on Aboriginal holistic views of mental health, incorporate an ongoing recognition of the past and history as well as mental, physical, emotional, spiritual, social, and environmental aspects of the present (Collard & Garvey, 1994).

It is a great tribute to the personal qualities and abilities of Aboriginal peoples that they have survived despite these assaults on their personhood, humanity, society, and psyche. Through their enduring strengths, they may have much to teach others of resilience and survival. It is their human right to have appropriate support and resources to overcome the effects of the present and the past, and to preserve an Aboriginal future for themselves and their children.

REFERENCES

Angus, G., & Woodward, S. (1995). *Child abuse and neglect Australia 1993–94.* Canberra: AGPS Australian Institute of Health and Welfare, Child Welfare Series No. 13.

Bowlby, J. (1979). *The making and breaking of affectional bonds.* London: Tavistock.

Brady, M. (1995). *The prevention of drug and alcohol abuse among Aboriginal people: Resilience and vulnerability.* Research Discussion Paper No. 2, Australian Institute of Aboriginal and Torres Strait Islander Studies.

Burdekin, B. (1993). *Human rights and mental illness.* Report of the National Enquiry into the Human Rights of People with Mental Illness. Canberra: Australian Government Printing Service.

Clayer, J. (1991). *Mental health and behavioral problems in the urban Aboriginal population.* Adelaide: South Australian Health Commission.

Collard, S., & Garvey, D. (1994). Counselling and Aboriginal people: Talking about mental health. *Aboriginal and Islander Health Worker Journal, 18,* 17–21.

Cummings, B. (1990). *Take this child . . . from Kahlin Compound to the Retta Dixon Children's Home.* Canberra: Aboriginal Studies Press.

Danieli, Y. (1985). The treatment and prevention of long-term effects and intergenerational transmission of victimisation: A lesson from Holocaust survivors and their children. In C. R. Figley (Ed.), *Trauma and its wake* (pp. 295–313). New York: Brunner/Mazel.

Danieli, Y. (1989). Mourning in survivors and children of survivors of the Nazi Holocaust: The role of group and community modalities. In D. R. Dietrich & P. C. Shabab (Eds.), *The problem of loss and mourning: Psychoanalytic perspectives* (pp. 427–460). Madison, CT: International Universities Press.

Dodson, M. (1994). The rights of indigenous people in the international year of the family. *Family Matters, 37,* 34–41.

Edwards, C. (1982). Is the ward clean? In B. Gammage & A. Markus (Eds.), *All that dirt: Aborigines 1938: An Australia 1938 monograph.* Canberra: History Project, Inc.

Eitinger, L., & Strom, A. (Eds.). (1973). *Mortality and morbidity after excessive stress: A follow-up investigation of Norwegian concentration camp survivors.* Oslo and New York: Humanities Press.

Gray, A. (1987). The *"death bird": Aspects of adult Aboriginal mortality.* Aboriginal Family Demography Study, Working Paper No. 7. Department of Demography, Research School of Social Sciences, Australian National University.

Gungil Jindibah Centre. (1994). *Learning from the past.* Aboriginal perspectives on the effects and implications of welfare policies and practices on Aboriginal families in New South Wales. Southern Cross University, Lismore, Australia.

Harkness, L. L. (1993). Transgenerational transmission of war-related trauma. In J. P. Wilson & B. Raphael (Eds.), *The international handbook of traumatic stress syndromes* (pp. 635–643). New York: Plenum Press.

Herman, J. L. (1992). Complex PTSD: A syndrome in survivors of prolonged and repeated trauma. *Journal of Traumatic Stress, 5,* 377–393.

Howson, R., Graham, T., Hall, R., & Jenkins, A. (1994). *Certificate in narrative therapy for aboriginal people.* A project of the Social Health and Counselling Team of the Aboriginal Community Recreation and Health Services Centre of South Australia Inc.

Hunter, E. (1990). Using a socio-historical frame to analyse Aboriginal self-destructive behavior. *Australian and New Zealand Journal of Psychiatry, 24,* 191–198.

Hunter, E. M. (1993). *Aboriginal health and history: Power and prejudice in remote Australia.* Melbourne and New York: Cambridge University Press.

Hunter, E. (1994, April 12). *"Freedom's just another word": Aboriginal youth and mental health.* The Bill Robinson Memorial Lecture, Perth, Australia.

Kamien, M. (1978). The dark people of Bourke: A study of planned social change. Canberra: Australian Institute of Aboriginal Studies and Atlantic Highlands, NJ: Humanities Press.

Kendall, C. (1994). The history: Present and future issues affecting Aboriginal adults who were removed as children. *Aboriginal and Islander Health Worker Journal, 18,* 18–19.

McFarlane, A. C., Blumbergs, V., Policansky, S. K., & Irwin, C. (1985). *A longitudinal study of the psychological morbidity in children due to a natural disaster.* Department of Psychiatry, Flinders University of South Australia. Unpublished paper.

McKendrick, J. H. (1993). *Patterns of psychological distress and implications for mental health service delivery in an urban Aboriginal general practice population.* Ph.D. thesis, University of Melbourne.

McKendrick, J. H., Cutter, T., Mackenzie, A., & Chiu, E. (1992). The pattern of psychiatric morbidity in a Victorian urban Aboriginal general practice population. *Australian and New Zealand Journal of Psychiatry, 26,* 40–47.

McKendrick, J. H., & Thorpe, M. (1994). *The mental health of Aboriginal communities.* Department of Psychiatry, University of Melbourne, The Victorian Aboriginal Health Service, Melbourne.

National Aboriginal Mental Health Conference. (1993, November 25–27). University of Sydney, New South Wales, Australia.

Oliver, J. E. (1993). Intergenerational transmission of child abuse: Rates, research, and clinical implications. *American Journal of Psychiatry, 150,* 1315–1324.

O'Shane, P. (1993). Assimilation or acculturation problems of Aboriginal families. Plenary address, Australian Family Therapy Conference, Canberra, July 7, 1993. *Australian and New Zealand Journal of Family Therapy, 14,* 196–198.

O'Shane, P. (1995). The psychological impact of white colonialism on Aboriginal people. *Australasian Psychiatry, 3,* 148–153.

Peters, L. (1995). The years that never were. *Australasian Psychiatry, 3*,154–157.

Read, P. (1981). *The stolen generations. The removal of Aboriginal children in NSW 1883 to 1969.* New South Wales Ministry of Aboriginal Affairs: Occasional Paper (No. 1). Canberra: Australian Government Printing Service, NSW L.O. 1102.

Royal Commission into Aboriginal Deaths in Custody (RCIADC). (1991). Nation report (5 volumes). Canberra: Australian Government Printing Service.

Sibthorpe, B. (1988). *"All our people are dying': Diet and stress in an urban Aboriginal community.* Ph.D. thesis, Australian National University, Canberra.

Secretariat of National Aboriginal and Islander Child Care Report. (1992). Aims and Objectives. Melbourne: SNAICC.

Swan, P. (1988, September). *200 Years of Unfinished Business.* Paper presented to the Australian National Association for Mental Health Conference. *Aboriginal Medical Service Newsletter,* pp. 12–17.

Swan, P., & Raphael, B. (1995). *"Ways Forward": National Aboriginal and Torres Strait Islander Mental Health Policy.* Report prepared for Office for Aboriginal and Torres Strait Islander Health Services, Commonwealth Department of Human Services and Health. Canberra: Australian Government Printing Service.

Tennant, C. C., Goulston, K., & Dent, O. (1993). Medical and psychiatric consequences of being a prisoner of war of the Japanese. An Australian follow-up study. In J. P. Wilson & B. Raphael (Eds.), *The international handbook of traumatic stress syndromes* (pp. 231–239).

21

Healing the American Indian Soul Wound

EDUARDO DURAN, BONNIE DURAN,
MARIA YELLOW HORSE BRAVE HEART,
and SUSAN YELLOW HORSE-DAVIS

INTRODUCTION

It was almost two decades ago that the authors became aware of the concept of a "soul wound," although knowledge of what is characterized as the "soul wound" had been an integral part of indigenous knowledge ever since Columbus landed in this hemisphere and Cortez arrived in Vera Cruz, Mexico. Native people who were asked about problems in the contemporary Native community explained that present problems had their etiology in the traumatic events known as the "soul wound." Knowledge of the soul wound has been present in Indian country for many generations. Current synonymous terms include historical trauma (Brave Heart, in press a), historical legacy, American Indian holocaust, and intergenerational posttraumatic stress disorder (Brave Heart & De Brun, in press). In addition, there has been academic literature documenting the American Indian holocaust, thus bringing some validation to the feelings of a community that has not had the world acknowledge the systematic genocide perpetrated on it (Brave Heart-Jordan & DeBruyn, 1995; Brown, 1971; Legters, 1988; Stannard, 1992; Thornton, 1987).

European contact brought decimation of the indigenous population, primarily through waves of disease, annihilation, and military and colonialist expansionist policies. The forced social changes and bleak living conditions of the reservation system also contributed to the disruption of American Indian cultures. This painful legacy includes themes of encroachment based on the *manifest destiny* doctrine and betrayal of earlier agreements and treaties (Limmerick, 1987). Armed conflict and removal of tribes from traditional lands became the norm. Numerous tribes faced "long walks" where many, if not the majority, died of disease, fatigue, and starvation. As the reservation system developed, tribal groups were often forced to live together in restricted areas. When lands were found to be valuable to the government and Whites, . . . more ways were found to take them away and resettle the

EDUARDO DURAN and BONNIE DURAN • First Nations, 4100 Silver SE, Albuquerque, New Mexico 87108.
MARIA YELLOW HORSE BRAVE HEART and SUSAN YELLOW HORSE-DAVIS • Graduate School of Social Work, University of Denver, Denver, Colorado 80208.

International Handbook of Multigenerational Legacies of Trauma, edited by Yael Danieli. Plenum Press, New York, 1998.

Native peoples elsewhere (Jacobs, 1972; Pearce, 1988; White, 1983; Brave Heart and De-
Bruyn, in press).

Historical trauma is more complex than surface exploration would reveal. Historical
trauma is trauma that is multignerational and cumulative over time; it extends beyond the life
span. Historical trauma response has been identified and is delineated as a constellation of features in reaction to the multigenerational, collective, historical, and cumulative psychic wounding over time, both over the life span and across generations (Brave Heart-Jordan, 1995; Brave
Heart, in press a). Mourning that has not been completed and the ensuing depression are absorbed by children from birth on (Shoshan, 1989). Unresolved trauma also has been found to
be intergenerationally cumulative, thus compounding the subsequent health problems of the
community (Solomon, Kotler, & Mikulincer, 1988; Brave Heart, in press b). Evidence suggests depressive and emotional breakdowns of children who are descendants of Holocaust survivors are always linked to Holocaust experiences (Solomon *et al.,* 1988).

> The survivor's child complex is a constellation of features resulting from the intergenera-
> tional transmission of parental traumatic experiences and responses (Bergmann & Jucovy,
> 1982/1990; Kestenberg, 1990a; Kestenberg & Kestenberg, 1982, 1990a). Bergmann and Ju-
> covy . . . concluded that, despite the possibility of adaptation and sublimation, the mental
> health of most children of survivors is at risk, and that they are scarred by the psychic real-
> ity of the Holocaust. Cardinal themes of parental survival, persecution, and deaths of rela-
> tives, at times unconscious, were manifested in the analyses of survivors' children
> according to Kestenberg and Kestenberg (1990a).
>   Rather than a syndrome, the Kestenbergs describe a "survivor's child complex," which
> includes the Holocaust's impact upon psychic structure, fantasies, and identification. . . .
> Post-Holocaust experiences of oppression were regarded . . . as further impacting parental
> survivorship and quality of transmission to offspring (Brave Heart-Jordan, 1995, pp.
> 76–77).

Some of the features associated with the complex include depression, suicidal ideation and behavior, guilt and concern about betraying the ancestors for being excluded from the suffering,
as well as obligation to share in the ancestral pain, a sense of being obliged to take care of and
being responsible for survivor parents, identification with parental suffering and a compulsion
to compensate for the genocidal legacy, persecutory and intrusive Holocaust as well as
grandiose fantasies, dreams, images, and a perception of the world as dangerous.

The features of the survivor's child complex were congruent with those identified by
Macgregor (1946/1975; Erikson, 1950) among the Lakota, including persecutory fantasies and
a perception of the world as dangerous; the fantasy of the return of the old way of life, analogous to compensatory fantasies; apprehension, shame, withdrawal, grandiosity in daydreams,
and anxiety about aggressive impulses (Brave Heart-Jordan, 1995; Brave Heart & DeBruyn,
in press). Dreams of community members were collected over a period of 4 years and their
content was analyzed. There were over 800 themes, with the overwhelming message of the
dreams being a hostile environment or hostile world.

> It is apparent that the psyche of the community recognized the wounding of the environ-
> ment, and that this awareness in turn was perceived as a wounding of the psyche. Harmony
> had become discord and the community's unconscious perception was that the world was
> unfriendly and hostile. The problems that were manifested and verbalized were merely
> symptoms of a deeper wound—the soul wound. (Duran & Duran, 1995, p. 195)

Historical trauma is also an ongoing process via pressures brought on by acculturative
stress. The concept of acculturative stress refers to one kind of stress in which the stressors

are identified as having their source in the process of acculturation, often resulting in a particular set of stress behaviors that include anxiety, depression, feelings of marginality and alienation, heightened psychosomatic symptoms, and identity confusion. Acculturative stress is thus a phenomenon that may underlie a reduction in the health status of individuals, including physical, psychological, and social health (Williams & Berry, 1991). While historical trauma included acculturative stress, it goes much deeper and encompasses the aftereffects of racism, oppression, and genocide.

HISTORICAL LEGACY

Since the arrival of Europeans on Turtle Island (also known by the colonial name "New World"), the so-called "Indian Problem" has taken on a paternalistic dispassion by dominant policymakers (Yellow Horse-Davis, 1994). In the treaty era, European settlers used treaty-making as a form of protection from "hostiles" whose lands they were invading (Deloria & Lytle, 1983). Instead of using force to seize lands, treaty-making provided an atmosphere of "civility and legitimacy" to the settlers (Deloria & Lytle, 1983, p. 3). Thus, according to Deloria and Lytle, treaty-making was used to establish "legal and political relationships" by the invading forces (1983, p. 3).

When the United States won independence from Great Britain, the first treaty signed was between the government and the Delaware Tribe (Deloria & Lytle, 1983). Over the next century, over "600 treaties and agreements" were made between Indian tribes and colonial interests (Deloria, 1983, p. 4). Many of the treaties were broken by colonists. In addition, most treaties were written in English, and Indians signed (many times by force) by thumbprinting documents, thus placing Indians at a clear disadvantage (Yellow Horse-Davis, 1994).

The resulting Treaty of Fort Stanwix of 1784 was a fraud. Native leaders were coerced at gunpoint into signing a document conceding large tracts of land. Many of the Native delegates left before the treaty was signed. The inability of the delegates to adequately represent the interests of their tribes led to the disintegration of the original Iroquois Confederacy.

To offer structure to a chaotic and painful set of events, Duran and Duran (1995) delineate a sequence of six phases in historical trauma. (A similar structure has been offered by Brave Heart-Jordan, 1995.) Any trauma to one phase of life resulted in trauma to other aspects, since these life activities were interconnected. These phases are as follows:

First Contact

At this point, there was a total environmental and "lifeworld shock."[1] The lifeworld of the Native people was systematically destroyed through genocidal military actions. Grief and bereavement for losses were not possible due to yet other traumatic events that quickly followed.

Economic Competition

During this phase, Native people suffered the losses of sustenance, both physically and spiritually. It is therefore improper to view these traumas as separate for Native peoples.

---

[1]*Lifeworld* refers to all aspects of being. These include the physical, spiritual, cultural, and emotional facets of existence.

Invasion War Period

In this era the U.S. government carried out a policy of extermination through military force. Many Native people who were not killed were removed from traditional homelands by force. Native people began to suffer from a refugee syndrome as they were displaced.

Subjugation and Reservation Period

Native peoples were forced to live within the confines of reservations. This imposition of boundaries that kept people from moving from one place to another was yet another event that exacerbated the soul wound.

Boarding School Period

Since Native people still retained Native identity, the U.S. government decided to attack systematically the core of Native identity (i.e., the family system). Removing children from parents and placing them in distant boarding schools became the policy. Within the boarding schools, children were forbidden to speak Native languages, practice Native religion, or to convey anything that might remotely resemble native subjectivity.[2] Children were forced into a colonial lifeworld, where the Native lifeworld was despised and thought of as inferior and evil.

Brave Heart-Jordan's (1995) examination of the historical, traumatic boarding-school experiences among the Lakota is generalizable to other tribes. Boarding schools were operated like prison camps, with Indian children being starved, chained, and beaten (Brave Heart-Jordan, 1995; Tanner, 1982). Furthermore, the poor standards at the boarding schools, the confinement in overcrowded reservation housing, the neglect of Indian health needs, and the deliberate undermining of traditional healers by the federal government resulted in poor health for approximately 80% of the population on some reservations (Tanner, 1982). More than one-third of the Lakota population over one year of age died of tuberculosis between 1936 and 1941 (Brave Heart, in press a; Tanner, 1982).

Forced Relocation and Termination Period

During the 1950s, many Native people were relocated from reservations into large metropolitan areas. The intent was similar to the previous one (i.e., to assimilate Native people and remove them from any connections to the remaining indigenous culture).

> Over 100,000 American Indians were sent to major urban centers throughout the United States (Bars, 1994; Sorkin, 1978). Many . . . returned to their respective reservations within a very short period of time. Others remained in the cities, often developing a lifestyle of going back and forth to the home reservation. . . . This situation created additional stressors on American Indian families economically, socially, and spiritually. As of 1995, over half of all American Indians live in urban settings where they face a concerted lack of economic and health resources (Brave Heart & DeBruyn, in press).

Genocide has taken different forms in the American Indian community. There is "growing attention to a less murderous form of genocide, sometimes labeled 'cultural genocide,' that is taken to cover actions that are threatening to the integrity and continuing viability of peoples and social groups" (Legters, 1988, p. 769, as cited in Brave Heart-Jordan & DeBruyn, in

---

[2]The term *subjectivity* infers the deeper experience of who a person is and how he or she define him- or herself.

press). Prohibition of religious freedom has been a form of cultural genocide that is ongoing even to this day. It was only in 1994 that Native peoples were allowed to practice some forms of religion without fear of reprisal by state and federal governmental policies.

SURVIVOR SYNDROME/SURVIVOR'S CHILD COMPLEX

Although some caution is urged in the assertion of a "Survivor Syndrome" (Marcus & Rosenberg, 1988; Weinfeld, Sigal, & Eaton, 1981), "the bulk of the literature acknowledges the existence of special features among the clinical population of survivors. The similar dynamics observed among the children of survivors and their descendants have been called a "survivor's child complex" (Kestenberg & Kestenberg, 1990; Brave-Heart & De Bruyn, in press). Addressing criticisms of the Survivor Syndrome, Fogelman (1988) asserts that although more empirical studies are needed, the pain and psychological impairment of survivors are not captured by standardized personality tests.

Brave Heart-Jordan (1995) outlines aspects of Jewish survivors that are relevant for American Indians, such as "the difficulty in mourning a mass grave, the dynamics of collective grief, and the importance of community memorialization" (p. 67). A specific example is the Lakota survivors and descendants of the Wounded Knee Massacre in 1890. Fogleman further "addresses the challenges for Jews in European countries, where [they] 'lived among the perpetrators and murderers of their families'" (p. 94). A comparison may be made to natives who live in a colonized country, suggesting that similar patterns of grief have emerged. Fogelman asserts that

> Jews in Europe have not found . . . effective means of coping, integration, and adaption. Most are in a stage of complete denial and stunted mourning of their losses. . . . They feel a great need to control their emotions, because they fear that if their intense emotions were given free reign, they might go insane. . . . Survivors feared the uncontrollable rage locked within them, they feared they would be devoured by thoughts of avenging the deaths of their loved ones. These repressions result in "psychic numbing." (1988, p. 93)

She also distinguishes the healthier, communal grief process of American Jews from the delayed and impaired grief of European Jews (Brave Heart & De Bruyn, in press; Brave Heart-Jordan, 1995, pp. 67–68).

For American Indians, the United States is the perpetrator of their holocaust. Whereas other oppressed groups have a place to immigrate to escape further genocide, Native people have not had this option (Brave Heart-Jordan, 1995; Brave Heart & DeBruyn, in press). Kehoe (1989) states, "Where was America for American Indians? No other country welcomed them as immigrants, no other country promised them what their native land had denied them" (p. 133).

Native problems brought on by the devastation of their holocaust are further complicated by a lack of validation and no escape route being offered by the world community. These dynamics make it necessary for a repressed psychology to manifest symptoms of the pain suffered. A 15-year-old Pueblo girl, referred for a suicide attempt from an aspirin overdose, manifests a protective attitude toward her parents and a sense of guilt about her own pain. "I just can't talk to my parents. I don't want to burden them with my problems and feelings. They have so much pain of their own. I just can't bring myself to do that, but I felt like I had no one to talk to" (Brave Heart & DeBruyn, in press).

In another case, a young man reported walking in a certain part of his homeland. As he was doing so, he found himself engulfed by horses and cavalry in the middle of a massacre. He saw old Indian women and children huddled against the river bank, trying to shield themselves from the sabers and the shooting. When he came out of this vision, he shared it with some of the elders of his community. They informed him that on that very spot, a massacre had occurred over 100 years ago (Duran & Duran, 1995).

Such cases are common in clinical settings where American Indians are seen for treatment. The pain is evident in both cases. In the second case, it is remarkable that there was a complete experience of the trauma of the young man's people in what may otherwise appear as a psychological breakdown. A similar phenomenon, *transposition,* has been observed among Jewish Holocaust descendants, where the past is simultaneously experienced with the present reality (Kestenberg, 1990, cited in Brave Heart & DeBruyn, in press, and Brave Heart, in press a). In many cases, there is a complete denial or shutdown of emotions, since the surfacing of these emotions would elicit extreme anger. The anger may be manifested externally or internally. The resulting need for anesthetic self-intervention, such as alcohol, drug abuse, domestic violence, and suicide, makes psychological sense.

CHRONIC AND ACUTE REACTIONS TO COLONIALISM

The title of this section underscores colonialism as the focus of people's reactions. This distinction is important to make since, in most instances, health providers prefer to label these problems with standardized diagnostic names. Labeling and naming are powerful methods of creating subjectivity and lifeworlds. If the authors were to utilize standard diagnosing practices, they would be contributing to the invalidation of the pain and suffering that is directly connected to the centuries of genocide.

In 1984, American Indians died due to alcoholism, alcohol psychosis, and cirrhosis of the liver at a rate of 30 per 100,000, which is 4.8 times the 1984 all-races rate of 6.2 deaths per 100,000 (Indian Health Service, 1987). Loss of life due to alcohol-related problems has affected the community over several generations. Although the problem of alcoholism is very complex, there can be very little argument that the genocidal legacy is a key factor in understanding it.

Alcohol was known by few Indians before colonization. Some tribes used it sparingly for either informal secular gatherings or religious ceremonies. Within this context, alcohol was strictly controlled and did not create social problems. White explorers such as Jacques Cartier and Henry Hudson noticed alcohol being used as a trading commodity in the late 1500s (MacAndrews & Edgerton, 1969). Captain Cook reported that when offered spirituous liquors, they rejected them as something unnatural and disgusting to the taste (MacAndrews & Edgerton, 1969).

Indian attitudes toward alcohol changed in time. They were distrustful of its effects early on but some learned to enjoy them. Explorers began to trade alcohol for furs, and alcoholic beverages became the ideal commodity for the conspicuous consumption that the traders needed to increase their business and profits. By the 1800s, liquor was the basic bartering item on the frontier, as colonists used deceitful tactics to make large profits. There are numerous reports of plying Indians with rum or whiskey as a show of friendship, then trading watered liquor of the most vile nature (often poisonous) for the valuable furs and other items that Indians gave away while intoxicated.

Suicide on some reservations is as high as 70.3 per 100,000, as compared with 11.6 per 100,000 for the general U.S. population (Claymore, 1988). Most of the studies on suicide neglect the effects of historical trauma caused by centuries of colonialism (Brave Heart, in press; Brave Heart & DeBruyn, in press). The Indian Health Service (1995) reports that suicide is a serious problem, particularly among younger age groups. Such deaths occur needlessly and are usually predictable and preventable. The lack of awareness of the historical legacy limits true understanding of American Indian health status and fosters the practice of blaming Indian people for alcohol-related and other health-related morbidity. The relationship between morbidity and trauma is examined in the literature (Brave Heart, in press b). Villanueva (1989) notes:

> The more recent literature shows both the suicidal adult and the suicidal adolescent as holding rapidly eroding tribal tradition; the developmental social structure which for centuries established roles and expectation and guided both through the life span is tottering—for many Native Americans it is no longer applicable, for others it is non-existent. For those pueblos, tribes and individual Native American families in cities for which their traditions are viable and workable, the suicide rates are the lowest. In other words, if the culture would have remained intact, we would not be experiencing the devastating problems that we are facing. The responsibility should be placed in the right place and some honesty shed on the issue and then perhaps we could begin to ameliorate the problem. (p. 30)

Krugman (1987) utilized the concept of intergenerational transfer of posttraumatic stress disorder (PTSD) and unresolved trauma in his clinical work with family violence. "He concluded that untreated family violence victims appeared to suffer from chronic or delayed PTSD, and that trauma appears to be the central organizing factor in these families across generations. The central role of trauma within the family implicitly influences its transfer to subsequent generations" (Brave Heart-Jordan, 1995, p. 89). Incidence of domestic violence is remarkably high in Indian country, although no systematic epidemiological studies have been conducted in this area.

Violence directed at family members or other Indian people can be understood through the internalized oppression model (Freire, 1968). The release of psychic tension is directed either at the self, as in suicide, or projected outward to someone who is close to the person (i.e., a family member). Curry (1972) states that "the explicit and conscious act of killing involves the affirmation of life, which is nourished by that which is killed. . . . Death belongs to life, perhaps not as specifically as the phrase destructive love suggests. But they are nevertheless related. The patient has not actually committed murder; he is, we may quickly conclude, only killing an image of himself" (p. 103). The acts of killing or hurting family members makes sense in light of the many generations of imposed lessons that focused on teaching Indians how unworthy they were of life.

Physical health has also been a historical problem among Indian people since the imposition of the reservation era (Erikson, 1950; Macgregor, 1975; Tanner, 1982). Indian Health Service (1995) statistics reveal high rates of coronary heart disease, hypertension, diabetes, and other life-threatening chronic diseases. Paternalistic views also create suppression and bureaucratic barriers that prevent Indians from receiving quality social and health services. Specifically, the problem is made manifest when the Indian Health Service expects urban Indians to access services through the local public mainstream. On the other hand, the public mainstream has a myth that urban Indians can access health services from the Indian Health Service, thus leaving urban Indians without the help they need (Yellow Horse-Davis, 1994). Considering the extremely numerous health problems and the large numbers of urban Indians, the case for ongoing trauma is obvious.

PRESENT ENVIRONMENTAL RISK FACTORS AND SOCIAL PROBLEMS AND POLICIES AFFECTING NATIVE AMERICANS

A broader understanding of present social problems can only be arrived at through scrutinizing environmental risk factors. Federal government policy has been the source of community instability in addressing the aforementioned problems (Yellow Horse-Davis, 1994). Some Indian policy researchers believe that some of the problems confronting Indian people today may be related to historical oversights by federal policymakers (Report to Congress, 1992).

Another environmental factor is institutional oppression. Literature on institutional oppression and its effect on Indian people is limited. Calling it cultural oppression, Latimer reports that American Indians continue to experience oppression as a result of forced dominant values in institutional settings (Indian Health Service Report, 1991). Paternalistic policymaking is an environmental risk factor that has exacerbated Indian social problems for centuries (Yellow Horse-Davis, 1994). Examples of this paternalistic attitude exist in the language embedded in the Indian Child Welfare Act of 1978, which states, "Congress has plenary power over Indian affairs" (Prucha, 1990, p. 293).

Although some progress has been made in policies toward Indians, there is still an overtone of paternalism in the delivery of health services. While the Indian Health Service is responsible for providing health services to tribal and urban communities, Congress has "inconsistently" provided funds for appropriate levels of functioning (Yellow Horse-Davis, 1994). Policymakers appropriate funds based on their conception of what is good for Indians, without considering needs assessment data. These decisions have a direct impact on the delivery of mental health services, which would address some of the healing of the trauma discussed in this chapter. In 1990, a meager 2% of the Indian Health Service budget was devoted to mental health, while the rest of the money went for upkeep of the bureaucracy and to support the Western medical model of dealing with health issues (Indian Health Service, 1991).

RESTORATION OF THE CIRCLE

> And as I looked and wept, I saw that there stood on the north side of the starving camp a Sacred man who was painted red all over his body, and he held a spear as he walked into the center of his people, and there he layed down and rolled. And when he got up it was a fat bison standing there, and where the bison stood a Sacred herb sprang up right where the tree had been in the center of the nation's hoop. The herb grew and bore four blossoms on a single stem while I was looking—a blue, a white, a scarlet and a yellow—and the bright rays of these flashed to the heavens. (Black Elk, quoted in Neihardt, 1959)

When the young Black Elk saw this vision, he understood it as the restoration of the nations' hoop—the healing of the Indian nations. Black Elk also understood that the healing would take place in seven generations—the youth today.

Contemporary philosophical and scientific advances inform us that theories do not mirror reality and, at best, they are tools. Sociocultural, behavioral, and disease theories are the leading approaches that public and Indian Health Service officials apply to interpret and intervene in some of the problems afflicting Indians.

> These approaches, however useful, are not neutral insights and assessments of native drinking patterns but rather venture to explain and predict behavior based on a very historically

and culturally specific mode of representation—realism—which erroneously assumes unity between the sensible and intelligible. Embedded within this Eurocentric mode of representation is a biased assessment of non-Western cultures. Behavioral theories decontextualize and individualize social problems and many sociocultural theories continue European representations of native peoples that have origins in the politics of the colonial and early American era. Insofar as these approaches are cultural products—a form of literature— we can say that they are hegemonic. By this we mean that they partake in ideological/cultural domination by the assertion of universality and neutrality and by the disavowal of all other cultural forms or interpretations. (Duran & Duran, 1995)

Hegemonic policy is reflected in the bureaucratic attempts at ameliorating the problems of Indian people. Indian Health Service programs are often forced to hire non-Indian clinicians who work under the belief that they know what's best for Indians (Yellow Horse-Davis, 1994). A roundtable panel reached a consensus that providers working in Indian country must make an effort to "understand and value the resilience of healthy traditions and cultural strengths" (Indian Health Service, 1991, p. 3). Usually, it is found that blame is placed on the patient instead of on a delivery system that is still ladened with 1800s Department of War policy: assimilation and/or termination of Indian people. Western attitudes must be approached with care, since many of these therapies are ways of colonizing the lifeworld, which results in the ongoing cultural hegemony over the Indian client seeking relief for the soul wound. Clinicians working with Indian people must develop cultural competence, which requires therapeutic congruence with the client's culture (Brave Heart-Jordan & DeBruyn, 1995).

Most therapies used in Indian country today are a direct derivative of psychoanalysis: client-centered, behavioral, and other European/Euro-American models. The fact that traditional indigenous therapies are completely disregarded is indicative of ongoing cultural hegemony within the therapeutic arena. As mentioned earlier, the therapeutic arena does not exist in a vacuum and is therefore suspect as a hegemonic tool. Foucault (1967) eloquently describes the mental health field as merely another tool of social control. Until traditional indigenous therapies are implemented and considered legitimate, there will be a struggle, and, sadly, the suffering of a historical legacy and ongoing trauma will continue.

It is interesting that many of the present-day interventions in some arenas within Indian country were recommended by our ancestors for centuries. Early in the 17th century, Handsome Lake had a series of visions in which he prescribed cultural revitalization as a way of counteracting the devastation of colonialism and its effects. The use of alcohol was seen as a prime force causing instability in Indian country (Wallace, 1969). "The second social principle was peace and social unity. This principle was institutionalized in 1801 when Handsome Lake became the moral censor and principal leader of the Six Nations" (Duran & Duran, 1995, p. 65). Tenskwatawa also urged tribal members to give up ideas of private property and to return to communal life and fight the acquisition of land by whites. He taught Indians to move away from white people's food, technology, and manner of dress. Tenskwatawa also cautioned against any close association with colonial Americans.

Interventions have been prescribed by our ancestors for many generations, and through the integrating and reviving of their teachings, some effective therapies have been developed. These therapies have moved from a colonized mind-set into a postcolonial paradigm. By postcolonial we mean "a social criticism that bears witness to those unequal processes of representation by which the historical experience of the once colonized comes to be framed in the west" (Bhabha, 1983, p. 8). Postcolonial therapies will not operate on the logic of equivalence—A:non-A—but rather on a logic of difference—A:B—thus celebrating all diverse ways of life rather than comparing others to what they are not (Duran & Duran, 1995).

Programs that have succeeded are programs that have utilized indigenous epistemology as the root metaphor for theoretical and clinical implementation. Once indigenous knowledge and therapies are in place, it becomes a simple task to integrate the healing with Euro-American models of therapy. This is remarkable, because the opposite is true in most situations where the bureaucracy seeks integrated treatment models. That bureaucratic model continues to place Western medical practitioners in charge, and any indigenous knowledge is therefore the handmaiden of the perceived superior Western model. It is obvious that this merely reifies ongoing colonial paradigms and serves to exacerbate the soul wound.

A protocol has been developed in which the movement of therapy in a postcolonial treatment paradigm can be seen. The program described has staff who are trained in both Western and indigenous treatment and epistemological systems, which allows them to have some understanding of the client's lifeworld. In addition, there are traditional medicine people who also participate in diagnosis, treatment, and other facets of therapy. A typical protocol for a client may be as follows:

1. The client is referred to either the traditional (indigenous therapist) provider or psychologist for intervention (both of these instances will have people who understand both Western and indigenous treatments).
2. The traditional counselor or psychologist makes an assessment of the client and immediately has a conference with the other providers.
3. The client then receives psychotherapy, as well as participates in traditional ceremonies as appropriate. If the client needs help from a medicine person, she or he is referred to one from her or his traditional belief system. The therapy that the client receives is designed to help the client understand the process itself. Many Native American clients have been so acculturated that, many times, the focus of the therapy is merely to reconnect them to a traditional system of belief and make sense of their lifeworld from a traditional perspective.
4. The client is evaluated and recommendations are made for ongoing therapy or participation in traditional ceremonies.

We have attempted to delineate an approach that has had significant success with people from many tribes. It is critical that the reader understand that this is not a technique taught in most counseling programs. The people intervening must themselves practice a lifestyle that reflects some indigenous teachings. If the practitioners do not live a lifestyle that follows some traditional forms, the interventions will be seen as caricatures and offensive by the community.

We must impress on the reader the importance of helping the client get in touch with indigenous identities and ways of being in the world. In so doing, the client's self-esteem and identity will be enhanced. In addition, by becoming aware of historical factors, the client will be able to rid him- or herself of the internalized oppressor. The exorcizing of the internalized oppressor is one of the biggest accomplishments that the client can make in the therapy process. Ridding the client of the oppressor can only be effected through the implementation of the integrated model of therapy. If there is no integrated model of treatment, then the client is once more hearing that only white models are valid, thus facilitating a deeper internalization of the oppressor.

There are approaches being used that address the trauma of a whole community. Brave Heart-Jordan (1995; see also Brave Heart, in press a) details, in her study, an intervention model of culturally syntonic grief resolution and healing from the historical trauma response among the Lakota. She identified and incorporated features congruent with treatment for Holocaust survivors and descendants such as the following: (1) facilitating mourning as the primary task (Danieli, 1989; Fogelman, 1991); (2) helping the patient tolerate affects that accompany the traumatic memories and the process of working through (Krystal, 1984; van der Kolk, 1987); (3) codifications in self- and object representations as well as world representations (Krystal, 1984); and (4) validation and normalization of the trauma response (Krystal, 1984; Lifton, 1988) and techniques such as visualization and pseudohypnotic suggestibility (Koller, Marmar, & Kansas, 1992). She also uses techniques involving exploration of pre-Holocaust family history (Danieli, 1989, 1993).

Brave Heart-Jordan (1995) describes her treatment as a group treatment model. The restorative factors of this modality incorporate sharing experiences, the provision of hope, collective mourning, and social support. Specifically, short-term group treatment models are also recommended. Advantages of group treatment include bonding through sharing common traumatic experiences and mutual identification. "The transmission of psychopathology is inhibited through developing awareness of the intergenerational transfer processes" (Danieli, 1989; Brave Heart-Jordan, 1995, p. 114).

The Lakota have implemented a communal memorialization through the Tatanka Iyotake and Wokiksuye (Sitting Bull Memorial and Bigfoot) Ride, which traces the path of the Hunkpapa and Miniconju massacred at Wounded Knee. "The Lakota intervention model includes catharsis, abreaction, group sharing, testimony, opportunities for expression of traditional culture and language, and ritual and communal mourning" (Brave Heart, in press a). Wounded Knee and the generational boarding-school trauma cannot be forgotten.

Brave Heart-Jordan (1995) found that

- Education about the historical trauma leads to increased awareness about trauma, its impact, and the grief-related affects.
- The process of sharing these affects with others of similar background and within a traditional Lakota context leads to a cathartic sense of relief.
- A healing and mourning process was initiated, resulting in a reduction of grief affects, an experience of more positive group identity, and an increased commitment to continuing healing work both on an individual and community level.

In the study conducted by Brave Heart-Jordan (1995), 100% found the intervention helped them with their grief resolution and 72.7% found it very helpful. Ninety-seven percent felt they could now make a constructive commitment to the memory of their ancestors; a majority found this to be very true. All respondents felt better about themselves after the intervention, with 75.8% expressing high agreement with this statement. In a qualitative study of a reservation Lakota parenting skills curriculum based on her historical trauma intervention model, Brave Heart (in press c) found that participants experienced improvement in their parenting. The Takini Network, a collective of Lakota historical trauma survivors, is furthering this type of research as well as community healing interventions and prevention curricula.

DISCUSSION

Many years of pain and grieving have gone into the concepts and thoughts presented in this chapter. All of the knowledge discussed has been passed in an oral manner from many elders in our communities. The knowledge imparted by the elders has been translated into a form that will make sense to academicians and other people interested in the topic. It is important to note that explanations of the soul wound are centuries old. This knowledge has been kept out of the mainstream due to the invalidating nature of Western gatekeepers of literature dissemination.

For the most part, the information available to the public in this regard has had to pass through colonial lenses, and by the time it is made available, the story has been distorted.

Intervention strategies that have been useful in dealing with the soul wound have been effective in many ways. People have engaged the healing process and have made use of traditional forms of healing. The fact that they integrate indigenous knowledge into their lives is a step in the creation of counterhegemonic discourse. Most of the people who became clients in our clinics and/or participants at our workshops engaged in this discourse. That made their lives more meaningful and helped to liberate them from the symptoms of ongoing neocolonialism that may have been imposed on them by other health systems that were not aware of the issues discussed in this chapter.

Soul-wound workshops and group interventions on healing from historical trauma and unresolved grief have been developed and given all over Indian country. Every time these workshops are given, many participants make it public that finally they understand why they have been feeling so bad, and why they have been symptomatic. We have seen many tears in the eyes of our elders as they feel the liberating touch of historical truth and the validation of their pain, grief, and anger. Through purification and other ceremonies, the pain can then be transformed into a powerful, life-giving force. As one healer states, "We have already paid the price. It's time to accept the many blessings that the Creator has in store for us. We must honor our people who sacrificed everything through honoring ourselves and healing ourselves. By healing ourselves, we will also heal the wounds of our ancestors and the unborn generations."

REFERENCES

Bergmann, M. S., & Jucovy, M. E. (Eds.) (1990). *Generations of the Holocaust.* New York: Columbia University Press. (Originally published 1982)

Bhabha, H. (1983). *The other question: The stereotype and colonial discourse. Screen, 24,* 6–23.

Brave Heart-Jordan, M. Y. H. (1995). *The return to the Sacred Path: Healing from historical trauma and historical unresolved grief among the Lakota.* Doctoral dissertation Smith College, School for Social Work, Northampton, Massachusetts. (Copies are available through the Takini Network, c/o the author, University of Denver Graduate School of Social Work, 2148 S. High Street, Denver, CO 80208.)

Brave Heart-Jordan, M., & DeBruyn, L. M. (1995). *So she may walk in balance: Integrating the impact of historical trauma in the treatment of Native American Indian women.* In J. Adleman & G. Enguidanos (Eds.), *Racism in the lives of women: Testimony, theory, and guides to anti-racist practice* (pp. 345–368). New York: Haworth Press.

Brave Heart, M. Y. H. (in press a). The return to the sacred path: Healing the historical trauma and historical unresolved grief response among the Lakota. *Smith College Studies in Social Work,* June 1998.

Brave Heart, M. Y. H. (in press b). Gender differences in the historical trauma response among the Lakota. *Journal of Health and Social Policy.*

Brave Heart, M. Y. H. (in press c). *Oyate Ptayela:* Rebuilding the Lakota Nation through addressing historical trauma among Lakota parents. *Journal of Human Behavior and the Social Environment.*

Brave Heart, M. Y. H., & DeBruyn, L. M. (in press). The American Indian Holocaust: Healing historical unresolved grief. *National Center for American Indian and Alaska Native Research.*

Brown, D. (1971). *Bury my heart at Wounded Knee.* New York: Holt, Rinehart and Winston.

Claymore, B. (1988). A public health approach to suicide attempts on a Sioux reservation. *American Indian and Alaska Native Mental Health Research, 1*(3), 19–24.

Curry, A. (1972). *Bringing of forms,* Colorado Springs, CO:Dustbooks. Distributed by Seventh-Wing Publications.

Danieli, Y. (1985). The treatment and prevention of long-term effects and intergenerational transmission of victimization: A lesson from Holocaust survivors and their children. In C. R. Figley (Ed.), *Trauma and it's wake* (pp. 295–313). New York: Brunner/Mazel.

Danieli, Y. (1989). Mourning in survivors and children of survivors of the Nazi Holocaust: The role of group and community modalities. In D. R. Dietrich & P. C. Shabad (Eds.), *The problems of loss and mourning: Psychoanalytic perspectives* (pp. 427–457). Madison, CT: International Universities Press.

Danieli, Y. (1993). Diagnostic and therapeutic use of the multigenerational family tree in working with survivors of the Nazi Holocaust. In P. W. Wilson & B. Raphael (Eds.), *International handbook of traumatic stress syndromes* (pp. 889–898). New York: Plenum Press.

Deloria, V. & Lytle, C. M. (1983). *American Indians, American justice.* Austin: University of Texas Press.

Duran, E. F. (1990). *Transforming the soul wound: A theoretical/clinical approach to American Indian psychology.* Berkeley, CA: Folklore Institute.

Duran, E. F., & Duran, B. M. (1995). *Native American postcolonial psychology.* Albany, NY: State University of New York Press.

Erikson, E. (1950). *Childhood and society.* New York: Norton.

Fogelman, E. (1988). Therapeutic alternatives of survivors. In R. L. Braham (Ed.), *The psychological perspectives of the Holocaust and of its aftermath* (pp. 79–108). New York: Columbia University Press.

Fogelman, E. (1991). Mourning without graves. In A. Medvene (Ed.), *Storms and rainbows: The many faces of death* (pp. 25–43). Washington, DC: Lewis Press.

Foucault, M. (1967). *Madness and civilization.* London: Tavistock.

Freire, P. (1968). *Pedagogy of the oppressed.* New York: Seabury Press.

Indian Health Service. (1987). *Chart series book.* Washington, DC: U.S. Department of Health and Human Services, Public Health Service, IHS, Office of Planning and Evaluation and Legislation, Division of program statistics.

Indian Health Service. (1995). *Trends in Indian health.* Washington, DC: Department of Health and Human Services.

Indian Health Service Report. (1991, December). *A roundtable conference on dysfunctional behavior and its impact on Indian health.* Final Report. Albuquerque, NM & Washington, DC: Kauffman.

Jacobs. (1972). *Dispossessing the American Indian: Indians and whites on the colonial frontier.* Norman: University of Oklahoma Press.

Jucovy, M. (1992). Psychoanalytic contributions to Holocaust studies. *International Journal of Psychoanalysis, 73,* 267–282.

Kehoe, A. B. (1989). *The Ghost Dance: Ethnohistory and revitalization.* Fort Worth, TX: Holt, Rinehart and Winston.

Kestenberg, J. S. (1990). A metapsychological assessment based on an analysis of a survivor's child. In M. S. Bergmann & M. E. Jucovy (Eds.), *Generations of the Holocaust* (pp. 137–158). New York: Columbia University Press. (Original publication 1982)

Koller, P., Marmar, C. R., & Kansas, N. (1992). Psychodynamic group treatment of post-traumatic stress disorder in Vietnam veterans. *International Journal of Group Psychotherapy, 42*(2), 225–246.

Krugman, S. (1987). Trauma in the family: Perspectives on the intergenerational transmission of violence. In B. A. van der Kolk (Ed.), *Psychological trauma* (pp. 127–151). Washington, DC: American Psychiatric Association Press.

Krystal, H. (1984). Integration and self-healing in post-traumatic states. In S. A. Luel & P. Marcus (Eds.), *Psychoanalytic reflections on the Holocaust: Selected essays* (pp. 113–134). New York: Holocaust Awareness Institute, Center for Judaic Studies, University of Denver and Ktav Publishing House.

Legters, L. H. (1988). The American genocide. *Policy Studies Journal, 16*(4), 768–777.

Lifton, R. J. (1988). Understanding the traumatized self: Imagery, symbolization, and transformation. In J. P. Wilson, Z. Harel, & B. Kahana (Eds.), *Human adaptation to extreme stress: From the Holocaust to Vietnam* (pp. 7–31). New York: Plenum Press.

Limmerick, P. N. (1987). *The legacy of conquest: The unbroken past of the American West.* New York: Norton.

MacAndrews, C., & Edgerton, R. (1969). *Drunken comportment: A social explanation.* Chicago: Aldine.

Macgregor, G. (1975). *Warriors without weapons.* Chicago: University of Chicago Press. (Original published 1946)

Marcus, P., & Rosenberg, A. (1988). A philosophical critique of the "Survivor Syndrome" and some implications for treatment. In R. L. Braham (Ed.), *The psychological perspectives of the Holocaust and of its aftermath* (pp. 53–78). New York: Columbia University Press.

Niehardt. (1959). *Black Elk speaks.* New York: Simon & Schuster.

Pearce, R. H. (1988). *Savagism and civilization: A study of the Indian and the American mind.* Berkeley: University of California Press.

Prucha, F. P. (1990). *Documents of the United States Indian policy* (2nd Ed. Expanded). Lincoln: University of Nebraska Press. (Original publication 1975)

Report to Congress. (1992). *National Indian Policy Center: Reporting to Congress, Recommendation for the establishment of a National Indian Policy Center.* Washington, DC: U.S. Government Printing Office.

Shoshan, T. (1989). Mourning and longing from generation to generation. *American Journal of Psychotherapy, 43*(2), 193–207.

Solomon, Z., Kotler, M., & Mikulincer, M. (1988). Combat-related posttraumatic stress disorder among second-generation Holocaust survivors: Preliminary findings. *American Journal of Psychiatry, 145*(7), 865–868.

Stannard, D. (1992). *American Holocaust: Columbus and the conquest of the New World.* New York: Oxford University Press.

Tanner, H. (1982). *A history of all the dealings of the United States government with the Sioux.* Unpublished manuscript. Prepared for the Black Hills Land Claim by order of the U.S. Supreme court, on file at the D'Arcy McNickle Center for the History of the American Indian, Newberry Library, Chicago.

Thornton, R. (1987). *American Indian holocaust and survival: A population history since 1942.* Norman: University of Oklahoma Press.

van der Kolk, B. A. (Ed.) (1987). *Psychological trauma.* Washington, DC: American Psychiatric Press.

Villanueva, M. (1989). *Literature review.* In E. Duran (Ed.), *Suicide handbook: Prevention and intervention with Native Americans* (pp. 13–36). Sacramento, CA: Indian Health Service.

Wallace, A. F. (1969). *The death and rebirth of the Seneca.* New York: Vintage Books.

Weinfeld, M., Sigal, J. J., & Eaton, W. W. (1981). Long-term effects of the Holocaust on selected social attitudes and behaviors of survivors: A cautionary note. *Social Forces, 60,* 1–19.

White, R. (1983). *The roots of dependency: Subsistence, environment and social change among the Choctaws, Pawnees, and Navajos.* Lincoln: University of Nebraska Press.

Williams, C. L., & Berry, J. W. (1991). Primary prevention of acculturative stress among refugees: Application of psychological theory and practice. *American Psychologist, 46*(6), 632–641.

Yellow Horse-Davis, S. F. (1994). Federal Policy Impact on Indian Mental Health Services. Unpublished manuscript.

22

The Role of Dependency and Colonialism in Generating Trauma in First Nations Citizens

The James Bay Cree

MARIE-ANIK GAGNÉ

INTRODUCTION

Research on trauma among First Nations citizens has focused primarily upon the psychological aspects of posttraumatic stress disorder (PTSD). The role of sociology in this area of research is different than that of psychology. This chapter elaborates upon a general sociological discussion of the legacy of colonialism and dependency and focus on the intergenerational effects of this trauma. Figure 1 illustrates the process by which the trauma is passed on, from the seed of colonialism to the outer layer, which represents the current traumatic events being experienced by First Nations citizens. The Cree of the James Bay region in Canada are utilized to describe this figure in more detail.

This chapter has three main sections. The first includes a discussion of trauma, with emphasis on PTSD and an explanation and elaboration of Figure 1. The second section discusses, from both psychological and sociological perspectives, solutions to the trauma experienced by First Nations citizens. The third section summarizes the process by which the effects of trauma have become intergenerational among First Nations citizens.

DEFINING TRAUMA

The concept of trauma figures more and more in the literature of First Nations (see, e.g., Manson *et al.,* 1996; Young, 1995). It appears that this concept, and, in particular, the experience

Some of the issues discussed in this chapter have been elaborated in more detail in Marie-Anik Gagné, *A Nation within a Nation: Dependency and the Cree.* Montreal: Black Rose Books, 1994.

MARIE-ANIK GAGNÉ • Health Systems Research Unit, Clarke Institute of Psychiatry, 250 College Street, Toronto, Ontario, M5T 1R8 Canada

International Handbook of Multigenerational Legacies of Trauma, edited by Yael Danieli. Plenum Press, New York, 1998.

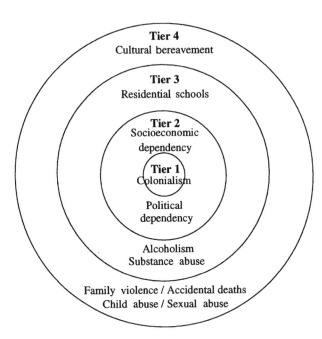

Figure 1. Cycle of traumatic events.

of PTSD, is employed as a form of metaphor for the consequences of economic and social dependence experienced by First Nations citizens. Later sections of this chapter explore how this concept can be accurately applied to the James Bay Cree and other First Nations citizens. Before embarking on a discussion of the cause and effect of trauma, it is important to define the concept of trauma itself.

The basic definition of trauma is that of a shock that is deemed emotional and substantially damages, over a long time period, the psychological development of the victim, often leading to neurosis. The discussion of the effects of trauma on First Nations citizens usually centers around PTSD. Even with this definition of trauma, one remaining question is: What constitutes a traumatic event? The third edition of the *Diagnostic and Statistical Manual of Mental Disorders* (DSM-III-R); American Psychiatric Association, 1987), defined a traumatic event as a nonordinary human experience that may lead to PTSD, and which would be distressing to most people, such as serious harm or threat to self, spouse, children, close relatives or friends; witnessing a serious accident or violence against another person, who, as a result, is either killed or seriously injured; or having one's home or community suddenly destroyed.

In order to receive the diagnosis of PTSD, an individual has to "persistently experience" the traumatic event, persistently try to avoid stimuli associated with the event, experience an increased arousal (i.e., trouble falling asleep, irritability, or hypervigilance) and, finally, suffer from these symptoms for at least 1 month. The exact criteria for diagnosis are listed in the fourth edition of the *Diagnostic and Statistical Manual of Mental Disorders* (DSM-IV; American Psychiatric Association, 1994). PTSD is, in fact, classified under anxiety disorders in the DSM-IV, as most manifestations of PTSD are also symptoms of anxiety. Symptoms accompanying anxiety disorders, such as dissociative, depressive, or somatic symptoms, arise when the body is having a conditioned emotional response to fear, severe stress, and loss.

Despite the fact that PTSD is discussed in the literature, actual data are scarce. The National Center for American Indian and Alaska Native Mental Health Research conducted three studies with the aim of further understanding trauma and PTSD in young Natives. Manson *et al.* (1996) summarized the findings of these studies conducted between 1989 and 1992. These were titled the Health Survey of Indian Boarding School Students, the Flower of Two Soils Reinterview, and the Foundations of Indian Teens Project. A total of 477 youths, ranging in age from 8 to 20, and from grades 2 to 12, were interviewed in various reserves and/or tribally controlled secondary schools in the United States and Canada. Examples of enumerated traumatic events involving the students were overdoses, shootings, car accidents, and rapes. Traumatic events not involving the students were shootings, stabbings, surgeries, beatings, car accidents, death by natural causes, suicides, murders, drownings, and auto–pedestrian accidents. Summarizing the results from all three studies, between 50.8% and 62% of the students had experienced at least one traumatic event. Of the students with a (past) history of traumatic events, between 50% and 87.4% met the DSM-III-R Criterion B (persistently reexperiences the traumatic event), 8% and 66.9% met Criterion C (persistently avoids stimuli associated with the trauma and/or psychiatric numbing), 16% to 72% of the students had persistent symptoms of automatic hyperarousal (Criterion D), and, 9% to 19% exhibited Criterion E (experiencing their symptoms for at least 1 month). In these studies, between 1.6% and 29.6% of the students met the criteria for PTSD. The latter figure is inflated due to the nature of a self-administered test distributed to the Foundation of Indians Teen Project study sample. However, Manson *et al.* (1996) report that the observed symptoms of PTSD may have been triggered by prior trauma; hence, an in-depth interview is necessary to determine the cause. Other reported mental disorders, such as anxiety and affective disorders, may have been experienced or may be comorbid to the PTSD symptoms. For example, in the Flower of Two Soils Reinterview, more than half of the students (52%, $n = 32$) who experienced a traumatic event also met the criteria for diagnosis of an additional or independent mental disorder. Manson *et al.* also found that there was a direct relationship between the number of reported traumatic experiences and the likelihood of diagnosis of a non-PTSD disorder.

To briefly summarize some of the findings, Manson *et al.* (1996, 1990) and O'Nell (1989) have, in general, found a disproportionately high percentage of First Nation citizens in the United States who suffer from anxiety disorders, exposure to traumatic events, and PTSD.

THE ROLE OF THE SOCIOLOGIST

As stated in the introduction, this chapter takes a sociological approach to trauma. The role of sociologists and anthropologists is to consider trauma as dramatically changing the system of human relationships, which will, as a consequence, directly affect future generations. Hence, sociologists must consider social trauma as influencing society as a whole (Rousseau & Drapeau, Chapter 28, this volume). This approach differs from the more individually oriented disciplines, which normally consider single individuals with a disorder related to trauma, who, in turn, transmit their behavior to the members of their family. Although Rousseau and Drapeau elaborated on this concept as a preface to studying the impact of culture on the transmission of trauma, this chapter utilizes this approach to illustrate how the James Bay Cree are continuously affected by trauma imbedded in their society.

TIER 1

Colonialism

This chapter hypothesizes that colonialism is the seed of trauma because it leads to dependency, then to cultural genocide, racism, and alcoholism. These in turn lead to sexual abuse, family violence, child abuse, and accidental deaths/suicides (Figure 1). Although colonialism is often said to be the primary source of the problems experienced by First Nations citizens, few studying PTSD among this population discuss the actual history of the people and by what means colonialism has led to dependency. O'Neil (1994) commented that it is remarkable that the Native culture has survived despite colonialism. Colonialism threatened oral traditions by decimating entire families and bands, causing the premature loss of elders who were responsible for passing on oral traditions, and creating economic dependency. Hence, First Nations had to depend on the external society in order to survive.

This section presents a discussion of the emergence of the James Bay region as a "periphery" and its people as dependents. This area was first discovered when Henry Hudson sailed his ship, *The Discovery,* up the Hudson river in 1611. To acquire valuable fur resources, Europeans built trading posts throughout the area. Rupert House, the first post of the Hudson's Bay Company (HBC), was established in 1668. In the spring of 1969, the first pelts acquired from Cree hunters were brought back to London. From the very beginning, the relationship between the Europeans and the Cree was not an equal one, with the HBC fixing the scales in its favor.

Debt plays a large role in determining the level of dependence of peripheral populations. Beginning in the first half of the 18th century, the HBC made the Natives dependent on particular trading posts by extending credit to them. As the Natives left the posts in the fall, they would be given quantities of supplies for the bush, the price of which would be deducted from the value of spring furs. The amount of credit was determined by their previous season's catch, an average of 20 pelts. The HBC did this to keep the Natives trading with the Company instead of with the inland competition. Most were given a credit of 10–12 beaver pelts. The HBC found that they could manipulate the Natives into trading with them by extending this credit. However, the Company was always careful not to give too much, so that the hunter would not move to the competition once his debt accumulated or die with a large debt that the Company would have to absorb. Decades later, the HBC introduced new regulations assigning Natives to a particular post, so that they could not avoid paying their debts, thus limiting the hunter's movements from that day onward.

In 1828, the HBC began assigning not only particular trading posts but also land to hunting families, thus ensuring control of each hunter's credit. This arrangement benefited only the Company and consequently rearranged the social organization of Natives. The HBC's division of land had little regard for previous traplines or for nonmonogamous families. In fact, as many as one-sixth of the families were polygamous at the time. The HBC redistributed the land to monogamous families, leaving numerous women and children, who had been the second and third wives and offspring of hunters, dependent.

James Bay Natives were now being controlled by economic arrangements that primarily benefited the HBC; they were assigned land that was previously defined, their family structure was altered, and their hunting habits were controlled. Finally, the HBC even sought to control the marriages of Natives at the posts—by requiring them to receive the postmaster's permission to marry. This provided economic benefits for the Company by creating fewer dependents. In addition, hunters had to leave 10% of their earnings as a security deposit, in case of death.

The War of 1812 marked a period of considerable change for First Nations citizens. After this war, Canada was no longer threatened by the United States, leading to a large migration of British in search of the promised agricultural land. The population in Canada increased from 95,000 to 952,000 in the decade from 1841 to 1851 (Janigan, 1992). Consequently, Natives were no longer a majority and were no longer needed for military or economic purposes. They quickly lost their power while the Canadian government proceeded in its attempt to assimilate them.

During the next century, many new laws were created by the government in the hope of assimilating Natives. In 1857, Canada gave the right to vote and 20 hectares of land to Natives who were debt-free, educated, and of good moral character. In exchange, Natives had to relinquish their aboriginal status. In 1869, federal bureaucrats were given the power to remove traditional Indian leaders from their positions for what the bureaucrats deemed as dishonesty, intemperance, or immorality. The same statute stipulated that Indian women who married non-Indians lost their status. The federal representatives replaced the traditional Native leaders with elected band councils. Those First Nations citizens who had agricultural products to sell required permits to do so; they also needed permits to leave the reserves in western Canada. Natives were not allowed to wear traditional dress off reserves. According to the Royal Proclamation of 1763, First Nations citizens could not mortgage their lands for capital to finance economic projects; they could only cede their lands to the Crown. From 1894 to the 1960s, Natives were forced to send their children to schools run by missionaries (the effects of this law on Natives are discussed in a later section). Until 1976, according to the first Indian Act, Natives lost their status if they practiced medicine, law, or entered the ministry.

To summarize and place this history in a sociological context, peripheral countries or regions are primarily viewed as exporters of raw materials. Whether the products are agricultural or mineral, these regions are exploited for the benefit of others. In the case of the James Bay area, the land was stripped of its animals to benefit the Europeans. In an analogous fashion, the Cree were stripped of their status, of their organizational process, and of their language, to name but a few of their losses.

The changes that the James Bay Cree experienced from the predependent era to after the colonizing period were tremendous. From the time the HBC first established trading posts, the lives of the Cree would never be the same. As their hunting patterns were altered by the HBC's policies, they began relying more on the posts and less on their previous hunting activities. Some argue that these changes are part of a natural evolution, that First Nations citizens in Canada could not continue to live in "teepees" year-round while sustaining themselves by hunting (as with most First Nations citizens around the world). Nevertheless, these changes would not have occurred so quickly without this process of colonialization, even though contact with the outside world was inevitable. The primary problem with these changes was that they made the James Bay area a periphery, and, by doing so, made its residents dependent on the "center." The actions of the HBC, the missionaries, and the government made the Cree dependent by removing their self-sufficiency. Both the HBC and the federal government found itself with more dependents after the implementation of new policy. Peripheral areas and countries are created by the core, not by the members of the periphery, and they are not a natural process of development.

TIER 2

The Dependent Theory

The previous section outlined how the James Bay area became a dependent periphery. It is important to have an understanding of the dependency theory when utilizing this concept to explain particular ailments in society. The concept of dependence has traditionally been employed when discussing the existing relationship between industrialized and underdeveloped countries. Dependency theory maintains that underdevelopment in the periphery is caused by obstacles placed by economic and political external structures, that is, those imposed by the center.

Before venturing further, it is interesting to note the origin of this theory. Hall (1981) describes the emergence of the dependency theory as one that was created by Native scholars in semiperipheral areas. It was not recognized until it was first denied and "reinvented" by the scholars in the center, who labeled it a world-system theory and reexported it to its point of origin.

Dependency theorists use the terms *center* and *periphery* to describe the developed and the underdeveloped, respectively, or to be more precise, the *controller* and the *dependent*. Interchangeable terms for the center are *core* and *metropole;* the periphery is also called *satellite* and *hinterland*. Since this theory was initially introduced to explain the differences between the industrialized and the nonindustrialized countries, they are often respectively grouped as North and South.

Dependency theory has been criticized for not examining the development of Third World countries independently of the development of the center or North. Dependency theorists (Dos Santos, 1973; Frank, 1973), viewing the world as a "single system," disagree with this criticism. They believe that one must look at how the underdeveloped countries were "inserted" into the world system and study how their historical positions and development were different from that of the North. Dependency theory was, in fact, created in response to imperialistic theories.

Dependency occurs when the economies of one group of countries are subjected to the development and expansion of other economies (Dos Santos, 1973). Furthermore, this dependency will alter the internal structures of underdeveloped countries. This is a good definition of dependency, because it takes into consideration both the internal and the external factors of dependency and recognizes the existence of interdependent relationships (between the North and the South). It states that the relationship is dependent when the dominant countries expand and are self-sustaining, while the dependent countries can only expand as a reflection of the dominant ones (Roxborough, 1983).

There is a direct relationship between the level of "underdevelopment" and dependency in countries (Bromley & Bromley, 1988). The more a country relies on foreign investment, political decisions, resources, and technology, the fewer important changes a country can make without the approval of outsiders, hence the increase in dependency. Even though there are several different lines of thought in the dependency paradigm, most theorists agree that currently underdeveloped countries were not always at this stage. Underdevelopment, rather, is a state that arose after contact with imperialist nations.

There is a clear distinction to be made between the terms *underdeveloped* and *undeveloped*. Development occurs in undeveloped countries when self-reliance is maintained during the process. Undeveloped countries have, perhaps, easier access to development because they are not controlled by outside economic and political powers. Underdeveloped countries, on the other hand, are dependent without self-reliance and in need of foreign investment and technology. Therefore, countries that are undeveloped can have access to development; their regions have fewer problems with social and economic inequalities and, thus, have a stronger balance. (Examples of this movement from undeveloped to developed are the United States and Britain; meanwhile, countries such as Trinidad and Haiti went from undeveloped to underdeveloped [Allahar, 1995].) For Bromley and Bromley (1988), self-reliance is the key indicator to determine whether a country or region is underdeveloped or undeveloped. They state that the simplest way to determine whether a region is underdeveloped is to examine its gross national product. Underdevelopment leads to extreme poverty and no growth; therefore, the poorest countries or regions within countries are the most underdeveloped.

The center and periphery theory states, in general, that the reason one region is developed is that another is underdeveloped (Sacouman, 1981). Furthermore, when using the center and periphery theory, it is important to understand how these regions were formed. Roxborough (1983) believes that such regions were created when societies changed from feudalism to capitalism. Three major changes took place with this transition: (1) conflict between landowners and peasants, (2) urbanization, and (3) the evolution of centralized states. He explains that for this chain of events to occur, there had to be a rapid increase in capital. Two methods have been employed to increase the capital in the center: the first was to strip the wealth of the peripheries by colonialists, the second was to confiscate land held by peasants and the Church. These methods of "freeing" capital also created a landless class.

Resources are exported from the peripheral countries or regions to where they are processed into finished products. They are then returned to their point of origin with an inflated price tag. Thus, capital is accumulated in the center, which benefits not only from the profits but also from the jobs created by the manufacturing industry. Employed workers of the center generally have more money to spend, hence the development for a service industry. Dependence theorists see this economic "rape" of a country's wealth as directly related to its continued dependence and backwardness. The peripheral regions become dependent because they neglect their internal markets, whereby most of their structures are developed for export. Part of their dependence stems from the fact that they have tailored "their economies to meet the needs of the advanced ones" (Allahar, 1989, p. 90).

Clement (1980), Matthews (1982) and Veltmeyer (1978) have used the dependency theory to explain economic and social regional differences within Canada. They claim that Canada became more dependent on the United States as it detached itself from Britain and traded more with its southern neighbor. This increase in dependence accentuated the regional disparities. This occurred because the "regional economies are tied to national economies and national ones to international ones," thus creating a chain reaction (Allahar, 1989, p. 90).

As discussed earlier, in the context of peripheral and central countries in the world, the South (e.g., Central and South America) had supplied inexpensive raw materials, while many countries in the North (e.g., United States and Canada) utilized these raw materials to manufacture final products. Because of this division, only the North directly and indirectly profited from the raw resources. As Canada is divided into an industrial region and a hinterland, Clement (1980) believes that this process has occurred in Canada as well (only here the center is southern and the peripheral regions tend to be northern). Industrial Canada can be found between Windsor, Ontario, and Montreal, Quebec. Even though there are other industrial pockets across the country, there are some regions that are clearly "underdeveloped," for example, areas of the Atlantic provinces and much of the North. These regions have wealth, but this wealth is primarily made up of natural resources as opposed to financial institutions and production plants. Since the main source of income is from raw materials, wages and employment rates remain low in these regions. The consequence of this underdevelopment is that infrastructures are substandard, social development is of low priority (Matthews, 1982), and "life chances" for those residing in the core are much better.

In conclusion, dependency theory essentially maintains that developed countries are such because there are underdeveloped nations, that the economy of an underdeveloped country is dependent on the center, and that consequences of underdevelopment include neglected social development and lack of social infrastructure. Applying dependency theory, the following section discusses concrete examples of economic and political dependence experienced by First Nations citizens, in particular the James Bay Cree.

Economic Dependency.   One way of determining the degree of dependence of First Nations citizens is to examine the origin of their major sources of income. In 1986, 50% of registered Indians residing on-reserve reported that their major source of income was government transfer payments, whereas only 20% of the general population reported the same major source (Quantitative Analysis and Socio-Demographic Research, 1989, p. 27). Only 55% of registered Indians residing off-reserve reported employment income as their major source of income, compared to 70% of the general population (Quantitative Analysis and Socio-Demographic Research, 1989, p. 27). Also in 1986, registered Indian women earned two-thirds of the income earned by registered Indian men (Indian and Northern Affairs Canada, 1990, p. 30). It is also important to realize that a given amount of income received does not have the same buying power in isolated communities (e.g., northern, as compared with southern reserves) because of the inflated price of goods.

As mentioned earlier, one of the consequences of living in a peripheral region is improper infrastructure; poor housing conditions are an example. Statistics Canada defines a crowded dwelling as a home that has more than one occupant per room. In 1986, 37% of registered Indians living on-reserve in Quebec reported crowded dwellings, compared to 4% of the non-Native population residing near reserves (Indian and Northern Affairs Canada, 1990, p. 20). Registered Indians living off-reserve in Canada were approximately 18 times more likely to live in crowded dwellings than the non-Native population (Indian and Northern Affairs Canada, 1990, p. 29). Some may argue that First Nations citizens choose to live this way, that it is part of their culture to live with their extended families and friends. However, it is not culture but poor income that determines if they will have heating systems in their homes.

In 1986, 38% of registered Indian dwellings located on-reserve in Canada reported not having a central heating system (Indian and Northern Affairs Canada, 1990, p. 31). A central heating system is defined by Statistics Canada as a steam or hot-water furnace, forced air, or installed electric heating system. Registered Indians living off-reserve were almost twice as likely to report having a home without a central heating system than the general population, while registered Indians in Quebec were more than three times as likely to report the absence of central heating (Indian and Northern Affairs Canada, 1990, p. 31). Overcrowding and/or inadequate heating systems increase the occurrence of fire, and where there are substandard firefighting facilities—as in remote northern areas—these fires often lead to death.

Political Dependency.   The center has also hampered the development of First Nations citizens by controlling their political structures. In the late 1800s, the Canadian government began replacing traditional Native leaders with elected band councils. In so doing, the center removed the existing political structures, which were already quite sophisticated. It was easier for colonizers to standardize all peripheral governments according to one model, thus diminishing the task of dealing with several different nations, each with its own culture and political idiosyncrasies. The "whites" were seeking to assimilate and "civilize" the Natives. They forced municipal-like political structures onto First Nations bands, causing the loss of culture and power.

The policies of the HBC and the laws governing the Cree created dependency. The James Bay region was exploited for its natural resources; hence, their economy was tailored to the needs of the South. The laws prevented them from adapting their social infrastructure in light of the sudden changes. This state of imposed dependence led to a cultural genocide by the dominant society through residential schools, and alcoholism among the Natives, just as colonialism led to dependency (Figure 1). The trauma was not only continued but it also became more prominent. The next section discusses the emergence and effects of residential schools and alcoholism in First Nations communities.

TIER 3

Residential Schools

Much of the family violence, alcoholism, and suicidal behavior among First Nations citizens has originated either directly or indirectly from the abuse inflicted on students in the residential schools. York (1990) reports Mandy Brown (a social worker on the Lytton reserve) to say that these are problems that are transmitted from generation to generation, like an inherited disease. She repeatedly tried to treat community members for these problems without any success. Examining the family trees of the victims, she finally noticed one connecting factor: St. George's School, an Indian residential school near the reserve. In December 1987, the former dormitory supervisor, Derek Clarke, pleaded guilty to numerous counts of buggery and indecent assault. Judge William Blair said that Clarke had been responsible for as many as 700 incidents of sexual assault. In this instance, an entire community was deeply affected by the sexual abuse that occurred at the residential school. This scenario is not unique to the Lytton reserve. The horror stories of child abuse and sexual assault in these schools are still coming to light.

Residential schools were founded and operated by Protestant and Catholic missionaries. As mentioned earlier, Native children were sent away from their families and communities to these institutions across Canada from the late 19th century until the 1960s. First Nations citizens in western Canada were forced to send their children to schools run by missionaries as early as 1894.

Many believe that the placement of children, often by force, in isolated residential schools was in fact cultural genocide. These schools were more often than not administered by a practicing religious group, so that the students were forced to practice a religion that was not their own. Native children were forbidden to speak their mother tongue or to practice ceremonial rituals. These children became caught between two cultures: "Whites" tried to assimilate them into a society that was not ready to receive them, while taking away all the skills necessary to function in their own society. They never received the informal education that was required to learn their Native language, religion, and skills such as hunting and gathering.

Residential schools did not affect just the students who attended them. At least two subsequent generations were also "lost." The children of these students became victims of abuse as their parents became abusers because of the residential school experience. Since their parents had lost much of their culture, the small amount of informal education these children could receive came from other relations who did not attend the schools. The loss of culture that occurred in the decades of the residential schools was enormous. At least four generations of First Nations citizens attended these schools. The lasting effects of residential schools have been so severe that psychologists deemed it necessary to coin the term "residential-school syndrome." The cycle of grief associated with a loss of culture is as intense as the loss of a loved one (York, 1990). Genocide on the basis of ethnicity and religion has a traumatic effect on the families concerned (Rousseau & Drapeau, Chapter 28, this volume).

Alcoholism/Substance Abuse

Substance abuse, especially alcoholism, is a problem often associated with First Nations citizens. There are high levels of alcoholism in many Native communities. According to several Native leaders, alcohol is the number-one community problem (York, 1990). The problem with alcohol did not become obvious until after World War II, when the federal government began establishing military bases in remote areas of the country. These bases were most often near reserves and introduced social programs, such as housing projects and welfare. This increased flow of money into reserves and allowed Natives to purchase readily available goods outside the reserve for the first time. Residential schools were also beginning to have their intergenerational effect on the communities during this time. The frustration and pain of losing one's identity and of being caught between two cultures was transmitted from one generation to the next. The list of causes that pushed First Nations citizens toward alcoholism is endless and continues to grow. Many Natives may have started drinking after World War II for some of the reasons listed earlier. Some Natives are drinking today because the habit has been passed on from one generation to the next.

Alcoholism is also linked to the trauma described in Tier 4. The far-reaching effects of alcohol abuse are as enormous as the causes of alcoholism in First Nations communities. Binge drinking is very common among First Nations Citizens. Drinking is implicated in many of the accidental deaths of Natives. Many congenital defects are caused by the consumption of alcohol by pregnant women. Recently, as many as 25% of the children born on a British Columbian reserve had birth defects caused by fetal alcohol syndrome (York, 1990, p. 195). York quotes Bea Shawanda's (of the National Native Association of Treatment Directors) comment that violence and alcoholism are reactions by her people to a loss of language and culture, substituting, in effect, for grieving.

Another serious problem faced by First Nations bands is gasoline sniffing. It was first noticed among Natives in the early 1970s and has since become more popular. In 1975, 62% of Cree and Inuit youths at Great Whale River in northern Quebec revealed that they had sniffed gasoline at least once in the last 6 months (York, 1990, p. 10). Some people were said to use gasoline to calm their infants. The greatest problem with this kind of substance abuse is finding ways to control access to gasoline. In the case of alcohol, many reserves have set up roadblocks and search incoming airplanes in order to confiscate all forms of liquor. Gasoline, on the other hand, is necessary for operating boats, trucks, and skidoos. Medical experts assert that gasoline sniffing is the most dangerous addiction in the world; children may become addicted after only a single inhalation, and it causes severe physical damage to the nervous system (York, 1990). The effects of sniffing are similar to those of LSD; it creates a state of euphoria and altered consciousness.

One of the effects of gasoline sniffing is extreme violence. Police and court officials have claimed that 60% to 70% of juvenile crimes involved gasoline sniffing (York, 1990, p. 10). The problem is so serious that the death it can cause has been given a name, "sudden sniffing death syndrome." Chemicals in the inhalant cause an irregular heartbeat. When the sniffer attempts to fight or run, increased adrenalin causes the heartbeat to become more irregular and uncontrollable, resulting in heart failure and death.

Many precautions have been attempted in order to stop the sniffing addiction among First Nation citizens. The Hudson Bay store stopped selling glue, wood filler, nail-polish remover, felt-tip markers, typewriter correction fluid, and aerosol sprays in the North. Some bands have imposed curfews and "gas patrols." Patrollers take down the names of children who are caught sniffing and provide a copy to the nursing station and the band council. But gasoline sniffing is not illegal; therefore, the gas patrols are quite powerless. Some children start sniffing as early as 4 years old, when they see their brothers and sisters doing it.

York (1990) reports Dr. Fornazzari's (a neurologist at the Addiction Research Foundation in Toronto and an expert on inhalant abuse) observation that gasoline sniffing predominantly afflicts members of minority groups. Many minorities, such as the First Nations citizens of Australia and the United States, Hispanics, children of migrant workers, and illegal aliens, have been found to be inhalant abusers. Through complete or attempted assimilation, the dominant culture has destroyed the traditional economy and social organization of these groups. The dependent members of these minority groups adopt self-destructive behaviors, such as gasoline sniffing and alcoholism, because their identity has been lost and their traditional way of life has been destroyed.

Alcoholism is a more recent threat to the Inuit, who only came into contact with the substance on a regular basis in the mid-1960s. This coincided with the implementation of the Northern Rental Housing Program and the introduction of public schools. Their nomadic lifestyle was shifted to that of a sedentary village society. Since villages were first inhabited by people from different "tribal" backgrounds from a large geographic area, there was initially no real sense of community (O'Neil, 1984). Although the problem of alcoholism is more recent in the farthest points of the Canadian North, the causes and consequences (loss and separation) remain the same.

As indicated in Figure 1, the social problems of First Nations citizens are interrelated. To give a specific example, alcohol was said always to be involved in domestic fights by 44% of respondents in the Ontario Native Women's Association survey (1989), while 37% stated that it was often present in incidents of family violence (p. 22). In total, 78% of respondents said that alcoholism was a main cause of domestic violence. Alcohol abuse has been found to increase the risk of car accidents, domestic violence, and other traumatic circumstances, and this in turn increases the risk of PTSD (Manson, 1997).

The following section discusses the items listed in the Tier 4 of Figure 1: family violence, child abuse, sexual abuse, suicide, and accidental deaths.

TIER 4

Suicide, sexual abuse, alcoholism, and family violence are among the recognized effects of trauma experienced by First Nations citizens (Manson *et al.,* 1996). This chapter maintains that items in Tier 4 of Figure 1 constitute not only the effects of tauma, but also that they are themselves traumatic events, capable of creating yet more trauma. This follows Kirmayer's (1996) contention that the onset of PTSD is not only caused by a catastrophic stress, but that it also may emerge as a consequence of the accumulation and/or continuation of milder stressors.

Therefore, once we reach Tier 4, its items can be classified as traumatic events that in themselves are significant stressors that can lead to PTSD. The following briefly discusses some thoughts in the trauma literature regarding child and sexual abuse, family violence, accidental deaths, and cultural bereavement.

Child Abuse/Sexual Abuse

There are countless examples of child abuse as it relates to residential schools and other institutions, as demonstrated in the section on residential schools. However, rates of abuse within families are more sensitive in nature and less readily available. This is a problem that is of significance but is usually dealt with in an ethnographic manner (e.g., Martens, 1988).

Child abuse and sexual abuse are events that have been deemed to be traumatic enough to initiate symptoms of PTSD. As demonstrated by the measures used to diagnose this disorder in teens, these primarily focus on the trauma of sexual abuse. Kirmayer (1995) indicated that adults who were victims of childhood abuse are often initially unaware of their traumatic experiences as memories. Moreover, these adults will often be diagnosed with dissociative disorders. Their trauma manifests itself through symptoms such as numbing, substance abuse, emotional and physical pain, changes of identity, and lapses of memory.

Family Violence/Accidental Deaths

In the 1986 census, Statistics Canada reported that accidental death rates for registered Indians on- and off-reserve had decreased since the previous census but were still higher than the national average (Indian and Northern Affairs Canada, 1990). It was also reported that First Nations women in Canada were four times more likely than non-Native women to die as a result of accidents or violence. The Ontario Native Women's Association (1989) reported that 84% of respondents were aware of family violence in their community (p. 3). Furthermore, 24% reported personally knowing of family violence that has led to death, primarily of women. Statistics are readily available in the areas of suicide, family violence, and accidental deaths, but the important point to remember here is not the great number of incidents but the link between the items in Tiers 2, 3, and 4. Prior to dependence and colonialism, family violence and alcoholism were not prevalent (Martens, 1988). Furthermore, as with sexual abuse and child abuse, family violence and accidental deaths are events that have been found to be traumatic, as discussed earlier, and may lead to PTSD.

Cultural Bereavement

In the trauma literature, the loss of one's culture constitutes a traumatic event that often leads to anxiety disorders. PTSD is quite common among refugee groups. The symptoms of these disorders, in these cases, are best understood as cultural bereavement. The notion of cultural bereavement must have a place in research and clinical practice, because it is through narrative traditions, which are transmitted through participation in communal life, that people come to value themselves (Kirmayer, 1995). Hence, the loss of such a narrative would lead to cultural bereavement.

First Nations citizens are then caught in a vicious cycle of continuous exposure to traumatic events. As is the case with most vicious cycles, it is difficult to break free. However, the answers are most likely to be found in the removal of colonialism and the resolution of dependency. If efforts are concentrated only on responding to the symptoms in the outer tiers, without solving what created the problems to begin with, that is, the effects of colonialism and dependency, then the cycle will only continue. The following section illustrates some ideas regarding solutions to the cycle of trauma among First Nations citizens.

SOLUTIONS

From a Psychological Point of View

In order to truly understand anxiety disorders, one should examine the factors that influence their intrapsychic and interpersonal mechanisms, along with the cognitive and physiological systems (Kirmayer, Young, & Hayton, 1995). Hence, situations, roles, cultural practices, and social meanings must be examined to fully comprehend such disorders. Behavior varies from culture to culture. These differences may either contribute to overdiagnosing particular disorders or masking them in various populations. Consider, for example, the custom of women rarely leaving the home in particular countries, and the accompaniment of the women when they do leave, and its relationship to agoraphobia (Kirmayer *et al.,* 1995). Manson *et al.* (1996) also stress the importance of cultural sensitivity when measuring PTSD in American Indians; for example, who is to say whether behaviors that seem to an outsider as lacking in emotion can be classified as psychic numbing, when these may express traditional stoicism and limited disclosure? With respect to diagnosing depression, Neligh (1988) noticed that social service providers have avoided labeling American Indian adolescents as depressive because of uncertainty about potential stigma in this cultural context.

Kirmayer *et al.* (1995) summarize that culture should be taken into account when treating individuals. They state that a professional needs to be culturally sensitive toward his or her patient to fully understand reactions and behaviors that are dictated by sociocultural norms. Furthermore, the individual attempting to give aid must factor in the issues of gender, race, power, and forces of oppression to facilitate a successful recovery.

Being culturally sensitive may mean adopting different ways of healing, or rediscovering traditional ways, such as "healing ceremonies" (Manson, 1997; Manson *et al.,* 1996). It also means offering appropriate services. For example, the "patchwork" solution to domestic violence, favored by the "central" society in Canada, has been shelters. Shelters for First Nations women are not only limited in number but also in cultural sensitivity. Furthermore, most victims of family violence must seek help in "nonaboriginal" shelters, which are, primarily, located in urban areas, far removed from the victim's community and family (Ontario Native Women's Association, 1989).

From a Sociological Point of View

The negative effects of the vicious cycle of traumatic events witnessed by First Nations citizens cannot be resolved without substantially diminishing their economic, social, and political dependence. A change in government policies is required in order to have any positive effects on the level of dependency of First Nations citizens. Meanwhile, there are smaller steps researchers should remain aware of when dealing with this complex issue. From a sociological perspective, one must be aware of the motives and the potential negative effects of public health surveillance systems. Involving Native researchers in trauma studies within their communities may prevent some of the negative effects of health studies. The knowledge generated about certain populations may reinforce the image of disorganized and sick communities, hence forging unequal power relationships and justifying paternalistic and dependent roles (O'Neil, 1994).

Some argue that the answer to the problem of underdevelopment in a peripheral region is economic growth. However, one must be careful, because there is a great difference between economic growth and economic development (Frideres, 1988). In communities that have experienced only economic growth, social problems have remained. For example, royalties from oil do not provide employment, education, and social services unless these funds are used for economic development. One needs power to create change, and power is out of reach when dependent.

Community health development needs to be founded on the basis of harmony and respect for all realms affecting aboriginal life (O'Neil, 1994). Therefore, communal health and policies concerning self-government, environmental protection, and socioeconomic management must be developed simultaneously. However, in the search to make First Nations peoples "healthier," it is important not to reconstruct their memory in terms of victimhood. This will only serve to alienate families, and, more importantly, oversimplify the problems that are, in fact, caused by a web of complex events. Ultimately, this would only institutionalize the notion of victim and remove power from those it aims to help.

Due to their dependent state, peripheries have little power to create change. For example, in 1989, the village of Chisasibi set up a roadblock on the road leading into the village, where alcohol was confiscated. Soon after, the Sûreté de Québec notified the Chief of Chisasibi, Violet Pachanos, that their actions were illegal, because the road was on Category II land and not within the jurisdiction of the village. However, by returning more control to Native communities, they become free to introduce laws that may help them combat particularly harmful behavior, such as alcoholism. The first documented initiative toward curbing the consumption of alcohol occured in Frobisher Bay, when it closed its liquor store in 1976. Since then, two Inuit communities have implemented, for their problem drinkers, systems of interdiction; two communities have instituted alcohol rationing systems; two have closed their liquor stores; and , a total of 10 communities have hired counselors. Since 1978, eight out of 24 villages with populations between 200 and 1,000 have prohibited alcohol completely (O'Neil, 1984; p. 340). Prohibition has decreased both substance and illegal substance abuse in these communities. Since prohibition, many observers have noted the low incidence of alcohol-related problems in these communities in comparison with other Northern communities without forms of prohibition (O'Neil, 1984). One of the main reasons why this ban has had these positive effects is that it is locally implemented. Villages are given the prohibition option by the government of the territory, and its implementation is negotiated by local institutions. Returning control to Native communities also promotes the rejuvenation of their culture. An example of such rejuvenation is the reestablishment of sweat lodges and elders.

CONCLUSION: HOW IS THIS TRAUMA DEEMED INTERGENERATIONAL?

The trauma described in this chapter is not intergenerational in the same way as that experienced by war survivors. In the case of war, the traumatic experience itself is experienced by the first generation only. This theoretically alters the behavior of the victim and consequently alters the behaviors of family members. In the case of First Nation citizens, several generations have been continuously exposed to the traumatic experiences of sexual abuse, family violence, child abuse, accidental death, and suicide. The trauma here is intergenerational in the sense that economic, social, and political dependence—the effects of colonialism—are intergenerational. As with the example of the residential schools discussed earlier, the sexual and physical abuse experienced by their pupils have led entire communities to become inundated with alcoholism and the aformentioned abuses.

The effects of trauma can also be transmitted to succeeding generations through culture. The ways in which cultures encourage or discourage people to deal with their negative emotions will, to some extent, determine the intergenerational effects of trauma. Encouragement to suppress emotional responses and limit the disclosure of events, viewed in particular cultures as a way to protect others and oneself, may nonetheless be harmful (Kirmayer *et al.,* 1995). An example of the effects of silence is provided by Rousseau and Drapeau, Chapter 28 in this book. They found that among Southeast Asians, a "return of the repressed" can occur through indirect allusions to past traumatic events. The silence regarding these events was originally intended to protect the children; however, allusions to rape appear to inflate the anxiety and depressive symptoms in girls who are going through puberty. When studying the effects of intergenerational trauma, one should examine the cultural rituals of communication and topics of conversation that are considered taboo. There is a social and cultural context to determine how a life story, or a narrative, will be registered and recalled (Kirmayer, 1995). How these memories are interpreted and encoded when registered is governed by cultural models that also dictate what is socially acceptable to be spoken of and acknowledged.

One should also remember that First Nations citizens suffer not only from the effects of dependency and colonialism, but also from being considered by many as second-class citizens. Racism plays a major role in elevated rates of anxiety disorders among Natives. Kirmayer *et al.* (1995) indicate that higher rates of phobia in particular minority groups, compared to nonminority groups, when sociodemographic variables were controlled, could be attributed to the fact that minorities experience more stressful events and suffer from racism, and from being labeled as members of a minority group.

It is important to note that despite having divided the items discussed in this chapter into four tiers, these traumatic events, among others, are all interrelated and have a cumulative effect on the individuals experiencing them. It is because First Nations citizens have experienced so many of these events in their lifetime that such a high percentage of their population suffers from PTSD and other anxiety disorders.

Finally, cultural sensitivity on the part of the professional is mandatory if the cycle of trauma is to be stopped. To prevent further intergenerational transmission, perhaps the most important goal should be to return political, economic, and social power to First Nations bands and to end this destructive dependence.

Acknowledgments: Special thanks to Dr. J. Sigal for introducing me to this new area of research, Dr. L. J. Kirmayer for his suggestions regarding literature on trauma, and L. Boothroyd, K., Dion, and Y. Danieli for their thorough editing.

REFERENCES

Allahar, A. L. (1989). *Sociology and the periphery: Theories and issues.* Toronto: Garamond Press.
Allahar, A. L. (1995). *Sociology and the periphery: Theories and issues* (2nd ed). Toronto: Garamond Press.
American Psychiatric Association. (1987). *Diagnostic and statistical manual of mental disorders* (3rd ed. rev.). Washington, DC: Author.
American Psychiatric Association. (1994). *Diagnostic and statistical manual of mental disorders* (4th ed.). Washington, DC: Author.
Amin, S. (1989). *La faillite du développement en Afrique et dans le Tiers-Monde.* Paris: L'Harmattan.

Beaulieu, D. (1984). *The Crees and Naskapes of Quebec: Their socio-economic conditions.* Direction des Communications du Governement du Québec, Québec, Quebec, Canada.

Berger, T. R. (1985). *Liberté fragile: Droits de la personne et dissidence au Canada. (1981).* Ville de la Salle, Québec: Editions Hurtubise.

Blomstrom, M., & Hettne, B. (1984). *Development theory in transition: The dependency debate and beyond: Third World responses.* London: Zed Books.

Brecher, I. (Ed.). (1989). *Human rights, development and foreign policy: Canadian perspectives.* Halifax, Nova Scotia: Institute for Research on Public Policy.

Bromley, D. F. R., & Bromley, R. (1988). *South American development: A geographical introduction.* Cambridge, UK: Cambridge University Press.

Cassidy, F. (1991). *Aboriginal self-determination.* Winnipeg: Oolichan Books and the Institute for Research on Public Policy.

Cassidy, F., & Bish, R. L. (1990). *Indian Government its meaning in practice.* Halifax: Institute for Research on Public Policy.

Chalk, F., & Jonassohn, K. (1990). *The history and sociology of genocide: Analyses and case studies.* London: Yale University Press.

Chance, N. A. (1970). *Summary report: Developmental change among the Cree Indians of Quebec.* Ottawa: Rural Development Branch.

Clement, W. (1980). A political economy of regionalism in Canada. In J. Harp & J. R. Hofley (Eds.), *Structured inequality in Canada* (pp. 268–284). Toronto: Prentice-Hall.

Clement, W. (1983). *Class, power and poverty.* Toronto: Matthew Publication.

Cree Housing Corporation. (1980). *Cree housing and infrastructure program: Five-year capital works program 1979–1984.* Rupert House.

Cumming, P. A., & Mickenberg, N. H. (Eds.). (1971). *Native Rights in Canada* (2nd ed.). Toronto: Indian–Eskimo Association of Canada in association with General Publishing.

Darnell, F. (1983). *Indigenous cultural minorities: Concepts pertaining to their education. The education of minority groups - An enquiry into problems and practices of fifteen countries.* Grower, Hampshire, UK: Organisation for Economic Co-operation and Development.

Delâge, D. (1989). L'alliance franco-amérindienne 1660–1701. *Recherches Amérindiennes au Québec, 19*(1), 3–15.

Delâge, D. (1991). *Le Pays renversé: Amérindiens et Européens en Amérique du nord-est: 1600–1664.* Quebec: Boréal, Compact.

Demmert, W. G. (1971). *An American Indian view on education for indigenous minorities. The education of minority groups - An enquiry into problems and practices of fifteen countries.* Grower, Hampshire, UK: Organization for Economic Co-operation and Development.

Dos Santos, T. (1973). The structure of dependence. In C. K. Wilber (Ed.), *The political economy of development and underdevelopment* (pp. 15–37). New York: Random House.

Dwyer, A. (1992, February). The trouble of Great Whale. *Equinox, 61,* 28–41.

Francis, D., & Morantz, T. (1983). *Partners in furs: A history of the fur trade in eastern James Bay, 1600–1870.* Kingston & Montreal: McGill-Queen's University Press.

Frank, G. A. (1973). *Sociology of development and underdevelopment of sociology.* London: Pluto Press.

Frideres, J. S. (1988). *Native peoples in Canada: Contemporary conflicts.* Scarborough, Canada: Prentice-Hall.

Gagné, M. A. (1994). *A Nation within a nation: Dependency and the Cree.* Montreal: Black Rose Books.

Glewwe, P., & Van der Gaag, J. (1990). Identifying the poor in developing countries: Do different definitions matter? *World Development, 18*(6), 803–814.

Hall, T. D. (1981). Is historical sociology of peripheral regions peripheral? *Studies in Political Economy: A Socialist Review: Rethinking Canadian Political Economy, 6.*

Harrington, M. (1977). *The development of underdevelopment: Why poor nations stay poor.* New York: Simon & Schuster.

Indian and Northern Affairs Canada. (1981). *Supplementary I: Briefing notes on the James Bay health crisis and epidemic.* Ottawa, Canada: Ministry of Supply and Services.

Indian and Northern Affairs Canada. (1982). *James Bay and Northern Quebec Agreement implementation review.* Ottawa, Canada: Ministry of Supply and Services.

Indian and Northern Affairs Canada. (1990). *Health of Indian women: Notes on socio-demographic conditions.* Ottawa, Canada: Ministry of Supply and Services.

Janigan, M. (1992). Lonely cries of distrust: Anger and pain fuel Native claims. *Maclean's, 105*(11), 22–24.

Kirmayer, L. J. (1995). Landscapes of memory: Trauma, narrative and dissociation. In P. Antze & M. Lambek (Eds.), *The subject of memory* (pp. 173–198). London: Routledge.

Kirmayer, L. J. (1996). Confusion of the senses: Implications of cultural variations in somatoform and dissociative disorders to PTSD. In A. J. Marsella, M. Friedman, E. Gerrity, & R. Scurfield (Eds.), *Ethnocultural aspects of posttraumatic stress disorders.* Washington, DC: American Psychiatric Press.

Kirmayer, L. J., Young, A., & Hayton, B. C. (1995). The cultural context of anxiety disorders. *The psychiatric Clinics of North America, 18*(3), 503–521.

Knight, R. (1968, March). *Ecological factors in changing economy and social organization among the Rupert House Cree.* Anthropology Papers National Museum of Canada, No. 15, Ottawa: Department of the Secretary of State.

Manson, S. M. (1997). Cross-cultural and multiethnic assessment of trauma. In J. P. Wilson & T. M. Keane (Eds.), *Assessing psychological trauma and PTSD* (pp. 267–290). New York: Guilford.

Manson, S. M., Ackerson, L. M., Wiegman Dick, R., Baron, A. E., & Fleming, C. M. (1990). Depressive symptoms among American Indian adolescents: Psychometric characteristics of the Center for Epidemiologic Studies Depression Scale (CES-D). *Psychological Assessment: A Journal of Consulting and Clinical Psychology, 2*(3), 231–237.

Manson, S. M., Beals, J., O'Nell, T., Piaseki, J., Bechtold, D., Keane, E., & Jones, M. (1996). Wounded spirits, ailing hearts: PTSD and related disorders among American Indians. In A. J. Marsella, M. J. Friedman, E. T. Gerrity, & R. M. Scurfield (Eds.), *Ethnocultural aspects of posttraumatic stress disorder: Issues, research, and clinical applications* (pp. 225–284). Washington, DC: American Psychological Association.

Manson, S. M., & Shore, J. H. (1981). Psychiatric epidemiological research among American Indians and Alaska Natives: Methodological issues. *White Cloud Journal, 2*(2), 48–56.

Martens, T. (1988). *The spirit weeps: Characteristics and dynamics of incest and child sexual abuse.* Edmonton, Canada: Nechi Institute.

Matthews, R. (1982). Regional differences in Canada: Social versus economic interpretations. In D. Forcese & S. Richer (Eds.), *Social issues: Sociological views in Canada* (pp. 82–123). Toronto: Prentice-Hall.

McCutcheon, S. (1991). *Electric rivers: The story of the James Bay Project.* Montreal: Black Rose Books.

Mohawk Council of Akwesasne and Mohawk Council of Kahnawake. (1986). *Declaration of intent on Mohawks self-government, self-determination.* Quebec: St-Regis.

Mohawk, J. (1990). *Indian economic development: The U.S. experience of an evolving Indian sovereignty.* Unpublished manuscript.

Neligh, G. (1988). Major mental disorders and behavior among American Indians and Alaska Natives. In S. M. Manson & N. G. Dinges (Eds.), *Behavioral health issues among American Indians and Alaska Natives: Explorations on the frontiers of the biobehavioral sciences* (pp. 116–159). Denver: University of Colorado Health Sciences Center.

O'Neil, J. D. (1984). Community control over health problems: Alcohol prohibition in a Canadian Inuit village. *Circumpolar Health, 84,* 340–343. Proceedings of the Sixth International Symposium on Circumpolar Health, edited by R. Fortune. Seattle: University of Washington Press.

O'Neil, J. D. (1986). Colonial stress in the Canadian Arctic: An ethnography of young adults changing. In C. R. Janes, R. Stall, & S. M. Gifford (Eds.), *Anthropology and epidemiology* (pp. 249–274). Norwell, MA: D. Reidel.

O'Neil, J. D. (1993). Aboriginal health policy for the next century. In Royal Commission on Aboriginal Peoples (Ed.), *Path to healing* (pp. 27–48). Ottawa: Ministry of Supply and Services.

O'Nell, T. (1989). Psychiatric investigations among American Indians and Alaska Natives: A critical review. *Culture Medicine and Psychiatry, 13,* 58–87.

O'Nell, T., & Koester, S. K. (1993). *Courage, excitement, unwanted sex and spiritual perils: A qualitative investigation of the costs and benefits of alcohol and drug use among American Indian adolescents.* Denver: National Center for American Indian and Alaska Native Mental Health Research, University of Colorado.

Ontario Native Womens Association. (1989). *Breaking free: A proposal for change to Aboriginal family violence.* Thunder Bay, Ontario: Author.

Quantitative Analysis and Socio-Demographic Research. (1989). *1986 census highlights on registered Indians: Annotated tables.* (Department of Indian and Northern Development) Minister of Supply and Services, Ottawa, Canada.

Richardson, B. (1991). *Strangers devour the land.* Vancouver: Douglas & McIntyre.

Roxborough, I. (1983). *Theories of underdevelopment.* London: Macmillan.

Sacouman, J. R. (1981). The "peripheral" maritimes and Canada-wide Marxist political economy. *Studies in Political Economy: A Socialist Review: Rethinking Canadian Political Economy, 6,* 135–151.

Tanner, A. (1979). *Bringing home animals: Religious ideology and mode of production of the Mistassini Cree hunters.* Social and Economics Studies No. 23, Institute of Social and Economic Research, Memorial University of Newfoundland. London: C. Hurst.

United Nations Development Program. (1990). *United Nations development program: World development annual report*. New York: Author.

United Native Nations. (n.d.). *After the ink dries: Will promises made be promises kept: Concerning James Bay Agreement Alaska Settlement, proposed CODE agreement*. Vancouver, BC: Legal Services Society of British Columbia.

Veltmeyer, H. (1978). The underdevelopment of Atlantic Canada. *Review of Radical Political Economics, 10*(2), 95–105.

Wright, J. V. (1979). *Quebec prehistory*. National Museum of Man. Toronto: Van Nostrand Reinhold.

York, G., & Pindera, L. (1991). *Peoples of the pines: The warriors and the legacy of Oka*. Toronto: Little, Brown.

York, G. (1990). *The dispossessed: Life and death in Native Canada*. London: Vintage.

Young, A. (1995). *Harmony of illusions*. Princeton, NJ: Princeton University Press.

23

Intergenerational Aspects of Ethnic Conflict in Africa
The Nigerian Experience

ADEBAYO OLABISI ODEJIDE, AKINADE OLUMUYIWA SANDA,
and ABIOLA I. ODEJIDE

INTRODUCTION

This chapter examines ethnic conflicts and their long-term consequences in Africa in general and in Nigeria in particular. At the outset, we need to outline our understanding of ethnic conflict.

In some cases, ethnic conflicts may be reflected in hostile interethnic stereotypes and prejudices that may derive from sociocultural contact or economic competition (Post & Vickers, 1973). In other cases, ethnic conflicts may be transformed into fierce political contests between ethnic groups over vital issues, interests, or objectives (e.g., census counts, rotational presidency) or violent interethnic internal wars.

Theories and research in the field of ethnic relations suggest that ethnic conflict may result from emergent forms of social stratification and collisions over power, especially when power, or what Post and Vickers (1973) termed "control capacity," becomes valued above anything else.

Ethnic conflict may also result in threats of secession, secession, or wars against or in favor of secession, as has been the case in Nigeria, Uganda, and Zaire. In all these cases, considerable violence and loss of life occurred and, as in all wars, there was also significant destruction of property in ethnic communities.

In essence, therefore, ethnic conflict, as conceived in this chapter, occurs to different degrees and in different forms, and can therefore be perceived within the context of a continuum:

Ethnopolitical contests		Secession	
Debates, controversies	Attempted secession		Interethnic warfare

ADEBAYO OLABISI ODEJIDE • Department of Psychiatry, College of Medicine, University College Hospital, Ibadan Nigeria. AKINADE OLUMUYIWA SANDA • Department of Public Administration, Obafemi Awolowo University, Ile-Ife, Nigeria. ABIOLA I. ODEJIDE • Department of Communication and Language Arts, University of Ibadan, Ibadan, Nigeria.

International Handbook of Multigenerational Legacies of Trauma, edited by Yael Danieli. Plenum Press, New York, 1998.

In order to appreciate the theoretical roots of ethnic conflict, it may be useful to examine both the theoretically assumed sources of conflict and the meaning of the ethnic group. These two preliminary exercises provide a useful understanding of how ethnic conflicts persist over generations and the consequences of this persistence.

The ethnic group has been variously defined in the literature (Sanda, 1976). Two definitions are, however, of particular interest. One, by Cohen (1969), underscores the common interest of members as the unifying factor. This is why he perceives the ethnic group as an *informal interest group,* whose member share some compulsory institutions that differentiate them from other groups in the society. Another definition by several authors (e.g., Olorunsola, 1972; Schwartz, 1965) emphasizes the unique social and cultural heritage that binds members of an ethnic group together and is transmitted from one generation to another.

When conflicts occur between ethnic groups, they tend to persist as a result of either cultural differences that are transmitted over different generations, or as a result of the type or nature of ethnic interest that is at stake. Such conflicts of interest often include power conflict or conflict of authorities, or economic conflict, as distinct from a conflict of cultures. In Africa, all these types of conflict (political, economic, class, and religious) often take on ethnic dimensions or become couched in ethnic terms.

Magnarella (1993) attempts to account for the genesis of the conflicts and the outcomes:

> European powers drew their boundaries with little regard for the political affiliations, or lack thereof, of encapsulated indigenous populations. Subsequently, many African leaders have relied on the support of fellow tribesmen or cultural affiliates to achieve and maintain positions of power. In return, these leaders have often favoured their supporters with privileged access to the limited available resources. Such tribal or ethnic politics, which favours the few over the many, has not and cannot generate the generality of legitimacy necessary for regime stability and internal security. (p. 331)

Our concern in this contribution, however, is with intergenerational aspects of ethnic conflict. According to the *Webster Encyclopedic Dictionary of the English Language,* a generation is "a single succession of the human race in national descent, calculated at thirty years" (1969, p. 362). In other words, while a set of people and activities may belong to one generation, another cohort of people that emerges after about 30 years constitutes a different generation. And the persisting consequences of events (ethnic conflicts) beyond 30 years represent intergenerational effects.

THEORY AND CONCEPT IN ETHNIC CONFLICT

Ethnic conflicts have been described and explained from a variety of theoretical viewpoints in the literature on ethnicity (Wolf, 1967). Some authors have explained such phenomena (ethnic conflicts) by reference to structural causes (Skocpol, 1985). Others have argued for the recognition of the place of *actions* (e.g., individual or group actions) in patterning responses to either structural preconditions or determining structural outcomes (Taylor, 1988). The exact relationship between *structure* of societies, *culture* of social groups, and *actions* of individuals remains controversial in the literature, especially in the ways in which each of the three variables influences social (or revolutionary) changes.

With particular reference to ethnic conflicts, while there may be some structural and cultural preconditions to ethnic tension in society, it seems plausible to suggest that individual or coercive state actions may function as the catalyst to the outbreak of conflicts (Sklar, 1963).

Some analyses of interethnic conflicts in Nigeria may have relied extensively on the assumed dominance of contradictory or conflicting political cultures (Olorunsola, 1972), or what Schwarz (1965) aptly described as being the dominant issues: my tribe, my faith, my culture. These were also described as pluralism, tribalism, or primordialism (Geertz, 1963; Olorunsola, 1972; Skinner, 1968).

Other analyses of ethnic conflicts have emphasised economic stratification (Bamishaiye, 1976; Kuper, 1971), political stratification and contests for political succession (Sanda, 1974b; Skinner, 1968; Sklar, 1976), or for control of scarce resources, such as land, or control of public offices (Ayoade, 1982; Sanda, 1982). The following observations by three different authors may illuminate these points.

According to Skinner (1968),

> The various groups in contemporary African societies are not competing for ancestral rights or privileges, but for the appurtenances of modern power. In most cases they seek to control the nation state where they find themselves or at worst they seek to prevent being dominated by other groups within the state. (p. 183)

Skinner's contention is that, rather than focus attention upon culture and tradition as possible sources of ethnic conflicts, we must direct our attention toward the various manifestations of power contests that have become transformed into ethnic conflicts.

While recognizing the great potential that an ethnically plural society has for transforming power and authority conflict into ethnic conflicts, Sanda (1974b) observed elsewhere that "non-elite political actors in our research area are as likely to transform intergroup competition for scarce goals into their ethnic conflicts as are elite members of the same society" (p. 518). Two closely related policy implications emerge from this: first, the strategy for distributing scarce values or goals in an ethnically plural society such as Nigeria and, second, and perhaps more important, the procedure for electing top political officials.

From the preceding statement, it would appear that interethnic conflicts are intrinsic to ethnically plural societies, owing to the ever-present issue of competition over scarce resources and positions of authority. But just as different types and scales of conflicts may be generated from experiences of ethnic hierarchy or domination, the effects of ethnic conflict may also vary, depending upon the type and scale of conflict.

In addition, since the segmentary structure of ethnic communities provides a basis for fission and fusion at different times (Otite, 1976), the consequences of interethnic conflicts may also vary. This is largely because of the possibility of changing alliances among ethnic groups in the ethnically segmentary and plural society.

It is nevertheless instructive to acknowledge Horowitz's (1985) social-psychological explanation of ethnic conflict and its basic derivation from the ascriptive traits that give the ethnic group its identity as distinct from other identities. Horowitz recognized the potential of ethnic elites for manipulating and mobilizing the masses in order to attain status-related or economic gains. However, in his view, the cultural, symbolic differences provide the roots for the ethnic groups' anxiety, or feeling of wrong, or perception of threat. According to him, "The sources of ethnic conflict reside above all in the struggle for relative group worth" (p. 143).

Perhaps the most illuminating part of Horowitz's contribution lies in his prescriptions for reducing ethnic conflict. These are (1) deliberate proliferation of power centers instead of a single power center; (2) conscious devolution of power and reservation of offices for ethnic groups, thereby fostering intraethnic conflicts that would reduce interethnic conflicts; (3) deliberate encouragement of interethnic cooperation through provision of inducements; (4) fostering of policies that promote assignments that are not based upon ethnicity (e.g., social class or territory); and (5) reduction of disparities between ethnic groups in order to reduce roots of disaffection.

While it has not been expressly stated by Horowitz, it could be inferred that the absence of these five measures or prevalence of the opposite trends in state policies may perpetuate interethnic conflicts across generations.

If not resolved, interethnic conflicts often result in traumatic events such as pogroms, civil wars, and destruction of property. Such significant human stressors create emotional problems described in the *Diagnostic and Statistical Manual of Mental Disorders* (DSM-III) of the American Psychiatric Association as posttraumatic stress disorder (PTSD) (Kaplan and Sadock, 1988). In this disorder, characteristic symptoms such as reexperiencing the traumatic event, numbing of responsiveness to or involvement with the external world, exaggerated startle response, difficulty in concentrating, memory impairment, sleep difficulty, guilt feelings, and depression occur after the experiencing of a psychologically traumatic event or events outside the range of normal human experience.

Apart from the direct effect of the disorder on the individual, PTSD may impact on the family and the family's attitude toward future generations, thereby creating intergenerational transfer of the trauma (Danieli, 1985). The transfer of the effects to future generations may imbue in them traits of aggression, anger, disillusionment, resignation, apathy, low self-esteem, guilt, and depression.

THE STATE OF KNOWLEDGE OF THE ROOTS OF ETHNIC CONFLICT IN NIGERIA

According to Aliyu (1975), intergroup conflicts and competition in Nigeria before 1966 reflected the interparty competition between the three dominant political parties in the society (i.e., the Northern People's Congress [NPC]; the National Congress of Nigerian Citizens [NCNC]; and the Action Group [AG]). The three political parties were ethnically or regionally based: The NPC was dominated by the Hausa-Fulani ethnic cluster; the NCNC was dominated by the Igbo ethnic group; and the AG was dominated by the Yoruba. Also, geographically, AG membership was concentrated in the old Western Region that later metamorphosed into six new states. The NCNC was largely an eastern regional party, while the NPC was a northern political party. It was therefore relatively easy for political competition among the three dominant parties to become transformed into ethnic conflict.

A pattern of ethnic politics did not, however, emerge until 1952. This was the year when Dr. Nnamdi Azikwe resigned his membership in the Western House of Assembly and retreated to the Eastern Region as a result of the failure of the Yoruba-dominated Western House (which functioned as the electoral college of the central legislature) to vote for him in the elections for the Central Legislature. Since that episode, ethnoregional political parties have emerged in different parts of Nigeria to ensure the success of aspirants to strategic national or state offices.

Two other contests for scarce resources preceded the 1967–1970 civil war. One was the struggle for the control of strategic bureaucratic positions (i.e., in the public service, including the civil service, parastatals, government corporations, banks, etc.). The other was the perennial struggle over the creation of new states.

While the former process resulted in the subsequent inclusion of the ethnic representation principle in the 1979 Constitution, the latter produced the progressive fragmentation of Nigeria from three regions to four regions, to 12 states, to 19 states, and to the current 30 states.

The agitation for the creation of more states from the nonviable ones already existing has continued unabated, thus increasing the pressures for the creation of new states such as Anioma, Oke-Ogun, Ijebu, and Ekiti. The arguments are predicated on perceived marginalization of the people from the federal government, nonlocation of key federal establishments in their areas, loss of revenue accruing to states, and exclusion from key government positions in charge of generating and managing the nation's wealth.

The year 1966 appears to be a more indicative time for the events that perpetuated interethnic conflicts across the generations in Nigeria. This is not to ignore the context provided by the artificial state boundaries and the structure and culture of ethnic pluralism in Nigeria, but it is meant to underscore the emergent definition of ethnic relations that started with the events of January 15, 1966, and culminated in the 1967–1970 civil war and the subsequent events.

On January 15, 1966, a group of young majors in the Nigerian army attempted a military coup to overthrow the civilian government of Sir Abubakar Tafawa Balewa, a northerner. The exact ethnic composition of the coup plotters has continued to be a subject of controversy (Ezeigbo, 1986), but the core group was made up of five officers from the southern part of the country (Ademoyega, 1981). After the initial confusion, the most senior officer in the army, Major General Aguiyi Ironsi, became Head of State.

The background to the outburst of hostilities was provided by the continuation of the colonial policy on army recruitment, which was based on the quota system, to the advantage of Northern Hausa-Fulani, the Tivs of the middle belt, and the Kanuri, but to the disadvantage of the Southern Igbo and Yoruba groups. Fifty percent of the army was recruited from the North while the Western and Eastern Regions (i.e., where Yoruba and Igbo ethnic groups were dominant) provided only 25% of army recruits (Barua, 1992). By January 1966, when the military took over the government, most of the army officers were of Igbo origin, whereas most of the noncommissioned officers and other ranks were largely of northern origin. To quote Barua (1992),

> In 1966, the Nigerian army was yet another manifestation of the numerous ethnic tensions that divided Nigerian society. Hence the structure of the Nigerian army, instead of contributing to the solution of the divisions in society merely reflected and reinforced them. It was the coincidence of military rank and ethnicity that made possible the coup or mutiny against military superiors who were also ethnic opponents. (p. 131)

General Obasanjo's account also outlined the existence of ethnic divisions and what he called "tribalism" in the army. However, he did not share the ethnic explanation of the coup. Obasanjo suggested that the coup leader was motivated by national patriotic concerns, but the implementation of the coup by the coup leader's accomplices led to misinterpretations. His biography of Nzeogwu, the coup leader, clearly depicted the ethnic political origin of the crisis that began with the Western Regional elections of 1965, the final precipitant. He (Obasanjo, 1987) asserted:

> All sorts of postulations have been made on the failure of the coup to bring about the "honest progressive new government" which would be closely watched and guided by the military but to my mind *the coup was heavily tribally based in its execution* in the South and that nailed its coffin. (p. 100, emphasis added).

Northern politicians and officers suffered a greater loss of their key members than the southern politicians and officers in the January 1966 coup. The June–July reprisals by northern soldiers were meant to avenge their initial loss and to prevent a "sudden change in the political equation" (Obasanjo, 1987, p. 100). The ethnic motivations in the Hausa-Fulani soldiers' attack on 180 officers were also emphasized by Barua (1992). Interpretations of the motivations for the coup have differed radically, ranging from those that explain it as an "Igbo coup" as in *Danjuma: The Making of a General* (Barrett, 1979) and Mainasara's *The Five Majors: Why They Struck* (1982) to that of Nnoli (1972), who attributed it to the imperialist and colonialist forces in the country, led by British monopoly capitalist interests.

The June–July 1966 massacres of Igbos in the cities and villages in the North resulted in the massive dislocation of the people—civil servants, teachers, traders, artisans, farmers, and university students from all over Nigeria—to the eastern part. Soyinka's (1972) *The Man Died,* the memoirs of his detention by the federal government during the period, reports some of the dilemmas of such Igbo victims. *Nigerian Crisis: Pogrom 1966,* an official publication of what was then Eastern Nigeria, was a potent propaganda weapon used internationally to portray to the outside world the reality of the horrors of the massacres. As Ezeigbo (1986) described the booklet, it contained "bizarre and horrifying pictures of the Northern massacres of Eastern Nigerians in 1966" (p. 90). It showed pictures of men, women, and children with maimed limbs, matchete cuts all over their bodies, and "eyes gouged out of the sockets" (p. 90).

Yet the federal government was "unable or unwilling to provide effective protection for Ibo civilians during the gruesome massacres" (Uwechue, 1971, p. xxii). Eastern Nigeria then declared itself a separate state named Biafra.

These were the events that set the stage for Nigeria's 3-year civil war to prevent the attempted secession. The war was marked by starvation and suffering among the Igbos, and indiscriminate bombings of civilians by the Nigerian Air Force (and reprisals by Biafrans). The figures of the Igbo casualties in the massacre range between 30,000 and 50,000 (the Biafran figures) and 5,000 and 7,000 (the Nigerian figures) (Ezeigbo, 1986). It was incontestable that Igbo losses in lives and property were massive enough to be devastating.

According to Odogwu (1985), the fear of extermination of the Igbo race was largely what "fired and sustained the Biafran resistance" (p. 253).

The tragedies of the wars left indelible marks on families, who lost children, and wives of dead husbands. The negative consequences were of such dimensions that Gowon's victorious government announced his policies of no victor and no vanquished, as well as the deliberate fostering of reconciliation, reconstruction, and rehabilitation.

INTERGENERATIONAL EFFECTS

It is significant that there are no studies on the psychological effects of the civil war on the combatants on both sides. However, there is a considerable amount of civil war literature that explores with varying degrees of literary expertise the horrors of living through the war and its posttraumatic effects. One could ascribe this phenomenon to one of the features of posttraumatic syndrome described by Kaplan and Sadock (1988), that is, "actual or preferred avoidance of circumstances resembling or associated with the stressor" (p. 321). The preference for its recreation in fictional forms may well be best described as a displacement reaction.

A host of accounts written by participants and observers, as well as some official histories, though showing bias in varying degrees, provide insight into the effects of the trauma suffered in the Nigerian civil war. Fictional writings for adults and young children by renowned Nigerian writers such as Achebe (1977), *Girls at War and Other Stories;* Emecheta (1980), *The Wrestling Match;* Nwapa (1975), *Never Again;* Ekwensi (1973), *Coal Camp Boy;* Okpewho (1976), *The Last Duty;* and, Ekwuru (1979), *Songs of Steel,* reveal a wide array of responses. Examples are numbness at the perceived injustice of the pogroms before the war, the savagery of the war period, intense yet muted anger at the Igbo's powerlessness as a vanquished people, and resentment of the rest of Nigeria and the world that stood by and let it happen. Odumegwu-Ojukwu (1989), the leader of the Igbo during the war years, captures the postwar mood succinctly: "The post–civil war Igbo historical vogue is to bemoan the material losses, the diminution of human dignity, an endemic economic retardation and the like" (p. 95).

Ekwuru's (1979) *Songs of Steel* reports in an unconstrained way the unmitigated horrors of the war. In this apparently fictional writing, a young boy is portrayed sitting, "holding the head of his capitated brother, . . . his face and hands covered in blood" (p. 97). In Achebe's (1974) short stories, *Girls at War and Other Stories,* these same kinds of experiences are transmuted into artistic forms through implied meanings and subtle nudges at the reader's sensibilities.

Achebe and Iroaganachi's (1972) *How the Leopard Got Its Claws,* published 2 years after the end of the Nigerian civil war, has been explored as an allegory of the traumatic experiences of the Igbo people and the Nigerian nation (Miller, 1981; Odejide, 1989). A fight over brazen inequity in the sharing of national assets results in the humiliation and ejection of the erstwhile king: the leopard. The allegory ends with the leopard arming itself with the most deadly weapons—claws, teeth, a thunderous roar—in order to reclaim its throne. Echoes of the civil war slogans abound—"We must stay together"—and so on.

The possibilities for drawing parallels are endless: the animal's hall and the nation's assets, the embattled leopard and the Igbo people, the vicious and unjust dog and the military leaders of the time, and the other conniving, inconsistent animals and the remaining Nigerian regions (Odejide, 1989).

One insidious but possible interpretation of the ending is the possibility of a resurgence of the fight for Igbo rights, a possibility that cannot be easily ignored in the light of recent undercurrents of Biafran agitation, especially in the wake of the annulment of the 1993 presidential elections in the country.

The degree of apprehension over the marginalization of the Igbos since the civil war has not diminished. It has been expressed in newspaper articles and public pronouncements by Igbo citizens. As Odumegwu-Ojukwu (1989) argues,

> Constant punishment, reproach or reminder has inhibited true Igbo participation in Nigeria's development efforts. . . . What they (the Igbos) feel and say today is that the speed of total reintegration is slow and that it should be faster to the mutual benefit of all Nigerians. . . . Today there is a yawning gap of non-Igbo presence in crucial organisations from which they withdrew in 1966. Properties are seized and regarded as abandoned. (p. 171)

This is articulated in the complaints about the paucity of senior officers of Igbo origin in the armed forces, premature retirement of the few in such positions, the paucity of Igbos in top civil-service positions, and recurrent attacks on them in northern cities. This is summed up by a feature writer in the newspaper *Vanguard* (Nwakanma, 1994), who, in the heat of the political crisis following the first anniversary of the annulment of the presidential elections, wrote that a "mixture of apathy, undefined empathy, 'siddon look' [pidgin for sit down, look] and an under-current of tension boiling steadily into a rage paints a blurred picture of the East, in the current logjam" (p. 13).

Odumegwu-Ojukwu (1989) had argued earlier that this kind of apathy could be one of the psychological and political hangovers of the civil war, a dilemma for the Igbo vanquished. Should they retreat into isolation or not? Which political party should they join?

It could, however, be argued that the "siddon look" attitude, the apathy, is limited to national politics, to activities in Abuja and Lagos, except where it touches on the economy. The preoccupation is primarily with individual and ethnic survival, through working aggressively to recover from the material losses of the civil war. The emphasis of the young Ibgo men appears to be on trading, and it is no wonder that they have a virtual monopoly on the trade in motor spare parts and building materials in several cities nationwide. The sheer size and great visibility of such a population of young Igbo traders led in the late eighties and early nineties to a widespread assumption that the ratio of school enrollment of boys vis-à-vis girls had shifted drastically in favor of the girls. However, a recent study commissioned by UNICEF (Women's Research and Documentation Centre, 1994) showed that, contrary to popular assumption, there were more boys in primary and secondary schools in Imo state. The difference was 1.34% in favor of the boys at the primary level, whereas, at the secondary level, the percentage difference had fallen to 0.06% (p. 210).

Although it is instructive to observe that in comparison with non-Igbo states, the percentage difference among the Igbo schoolboys and -girls, especially at the secondary level, is low, the greater significance is in the decline of the enrollment for boys. In the long term, a situation might be created in which a people who had prided themselves on their intellectual achievement since the 1930s, with the graduation of Nnamdi Azikwe from Lincoln University, would now become disadvantaged academically.

The apparent loss of faith in academic achievement among the Igbo males could be regarded as one of the intergenerational effects of the civil war. Their emphasis during the immediate post–civil war period was on rebuilding their towns and their ravaged economy. The acquisition of Western education to a high level was not a prerequisite for their kind of trading, so apprenticeship to established traders became the norm for young boys.

In addition, this refusal to obtain qualifications that would enable them to enter into the civil service and become part of the administration of the government could reflect a deliberate distancing of themselves as a group from a state apparatus that had been unable or unwilling to protect them at a time of need. This highlights a decline in their feeling of national identity.

PSYCHOSOCIAL EFFECTS

The psychological fallout of the experience of a civil war does not elude children, as seen in Okpewho (1976), who re-creates the chaos and dislocation of the war as seen through the eyes of a young boy. His thoughts are revealed in a free flow of language, lacking the constraints of adult conventions of punctuation but exhibiting an uncanny insight into the concept of the spoils of war: "The soldiers don't like people to steal anything because they want to keep it all to themselves" (p. 114). An entire family's life is blighted by the civil war experiences, and the last picture of the boy is a poignant one: frightened, powerless, unable to comprehend the full tragedy of the wasting of his entire family.

In contrast, emotional rehabilitation is the theme of Ekwensi's (1973) *Coal Camp Boy.* The major problem is the rediscovery of the self, the individual as well as group psyche, in the aftermath of a war that had shattered the closely knit urban community built around the Enugu coal mines. The disruption of their economic and social lives had bred a new kind of morality in some of the returnees, that is, survival by all means: the "win the war" mentality. However, the author, in his usual commitment to morality, optimism, and belief in the regeneration of man, no matter the level of debasement, advocates a sense of optimism, disregard of bitterness, and rugged resilience of the people epitomized in the staging of a festival of masquerades as soon as they settled down. For them, life had started again, and their creativity was an affirmation of the continuity of life.

Yet ripples of the war are evident in the consequent disregard of social values exhibited by the "Omu aya Biafra," an age group born during the civil war, as recreated in Buchi Emecheta's (1980) *The Wrestling Match*. This subculture, exhibiting disruptive behaviors such as muggings, lawlessness, and disregard for elders, was a creation of the social and educational limbo occasioned by the war. Semiliterate, unemployed, and lacking a sense of direction, the boys could not be accommodated in a society that was trying to exhibit the national postwar affirmation of "No victor, no vanquished." The elders arranged a placebo treatment, a farcical wrestling match with young men from a neighboring village. At the end, the author appears to reiterate the slogan: "In all good fights, just like wars, nobody wins" (p. 73).

The immediate post–civil war trauma is re-created in Ekwensi's (1976) *Survive the Peace,* a fictional work that presents the chaos and lawlessness of the former Biafra. It was a situation in which people in army uniforms paraded on the highways, posing as genuine military officers, and carried out brazen armed robbery—events completely alien to the community before the war. Traumatized, young, demobilized men took to robbery and unleashed terror on their own kith and kin.

Iroh's (1982) *The Siren in the Night* examines in fictional form a new kind of terror imposed on the vanquished: the sadism, the psychologically dehumanizing attacks on their psyche. The much-touted reconciliation, especially the question of the general amnesty given to the "rebel officers" by the federal government, did not preclude the use of torture by military intelligence. Anarchy, uncertainty, an unprecedented increase in the crime rate, and chaos were the fallout of the war. Immediately after the war, the people who had lost were still suspects, subject to accusations of fueling rebel resurgence.

The placatory pronouncements quoted in *The Wresting Match* (Emecheta, 1980), however, mask growing tension among the three dominant ethnic groups as well as between the minority groups and the dominant ethnic groups. The former has been discussed in the earlier sections of this chapter. The latter is reflected in the current struggles for self-determination by such groups as the Ogoni in the Rivers state, who have taken their case against Nigeria and the multinational oil companies over the devastation of their environment to the United Nations. Continuous agitation over the mismanagement of resources derived from the oil-producing areas in Rivers, Delta, and lately Ondo states have increased the presence of military personnel there to protect the pipelines against sabotage. Allegations have been made of destabilization and promotion of ethnic rivalries in such areas. The consequence is the prevalent feeling among the indigenes that they are under an army of occupation. The trials and executions of their leaders such as Ken Saro Wiwa by military tribunals have exacerbated the tension. This corroborates Sivard's finding that "military governments are more than twice as likely as other Third World governments to frequently employ torture and other violent forms of repression against the populace" (Magnarella, 1993, p. 332).

Lingering mutual mistrust fueled by statements about the belief of particular sections of the country that they are destined to continuously produce political leadership has led to calls for confederation or even a complete breakup of the country into smaller states. The "Sabongeri," "settler stranger" syndrome, whereby indigenes from other ethnic groups live in distinct areas of towns among the host communities, inhibits full integration and prevents them from feeling that they have a stake in the progress of the community. Institutional and procedural mechanisms such as the "nonindigene" label, different school fees for "nonindigene" children, different examination cutoff marks for secondary and tertiary institution candidates based on their states of origin, and preference for expatriates in appointments into the civil service rather than Nigerians from other states accentuate, amplify, and reinforce the feeling of alienation. As Obasanjo (1994), a former leader of Nigeria, convincingly argues,

> For as long as our leaders and sponsors of leaders lead and sponsor for personal, ethnic, geographical, sectional, religious and purely economic interests, for so long will problems (i.e., the politics of prebendalism) remain with us, no matter the sophistication of our constitution or the frequency of change. How do we provide a stake in Nigeria for every Nigerian if Nigerians from one part of the country can be told that God has ordained people from another part of Nigeria for permanent political leadership and the others for followership? (p. 31)

Odumegwu-Ojukwu (1989) may be correct in his conjecture that without the reintegration of disadvantaged groups, there might grow "a sense of apathy, anger, and disillusionment in the minds of future generations who did not know anything about the war" (p. 172). He concludes that "the aim should not be to create intellectual Bantustans in our polity" (p. 172).

Intergenerational effects have continued to linger. The report of an assembly of Nigerian elites at the Azikwe-Gowon Forum held in 1994 in Nigeria was aptly termed "A Babel of Tongues" by a leading Nigerian newspaper (now proscribed). It was marked by accusations and counteraccusations of political dominance, lopsided revenue allocation formulae, unfaithful implementation of the federal character policy, neglect and oppression of minority peoples, and militarization of politics. The conclusion was, however, an affirmation of the continued corporate existence of Nigeria as a federation predicated on justice, fairness, and equity.

A most telling repartee was a quote from John F. Kennedy by David-West, a former Petroleum Resources Minister and a member of a minority: "If you say there is no discrimination in America, which of you whites are willing to change their complexion?" (Odivwri, 1994, p. A7).

INTERGENERATIONAL EFFECTS: SUMMARY AND CONCLUSION

From the preceding sections, it is easier to appreciate the increasing significance and multidirectional manifestation of the effects of ethnic conflicts in Nigeria. On January 15, 1996, it was 30 years since the first coup, which epitomized the first major interethnic violence of great proportions, took place. Yet today, the level of interethnic tension, which has become intensified as a result of the mishandling of the June 12, 1993, presidential elections, suggests that there has been an increase in the negative effects of interethnic conflicts.

First, because of the experience of non-Hausa victims and survivors of the 1966 interethnic conflicts, there has been an increase in the private arming (with guns and other dangerous weapons) of individuals in many northern cities. Igbos in Kano and Kaduna, Christians in all northern cities, and Hausa in the "Sabongeris," "the stranger areas," of many southern cities, are now in a state of preparedness in the event of an outbreak of interethnic conflict. The federal government reacted about a year ago by asking all private owners of firearms to submit them to the police for relicensing, and this year, all private licenses for arms importation have been revoked and private dealers' depots sealed all over the country.

Second, agitation for the creation of new states as a means of fostering social, political, and economic development of ethnic areas has intensified. Although it is recognized that the elites have benefited significantly from such exercises in the past, the fragmentation of the nation into 30 states and Abuja has not reduced the intensity of demands for new states based upon ethnogeographical affinity, solidarity, and ethnogeographical contiguity.

The third and perhaps the most important effect of interethnic conflict lies in enhanced ethnic consciousness, the consequent proliferation of ethnic associations (for ethnic members in search of political, social, and economic security), and the corresponding decline in national integration. The national identity crisis is manifested in the failure of the Nigerian mil-

Table 1. Variables in Intergenerational Effects of Ethnic Conflicts

Independent variable	Intervening variable	Dependent variables (effects)
1. Ethnic pluralism	1. Leadership a. Quality b. Style (e.g., dictatorial) c. Legitimacy	1. Persistence or periodic resurgence of ethnic conflicts .or hostilities
2. Contest over scarce resources (e.g., political power)	2. Institutional patterns a. The military and ethnicity b. The civil service and federal character c. The universities and quotas	2. Identity crisis, intensity of ethnic awareness, and ethnic solidarity
3. Structure/pattern of inequality or ethnic stratification or domination	3. Policy instruments a. On equal citizenship b. On democratization c. On coercive strategies to national unity	3. Persistence of ethnic stereotypes and interethnic prejudices
4. Traumatic interethnic historical experiences: genocidal war or pogrom	4. Reward structure	4. Declining national identity or integration: the domination of politics by ethnicity, continued relevance of ethnic associations

itary in the political arena in spite of their domination of the political arena over the last three decades.

Table 1 shows the tabulation of the interrelationship of factors that have interacted to produce different consequences of interethnic relations over the years. A positive change from the current pattern will be dependent upon how the intervening variables (leadership, institutional pattern and processes, policy instruments, and reward structure) operate to impact upon the independent variables, especially through appropriate policy instruments and a legitimate corps of leaders.

From Table 1, it can be observed that four major categories of intergenerational effects have been highlighted. It is, however, necessary to ascertain the degree of significance, or the salience of any or all of these effects, through empirical research. The absence of such research in Nigeria is a major limitation on the present state of knowledge in this most important area of behavioral sciences.

REFERENCES

Achebe, C. (1974). *Girls at war and other stories*. London: Heinemann.

Achebe, C., & Iroganachi, J. (1972). *How the leopard got its claw*. Enugu: Fourth Dimension Publishers.

Ademoyega, A. (1981). *Why we struck: The story of the first Nigerian Coup*. Ibadan: Evans Brothers.

Aliyu, A. Y. (1975). Intergroup conflict and integration. In E. O. Akeredolu Ale (Ed.), *Social Research and National Development: Proceedings of the Conference on Social Research and National Development*. Ibadan: Nigerian Institute for Social and Economic Research.

Ayoade, J. A. A. (1982). Constitutional containment of ethnicity: The Nigerian case. Paper presented at the Twelfth World Conference of the International Political Science Association, Rio de Janeiro, Brazil, August 9–14.

Bamishaiye, A. (1976). Ethnic politics as an instrument of socio-economic development in Nigeria's First Republic. In A. O. Sanda (Ed.), *Ethnic relations in Nigeria* (pp. 71–91). Ibadan: Caxton Press.

Barrett, L. (1979). *Danjuma: The Making of a General.* Enugu: Fourth Dimension Publishers.

Barua, P. P. (1992). Ethnic conflict in the military of developing nations: A comparative analysis of India and Nigeria. *Armed Forces and Society, 19*(1), 131–137.

Cohen, A. (1969). *Custom and politics in Urban Africa.* London: Routledge & Kegan Paul.

Danieli, Y. (1985). The treatment and prevention of long-term effects and intergenerational transmission of victimization: A lesson from Holocaust survivors and their children. In C. R. Figley (Ed.), *Trauma and its wake* (pp. 299–312). New York: Brunner/Mazel.

Diamond, L. (1987). Ethnicity and ethnic conflict. *Journal of Modern African Studies, 25*(1), 125.

Ekwensi, C. (1973). *Coal camp boy.* Lagos: Longmans.

Ekwensi, C. (1976). *Survive the peace.* London: Heinemann.

Ekwuru, A. (1979). *Songs of steel.* London: Rex Collings.

Emecheta, B. (1980). *The wrestling match.* Ibadan: Oxford University Press.

Ezeigbo, T. A. (1986). *Fact and fiction in the literature in the Nigerian civil war.* Unpublished Ph.D. thesis, University of Ibadan.

Geertz, C. (1963). The integrative revolution: Primordial sentiments and civil politics in the new states. In C. Geertz (Ed.), *Old societies and new states* (pp. 105–157). New York: Free Press of Glencoe.

Horowitz, D. L. (1985). *Ethnic groups in conflict.* Berkeley: University of California Press.

Iroh, E. (1982). *The siren in the night.* London: Heinemann.

Kaplan, I. H., & Sadock, B. J. (1988). *Synopsis of psychiatry* (5th ed.). Baltimore: Williams & Wilkins.

Kuper, L. (1971). Theories of revolution and race relations. *Comparative Studies in Society and History, 13*(1), 87–107.

Magnarella, P. J. (1993). Preventing inter-ethnic conflict and promoting human rights through more effective legal and political aid structure: Focus on Africa. In *GA Journal International and Comparative Law, 23,* 327–345.

Mainasara, A. M. (1982). *The five Majors: Why they struck.* Zaria: Hudahuda.

Miller, J. (1981). The novelist as teacher. *Children's Literature, 9,* 7–18.

Morrison, D. G., & Stevenson, H. M. (1972). Cultural pluralism, modernisation and conflict: An empirical analysis of the sources of political instability in African nations. *Canadian Journal of Political Science, 5*(1),.

Nnoli, O. (1972). The Nigeria–Biafra Conflict: A political analysis. In Joseph Okpaku (Ed.), *Nigeria: Dilemma of nationhood.* New York: Third Press.

Nwakanma, O. (1994). Stop these ethnic wranglings. *The Vanguard,* July 6, 1994, p. 13.

Nwapa, F. (1975). *Never again.* Enugu: Nwamife Publishers.

Obasanjo, O. (1980). *My command.* Ibadan: Heinemann.

Obasanjo, O. (1987). *Nzeogwu.* Ibadan: Spectrum Books.

Obasanjo, O. (1994, February 2). *State of the nation: Which way forward?* Keynote Address at the Arewa House Conference, Kaduna.

Odejide, A. (1985). *Nigerian children's literature: From oral to written forms.* Seminar paper, Institute of African Studies, University of Ibadan.

Odejide, A. (1989). *Children and war in Nigerian children's and adult literature.* Seminar paper, Department of Communication and Language Arts, University of Ibadan.

Odivwri, E. (1994, April 3). A Babel of tongues at the Azikwe/Gowon Forum. *The Guardian,* p. A7.

Odogwu, B. (1985). *No place to hide: Crisis and conflict inside Biafra.* Enugu: Fourth Dimension Publishers.

Odumegwu-Ojukwu, E. (1989). *Because I am involved.* Ibadan: Spectrum Books.

Okpewho, I. (1976). *The last duty.* London: Longman.

Olorunsola, V. (1972). *The politics of cultural subnationalism in Africa.* New York: Doubleday.

Otite, O. (1976). The concept of Nigeria Society. In A. O. Sanda (Ed.), *Ethnic relations in Nigeria* (pp. 3–16). Ibadan: Caxton Press.

Post, K. W. J., & Vickers, M. (1973). *Structure and conflict in Nigeria 1960–1966.* Ibadan: Heinemann.

Sanda, A. O. (1974a). A comparative analysis of political leadership and ethnicity in Nigeria and Zaire. *Journal of Eastern African Research and Development 4*(1), 27–48.

Sanda, A. O. (1974b). Ethnicity and intergroup conflicts: Some insights from non-elite actors in a Nigerian city. *Nigerian Journal of Economics and Social Studies, 16*(3), 507–518.

Sanda, A. O. (1976). *Ethnic relations in Nigeria.* Ibadan: Caxton Press.

Sanda, A. O. (1992). National integration and national development. In A. O. Sanda, *Lectures on the Sociology of Development* (pp. 57–67). Ibadan: Fact Finders International.

Schwarz, F. A. O. (1965). *Nigeria: The tribes, the nation or the race, The Politics of Independence.* Cambridge, MA: MIT Press.

Skinner, E. (1968). Group dynamics and the politics of changing societies: The problem of tribal politics in Africa. In J. Helm (Ed.), *Essays on the problem of tribe* (pp. 170–185). Seattle: University of Washington Press.

Sklar, R. L. (1963). *Nigerian political parties: Power in emergent African nations.* Princeton, NJ: Princeton University Press.

Sklar, R. L. (1976). Ethnicity and Social Class. In A. O. Sanda (Ed.), *Ethnic relations in Nigeria* (pp. 146–157). Ibadan: Caxton Press.

Skocpol, T. (1985). Cultural idioms and political ideologies in the revolutionary reconstruction of state power: A rejoinder to Savell. *Journal of Modern History, 57,* 86–96.

Soyinka, W. (1972). *The man died: Prison notes of Wole Soyinka.* London: Rex Collings.

Taylor, M. (1988). "Rationality and revolutionary collective action." In M. Taylor (Ed.), *Rationality and revolution,* Cambridge: Cambridge University Press.

The Webster Encyclopedic Dictionary of the English Language. (1969). International Edition. New York: Grolier.

Women's Research and Documentation Centre (WORDOC). (1994). *Situation analysis of the girl-child.* Project commissioned by UNICEF and executed by the Women's Research and Documentation Centre, Institute of African Studies, University of Ibadan.

Uwechue, R. (1971). *Reflections on the Nigerian civil war.* New York: Africana.

Wolf, A. (1967). "Language, ethnic identity and social change in southern Nigeria. *Anthropological Linguistics, 9*(1), 18–25.

24

Black Psychological Functioning and the Legacy of Slavery
Myths and Realities

WILLIAM E. CROSS, JR.

INTRODUCTION

The collective or group trauma model being explored in this volume requires that we first identify a group that has experienced a jolting, unpredictable, and monstrous assault. Second, we must be able to identify an unambiguous period that marks the termination of the trauma, for then, and only then, can we establish a before-and-after frame of reference. More specifically, the experiences of the group following the trauma must be more normative or nontraumatic in nature. When these conditions are met, we document the trauma and its termination, and then try to determine whether attitudes and behaviors originally elicited by the trauma have been passed down to the immediate and extended kin of the original victims, even though the survivors and their progeny live under conditions that are a far cry from the period of trauma. When such transcendence is confirmed across several decades or longer, we speak of the intergenerational legacy of the trauma.

The *trauma–transcendence–legacy model* is not easily applied to the black encounter with American slavery. In the first place, how does one align the notion of a sudden and unpredictable event to an institution that lasted nearly 400 years? Trauma conjures images of victims, pain, and damage; however, slavery was a long-term, multidimensional experience involving black victimization as well as effective black coping. More will be said shortly about the legacy of effective coping. Second, even if we could find a way to depict slavery in grossly traumatic terms, how does one draw a straight line between slavery and, say, contemporary expressions of black "racial" anxiety, without necessarily trivializing the instances of oppression faced by blacks since slavery?

My father, a black Southerner born and raised in segregated Virginia, suffered from a certain racial anxiety, but he never gave evidence that slavery accounted for its origin. Instead, he mentioned the memory of a particularly gruesome lynching in which the stomach of a pregnant,

WILLIAM E. CROSS, JR. • School of Education, University of Massachusetts, Amherst, Massachusetts 01003-4160.

International Handbook of Multigenerational Legacies of Trauma, edited by Yael Danieli. Plenum Press, New York, 1998.

black female victim was pierced to reveal the unborn fetus. At other times, he reflected on the tragedy that befell one of his uncles. My Dad's uncle had a marvelous team of work horses, and when he received word of the need for such teams in the building of the New York City subways (circa 1900), he journeyed to New York. He and his horses quickly became part of the tunnel construction crew, but soon thereafter, so the story goes, the white workers poisoned all of his horses. Dad said that, in the aftermath, his uncle went insane, and the family lost touch with him. These stories always lie just below the surface of my father's worldview. Along the same lines, my mother recalled an evening from her youth, when men dressed in white sheets and ghostly hoods surrounded her family's home, because earlier in the day her father had accidentally dropped a brick on the foot of a white coworker. After that evening, Granddad would never again work as a mason. As was the case with my father, my mother's racial anxiety had a very contemporary ring to it.

My own moments of racial uncertainty are traceable to contemporary rather than transcendent anxiety. Upon completing my doctorate at Princeton in 1976, I recall wondering whether the doors to equal opportunity would really be open, or would I be stopped at the receptionist's desk? My concerns were framed by the story of William R. Ming, Jr., the attorney who became the primary legal advisor to Martin Luther King, Jr. He took his law degree from the University of Chicago in the 1940s, and he graduated third in his class. Despite this, he was neither recruited nor interviewed by a single law firm of repute. Ironically, Ming would later provide advice and counsel to former classmates who graduated far below his rank. He would help them with difficult cases, they would pay him a modest sum, and then they would use his strategy to win the case and pocket a fee worth many times the amount paid Ming, even though their cases were argued in accordance with Ming's outline.

Ming's story was relayed to me by my brother-in-law, Robert L. Tucker, who graduated from the Northwestern Law School in 1955. He, too, was given scant attention by law firms, though he placed in the top one-fourth of his class. It was from Robert that I first heard the expression: "The first hurdle is to get past the receptionist." Even more foreboding were the race-tainted legal difficulties Robert encountered during the prime of his career. He was falsely accused but nevertheless convicted of fraud, and he spent several years in prison. For the first 2 years after his release, he was one of the most bitter persons I had ever encountered. In asking the Illinois Supreme Court to reinstate his right to practice law within the State of Illinois, he was finally able to present all of the evidence that should have been admissible at his trial and subsequent appeals. So convinced was the high court that an injustice had been committed, they voted unanimously to reinstate Robert to the Illinois Bar. The details of Robert's case indicated that "race" played a significant role in what had transpired at the original trial. "Race" was also behind the poor medical treatment my brother, Charles Cross, received at the University of Chicago Medical Hospital, the consequences of which left him permanently paralyzed from the waist down. Some years later, Chuck would win his lawsuit against the doctors who "treated" him, but, as in Robert's return to the Illinois State Bar, Chuck's legal victory could not undo the damage already done. These *contemporary* encounters with racism, and not some transcendent racial anxiety from the past, are at the basis of my own racial anxiety.

The point to be made from all of these examples is that the oppressive episodes that followed American slavery, and that continue today (e.g., the Rodney King episode, as a case in point), have trauma potential in their own right. This makes it a scientific nightmare to design a strategy capable of disentangling transcendent racial anxiety from racial anxiety grounded in postslavery or contemporary encounters with discrimination and injustice.

SLAVERY AND BLACK CULTURE

Another shortcoming of the slavery-as-trauma schema is that little consideration is given to the efficacious coping strategies blacks were able to fashion during slavery, and that, had they encountered less resistance, would likely have facilitated their rapid social mobility into the larger social order after slavery. Slavery was evil, but the plantations were not operated like World War II German concentration camps (Thomas, 1993). The objective was not the creation of death factories, but the running of "factories" in the more literal sense (Fogel & Engerman, 1974). Plantation owners were in the business of manipulating the forced labor of black human beings in a manner that would result in the production of greater personal wealth for the white owner's family. In running the plantation, one option was to work a group of workers to death and replace them with another group of imported slaves. However, for much of the history of American slavery, owners had limited access to recent captives and were forced to consider ways whereby the slave population could reproduce itself. As part of this economic need for a predictable labor force, the owners were forced to provide a certain degree of social latitude or "lifespace" to the slaves; that is, the slave owner had to design a system that not only allowed for the exploitation of the slave's labor, but also made possible a level of social affiliation and intimacy between the slaves that would result in the birth, development, and socialization of replacement workers.

The resulting operation juxtaposed three overlapping circles of human activity: (1) the circle defining the world of the plantation owner, his wife, and their children; (2) the daytime world of work, which daily recorded the drudgery, banality, sadism, and general insanity of the forced-labor "enterprise"; and (3) the world of the black community, consisting of a series of hut-like structures set off some distance from the owner's home. It was during the daylight hours that each slave might be brought to his or her breaking point, that family members might be sold or exchanged, that children might be forced prematurely into adult work roles, that calculated or whimsical displays of violence might be heaped on the slaves—men, women, and children alike. The evening held its moments of sexual terror for black women, as it was commonplace for the owner, his sons, or his white employees to sexually savage black women. For the most part, however, the evening provided a buffer during which the slaves retreated into the lifespace so begrudgingly provided by the owner. Recent advances in the historical record reveal that the slaves exploited this lifespace in accordance with their own interests, resulting in a level of humanity and cultural cohesiveness never intended, and seldom appreciated, by the owners. Note that I am not saying that slavery was "nice." Instead, I am marking the systems unintended consequences (Bullock, 1967). In meeting the evil and inhuman objectives of the slave owners, *certain gaps and contradictions were exploited by the slaves themselves, resulting in efficacious, functional, and deeply human marriage, family, cultural, and personal psychology patterns* (Gutman, 1976, 1987).

The slave lifespace made it possible for the slaves to develop a multidimensional mind-set (Webber, 1978). This mind-set allowed one to oppose certain features of the American culture, while engaging and even incorporating into black culture other dynamics. This acculturation, which transformed Africans into African Americans, included mechanisms for protection against racism. In *Deep Like the Rivers*, Thomas Webber demonstrated that slaves evolved a worldview that let them discover and manipulate aspects of the owner's world, while filtering those aspects that were denigrating and dehumanizing. The slaves found ways to defend and protect themselves at the same time that they engaged and selectively embraced the more "race neutral" aspects of European-American culture.

One of the most powerful examples of this process involves the slaves' religious beliefs. We have already noted that slavery lasted almost 400 years, and while the earliest of captive Africans entered slavery with religious orientations very different from Christianity, over time, the majority of slaves grew comfortable with Christian concepts. However, though the slave owners stressed an interpretation of the Bible that validated slavery and the black group's lowly status, the slaves secretly countered that "real" Christians would not own slaves in the first place. More often than not, slaves saw themselves embracing a *superior* interpretation than that they judged the owners to hold. Following slavery, and into the present, the black church has had a long history of assisting in the black struggle against racism (themes of protection). However, the very fact that the overwhelming majority of black Americans express Christian beliefs is confirmation of the cultural fusion that first took place during slavery (acculturation).

Another example of the protection–acculturation mind-set developed by the slaves is revealed by their attitudes toward education. Keeping in mind that the average white Southerner was desperately poor and uneducated, the ex-slaves did not take their cues from this group. Rather, independent even of whites and black elites who would eventually befriend them during Reconstruction, the ex-slaves instantly evidenced social attitudes toward education and social mobility that might be expected of a more socially advanced group. Clearly, the slaves derived their educational stance from their observations of the advantages education accorded the slave owners and their family members. As a result, the slaves exhibited and anticipated the kind of highly charged achievement motivation more typically associated with white immigrant groups entering the United States some 40 years later at the turn of the century. As documented 60 years ago by W. E. B. Du Bois (1935) in *Black Reconstruction,* and more recently by James Anderson (1988) in his wonderful work, *The Education of Blacks in the South, 1860–1935,* the ex-slaves were at the vanguard of a social movement for public education in the South, between the end of the Civil War and the late 1870s. In this movement, the positive educational attitudes of the majority of uneducated ex-slaves were given greater articulation and direction by a small but critical mass of educated, free blacks, and in short order further assistance was provided by agents of the federal government and progressive whites. Ronald Butchart (1980) has shown that, for the ex-slaves, this movement was founded on themes of protection (education that helps one avoid exploitation and oppose racism), ethnicity and pride (education that explores African and African American history), and acculturation (education that encourages participation in the larger social order).

James Anderson (1988) has documented the legacy of the ex-slaves' high achievement motivation for the generation of blacks living in the Deep South between 1900 and 1935. During this period, poor rural blacks joined forces with black elites to double-tax themselves in support of the "public" education of their children. They paid taxes for which they received little return (this was the historical period during which white society funneled a disproportionate amount of public resources to support "white" education, while radically underfunding the education of black children) and then taxed themselves again in the form of special collections and school-building projects (blacks supplied the labor and materials, and in some cases, even the land). Anderson presents a strong case that the group unity and cultural cohesiveness displayed in the 1930s by both poor and educated blacks can be traced to the behavior, psychology, values, and worldview that their ancestors carried forward out of slavery.

Anderson's analysis ends in 1935. However, the reflections of Kathryn Morgan (1980; *Children of Strangers*), Clifton Taulbert (1989; *Once Upon a Time When We Were Colored*), Chalmers Archer, J. (1992; *Growing Up Black in Rural Mississippi*), and James Comer (1988; *Maggie's Dream: The Life and Times of a Black Family*), to mention a few, give powerful testimony that after slavery and into the late 1950s, normative black culture stressed not only education but also marriage, nuclear family life and strong kinship bonds, linkages to community through leisure, sports, religious and educational activities (in addition to a broad spectrum of nonreligious affiliations), and an aesthetic capable of creating and sustaining gospels, rural blues, dance, drama, literature, poetry, and sophisticated jazz. The fact that this culture was able to evolve continuously from 1865 through the late 1950s, while keeping manageable the levels of social pathologies that are inevitable with oppression, represents one of the most remarkable social histories in the annals of Western civilization.

In summary, the new historical research on slavery indicates that the ex-slaves had the wherewithal to be competitive with the *average* white workers of the day, who, as it turns out, were poor, landless, and uneducated themselves. On certain dimensions, such as education and achievement motivation, the ex-slaves stood *ahead* of the average white worker. Psychologically speaking, the ex-slaves had the same kind of positive mind-set generally associated with the mass of white ethnic immigrants who appeared on our shores some years later. This means that contemporary black problems are just that, problems traceable to contemporary circumstances and not dysfunctional attitudes transported out of slavery and projected into the present as a legacy of the trauma of slavery. In summary:

- Ex-slaves showed high achievement motivation, were quick to support the education of their children, and helped forge the establishment of public education in the South; *those black youth of today who show an estrangement from educational activities are not carrying on a black tradition; they are, in fact, at odds with it.*
- Ex-slaves centered their worldview on the value of the family and the need for close ties with kin, and from the late 1860s to the early 1950s, the overwhelming majority of black children were born to intact black families and highly functional kin networks; *that black birthing and marriage patterns have followed a reverse pattern since the 1950s has practically nothing to do with slavery and everything to do with institutionalized racism, discrimination in the workplace, and diminished employment opportunities.*
- Ex-slaves were cautious about their interactions with whites, but for the most part, their aim was to become a key group in the American economy and culture. The civil rights movement of the 1960s, a hopeful and militantly integrationist movement, was built on the integrationist themes easily traceable to the worldview of the ex-slaves; *the oppositionalism and nihilism to be found among many of today's black youth has little to do with this legacy of hope, struggle, and integration.*

THE ORIGINS OF CONTEMPORARY BLACK PROBLEMS: IF NOT SLAVERY, WHAT?

If African Americans exited from slavery with cultural patterns that might well have facilitated their successful social mobility over a period of two or three generations, how does one explain the deterioration in black life, especially since the late 1960s? To answer this question, I must turn to the real legacy of slavery, which is not black deficits, but white racism. Looking back through history, one can identify a series of "missed opportunities." Had America responded differently to the needs of its black citizens in the past, the poverty rate for blacks today would likely be greatly diminished. I will mention a few. First, after slavery, there were no reparations, and there was no attempt to redistribute land to any significant number of blacks, let alone a critical mass. Even worse, as Stephen Steinberg (1992) has pointed out in his book *Ethnic Myths,* federal agencies set up to "help" the former slaves did so by literally forcing them to sign patently unfair "tenant farm contracts" with their former masters! Thus, between 1865 and 1900, the inability of the black community in the South to produce a generation of prosperous farmers had almost nothing to do with motivation, imagination, or ability, and everything to do with a form of tenant farming that current historians correctly call an extension of the former slave system (Jayes, 1986). A second example involves the failure of labor unions to use nonracist recruitment tactics. Robert Allen noted in *Black Awakening in Capitalist America* (1969) that between 1880 and 1930, unions closed their doors to black membership, and, more often than not, the only access blacks had to manufacturing jobs and employment in mines was as strike breakers. As significant as the labor movement has been to American life, one cannot help but wonder how much more the union movement could have accomplished had it included black membership. One thing is certain: Given union access, an unknown but likely significant portion of today's poor blacks would have used such membership as a stepping-stone out of poverty, putting middle-class status within reach of their progeny. The union example is replicated in the history of sports, the entertainment industry, higher education, government, and the armed services. Each of these important sectors of American life made employment and participation *entitlements* for white (males) only.

Finally, as a last example, had the South, between 1900 and 1960, not established and maintained a social policy of deliberately underdeveloping its black citizens in terms of housing, and educational and employment opportunities, there would have been fewer undereducated and desperately poor blacks moving to the North over the last 50 years. I say what appears to be the obvious because, in commentaries about the origin of contemporary black urban poverty, one would think that poor blacks who migrated to such cities as New York, Detroit, or Chicago came from the planet Mars rather than the South. Instead, it is important for us to remember that they came from Mississippi, Alabama, Georgia, or other *American* states, if you will, states that for nearly 60 years established rather elaborate judicial, educational, and commercial infrastructures whose primary aim, according to James Anderson (1988) in *The Education of Blacks in the South, 1860–1935,* was the systematic underdevelopment of its black citizens. We must remember that segregation was not "separate but equal." It was a system that made possible the exaggerated and accelerated development of one group (whites) at the expense of the exaggerated and accelerated underdevelopment of blacks. Given every $100 in school taxes, "separate but equal" called for $50 to be spent on white and black children alike. What actually happened was that $80–90 might be spent on a white child and only $10–20 on a black child. This meant that an exaggerated amount ($80–90) dollars instead of ($50) was spent on each white child, thus, over the years, *accelerating* their educational development, while the fractional amount for black children produced, over time, an aggressively negative growth curve ($10–20 instead of $50). Also, keep in mind that just as was the case in the aftermath of slavery, the South paid no reparations to blacks for the consequences of state-supported segregation and racial underdevelopment. We need to remind ourselves that had Southern history followed a more enlightened track, the level of black poverty might be more manageable today. As it is, Americans have yet to come to grips with the past racial crimes of such states as Mississippi and South Carolina, yet when contemporary commentators discuss the origins of contemporary urban black poverty, they make it appear as though blacks *invented* their own poverty while living in the South.

Historians Dennis Dickerson (1986; *Out of the Crucible: Black Steelworkers in Western Pennsylvania, 1875–1980*) and Joe William Trotter (1985; *Black Milwaukee: The Making of An Industrial Proletariat, 1915–1945*) have revealed that when Southern blacks eventually did move north, they experienced fleeting success. From 1945 to the early 1960s, whites left the great urban factories for middle-class jobs, thus opening well-paying factory jobs to blacks. The children of these black factory workers went on to college, became the backbone of the civil rights movement, and started the expansion of today's black middle class, points underscored by Audrey Edwards and Craig Polite in *Children of the Dream: The Psychology of Black Success*. Had America's industrial sector remained healthy, the process of stable, working-class families producing tomorrow's black middle class would still be under way. However, these industrial jobs began to shrink, and most urban black communities have been in the midst of an economic depression since the mid-1960s.

At the onset of the Great Society Programs (circa mid-1960s), which were designed for the *transition* of poor blacks and poor people into the general economy, *entry level jobs in heavy industry that paid a meaningful wage began to dry up or were shifted overseas*. Ironically, the failure in the 1960s and 1970s of private industry to provide meaningful employment opportunities for all who work could has been blamed not on industry but on welfare programs designed to transition workers into these declining industries. The idea that the current malaise of poor people in general, and black people in particular, results from the welfare system and the failure of individuals to take personal responsibility is one of the great intellectual hoaxes of the 20th century (Coontz, 1992).

As it is, we tend to "see" and "explain" poverty differently, according to the race of the group. Rather than discuss poverty in America, we try to differentiate "black" poverty from "white" poverty. When African Americans are the focus, a moralistic measuring rod is often applied to some of the more sensational behavior of poor people who are black, leading to the impression that poor blacks are amoral, bizarre, and undeserving of assistance. These "black deficits" are called "legacies of slavery" or the consequences of IQ inferiority. However, when the unemployed in question are white people, scholars, policymakers, and people in the media often commence their analyses, not with issues of morality, *but with the complex chain of events that followed protracted unemployment*.

In a *systems perspective* that is more likely to be applied to unemployed white workers than blacks, the individual worker's predicament is typically traced to a larger scenario that connects factories, employment, the community tax base, the quality of schools, family functioning, and individual mental health. Following the closing of a factory in Perry, Florida, Andrea Stone wrote a story for *USA Today* (February 28, 1992) that was accompanied by a full-page graph, including personal photographs of 11 recently unemployed workers (10 of whom were white), that traced the economic fallout (ripple effect) of the factory closing to no less than 31 local commercial establishments (bank, hairdresser, jewelry store; cable television company, health spa, ice-cream shop, volume of advertisements for local newspaper, etc.). Along with the accompanying written stories, the reader was given a three-dimensional perspective about the negative consequences of unemployment. As importantly, the humanity and sense of worth of the people caught in this vicious cycle were never called into question. There was no mention that in the face of continued unemployment, such people might become "lazy," "unmotivated," or subject to sinking into a culture of poverty.

Around the same time of the Perry factory closing, the *New York Times* (July 5–10, 1992) was running a series of stories on the need to change the American welfare system. Here, the focus was often on black people. Though the connection between meaningful employment, and community and family functioning did not escape the writer, the emphasis was clearly on the "peculiar" pathologies of black communities, the "undeserving poor," and the "bizarre" behavior of black children. The theme of the *USA Today* article about white workers was the need to create jobs, whereas the *NY Times* series focused on the need to "get people off welfare."

SLAVERY AND BLACK IDENTITY

We have seen that the *legacy-of-slavery* model that emphasizes victimization and pathology can greatly distort the discourse on the evolution of black culture. This is not to suggest that there were no lasting, negative psychological effects caused by slavery, although, even here, framing the issue in positive or negative terms is too simplistic. We can say, with some degree of certitude, that at the beginning of slavery, the captive Africans were, if you will, "African" in their identities and worldview. One African was not a cultural carbon copy of the next, because, though frequently captured from the same geographic region of Africa, the historical record shows that the Africans consisted of a variety of African ethnicities, just as being French, English, Italian, or Spanish represent variability in European ethnicity. Nevertheless, if the Africans, in a plural sense, entered slavery as Africans, they left slavery with frames of reference that were decidedly not African. Taking a sledge-hammer approach, one can conclude that slavery stripped Africans of their true heritage and forced them to become a shallow imitation of white people. From this vantage point, one stresses the fact that the slave owners designed the slavery system to deracinate the Africans and make them pliable. They forced the slaves to see themselves as the slave owner wanted them to be seen: inferior Sambos suffering from self-loathing and a sense of cultural inferiority, divided by a skin-color hierarchy, and driven by an intense desire to find acceptance by the majority group, on terms dictated by the majority group.

This pejorative interpretation has a long history in the discourse on slavery and black identity (Clark, 1955; Frazier, 1939; Kardiner & Ovesey, 1951). It has subsequently fallen out of favor because the evolving historical record does not sustain the notion that the average black slave suffered from self-hatred (Kolchin, 1993). Along the same line, the history of the behaviors, activities, and organizational accomplishments of the slaves immediately after slavery and well into the early part of the 20th century, about which this author has already commented, suggests that to the extent it can be inferred, the ex-slaves seemed to exit slavery with far more psychological strengths and resources than psychological deficits and dysfunctionalities.

The record shows that the ex-slaves did not exit slavery with one type of identity, be it self-hating or self-accepting. Rather, it appears that they evidenced a broad spectrum of identities, none of which resembled the African identities with which their ancestors entered slavery. True, below the surface, residual Africanity was embedded in their language behavior, food preferences, musical aesthetic, naming practices, and family and kin ties. However, at each of these levels and more, one could also detect the presence of Irish, English, Native American, Spanish, and French influences, for slavery had transformed the Africans into a cultural and psychological mosaic.

If not Africanity, their exit-identities reflected various degrees of adjustment, coping, assimilation, and acculturation to what it means to be a "black" person in a predominantly "white-controlled" country. The types of adjustment patterns that Houston Baker, Jr. (1980) linked to literate slaves from the 1700s, and John Blassingame (1972) linked to common field slaves for the same time period are remarkably similar to the identity frames St. Clair Drake and Horace R. Cayton uncovered in their 1945 study of black life in Chicago, which McCord, Howard, Friedberg, and Harwood present in their 1969 text on lifestyles in the black ghetto, and which Gerald Early (1993) captured in a recent book of essays on the meaning of blackness written by 19 contemporary black men and women. Some of the more important identities that seem to continuously appear across black history are assimilationist, ambivalent, militant, self-hating, and internalizing or synthesizing. Persons with the assimilationist frame tend to play down the importance of race in their everyday conception of themselves, and they stress, instead, their sense of connection to the larger, dominant society. Ambivalent blacks seem openly perplexed about whether to stress their blackness or their Americanness in every-day life. Militants display a blind-faith commitment to all things black and a strong aversions to all things white. The self-hating types experience intense self-loathing, which they trace to being black. The internalizers or synthesizers operate with a multidimensional mind-set about blackness that allows them to be functional, proactive, and productive.

As fascinating as the discovery that certain black-identity categories transcend black his-tory is the discovery that, under certain circumstances, blacks may move from one identity frame to another, resulting in an identity conversion experience. The conversion results in a sense of black-identity *renewal and awakening.* The renewal theme was recorded during slav-ery, as in Nat Turner's identity conversion just before his well-known slave rebellion, and after slavery, as in W. E. B. Du Bois's oceanic awakening to his blackness when he was an under-graduate at Fisk University. This mapping of conversion continues during the early part of the 20th century (Lewis, 1993), when Alain Locke (1925) harked that the "New Negro's" renewal was the psychological infrastructure for the Harlem Renaissance. Moving closer to our times, we find identity renewal was a major theme in the lives of such figures as Malcolm X (1964) and Elaine Brown (1992), and it was a driving force in the Black Power Movement of the late 1960s and early 1970s (Van Deburg, 1992).

During the renewal process (Cross, 1971, 1991, 1995; Milliones, 1973; Thomas, 1971), some of the identity types (assimilative, ambivalent, militant, and internalizing) become mark-ers or "stages" of identity change. The identity to be changed tends to be assimilationist in na-ture (Stage 1). It accords little salience to race, either out of denial and self-hatred, or in a more positive light, because the person has an identity grounded in something *other* than race, as in one's religious orientation; that is, the person may have an intact and functional identity, but one which, in the overall scheme of things, makes being black somewhat insignificant. This is what ultimately makes the person susceptible to change, because something may happen, an *encounter,* if you will, that causes the person to feel she or he has been *miseducated.* From the *encounter* (Stage 2), the person may conclude that an assimilationist identity is clearly *not black enough,* and his or her first response may be a profound sense of confusion (ambivalent identity). The thought of having to change may even lead to a sense of loss and depression.

When the person recovers enough to continue to move forward, he or she enter a stage of militancy (Stage 3). All the fireworks of identity metamorphosis are contained in this mili-tancy stage, for within its boundaries, the old and emerging identity do battle. For the person who undergoes a particularly intense conversion, it is a period of extreme highs and lows, re-flecting the perturbation that comes from first feeling "I think I'm getting this right," to the next moment, when one falls flat on his or her face, mired in confusion. It is a period of high energy, risk taking, racial chauvinism, hatred, joy, and extreme certitude, interspersed with mo-ments of profound self-doubt. This high energy literally compels the person to seek self-expression, leading to poetry, art, or in more vulgar expressions, fantasies about the defeat and destruction on one's enemy (i.e., white people and white society). When the conversion is blan-keted in military themes, the person may feel he or she is a soldier for the people, ready for any show of commitment, including being placed in harm's way.

Given that things progress in a predictable fashion, the person eventually develops greater comfort (synthesis identity), and the new identity becomes internalized (Stage 4). Of course, not everyone moves "forward." People regress, they become "stuck" in transition—consumed by hatred—they become disillusioned, or may spin-off into still another cause and another identity "conversion." Or they become entrapped in the everyday dysfunctionalities and private demons that go with being human. Many therapists have notes on black clients who came to them with "blackness" issues, only for it later to be revealed that sexual problems, problems of repressed anger, or problems of low self-esteem, all unrelated to race, were at the core of their misery.

WHAT DOES IT MEAN TO HAVE A BLACK IDENTITY?

The linking of the different types of identity frames during the renewal process suggests that having a fully developed black identity involves the development of a multidimensional mindset, a point raised earlier in this chapter. In this sense, a fully mature sense of blackness borrows and reticulates aspects from a number of the different identity stances. Across history, blacks have attempted to experiment with a broad range of identities, and the legacy of this trial and error is a contemporary perspective that weaves dimensions from a number of these perspectives. From the assimilationist is borrowed a sense of hope and acceptance; however, from the militant, one notes the need to be careful and skeptical. From the culturally focused person, one heeds the need to know and relish black history and culture, and from the internalizer is discovered a way to feel comfortable with an identity that is complex rather than simplistic. Putting this all together, it becomes possible to approach black identity as a complex mind-set that helps a person better function in a variety of situations (Cross, 1991, 1995; Cross, Paarham, & Helms, 1996).

As part of the legacy of black coping strategies, the fully developed black identity of today serves at least three functions in a person's daily life: (1) to defend the person from the stress that results from having to live in a racist society; (2) to provide a sense of purpose, meaning and affiliation; and (3) to establish mechanisms that make possible productive interactions with people, cultures, and human situations that do not spring from the black experience.

The Defensive Functioning of Black Identity

The defensive function of black identity provides a psychological buffer during racist encounters. It is a translucent psychological filter that protects against the harmful effects of racism while letting the person process nonthreatening (race neutral) information and experiences. The structure of the protective function seems to involve five components: (1) an awareness that racism is a part of the American experience; (2) an anticipatory mind-set that, regardless of one's station in life, one could well be the target of racism; (3) keenly developed ego defenses that the person can employ when confronting racism; (4) a system blame and personal efficacy perspective in which the person is predisposed to find fault in one's circumstance and not one's self; and (5) a religious orientation that prevents the development of a sense of bitterness and the need to stigmatize whites.

The first two components constitute the heart of the protective capacity, for one cannot defend against something the existence of which is denied or minimized. For example, if one sees oneself as a special Negro who is beyond the reach of racism, then one will hardly be in a position to anticipate being the target of a racist assault. For a black person with a well-developed defensive shield, racism is a given, and one understands that he or she may well be the focus of racism. The third factor refers to the behavioral and attitudinal repertoire one can employ in negotiating racist situations (withdrawal, assertion, counteraggression, passivity, avoidance, etc.). The stronger, more mature, and more varied one's ego defenses, the greater one's capacity to handle a variety of racist interactions. Because blacks frequently find themselves living in poor and degrading circumstances, the fourth factor helps one to maintain a sense of perspective and personal worth in the face of racism. In this way, the person is able to distinguish between what is an extension of one's self-concept (that which one deserves and should be given credit for) versus what is a reflection of the racist and oppressive system against which one must endure, struggle, and survive. Finally, the fifth factor, the spiritual and religious one, helps the person to avoid becoming embittered and filled with hatred toward whites. This is important, because, time and again, hatred originally directed at whites will spill over and poison aspects of black-on-black relationships.

The defensive function also helps a person deal with the "hassle" of being black. It operates to minimize the hurt, pain, imposition, and stigma that comes when one is treated with disrespect, rudeness, and insensitivity. Rather than being unduly hurt and caught off guard, the defensive mode allows the person to maintain control and avoid overreacting. Highly motivated blacks apply the shield as they forage through the American experience for race-neutral opportunities, "open doors," and find resources that can improve their personal fortunes and the lives of their family and kin. The content of what a black person must guard against differs by gender. Consequently, while both black women and black men must defend against racist stereotypes, the content and dynamics of these stereotypes differ, as in the "Aunt Jemima" and sexually loose images heaped on black women, and the "lazy Sambo" or drug-crazed criminal images used to stigmatize black males.

It should be noted that the defensive function can become dysfunctional in a variety of ways. In one instance, the person may underplay the importance of racism, in which case the defensive function will be inadequately developed, and the person's identity will provide little protection against racism. The lack of a defensive modality can also result from the person having internalized the racist images of him- or herself (self-hatred) and/or from accepting as true the negative images directed at blacks as a group (group rejection). As is well documented, internalized racism can lead to color phobias, depression, drug and alcohol abuse, anger and rage, and black-on-black crime (Oliver, 1994; Russell, Wilson, & Hall, 1992). Finally, defensive dysfunctionality occurs when the person is oversensitive or even paranoiac, "seeing" racism where it does not exist. Instead of engaging the larger society and using one's defensive mode to filter out racist from race-neutral content, the person simply opposes contact or interaction with anything thought to be linked to the "white" experience. This can be disastrous in school-age black youth, who, in defining academic achievement as "white-behavior," disengage from academic pursuits.

The Group Affiliation Function of Black Identity

To function effectively, every human being needs to feel wanted, connected, accepted, and affiliated, although the group or groups from which one may derive a sense of well-being need not be the group to which one is socially or publicly ascribed. For example, many blacks derive their sense of affiliation from groups that have little to do with a black-oriented identity. Instead, some may achieve personal fulfillment, status, and happiness through their religious affiliation, their occupational status, or their sense of American patriotism. Such people cannot be said to have a black identity, because their sense of personal well-being is anchored to something other than their blackness.

Having a black identity means that one's group-affiliation needs are met through one's sense of connection to black people and black culture. The individual's feeling of being valued, accepted, appreciated, and affiliated is deeply rooted in black people, black culture, and the general black condition. One's values, cultural preferences, artistic tastes, leisure activities, cooking styles and food choices, secular and religious musical tastes, church affiliation, organizational memberships, and social network or intimate friends are all influenced by one's perceived connection to black people.

The affiliation functions of black identity can lead to the celebration and study of black accomplishments, the search for ways to solve black problems, and a desire to discover, protect, and disseminate information about black culture and history. When taken too far, as in racial chauvinism, it can result in intense social conformity, polarized "we–they" perceptions, and the stereotyping and demonization of nonblacks.

Bridging or Transcendent Function of Black Identity

When combined, the first two functions form the type of ethnic identity that is fairly typical of people whose lives revolve around a particular culture, religion, or ethnicity. Not only may such persons see the world primarily from the perspective of "their group," they may actually show little interest in learning about or interacting with persons from other groups. As long as a black person operates (work, play, marriage, religion, etc.) in an all-black or predominately black community, the need to have as part of one's identity the functional skills and sensitivities that make one competent in multicultural or multiracial situations may be a low priority. However, the omnipresent paradox of black life is that whether one lives in or out of the black community, it is nearly impossible to avoid intense social and commercial intercourse with ethnic whites, including Jews, Asian Americans, Latinos, and Native Americans.

Consequently, a third function that defines the multiple mind-set we call black identity is a *bridging function,* which, when developed, results in varying degrees of multiracial and multicultural competence. Some blacks are chagrined at the necessity for this third function and may take a minimalist attitude toward its development. Others may work hard at being both black and American, in a bicultural sense, while still others may relish a quite expansive bridging capacity that is multicultural in nature. This helps explain why black people who embrace a black identity do not represent one ideological position. Black nationalists may take a minimalist approach to the bridging function, persons who focus on black–white interactions may evidence a biracial salience, and multicultural blacks may be those who bridge to at least three or more cultural dimensions of the American experience.

Transracial and, especially, black–white bridging activities can lead to conflicts within the black community. Black nationalists may interpret bridging other than the Pan-African variety as a waste of limited time and resources, while those involved in transracial connections may counter that black life is inherently bicultural, if not multicultural. Other blacks see any debate about "to bridge or not to bridge" as not grounded in reality, since their workplaces, schools, and community environments are already cultural kaleidoscopes; they see the development of the bridging functions of black identity as a necessity. Black women argue that the sexism of both white and black men makes it necessary to constantly bridge between their gender and blackness orientation. Finally, bridging adds a crucial element of flexibility to black identity that allows one better to assimilate rapid culture and technological innovation. Black Americans, like all Americans, must be able to keep pace with change in American society, and a constricted, provincial, identity structure cannot handle innovation.

CONCLUSION

In 1951, two psychiatrists, Abraham Kardiner and Lionel Ovesey, published what at the time was thought to be a state-of-the-art psychological investigation of the mind and personality of the Negro. They concluded that middle-class and poor blacks alike suffered from a "Negro-self-hatred" syndrome that likely had origins in the slavery experience. They called this slavery legacy the "mark of oppression." With the unfolding of the civil rights and Black Power movements of the 1950s and 1960s, scholars took renewed interest in the study of slavery, and by the late 1970s, the "mark of oppression" legacy had been proven false. It is now understood that over the course of nearly 400 years of slavery, the slaves were able to exploit various gaps and contradictions in the way the slavery system operated to produce a level of humanity and cultural development never intended by the slave owners. Blacks exited from slavery with personality and cultural strengths that allowed them to navigate continued experiences with oppression from 1865 to the late 1950s. Over the last 30 years, this legacy of strength has met its match in black nihilism, stemming from the massive and protracted unemployment of black workers. That black and white observers alike have seen in this nihilism a "legacy of slavery" constitutes a form of intellectual denial of the psychological consequences of economic redundancy in the 1990s. In the past, as long as blacks were able to find linkages to the mainstream economy, they converted their meager earnings into fuel that sustained their culture and their protective psychology. In today's world, the employment links to the larger society have been severed completely for hundreds of thousands of blacks, and the resulting nadir may prove to be as grim a challenge as that faced by blacks after slavery or during the Depression.

Over the course of history, blacks have experimented with different identity frames that might provide relief from their predicament. I discussed the distinctive features of a number of these identity options. Furthermore, during attempts at identity self-renewal, blacks go through an identity conversion experience that requires leaping from one type of identity to another, as in a progression of stages, until a new identity resynthesis has been achieved. I concluded by looking at the way in which a modern conceptualization of black identity reflects a *multidimensional mind-set* that protects or shields against racism, provides a sense of group affiliation, and establishes links to the larger, nonblack or multicultural world within which most blacks are located.

REFERENCES

Allen, R. (1974). *Reluctant reformers: Racism and social reform movements in the United States.* Washington, DC: Howard University Press.

Anderson, J. D. (1988). *The education of blacks in the south, 1860–1935.* Chapel Hill: University of North Carolina Press.

Archer, C., Jr. (1992). *Growing up black in rural Mississippi.* New York: Walker.

Asante, M. (1993). Racism, consciousness and afrocentricity. In G. Early (Ed.), *Lure and loathing: Essays on race, identity, and the ambivalence of assimilation* (pp. 127–144). New York: Allen Lane/Penguin Press.

Baker, H. A., Jr. (1980). *The journey back: Issues in black literature and criticism.* Chicago: University of Chicago Press.

Blassingame, J. (1972). *The slave community.* New York: Oxford Press.

Brown, E. (1992). *A taste of power: A black woman's journey.* New York: Pantheon Press.

Bullock, H. A. (1967). *A history of Negro education in the South.* Cambridge: Harvard University Press.

Butchart, R. E. (1980). *Northern schools, Southern blacks, and reconstruction.* Westport, CT: Greenwood Press.

Clark, K. B. (1955). *Prejudice and your child.* Boston: Beacon Press.

Comer, J. P. (1988). *Maggie's Dream: The life and times of a black family.* New York: Plume.

Coontz, S. (1992). *The way we never were.* New York: Basic Books/HarperCollins.

Cross, W. E., Jr. (1971). The Negro-to-black conversion experience. *Black World, 20,* 13–27.

Cross, W. E., Jr. (1991). *Shades of black.* Philadelphia: Temple University Press.

Cross, W. E., Jr. (1995). The psychology of Nigrescence: Revising the cross model. In J. Ponterotto, J. Casa, L. Suzuki, & C. Alexander (Eds.), *Handbook of Multicultural Counseling.* Thousand Oaks, CA: Sage.

Cross, W. E., Jr., Parham, T. A., & Helms, J. E. (1996). Nigrescence revisited: Theory and research. In R. L. Jones (Ed.), *Advances in black psychology* (pp. 1–69). Los Angeles: Cobb & Henry.

Dickerson, D. (1986). *Out of the crucible: Black steel workers in western Pennsylvania, 1875–1980.* Albany, NY: State University of New York Press.

Drake, S., & Cayton, H. (1945). *Black metropolis: A study of Negro life in a Northern city.* New York: Harcourt, Brace.

Du Bois, W. E. B. (1936). *Black reconstruction.* New York: S. A. Russell.

Early, G. (1993). *Lure and loathing: Essays on race, identity, and the ambivalence of assimilation.* New York: Allen Lane/Penguin Press.

Edwards, A., & Polite, C. (199?). *Children of the dream: The psychology of black success.* New York: Doubleday.

Frazier, E. F. (1939). *The Negro family in the United States.* Chicago: University of Chicago Press.

Fogel, R., & Engerman, S. (1974). *Time on the cross.* Boston: Little, Brown.

Gutman, H. (1976). *The black family in slavery and freedom, 1750–1925.* New York: Pantheon.

Gutman, H. (1987). *Power and culture.* New York: Pantheon.

Jaynes, J. (1986). *Branches without roots: Genesis of the black working class in the American South, 1862–1882.* New York: Oxford University Press.

Kardiner, A., & Ovesey, L. (1951). *The mark of oppression.* New York: Norton.

Kolchin, P. (1993). *American slavery: 1619–1877.* New York: Hill & Wang.

Lewis, D. (1993). *W. E. B. Du Bois.* New York: Holt.

Locke, A. (1925). *The new Negro.* New York: Albert & Charles Boni.

Malcolm X, & Haley, A. (1964). *The Autobiography of Malcolm X.* New York: Grove Press.

McCord, W., Howard, J., Friedberg, B., & Harwood, E. (1969). *Life styles in the Black ghetto.* New York: W. W. Norton.

Milliones, J. (1973). *Construction of the developmental inventory of black consciousness.* Doctoral dissertation, University of Pittsburgh, Pittsburgh, PA.

Morgan, K. L. (1980). *Children of strangers.* Philadelphia: Temple University Press.

New York Times (1992, July 5–10). Rethinking welfare (six-part series).

Oliver, W. (1994). *The violent social world of black men.* New York: Lexington Books.

Russell, K., Wilson, M., & Hall, R. (1992). *The color complex: The politics of skin color among African Americans.* New York: Harcourt, Brace, Jovanovich.

Steinberg, S. (1992). *The ethnic myth: Race, ethnicity, and class in America* (2nd ed.). Boston: Beacon Press.

Taulbert, C. L. (1989). *Once upon a time when we were colored.* Tulsa, OK: Council Oak Books.

Thomas, C. W. (1971). *Boys no more.* Beverly Hills, CA: Glencoe Press.

Thomas, L. (1993). *Vessels of evil: American slavery and the Holocaust.* Philadelphia: Temple University Press.

Trotter, J., Jr. (1985). *Black Milwaukee: The making of an industrial proletariat, 1915–1945.* Urbana: University of Illinois Press.

Stone, A. (1992). The recession's ripple effect. *USA Today,* February 28, 1992, p. 6A.

Van Deburg, W. L. (1992). *New day in Babylon: The Black Power movement and American culture, 1965–1975.* Chicago: University of Chicago Press.

Webber, T. L. (1978). *Deep like the rivers.* New York: Norton.

VII

Repressive Regimes

25

Stalin's Purge and Its Impact on Russian Families
A Pilot Study

KATHARINE G. BAKER and JULIA B. GIPPENREITER

INTRODUCTION

This chapter describes a preliminary research project jointly undertaken during the winter of 1993–1994 by a Russian psychologist and an American social worker. The authors first met during KGB's presentation of Bowen Family Systems Theory (BFST) at Moscow State University in 1989. During frequent meetings in subsequent years in the United States and Russia, the authors shared their thoughts about the enormous political and societal upheaval occurring in Russia in the 1990s. The wider context of Russian history in the 20th-century and its impact on contemporary events, on the functioning of families over several generations, and on the functioning of individuals living through turbulent times was central to these discussions.

How did the prolonged societal nightmare of the 1920s and the 1930s affect the population of the Soviet Union? What was the impact of the demented paranoia of those years of totalitarian repression on innocent citizens who tried to live "normal" lives, raise families, go to work, stay healthy, and live out their lives in peace? What was the emotional legacy of Stalin's Purge of 1937–1939 for the children and grandchildren of its victims? Does it continue to have an impact on the functioning of modern-day Russians who are struggling with new societal disruptions during the post-Communist transition to a free-market democracy?

These are the questions that led to the research study presented in this chapter.[1] Fifty grandchildren of Stalin's Purge victims were interviewed in depth about their family experiences: What had happened to their grandparents, when had they found out about it, and what was the impact of these events on their own development and functioning? What was the

---

[1]Preliminary findings of this study appeared under the title "The effects of Stalin's purge on three generations of Russian families," in *Family Systems: A Journal of Natural Systems Thinking in Psychiatry and the Sciences* (Spring/Summer, 1996) 3(1), 5–35.

KATHARINE G. BAKER • 3 Chesterfield Road, Williamsburg, Massachusetts 01096. **JULIA B. GIPPENREITER** • Moscow State University, Psychology Faculty, Moscow, Russia 117463.

International Handbook of Multigenerational Legacies of Trauma, edited by Yael Danieli. Plenum Press, New York, 1998.

emotional atmosphere in a family that had experienced "the knock on the door in the middle of the night?" Did the surviving family stay together, or did it break up? What did parents share or hide from their children? How were children affected by knowing that they were "enemies of the people"? How did the family trauma of the Purge compare with other traumatic historical events in Russia, such as the loss of relatives in World War II or the "stagnation" of 20 years of Brezhnevism following Khrushchev's ouster from leadership in 1964?

The research was grounded in Bowen Family Systems Theory (BFST), which postulates that a multigenerational transmission process provides a continuity of emotional functioning in families, as well as the communication of values and beliefs across generations. According to this theory (Bowen, 1978), those who maintain a sense of connection with past family values, beliefs, and experiences, and have a sense of real relationship with family members who have preceded them, will manage the stresses of their own lives more effectively than those who have drifted away from their families. If this is true, it could have significant implications for societies, families, and individuals who have survived such catastrophic experiences as the Purge, or who may face unknown traumas in the future. The research was undertaken in order to test whether this concept from BFST could be useful in understanding a massive societal rediscovery of its past, as the Soviet archives on the Purge began to open up and the grandchild generation had the opportunity to discover what had really happened two generations ago.

The authors collaborated in planning the research, identifying a sample for interviews, creating a questionnaire, training Russian graduate students of psychology to conduct the interviews, analyzing the data that came from the interviews, and writing reports of the findings. The effort has been a beginning attempt to understand some of the madness that swept through all levels of Soviet society more than 50 years ago and has left scars that may never completely heal in millions of families.

THE HISTORICAL CONTEXT

The period in the Soviet Union between the two world wars has been the subject of an extensive literature in history and political science (e.g., Arendt, 1966; Conquest, 1990; Daniels, 1985; Gleason, 1995; Malia, 1994; Treadgold, 1995; Tucker, 1971; Ulam, 1989; Volkogonov, 1992; etc.). Stalin had inherited the Bolshevik Revolution from Lenin after Lenin's untimely death from a stroke in 1924. Shortly after his first stroke in 1921, Lenin had composed a "Testament" in which he expressed his thoughts on leadership succession in the Communist Party in the new Soviet Union. In Lenin's view, his two most talented deputies were Leon Trotsky and Joseph Stalin, but Lenin had reservations about Stalin because he had "concentrated an enormous power in his hands," and Lenin was not sure that Stalin would use this power with "sufficient caution" (Conquest, 1990, p. 4). This was a strange reservation from the man who had expanded Karl Marx's concept of proletarian revolution to include the violent overthrow of the Romanov dynasty and the establishment of a "dictatorship of the proletariat" through one-party rule. But Lenin knew how tenuous Communist Party control really was in the Soviet Union in the early 1920s, and he had even initiated a new economic policy (NEP) in which a limited return to a free market economy was permitted in order to assuage the wrath of a disrupted and exhausted Russian population still suffering from the losses of World War I, the Revolution, and a protracted civil war, which had only begun to wind down in 1921.

During the period between Lenin's death and the start of World War II, a vicious succession struggle took place in which millions of people died as Stalin established his control over the government apparatus, the Party, and through "collectivization" of the relatively affluent stratum of the agricultural population (*kulaki*). In an attempt to root out all manifestations of Trotskyism, tracking down Trotsky himself and ultimately having him murdered in Mexico in 1941, Stalin generated nationwide waves of hysteria that led to massive societal xenophobia, paranoia, and denunciations, culminating in the Great Purge from 1937 to 1939. During the Purge, millions were arrested as "enemies of the people," tortured, sent to concentration camps in Siberia, or instantly shot. Hitler's invasion of the Soviet Union in June 1941 slowed the fervor of the Purge, but it picked up again after the war with new denunciations of those who had "cooperated" with the Germans while interned in German prisoner-of-war camps. The Purge only truly ended with Stalin's death in March 1953.

For many Sovietologists, the Purge can only be explained as the madness of a single man, Joseph Stalin. Conquest (1990) describes the process by which "Stalin's blows were struck at every form of solidarity and comradeship outside of that provided by personal allegiance to himself" (p. 255). Conquest holds Stalin responsible for taking on "the disintegration of family loyalty" (p. 252) as a conscious aim: "In cold blood, quite deliberately and unprovokedly, . . . [he] started a new cycle of suffering" (p. 251). Conquest further notes that "Stalinist totalitarianism on the whole automatically encouraged the mean and malicious. The carriers of personal or office feuds, the poison-pen letter writers, who are a minor nuisance in any society, flourished and increased" (p. 253). Conquest not only holds Stalin personally responsible for the Purge but also describes a kind of mass hysteria in which "lunatic denunciations" rolled like waves throughout the society, through widening circles of colleagues, acquaintances, and neighbors, to envelop the entire society in a mass terror. Although the purges started out in the Party, "by mid-1937 practically the entire population was potential Purge fodder. Few can have failed to wonder if their turn had come" (p. 258).

Arendt (1966) comments that "drunkenness and incompetence . . . loom large in any description of Russia in the twenties and thirties" (p. xi), and she also describes the

> gigantic criminality of the Stalin regime which, after all, did not consist merely in the slander and murder of a few hundred or thousand prominent political and literary figures, whom one may 'rehabilitate' posthumously, but in the extermination of literally untold millions of people whom no one, not even Stalin, could have suspected of 'counter-revolutionary' activities. (p. xiii).

She notes further that it was Stalin's personal ruthlessness that introduced "into Bolshevism the same contempt for the Russian people that the Nazis showed toward the Germans" (p. 249). But beyond Stalin, Arendt describes the absolutism of totalitarianism in which the individual becomes

> submerged in the stream of dynamic movement of the universal itself. In this stream the difference between ends and means evaporates together with the personality, and the result is the monstrous immorality of ideological policies. All that matters is embodied in the moving movement itself; every idea, every value has vanished into a welter of superstitious pseudoscientific immanence. (p. 249)

Malia (1994) also addresses the sociopolitical system of Stalinist socialism in attempting to understand the Purge. He observes that "the need to salvage something of Stalinism will endure so long as belief exists in the instrumental program of integral socialism—namely, the end of private property, which was achieved for the first time in history under Stalin" (p. 229). He also describes an underlying purpose for the Purge as an attempt to bring all thought and art into the "totalizing logic" of the political system.

As described by Hochschild (1994), the Purge went beyond other human maladies in its scope:

> The Purge . . . seems almost totally unfamiliar. It went beyond ideology, beyond reason, beyond factional strife, and beyond even the self-interest of the Soviet Union's rulers. So many engineers and managers were killed that the economy slowed down; so many railway workers were killed that trains failed to run; so many Red Army officers were killed that, a few years later, the Soviets almost lost World War II. The Great Purge reached the realm of madness. (p. 96)

Hochschild (1994) also compares the Purge to the great witch-hunts of early modern Europe. He comments that

> part of the problem of explaining mass hysteria is that it has momentum: any outbreak seems quickly to become independent of the causes that triggered it. The hysteria touches an inflammable part of the human psyche, which, once ignited, is hard to put out. Belief in a devil can be as attractive as belief in a god. Even in the best of times, we have plenty of nameless frustrations and fears it is useful to have someone to blame for. And so mass hysteria takes on a seductive life of its own once a class of scapegoats for all problems is officially designated: Witches! Enemies of the people! Off with their heads! The contagion then often lasts long after the specific fears that caused it have disappeared or been replaced by others. (p. 172)

Contemporary Russian fiction also attempts to provide some explanation for the events of the interwar period. Vassily Aksyonov, a Russian writer whose parents were Purge victims, speaks through a 1930s character in his historical novel *Generations of Winter* (1945):

> All of modern Russian history looks like a series of breakers—waves of retribution. The February Revolution was retribution for our ruling aristocracy's arrogance and narrow-minded immovability in relation to the people. The October Revolution and the Civil War were retribution against the bourgeoisie and the intelligentsia for their obsessive summons to revolution, for the stirring up of the masses. Collectivization and the campaign against the kulaks were retribution against the peasants for their cruelty in the Civil War, for beating up clergymen, for the bloodthirsty anarchism. The current purges are retribution against the revolutionaries for the violence they wreaked upon the peasants. . . . As for the future, it's impossible to predict. (268)

Primary source materials from survivors of the Purge have exploded in the former Soviet Union in recent years and have provided validation for this research. These memoirs and fictional accounts (e.g., Adamova-Sliozberg, 1993; Babel, 1969; Chukovskaya, 1994; Forche, 1993; Ginzburg, 1967; Grossman, 1972; Mandelstam, 1970, 1972; Razgon, 1989; Shalamov, 1982; Solzhenitsyn, 1992; Tertz, 1960, 1989; Vilyenskiy, 1989; Volkov, 1989) describe the authors' personal experiences during the Purge, in concentration camps and in exile.

The memoir literature is very similar to verbal accounts given by this study's subjects with regard to events around the arrest and the subsequent fate of Purge victims in their own families. Both in the memoirs and in the research, the majority of those arrested were men. They were Party leaders, officers of the Tsar's army who had joined the Red Army, priests, scientists, engineers, railroad workers, Komintern officials, managers of plants and construction companies, ministers of the NKVD (secret police), and people with relatives abroad. Usually, the victims believed that the arrest was an error and that they would return home very soon. Yet most of those who were arrested were never again seen by their wives and children.

The arrests usually took place during the night. In some cases, most commonly when neighbors or colleagues had already been arrested, the victims and their families knew that arrest was imminent and tried to prepare for it. Many adults and children reported sleepless nights and an intense atmosphere of fear. A car, or sometimes a disguised commercial van, would park in the street in front of the building. Several officers of the NKVD would knock on the door, enter (usually without resistance from the family), and show an arrest order. There was a general search of the apartment that ignored family reactions (Remnick, 1993). Then, the victim was taken away. What he was permitted to take with him depended on the whims of the arresting officers. Small items such as toothbrushes were sometimes permitted, while extra sweaters may have been forbidden.

Aksyonov (1995) describes the atmosphere in families during the period when the arrests were taking place:

> It was only at night that fear began to creep along the streets; scores of Black Marias emerged from the iron gates of the Lubyanka [the central Moscow prison where political prisoners were taken for interrogation and torture] and drove to different buildings throughout the city. All in Moscow averted their eyes at the sight of these vans, the same way any man drives the thought of the inevitability of death from his mind. Please, God, don't let them come for me, or any of our family—ah, thank the Lord, they've passed by! The Black Marias stopped where the orders said they were supposed to, and the agents of the secret police entered homes unhurriedly. The sound of footfalls on the stairs or the noise of an elevator rising in the middle of the night became the habitual background of Moscow's nocturnal terror. People pressed close to the doors of their communal apartments and trembled in their rooms. "They aren't coming to our floor, are they?" "No, they're going higher. . . ." Sometimes in the home of the arrestee there would be sobbing—muffled, suppressed, of course, at first, but turning into hysteria that was unseemly in Soviet society but still very much alive. (p. 178)

The female Purge victims were most commonly arrested because they were the wives of arrested men (see, e.g., Adamova-Sliozberg, 1993; Ginzburg, 1967; Vilyenskiy, 1989). Very few women were arrested independently. If both parents were arrested, their children were often cared for by relatives or sent to special orphanages. Grandmothers were important to the survival of many of these children. Children over 18 were often sent into exile. Some younger children were permitted to join their mothers in exile after their mothers were released from the camps.

Male Purge victims were usually shot immediately after they were arrested or sent directly to concentration camps, where large numbers died because of conditions there. Their families usually did not know for many years what had happened to them or where they were (see, e.g., Akhmatova's *Requiem* in Forche, 1993, p. 101). Families of the men who were shot immediately were told that the sentence had been "10 years without the right to correspondence." After the general amnesty in 1956, families learned that this sentence was a euphemism for the men having been shot. Occasionally, after World War II, families were sent further misinformation about relatives who had been purged. Only later did they learn that they had been told lies.

Few Purge victims ever returned to western Russia (Grossman, 1972). Those who did return to the west after the war were usually rearrested at the end of the 1940s and remained in the camps until the general amnesty in 1956 (Adamova-Sliozberg, 1993; Volkov, 1989). Before their rearrest, Purge victims were forbidden to live with their families in large cities (Grossman, 1972). They met their families surreptitiously and secretly, while anxiously awaiting rearrest at any moment.

Surviving family members of Purge victims were often evicted from their apartments by the State. They were also fired from the jobs, expelled from universities and the Komsomol

(Communist Youth League), and often were unable to find employment. Highly qualified children of Purge victims were turned down by universities. They were officially labeled "Members of Families of Betrayers of the Fatherland" (Ch-S-I-R), or children of "Enemies of the People" (VNs). Being the family of a VN "carried a great stigma, and sometimes meant prison for the wife and an orphanage for the children" (Hochschild, 1994, p. 13). Between 1949 and 1950, some of the grown children of Purge victims were arrested in a campaign called Fragments (*Oscolki*), which aimed to collect and eliminate the remaining family members of Purge victims. After Stalin's death and the 1956 amnesty, many members of these families still had difficulty getting jobs.

The memoir literature describes a range of reactions among family members of the Purge victims. The spouses of Purge victims were generally despairing and frightened, and they withdrew from social contact. Friends and relatives avoided them. Sometimes politically secure friends would continue to visit or help, but this was the exception. Some families tried to use high-level political connections to try to protect themselves, but this could be risky for the helpers. Most families tried to hide the fact that a relative had been arrested. Sometimes families did not tell their very young children the truth about what had happened to a missing relative. Children and grandchildren born after the Purge might be told that their father or grandfather had died in the War. Usually, the surviving spouses raised their children alone. Some remarried when they had not heard from a purged husband for many years. If he then returned from prison camp after the general amnesty in 1956, wives faced terrible dilemmas of loyalty, love, and family definition (Grossman, 1972).

The children of VNs also suffered from profound identity confusion. Young men whose parents had been arrested would volunteer for the Front during the war in order to demonstrate their loyalty and innocence. Children of the VNs tried to avoid joining Communist Party organizations because they were frightened that they would be questioned about their families' political organizations because they were frightened that they would be questioned about their families' political reliability. Daughters of the VNs would try to marry when very young in order to change their names, but they often had trouble finding suitors. Prospective husbands (who were not the sons of VNs) wanted to "keep their resumes clean." If they married these young women, they would share the social–political shame of their wives and could themselves be vulnerable to political repression at the end of the 1940s.

The experiences of the grandchildren of Purge victims have so far not been explored in the memoir literature. Reference is sometimes made to a family's Purge experiences, but these family histories have not been linked with contemporary issues for members of the grandchild generation who are now establishing their own families.

THEORETICAL/CONCEPTUAL FRAMEWORK

Bowen Family Systems Theory was chosen as the theoretical foundation for this research project because it provides a useful framework for understanding family functioning across several generations. BFST addresses aspects of variability in human functioning within family relationship systems. These concepts are not culture-bound, but apply to some extent to all members of the species. The study used two principal concepts from BFST: (1) the multigenerational transmission process and (2) cutoff.

The BFST concept of the multigenerational transmission process describes fluctuations in functioning and emotional relationships through the generations of a family. As described by Kerr and Bowen (1988), BFST "assumes that individual differences in functioning and multigenerational trends in functioning reflect an orderly and predictable relationship process that connects the functioning of family members across generations" (p. 224). Variations in the functioning of family members are usually not dramatically discrepant over such a brief period as three generations, although "every family, given sufficient generations, tends to produce people at both functional extremes and people at most points on a continuum between these extremes" (p. 221). Anxiety and other behavioral and emotional patterns are transmitted from one generation to the next through relationships between grandparents, parents, and grandchildren.

This study looks at Russian families across three generations, including grandparents, parents, and grandchildren, but its interview subjects were drawn from the grandchild generations. According to BFST, the functioning of the grandchild generation in present-day Russia would be fairly consistent with patterns of family response to prior historic catastrophes such as the Great Purge. Families that had maintained a stable level of functioning during and after the Purge might be expected to produce grandchildren who would manage themselves effectively in post-Soviet Russia. Families that were unstable in the aftermath of the Purge might be expected to produce lower functioning grandchildren.

"Cutoff" is a component of the multigenerational transmission process. It describes the nature of connection across generations in a family. It can be part of vertical relationships between generations, as well as of horizontal relationships within the same generation. It is part of the natural process in which children move toward autonomy in relation to their parents, so that they can establish their own adult families and reproduce (Illick, 1993). Cutoff can be geographic or physical, as when family members move away from each other and lose touch. It can be also be emotional. Intense emotional cutoff is defined as a complete emotional withdrawal from important family members, which is driven by anxiety. Kerr and Bowen (1988) note that "people cut off from their families of origin to reduce the discomfort generated by being in emotional contact with them" (p. 271). In the opinion of these authors, cutoff may also be driven by societal forces that make family connection dangerous and may even threaten family survival.

Cutoff is associated with a wide range of human functioning. Mild cutoff is a part of a natural movement toward autonomy between generations. Some cutoff may represent a responsible effort to cope with internal family stressors. Intense emotional cutoff, however, can be said to be pathogenic and is associated with the more severe human psychological, social, and chronic physiological problems. In other words, families that manage anxiety through distancing from each other tend to be vulnerable to a variety of symptoms. Families that manage anxiety through a balance of autonomy and connection across generations tend to have fewer severe problems (Kerr & Bowen, 1988, p. 271). The relationship between cutoff and functioning is not causal or linear, but there is a strong association between the two factors.

In the Soviet Union during the 1930s, cutting off from family members who had been purged was often the most "sensible" course of action. Purge victims had been physically removed from their families through arrest, imprisonment, torture, assassination, and exile. The state then declared it a crime for family members to maintain relationships with these VNs. In addition, the family members themselves were cut off from the wider society, since they were officially labeled "relatives of VNs." In response to these State policies, many changed their names, went into hiding, and never mentioned their purged relatives again. But others kept the memories of lost family members alive and retained a sense of pride in those memories in spite of State policies.

The central hypothesis of this research was that cutoff was a pathogenic force for families of Purge victims. It was hypothesized that families who cut off physically or emotionally from their purged relatives during the late 1930s would manifest lower functioning in the grandchild generation. A related hypothesis was that avoidance of cutoff could provide a buffer against societal trauma. In other words, maintaining a sense of connection with lost family members could enhance the functioning of succeeding generations. The study proposed that an internal continuity of family identity, values, and beliefs across three generations might enhance the functioning of grandchildren living under the stressful conditions of Russian society in the 1990s.

A correlate of BFST hypothesizes that human societies, like human families, function along a continuum. At the lowest end of the continuum are extremely regressed societies that are unable to take care of their members, have ineffective leadership and chaotic internal structures, and are in conflict with their neighbors and the natural environment. At the highest end of the continuum are societies that are able to promote optimal functioning in their members, have orderly internal structures and processes for decision making and productivity, and exist in harmony with their neighbors and the natural environment.

At a societal level, cutoff could manifest itself externally in foreign relations or internally in the society's connection with its own history. According to BFST, a society that truly knows, understands, and maintains a connection with its own past (including both good and bad events) will most effectively manage the social, economic, and political challenges it confronts in the present and future. This aspect of BFST is particularly relevant to present-day Russia as it begins to open up the archives from the Soviet period and acknowledge the events of its past.

DESCRIPTION OF THE SAMPLE

The investigators utilized both probability and nonprobability sampling in selecting grandchildren of Purge victims for interviews. The total population for the study included all the grandchildren of all the millions of people arrested, tortured, killed, or imprisoned in the Soviet Union between 1937 and 1939. Because random sampling of this vast group was impractical, nonprobability or convenience sampling was used to identify an accessible subgroup of the population. The sample population that was selected consisted of grandchildren of Purge victims who were directly or indirectly associated with Memorial.

Memorial (Adler, 1993) is a Russian nongovernmental organization established in 1987 in order to erect a monument to the victims of the Purge. It quickly became a repository for information about these victims. Originally, it was a grassroots organization. But after the end of the Soviet Union in 1991, Memorial was officially registered with the Russian government and began to receive some government support. Its central office is in Moscow, but it has branch offices throughout the former Soviet Union. A high percentage of its members are the daughters and grandchildren of Purge victims.

The investigators wrote a letter to the director of Memorial describing the proposed study and requesting access to Memorial's membership list. The director reacted positively to the request and provided names, addresses, telephone numbers, ages, and other demographic information about its membership.

Within this convenience sample, the investigators used a stratified random sampling method to identify 50 subjects who were grandchildren of Purge victims. All were born between 1948 and 1958, had university or technical institute education, and currently lived in Moscow. An even number of men and women were selected. The decision to control for these variables was made for a number of reasons. Moscow was chosen for convenience in conducting the interviews. Subjects between the ages of 35 and 45 were chosen because they would have had time to establish their own families. About half were born before Stalin's death in

1953, and about half were born after. Approximately the same number of males and females were chosen in order to facilitate male–female comparisons. Nearly all of the subjects were university educated, since it was assumed that they would be optimally thoughtful about their family life experience.

Although controlling for these variables limits the generalizability of the study's findings, the investigators believe that the positive aspects of the selection protocol outweighed most disadvantages for the purpose of a small pilot study.

METHODOLOGY

Using an ex post facto design with in-depth interviews from a questionnaire as the data collection and measurement instrument, the investigators and their assistants interviewed 50 grandchildren of Purge victims in Moscow during the winter of 1993–1994. The research focused on the variation in family response to the Purge and on how this variation had manifested itself in the grandchild generation. There was no control group, but comparisons were made within the sample.

Four interviewers[2] were selected from among the psychology graduate students of coinvestigator Julia Gippenreiter. Gippenreiter was the fifth interviewer. Each interviewer interviewed 10 subjects. The interviewers were trained by Gippenreiter and Baker in Moscow in October 1993. The training included a detailed review of the questionnaire, with a focus on the significance of each question; an explanation of Bowen theory and its relevance for the study; and techniques for interviewing, including neutrality, encouragement of response to open-ended questions, and coding. Interviewers conducted test interviews before contacting study subjects. In addition, all interviewers practice-interviewed the same subject in order to test for interrater reliability.

Through in-depth interviews, the study gathered subjective observations, memories, general information, and measures of self-reported present functioning of the subjects. The subjects were asked about their factual knowledge of the events of the Purge and the experiences of their grandparents and parents at that time. They also reported their own emotional "memories" of those events (e.g., fear), as transmitted to them through their parents. They described their relationships with their parents and grandparents, their parents' and grandparents' values and guiding principles, and how these had or had not been incorporated into their own lives. Through these interviews, the study attempted to discover the multigenerational process of transmission of values, guiding principles, behaviors, coping mechanisms, and the ability to utilize resources, as well as relationship and emotional patterns. It also attempted to understand the reciprocal, three-way nature of the grandparent–parent–grandchild relationship system.

The Research Instrument

The data collection instrument, created by the coinvestigators in Washington, D.C., and Moscow, was a 58-item Russian-language interview questionnaire that included both closed and open-ended questions (see Appendix). The interviews were used to gather two kinds of responses: (1) objective information, such as dates, health status, education, and profession of the subjects, their parents, and grandparents; and (2) subjective information, such as the

[2]The authors appreciate the assistance of G. N. Vorobyevaya, A. A. Rudakov, M. L. Soroka, and A. V. Terentyevaya, who conducted in-depth interviews with the study subjects.

subjects' satisfaction with their career and life, attitudes' toward the future, and relationships with family members.

The interviews included four categories of questions: (1) basic demographic information; (2) questions relating to the functioning of the subject, his or her parents, and grandparents; (3) questions relating to the guiding principles of the subject; and (4) questions relating to the subject's degree of cutoff from the grandparent generation. Questions relating to functioning included such areas as physical and psychological health, marital status, education, and career path. Cutoff was measured through an assessment of how much the grandchildren knew about their grandparents.

Conduct of Interviews

Gippenreiter first established contact with the parents of the selected subjects, explained the research, and asked for help in contacting their children. The interviewers then telephoned the subjects directly, described the research, and arranged interview appointments. Interviews took place in the subject's apartment or office, or the interviewer's apartment. The interviews ranged from 50 minutes to 4 hours; the average length of the interviews was 1 hour and 20 minutes.

There was a range of responses to the interviews. Some subjects were formal, distant, nervous, and cautious during the interviews, showing anxiety about the "correctness" of their answers. Almost all of them became intensely emotionally involved in their responses to the questions. Many subjects smoked continuously. Several became flushed and exhibited dermatological splotches on the face and neck during the interview. Several subjects wanted to receive the results of the study when it was completed.

The interviewers coded the subjects' responses immediately following each interview. Answers were grouped into the four categories that reflected the hypotheses of the study: demographic information, functioning, guiding principles, and cutoff. Answers to questions that were relevant to more than one category were coded as responses in each relevant category. In coding the open-ended questions, the interviewers developed additional variables to identify varying family responses to the Purge, including material and career loss, anxiety, adherence to moral values, and the active search for information about the Purge and family members who were purged. This coding of open-ended variables was reviewed by a panel of BFST experts to establish its validity. Additional composite variables were developed during the data-analysis process.

FINDINGS

Initial data analysis was done in Moscow in the spring of 1994. Replication, follow-up analysis, and further extension of the findings were completed in Washington, D.C., in the summer.[3]

Frequencies

Simple frequencies were run on all descriptive variables. Variation within the sample was described in a number of specific areas. The *professions* of the subjects reflected their high level of education. Ninety-two percent described their work as "professional," while 2% de-

[3]The authors would like to express appreciation to Susan A. Weigert, M.A. (Washington, D.C.), A. N. Rudakov, and A. T. Terekhin (Moscow) for assistance in data analysis, and to the Georgetown Family Center for providing computer support.

scribed themselves as supervisors and managers, and 4% as engineers. Fifty-six percent were *only children,* 34% were the oldest, and 10% were the youngest. There were no middle children among the subjects. This is an accurate reflection of the small family size in this generation in the Soviet Union. Eighty-two percent of the subjects had *lived with a grandparent* while they were growing up, and of those, 83% had lived with the grandparent for more than 3 years. Eighty-eight percent of the subjects were *married,* with 68% of those married only once. Twenty-eight percent had divorced and remarried. None was widowed. Forty-four percent of the subjects lost one or more close relatives in *World War II.* About half of the family members lost were grandparents. Thirty percent of the subjects' fathers were deceased, but all the mothers were alive at the time the study was conducted. Sixteen percent of the subjects had been *members of the Communist Party,* and 12% of those were Party functionaries. Ninety-six percent of the subjects *lived in a household with other people.* Nearly 80% lived with a spouse or other partner. Forty percent lived with their mother. Seventy-four percent had four or five people in their household. Seventy percent of the subjects had *children;* of those, about 60% had only one child. Twenty-eight percent were sufficiently optimistic about the future in Russia to have had a child born in the past year or to have made plans to have another child. The *Purge victims* in the subjects' families included maternal grandfather (86%), maternal grandmother (34%), paternal grandfather (20%), and paternal grandmother (8%). This discrepancy between paternal and maternal victims apparently reflects the membership of Memorial, which includes a high percentage of daughters of Purge victims. Relatively few of the subjects' parents (4% of the fathers and 14% of the mothers) had been purged, since they were too young in the late 1930s to be involved in politics. Two subjects reported that four family members (both maternal grandparents and both parents) had been victims of the Purge. Six subjects reported that three family members had been purged, and 10 subjects reported that two members had been purged.

Seventy percent of the maternal grandfathers and 50% of the paternal grandfathers were shot immediately following their arrest. A majority of the grandfathers who were not killed did not return to their families even after the amnesty of the 1950s, since they were forbidden to enter the large western cities where most of their families lived (see Grossman, 1972, for a description of this experience). Most of the purged grandmothers were deported, imprisoned, or sent to concentration camps. None of the arrested grandmothers in the study was shot, but 18% of them died in the camps or in exile. Most of the grandmothers survived the camps and exile until the amnesty of 1956, and then returned to western Russia to reconnect with their children and grandchildren, passing on to them their living memory of the experience of the Purge.

Factor Analysis

Based on the original hypothesis of the study, the principal variables that were analyzed were (1) cutoff, and (2) functioning in the grandchild generation. An additional variable that emerged from responses to the interview questions measured the subjects' degree of loyalty to the Soviet regime.

In order to identify the most useful subset of variables for the data analysis, the researchers performed factor analysis and cluster analysis using average linking and dendograms of questionnaire items. The results suggested a 10-factor model to describe the principal variables.

Through the use of computer-generated dendograms, a large number of related variables were clustered to produce composite variables for cutoff and functioning. These clusters formed two separate groups of highly correlated variables for cutoff and functioning. Cutoff divided into two variables: *maternal*-line cutoff and *paternal*-line cutoff. Maternal-line cutoff was measured by the subjects' knowledge of basic demographic information about their mothers' families, as well as their knowledge of the Purge and of family memories. Paternal-line cutoff was measured by the subjects' knowledge of basic demographic information about their fathers' families, including knowledge about prior generations.

The same cluster-analysis procedure was followed for variables measuring functioning. These variables also divided into two highly correlated groups: (1) basic functioning, which included the number of marriages, divorces, general health, and physical and psychological symptoms; and (2) social functioning, which included financial stability, standard of living, and other social variables.

The third major variable, loyalty to the Soviet regime, was also divided into two subvariables through cluster analysis. The first group measured *active protest* against the Soviet regime, including a range of protest activities, motivations for engaging in those activities (ranging from impulsive decision to a struggle for personal rights), and family stories of the Purge victims. The second group of loyalty variables measured *passive protest* against the regime, including not joining the Communist Party and not receiving the special privileges granted to Party members.

The two cutoff variables (maternal- and paternal-line cutoff) were then analyzed in relation to the Purge on the mother's and father's sides of the family. Interestingly, the phenomenon of grandchild cutoff from grandparents was *not* associated with whether the grandparents had been purged. The authors had anticipated that the grandchildren might be more cut off from the side of the family that had been purged. However, it appears that cutoff, as a family relationship phenomenon, was rooted in factors other than the political–historical experience of the Purge. There was, however, a significant difference between the degree of cutoff in the maternal and paternal family lines, with grandchildren reporting more cutoff from their father's line than from their mother's line.

Another interesting finding related to differences in the parent and grandchild generations with regard to passive and active protest against the Soviet regime. The grandchildren were more likely than their parents to be engaged in protest activities. In addition, a significantly higher number of women than men in all generations were *passively* disloyal to the Soviet system (e.g., through not joining the Communist Party). A significantly higher number of women than men in the parent generation (mothers of subjects) were *actively* disloyal and took more personal risks in opposing the Soviet system.

Open-Ended Responses

Each interview concluded with two open-ended questions that were intended to encourage the subjects to express their thoughts in greater detail. The questions posed were these: (1) Do you think there are any connections between the events your family experienced in the period of the Purge at the end of the 1930s and the way your life developed for you? (2) Have you been actively involved in collecting information about your family members who were victims of the Purge?

Sense of Connectedness to the Purge. The following excerpts came from the wide range of responses to the first of the two open-ended questions: "positive influence on my personality," "inherited moral values from my grandparent," "a feeling of support from my family roots," "a critical relationship toward the totalitarian regime," "psychological problems such as anxiety, fear, and mistrust," and "impediments to my career development." Through cluster and factor analysis, these diverse responses were divided into four groups: those who saw the

Purge as having had a negative influence, positive influence, mixed negative and positive influence, or no influence on their own lives. Table 1 presents the distribution of responses to this question.

Negative Influence. Among the subjects who felt that the Purge at the end of the 1930s had a negative influence on their own lives were the following:

A 37-year-old doctor who lived with her husband, two children, and her mother. Her maternal grandfather, an officer, had been a victim of the Purge. Only the previous year, the family had learned that he had been shot without any charges being brought against him. His wife was German. The subject's mother, who was 18 years old at the time her father was purged, remembered being anxious and not sleeping the night of her father's arrest. They were awaiting the arrest, because all the other military people in the building had already been arrested. After the arrest, the family was evicted from their apartment, and the daughter was expelled from the university. She soon married (in order to change her name), but her husband volunteered for the Front and was killed in the first month of the War. Her second marriage, in order to escape persecution and starvation, was to the son of an NKVD official. After divorcing him, she married again. The subject (the granddaughter of the Purge victim) said, "I knew that I should not talk about my family with other people, although I was born in the year of Rehabilitation, 1956. I haven't gotten rid of this feeling even now. I know that I could find myself in the same situation [that is, a purge could occur again in Russia]."

A 40-year-old artist, who lived with her husband and daughter in Moscow, said, "The influence [of the Purge] is deep in my character. I can't take any initiative for myself. I am afraid. I fear official relationships. When *perestroika* began, I thought that all active people would [eventually] be arrested, all the same, or shot."

A 37-year-old librarian and translator, living with her husband, daughter, and mother, said: "There is some kind of anxiety in me. In this country, anything can happen to you. It's a kind of genetic memory for the Soviet people and for Jewish people."

A 42-year-old engineer described how her maternal grandfather was purged. He was sent into exile in 1923, and from that time on, his wife lived in different exile locations until she died in 1935. Her grandfather was shot in 1937. An uncle and aunt took the two children (one of whom was the subject's mother) and raised them after their mother's death. The subject said, "In the family, fear remains and also the impossibility of learning anything about our relatives. This had a great impact on the nervous system. All family members are closed, with heavy characters. My mother is very hypersensitive about these issues. My father was not able to work in his field, although he is very talented."

A 38-year-old teacher, who lives with his wife and daughters, said, "Yes, of course the Purge has affected me. If my grandfather were still alive, he would have had a much higher position. My mother had been studying and getting A's, but she was not accepted at law school. In my life, problems escalated and have increased like an avalanche."

**Table 1. Subjects' Perception of
How the Purge Influenced
Their Own Lives**

Negative influence	40%
Positive influence	26%
Mixed influence	18%
No influence	16%

A 39-year-old man, an alcoholic and former Komsomol functionary, had been married three times, divorced three times, and was living alone. He and his maternal grandparents were Party members. His father was also an alcoholic. The subject said, "Everything would be different if my grandmother and grandfather had not been purged. My parents would be living in a different way and relationships would be different. I would be different. It influenced my decisions in the field of political activity. Sometimes I couldn't afford to be active—for example, in the Komsomol, since I knew that my grandfather had been purged. He was rehabilitated, but all the same, at that time, the attitude toward this event was not very good. I had problems getting access to secret information. I tried not to be very active on the whole. There was a closedness and fear in the whole family that someone would reveal something by blabbing it [speaking out]. All questions about the Purge were discussed only inside the family and were kept quiet. When I was small, they did not trust me. About my grandfather I knew from my mother but not directly. We never discussed the political situation in the country in our family. I always had to conceal who my grandmother and grandfather were. I had always been controlling myself. This influenced my career and promotion in my work."

A 43-year-old manager of a trade firm lived with her husband, son, and mother. Her maternal grandfather, a vice-minister, was purged in 1938. He was sent to prison camp and then was exiled; he returned after 16 years (in 1954) and died of cancer in 1974. The subject's father refused to marry the subject's mother because her father (the subject's maternal grandfather) was an "Enemy of the People." The subject said, "There is a connection, of course. My mother and I graduated from university very late—in our 30s and 40s. It didn't go normally for us. The Purge disrupted our education and our social standard of living. If grandfather had not been taken, we would have had a much higher position."

Positive Influence.   In answering the question about what connection they saw between the tragic events their family experienced during the Purge and the way their own life developed, about one in four subjects described ways in which those events had a positive influence on their lives.

A 35-year-old man said, "Yes, there was an influence, not in the material sense, but in the spiritual sense. It had an impact on my understanding of values in my life, close people, and the meaning of life. I have the feeling that I should tell people about my grandmother and give her [memoirs] to people to read. I have a feeling that I should be worthy of her memory. When I come to a moral turning point or choice, then the very choice of my grandmother and her life help me to come to a moral decision. That has become very simple and natural for me. If I were to lose material possessions because of my decision, these losses would not be comparable to the material losses people in the camps had undergone. They lost a lot, but they saved their spiritual sense of self-worth. They are a moral model for me. I have the impression that the choice between the spiritual or pragmatic way of raising children is getting more and more challenging. We have to have very strong family roots in order that one should not think too much while bringing up children in the atmosphere of the Russian intelligentsia. Many people do not know what spiritual joy means. A person who knows it already has understood that everything else is worthless in comparison."

A 44-year-old Jewish radiophysicist lives with his wife and son. His maternal grandfather, who had been the chief engineer of a factory, was a victim of the Purge. He left behind a wife and three daughters. In the evacuation during the war, their relatives helped a lot because they were all together. The subject lived with his grandmother from birth until age 18. His father was a disabled World War II veteran who graduated from law school. In 1948–1949, the family lost their apartment in Moscow, and lost their permits to live in Moscow, because of the

Doctors' Plot (both the subject's grandmother and an aunt were doctors; the Doctors' Plot was an anti-Semitic drive launched by Stalin shortly before his death). Until 1956, they lived outside Moscow and worked only occasionally at part-time, temporary jobs. In 1956, they were allowed to return to Moscow to live in a communal apartment. The subject's father later published two books and received the title "Honored Lawyer" and a personal pension from the republic. The subject said, "I think, yes, there is an influence. If there are no hardships, I wouldn't be protected from being spoiled by corruption through the privileges my father had (nor would he). My father would say that because he was a good professional, he got what he deserved, but he never took advantage of his right as a disabled World War II veteran. For example, he did not break the line in purchasing a car. He could give up his vacation ticket for the sanitarium. This hard life and the losses he experienced made my father wise in perceiving life and its circumstances. In electricity, the current may pass along an electromagnetic field through an electric wire or through air. In our family it passed through air."

A 37-year-old engineer lived with his grandmother until he was 14. His father, a colonel in the Red Army, married the daughter of a Purge victim in 1953. The KGB didn't know how to react to this marriage, but nothing happened because it was the year of Stalin's death. The purged grandfather was from a noble family and had been on the faculty of the Military Academy. He had been an officer in the Tsar's army before transferring into the Red Army. His wife (the subject's grandmother) told the subject that her husband was a typical member of the old Russian intelligentsia, with a calm, reserved character. The interview subject said, "Of course, yes. Knowing about my grandfather, I could not understand how such a valuable person who had worked for the system could have been purged by it. In our family, everyone read Solzhenitsyn (even though father was a member of the Communist Party). When I got older, I started to understand what was what and how it could happen; that is, these experiences stimulated the capacity to reflect and search for answers to questions. For this, I read a lot, investigate a lot. I consciously prefer to have a moral orientation. That's the main thing. The same as my grandfather. He was never commercial or materialistic. And my grandmother never had any savings. In our family, there were books, a piano; we spent all our money on things of the spirit."

When asked what losses he experienced because of this, he responded, "A person who stands on moral principles cannot count on material well-being. But if we speak about family losses, I think it couldn't have happened if our country had had a different history. With our history, it would have happened all the same."

In thinking about the influence of the Purge on the country and on himself, the engineer said, "For me, everything is horrible! I consider that the Purge was a catastrophic, awful, inhumane experiment. I try not to read this literature about the Purge and the camps. It leads me to repressed rage. I haven't read all the writings of Solzhenitsyn. I tried to read Shalamov, but I couldn't. I glanced through it but wasn't able to read it. I have a wound that will never heal. It's necessary to find out what they did, and on the whole, I understood and I don't need any more details."

He continued, "It forces me to follow moral principles, especially in our confused time. I have no wish to rush to set up a kiosk or to organize a trading firm. I'll try (at the end of my military service) to work in a field that is interesting to me and is moral in the sense that it creates something (like a documentary film). I also am raising my children based on these same moral principles."

A 45-year-old English teacher lives with her mother, grandmother, husband, her daughter, her husband's daughter, and their son (seven people in all). Her maternal grandfather was purged and spent 15 years in prison. Afterwards, he returned to live with his family. She said, "Our grandfather was everything for me; my love of nature, of Russia, comes from him. We try to keep our family roots. Suffering creates faith. The system of values in our family is unshakable. More spiritual than material. There was no hate. Our country is important, but not the political system. Grandfather left memoirs. I am looking for an opportunity to publish them."

Mixed Influence.   Other respondents felt the Purge had both a positive and negative influence on their own lives.

A 42-year-old librarian, divorced with no children, lives with her parents. Her maternal grandfather was purged. He was shot when the subject's mother was 19, and she was sent into exile in Kazakhstan. There, she met her husband and married. The subject was born in exile in 1951. Her family lived in an underground cave. Her parents worked under very difficult conditions. As a child, the subject stayed alone with the dog and was frequently sick. She lost her health in childhood. She said, "There were very good people around us who had also been sent into exile. They helped each other a lot. I learned about the Purge from my parents because in exile no one covered up this fact. In a prison cell, a person is free in spirit. A human who goes through this 'school' is never caught by materialistic values. In spirit, I am very close to my grandfather. He was very generous, attentive, open to other people, unconcerned with money. In our home there was a 'grandfather cult.' We all searched for information about him. On the wall his photograph hangs. Laziness and fear have prevented me from developing my life as I would have wished."

A 35-year-old divorced engineer lives with her daughter and mother. Her maternal grandfather, the director of a construction firm, was shot in 1938. His wife had divorced him not long before his arrest. She was a doctor and went to the war. He subject lived with her grandmother from age 21 to 24—the last 3 years of her grandmother's life. Her grandmother, her mother, and her father were members of the Party. They did nothing after the war, for which they might have been punished. She said, "It is connected somehow, but I don't think in a serious way. It wasn't directly harmful, because at that time there were no information lists. I was born in 1957, after the rehabilitation began. My grandmother got the documents. But until I was an adolescent, I was told only that my grandfather had died. We had been living mainly by believing in the 'rosy future' promised by the government, but it was dangerous to dig out our roots. You could accidentally find out something that you should know—for example, you might run across a *kulak* or a merchant in your roots. It's a pity that I lost information about my great-grandparents. It is unrecoverable now."

No Influence.   Another group of subjects reported that the Purge had no influence on their lives.

A 45-year-old man lives with his wife, two children, and his mother. Formerly a polar pilot, he is now a supervisor in an industrial factory. He is a master of sport (in basketball, the Dynamo team—the old NKVD-KGB team). The subject's maternal grandfather was purged. He knows little about him—only that he was a deputy of Dzerzhinsky (founder of the CHEKA [forerunner of the KGB]). An uncle (his mother's brother) worked in the NKVD. The subject said, "There is absolutely no connection, except for little things. Nobody prevented me from becoming a sportsman. I achieved a master of sport degree and nobody prevented me. No one prevented me from fulfilling my plans."

A 42-year-old college teacher, a member of the Party, is married with four children. His father was also a Party member. His maternal grandfather, a Comintern officer, was purged. In 1932, he was sent to a prison camp and was shot in 1937. The family was moved to a smaller apartment and closed themselves off because of fear. His grandmother changed her work. Both his mother and grandmother are reserved but get angry very easily (he described them as having explosive personalities). His mother hid the Purge, but within the family they talked of it constantly. He himself is quite closed and lives for the family. No photos, no memorabilia exist at home. He has not gathered information about the Purge. Although he lived with his grandmother for 7 years, he knows nothing of his ancestors on either side. The subject said, "I don't feel any harmful influence, except some little sense of disturbance and discomfort. Objectively the Purge did not influence me at all."

A 45-year-old economist lives with her mother and stepfather. She is very sick with thrombosis and lymphostatic disease. Her maternal grandfather was purged, leaving his wife and two children. The children were taken in by their maternal grandparents. The subject's mother (who was 14 when her father was arrested) became a dressmaker who went from house to house. The subject said, "The Purge had no impact at all. My life is completely different from their lives (in previous generations)." She says she knows nothing about the Purge and has not looked at the documentation of her grandfather's rehabilitation.

A 43-year-old Party member lives with his wife and two children. Although he is an engineer/mechanic, he works as a carpenter and is angry because he is not working at the level of his education. His paternal grandfather, a Party member and an accountant, was purged. According to the subject, his grandfather was socially an "insignificant person." His grandmother, who is still alive, was very frightened; she married for the second time in her fifties. The subject never lived with her. His father, also a Party member and vice–chief engineer, survived because of his Party membership. The subject said, "There is no connection. If my grandfather had lived, nothing would be different. He was too small a person. . . . No, I did not investigate what happened in the Purge, since I'm not interested."

A 43-year-old music teacher hates her work. She lives with lots of Siamese cats. She asked by telephone, "What privilege will I get for doing the interview?" (She agreed to be interviewed when told she would be paid $15.) Her maternal grandfather, an engineer, was purged. The subject's mother, a movie actress, said, "Nobody ever knew that I am the daughter of an Enemy of the People, and I am proud that I hid it so well." Recently, her mother had a party at her home. At the party, she asked her friends, "Do you know that you are sitting and eating at the table of an Enemy of the People?" Everyone said, "Congratulations for hiding it so well." The subject said, "There is no connection between the Purge and my present life."

A 36-year-old linguist is married but living alone. He sees his children twice a week. His maternal grandfather, an engineer from a long family line of priests, was arrested in 1932 while he was working on Belomor Kanal. He was arrested again in 1936 and sent to prison, camp, and exile before being granted amnesty in 1956. The subject lived with his rehabilitated grandfather for 8 years. His own father was a Party member, an engineer, and a professor. The subject said, "How could it influence my life? No, it didn't. I can't imagine another life. Evidently, it did not influence me."

Involvement in Purge-Related Research. Another variable, labeled *research effort*,[4] was developed from an analysis of responses to the final question, which asked the subjects whether they had been actively involved in collecting information about their family members who were victims of the Purge. Responses to this question were coded according to a 5-point scale that reflected a continuum of involvement from *Learning from my parent(s)' investigation* (1 point) to *Searching the KGB archives myself* (5 points).

---

[4]Research effort as it is used in this study implies an informal personal effort to find out more about the extended family.

Correlations

Table 2 displays the correlation matrix for all the variables derived from cluster and factor analysis, as described earlier. As can be seen, the cutoff variable for *both* family lines (mother's and father's) was highly negatively associated with the derived factor *basic functioning* ($r = -.33$ and $-.40$; $p = .018$ and $.004$, respectively). *Social functioning* was positively associated with extended family research effort ($r = .42$; $p = .002$), active protest ($r = 0.25$; $p = .077$), and positive influence of the Purge ($r = 0.30$; $p = .034$). Research effort was also strongly positively correlated with positive influence of the Purge. Interestingly, passive protest did not correlate with any other factor, possibly because passive protest was so widespread throughout the population that it could not have statistical significance.

Regression Analysis

The outcome of these correlational analyses suggested the advisability of simple linear and multiple regression analysis for evaluating the predictive value of a composite *cutoff* variable for the functioning related variable, basic functioning. Table 3 displays the results of this regression procedure between standardized variables.

The initial hypothesis predicting that higher levels of cutoff would be negatively associated with basic functioning was supported by the results of the regression analysis displayed in Table 3 ($R^2 = .26$, $F = 16.56$, and $p < .0002$). In other words, the more cut off the grandchildren were from their grandparents, the lower their functioning was in certain basic areas, such as health.

Table 2. Correlation Matrix for Variables Derived from Cluster and Factor Analysis

	Basic function	Social function	Cutoff (mother)	Cutoff (father)	Active protest	Passive protest	No effect	Negative effect	Positive effect	Research effect
Basic function										
Social function										
Cutoff (mother)	$p = .018*$									
Cutoff (father)	$p = .004*$									
Active protest		$p = .077$								
Passive protest										
No effect		$p = .054$	$p = .000$		$p = .071$					
Negative effect							$p = .002*$			
Positive effect		$p = .034$								
Research effect		$p = .002*$	$p = .015$		$p = .001**$		$p = .012$		$p = .000$	

*$p < .01$
**$p < .001$, two-tailed significance

Table 3. Simple Linear Regression Analysis Predicting Basic Functioning

Variable	R^2	F-Ratio for R^2	Significance of F
Cutoff	.26	16.56	.0002

DISCUSSION

The major finding of the study is the strong *negative correlation* between *cutoff* (for both the maternal and paternal lines) and *basic functioning* in the grandchild generation. This finding validates the hypothesis that cutoff is a relationship phenomenon rooted in basic human functioning and is transmitted from one generation to the next. The lack of significant correlation between cutoff and the experience of the Purge raised interesting questions about the nature of cutoff. If emotional cutoff is viewed as a multigenerational family relationship response to anxiety, then many of these families probably *already* used emotional cutoff as a technique for managing anxiety. They would have automatically resorted to cutoff at the time of the Purge in order to manage the intense stress and anxiety of losing a family member under violent circumstances. But other families would *not* have responded in this way to a traumatic family event, because cutoff was not in their emotional response repertoire. But there clearly is not a linear, causal relationship between cutoff and the experience of the Purge.

It may seem paradoxical that the grandchildren's *social functioning* correlates positively with *active protest,* efforts to research a family member's experience of the Purge, and the perception that the Purge had a *positive influence* on their own lives. However, all of these factors indicate energy, purposefulness, and responsibility, which, according to BFST, are associated with higher levels of functioning. Higher functioning families apparently survived the tragedy of the Purge through finding a positive framework for the experience and transmitting this positive view to their grandchildren. Family emotional resources such as courage, firmness in critical situations, the ability to protest actively against social coercion, and a commitment to high moral values and ideals were passed on to the grandchild generation. This pattern in families is also fully congruent with the theories of Satir (1972), who refers to the "nurturing" strength of family roots and the importance of connections across generations.

The special role of women in preserving and passing on family memories came across clearly in the findings. There was less evidence of cutoff from the maternal line than from the paternal line. Daughters of Purge victims seemed to take a more active role than sons in researching family information through their membership in Memorial. Members of the grandchild generation typically reported their grandmothers and mothers as resources and communicators of family memory and tradition. This does not mean that the men in these families were less emotionally involved with their families than the women. In fact, grandfathers were often described as family heroes and as people who had provided strong personal examples. But higher percentages of men than women were killed in the Purge, and those men who survived faced greater obstacles and died younger. In this study, the women took on the role of *messenger* of family values, traditions, and memories.

Another finding had to do with the significant tendency of the grandchild generation to move in the direction of higher functioning, as evidenced by a decrease in Party membership and an increase in active protest. This shift may have been associated with societal changes in relation to the Party that were taking place when our subjects were young adults. Nevertheless,

Table 4. Regression Analysis Predicting Social Functioning

Variable	R^2	F-Ratio for R^2	Significance of F
Research effort	.19	10.88	.0018

the pressure to conform by joining the Party continued to exist, yet more grandchildren of Purge victims chose not to join than in their parents' generation.

A final observation has to do with the conflict within families with regard to the Communist system. Not surprisingly, most victims who survived the Purge became disaffected with the Communist Party because of their personal experience. The middle generation, however, often developed intense ambivalence about the Party. The Party had destroyed the lives of their parents, but their own membership in the Party could also be a means for survival, for keeping the family safe, and even for gaining some privileges in a period of disastrous societal disorder. If they protested against the Purge too strongly or openly disagreed with Party policies, they themselves could become the victims of later purges.

Interestingly, the children of these middle-generation Party members did not try to hold onto their parents' privileges. In fact, higher social functioning in the third generation was correlated with active protest in the middle generation. The grandchildren whose parents were Party members often disassociated themselves from the values of their parents and, jumping back a generation, felt a stronger emotional and spiritual bond to their victimized grandparents.

CONCLUSION

The study was undertaken in order to gain some understanding of the multigenerational impact of widespread catastrophic loss of significant family members during a period of societal trauma. Russia was selected as the society in which to study the long-term impact of this kind of loss because the events of the Purge—including execution, murder, torture, exile, and separation of millions of family members—took place there during a discrete period of time (1937–1939) that can be specifically identified by succeeding generations. In addition, Russian society has now evolved politically to the point that many catastrophic episodes in the past are being rediscovered and explored. Archives are opening up, and memoirs of the period are flooding the literary marketplace. Organizations such as Memorial are being established that bring together survivors and the families of those who were killed in the Purge in a new spirit of respect, fact gathering, and attempts to understand what happened.

The investigators hypothesized that families who were unable to maintain some sense of connection and continuity with their lost grandparents would experience a negative impact on functioning in succeeding generations; that is, those who were cut off emotionally as well as physically from their grandparents would experience a decline in functioning. The study confirmed this hypothesis. It showed that the way families dealt with the trauma at the time of its occurrence profoundly affected later family functioning. Those who kept a sense of connection with lost family members fared better than those who intentionally or unintentionally let those family members slip into oblivion. Whether the grandparents actually physically survived the Purge was less important than the strength and values passed on to their grandchildren through the knowledge of what had happened to them. Connected grandchildren had a sense of identity firmly rooted in family experience, and many of them continued to enhance their connections through family research into the past. Disconnected grandchildren were less clear about who they were or where they were going as they attempted to function in the Russia of the 1990s.

FUTURE RESEARCH

This was a relatively small pilot study with a stratified random sample, and therefore, the findings cannot be fully generalized to the wider population of Russia. Nevertheless, the findings indicate potentially significant directions for future research. The concept of cutoff as an aspect of multigenerational process and extended family relationships may prove useful in describing and defining family and societal response to mass trauma, not only in larger samples of the Russian population but also in other societies that have experienced extensive losses of significant family members in past generations. Solid, replicated findings could also have value in predicting the basic functioning of future generations in other traumatized societies. In addition, knowledge about the impact of cutoff on the functioning of succeeding generations may lead to the development of clinical interventions with currently at-risk populations, such as persons in refugee camps.

The phenomenon of cutoff at the societal level is also deserving of future research. When deeply hidden secrets and the shames of the past, as well as access to knowledge and understanding of historical events, are "cut off" from succeeding generations, there may indeed be significant impact on societal functioning, on the ability of that society to care for its members, to generate effective leadership, and to keep a principled course in wider international political and environmental arenas.

Conversely, as cutoff is bridged, as societies uncover, understand, accept, and learn from past catastrophe, they may strengthen themselves for future adversity. As the new Russian government permits an opening up of its archives and an examination of the traumas of the past, the society itself may begin to heal from the atrocities of the Stalin period.

ACKNOWLEDGMENTS: Research for this study was supported by a grant from the International Research and Exchanges Board (IREX), with funds provided by the U.S. Department of State (Title VIII). Neither of these organizations is responsible for the views expressed in this chapter.

REFERENCES

Adamova-Sliozberg, O. L. (1993). Put' [Way]. Moscow: Vosvrashcheniye.
Adler, N. (1993). Victims of Soviet terror: The story of the Memorial movement. London: Praeger.
Aksyonov, V. (1995). Generations of winter. New York: Vintage International.
Arendt, H. (1966). The origins of totalitarianism. New York: Harcourt, Brace & World.
Babel, I. (1969). You must know everything: Stories 1915–1937. New York: Farrar, Straus & Giroux.
Bowen, M. (1978). Family therapy in clinical practice. New York: Jason Aronson.
Chukovskaya, L. (1994). The Akhmatova journals: Volume 1. 1938–41. New York: Farrar, Straus & Giroux.
Conquest, R. (1990). The Great Terror: A reassessment. New York: Oxford University Press.
Daniels, R. V. (1985). Russia: The roots of confrontation. Cambridge, MA: Harvard University Press.
Forche, C. (Ed.). (1993). Against forgetting: Twentieth-century poetry of witness. New York: Norton.
Ginzburg, Y. S. (1967). Krutoi marshrut [Journey into the whirlwind]. Moscow: Kniga.
Gleason, A. (1995). Totalitarianism. New York: Oxford University Press.
Grossman, V. (1972). Forever flowing. New York: Harper & Row.
Hochschild, A. (1994). The unquiet ghost. New York: Viking Penguin.

Illick, S. D. (1993, May). *The process between generations: Emotional cut-off and degree of unresolved emotional attachment in human and animal behavior.* Paper presented at the Midwest Symposium on Family Systems Theory and Therapy, Chicago, IL.

Kerr, M. E., & Bowen, M. (1988). *Family evaluation: An approach based on Bowen Theory.* New York: Norton.

Malia, M. (1994). *The Soviet tragedy: A history of socialism in Russia, 1917–1991.* New York: Maxwell Macmillan International.

Mandelstam, N. (1970). *Hope against hope.* New York: Atheneum.

Mandelstam, N. (1972). *Hope abandoned.* New York: Atheneum.

Razgon, L. E. (1989). *Nepridumanoye* [Not invented]. Moscow: Kniga.

Remnick, D. (1993). *Lenin's tomb: The last days of the Soviet empire.* New York: Random House.

Satir, V. (1972). *Peoplemaking.* Palo Alto, CA: Science and Behavior Books.

Shalamov, V. (1982). *Kolyma tales.* New York: Norton.

Solzhenitsyn, A. (1962). *The gulag archipelago.* New York: Harper & Row.

Tertz, A. (1960). *The trial begins.* New York: Pantheon.

Tertz, A. (1989). *Goodnight!* New York: Viking Penguin.

Treadgold, D. W. (1995). *Twentieth-century Russia.* Boulder, CO: Westview Press.

Tucker R. C. (1971). *The Soviet political mind.* New York: Norton.

Ulam, A. B. (1989). *Stalin: The man and the era.* Boston: Beacon Press.

Vilyenskiy, S. S. (Ed.). (1989). *Dodnes'tyazhoteyet* [It's still hard]. Moscow: Sovietskiy Pisatel'.

Volkogonov, D. (1992). *Stalin: Triumph and tragedy.* Rocklin, CA: Prima Publishing.

Volkov, O. (1989). *Pozhruzheniye vo t'my* [Immersion in darkness]. Moscow: Molodaya Gvardiya.

APPENDIX: QUESTIONNAIRE FOR INTERVIEWS WITH RUSSIAN SUBJECTS, FALL–WINTER, 1993–1994

A. DEMOGRAPHICS

1. Please give the birth year of the following people:

    (a) Yourself _____

    (b) Your mother _____

    (c) Your father _____

    (d) Your maternal grandmother _____

    (e) Your maternal grandfather _____

    (f) Your paternal grandmother _____

    (g) Your paternal grandfather _____

2. What is your gender? _____

3. What is your family religion? _____

    (a) Yours _____

    (b) Your parents' _____

    (c) Your maternal grandparents' _____

    (d) Your paternal grandparents' _____

4. What is the level of education completed by the following members of your family? (*Primary, secondary, university*)

    (a) Yourself _____

    (b) Your mother _____

    (c) Your father _____

    (d) Your maternal grandmother _____

    (e) Your maternal grandfather _____

(f) Your paternal grandmother _____

(g) Your paternal grandfather _____

5. What is/was the main occupation of the following people? (*Create categories*)

   (a) Yourself _____
   (b) Your mother _____
   (c) Your father _____
   (d) Your maternal grandmother _____
   (e) Your maternal grandfather _____
   (f) Your paternal grandmother _____
   (g) Your paternal grandfather _____

6. How is the current health of the following people? (*Choose from the following: excellent = 5, good = 4, fair = 3, poor = 2, very poor = 1, deceased = 0*)

   (a) Yourself _____
   (b) Your mother _____
   (c) Your father _____
   (d) Your maternal grandmother _____
   (e) Your maternal grandfather _____
   (f) Your paternal grandmother _____
   (g) Your paternal grandfather _____

7. If any of the following people have died, what was the year and cause of their death? (*List cause*)

   (a) Yourself _____
   (b) Your mother _____
   (c) Your father _____
   (d) Your maternal grandmother _____
   (e) Your maternal grandfather _____
   (f) Your paternal grandmother _____
   (g) Your paternal grandfather _____

8. What chronic physical symptoms do the following people have or did they have before they died? (*List any and all physical symptoms, for example: heart disease, high blood pressure, intestinal upset, ulcer, migraines, diabetes, arthritis, cancer, etc. Indicate how much this disrupts/disrupted daily living: 5 = very little; 1 = a lot*)

   (a) You _____
   (b) Your mother _____
   (c) Your father _____
   (d) Your maternal grandmother _____
   (e) Your maternal grandfather _____
   (f) Your paternal grandmother _____
   (g) Your paternal grandfather _____

9. What psychological or emotional symptoms do these people have or did they have before they died? (*List symptoms such as anxiety, depression, difficult personality, irritability, rages, alcoholism, etc. Indicate how much this disrupts/disrupted daily living and close relationships: 5 = very little, 1 = a lot*)

   (a) You _____

(b) Your mother _____

(c) Your father _____

(d) Your maternal grandmother _____

(e) Your maternal grandfather _____

(f) Your paternal grandmother _____

(g) Your paternal grandfather _____

10. How many pregnancies have the following people had?

(a) Yourself (if female) _____

(b) Your wife from this marriage (if male) _____

(c) Your mother _____

(d) Your maternal grandmother _____

(e) Your paternal grandmother _____

11. How many live births resulted from those pregnancies? *List the number of living children each of these people has*)

(a) Yourself (if female) _____

(b) Your wife from this marriage (if male) _____

(c) Your mother _____

(d) Your maternal grandmother _____

(e) Your paternal grandmother _____

12. How many of each of these people's children did not survive early childhood?

(a) Yourself (if female) _____

(b) Your wife from this marriage (if male) _____

(c) Your mother _____

(d) Your maternal grandmother _____

(e) Your paternal grandmother _____

13. What is the birth position in the family for the following: (*List oldest, middle, youngest, only child, or twin*)

(a) Yourself _____

(b) Your mother _____

(c) Your father _____

(d) Your maternal grandmother _____

(e) Your maternal grandfather _____

(f) Your paternal grandmother _____

(g) Your paternal grandfather _____

14. The number of times that home was moved during childhood (up to age 17) for the following people:

(a) Yourself _____

(b) Your mother _____

(c) Your father _____

(d) Your maternal grandmother _____

(e) Your maternal grandfather _____

(f) Your paternal grandmother _____

(g) Your paternal grandfather _____

15. The number of times that home (or apartment) was moved during adult life (after age 17) for the following people:

    (a) Yourself _____

    (b) Your mother _____

    (c) Your father _____

    (d) Your maternal grandmother _____

    (e) Your maternal grandfather _____

    (f) Your paternal grandmother _____

    (g) Your paternal grandfather _____

16. Did you ever live with a grandparent whose husband/wife was a victim of the purges? (*Circle one*)   YES   NO

    How about on the other side of the family?   YES   NO

17. If YES, for how many years? _____

    On the other side of the family _____

18. How many marriages have the following people had?

    (a) Yourself _____

    (b) Your mother _____

    (c) Your father _____

    (d) Your maternal grandmother _____

    (e) Your maternal grandfather _____

    (f) Your paternal grandmother _____

    (g) Your paternal grandfather _____

19. How many divorces have the following people had?

    (a) Yourself _____

    (b) Your mother _____

    (c) Your father _____

    (d) Your maternal grandmother _____

    (e) Your maternal grandfather _____

    (f) Your paternal grandmother _____

    (g) Your paternal grandfather _____

20. How many times have the following people been widowed?

    (a) Yourself _____

    (b) Your mother _____

    (c) Your father _____

    (d) Your maternal grandmother _____

    (e) Your maternal grandfather _____

    (f) Your paternal grandmother _____

    (g) Your paternal grandfather _____

21. Do you know anything about the life of your family in generations before your grandparents? (*Circle one*)   YES   SOME   NO

22. If you answered "yes" or "some" to the preceding question, what do you know about your family roots? (Open-ended)

23. How would you describe the general standard of living of your family?

  A. Standard of living (*indicate the following range using numbers: 1 = very poor, hard life; 5 = rich, high status*)

   (a) Yourself _____
   (b) Your parents _____
   (c) Your maternal grandparents _____
   (d) Your paternal grandparents _____

  B. Did anyone in your family receive any special privileges? (*Such as property, positions, trips abroad, special government apartment or car, country house, etc.*)

   (a) Yourself _____
   (b) Your parents _____
   (c) Your maternal grandparents _____
   (d) Your paternal grandparents _____
         If so, please describe:

B. EVENTS AT THE END OF THE 1930s

24. Did your parents/grandparents directly experience repression at the end of the 1930s in the USSR? (*Circle one*)   YES   NO

25. Which family members were affected by which types of repression and for how many years?
  A. Who? (*Write "yes" by all affected family members*)

   (a) Your mother _____
   (b) Your father _____
   (c) Your maternal grandmother _____
   (d) Your maternal grandfather _____
   (e) Your paternal grandmother _____
   (f) Your paternal grandfather _____

  B. What happened? (*Indicate arrested, imprisoned, sent to a death squad, sent to a concentration camp, tortured/shot*)

   (a) Your mother _____
   (b) Your father _____
   (c) Your maternal grandmother _____
   (d) Your maternal grandfather _____
   (e) Your paternal grandmother _____
   (f) Your paternal grandfather _____

  C. Did he/she return to the family (through amnesty or for other reasons)? (*Write "yes" or "no"*)

   (a) Your mother _____
   (b) Your father _____
   (c) Your maternal grandmother _____
   (d) Your maternal grandfather _____
   (e) Your paternal grandmother _____
   (f) Your paternal grandfather _____

D. If he/she returned to the family, how many years had gone by?

(a) Your mother _____

(b) Your father _____

(c) Your maternal grandmother _____

(d) Your maternal grandfather _____

(e) Your paternal grandmother _____

(f) Your paternal grandfather _____

26. Do you know why they were victims of repression? (*Describe in a few sentences*)

27. When did you first learn that repression had occurred in your family? (*Check one*)

(a) As a young child

(b) As an adolescent

(c) As an adult

28. Who told you what had happened? (*Check one*)

(a) The actual victim of repression

(b) The husband or wife of the victim, or your parents

(c) Other family members

(d) Nonfamily members

29. How did the victim's spouse continue to function after the victim was taken away? (*Choose the answer which most nearly reflects the functioning of the victim's spouse. Circle the answer if the respondent knows, write a "?" if he is unsure, and leave blank if he doesn't know.*)

a. Continued with previous work	b. Changed work
a. Remained healthy	b. Developed health problems
a. Stayed in same home	b. Moved
a. Stayed with other family members	b. Left them
a. Lived openly	b. Hid from the authorities
a. Remained married to the victim	b. Divorced the victim

Other examples of spouse functioning (list)

30. How did the victim's children continue to function after the victim was taken away? (*Choose the answer which most nearly reflects the functioning of the victim's children. Circle the answer if the respondent knows, write a "?" if he is unsure, and leave blank if he doesn't know*)

a. Continued with education/work	b. Education/work interrupted
a. Remained healthy	b. Developed health problems
a. Stayed in same home	b. Moved
a. Stayed with other family members	b. Left them
a. Lived openly	b. Hid from the authorities

Other examples of children's functioning (list)

31. In the years right after the repressions of the late 1930s how did the spouse relate to the victim? (*Check the answer which is closest to the spouse's behavior in relation to the victim*)

    (a) Spoke of him/her regularly with pride and love, maintained a belief in the victim's innocence, tried to obtain justice for the victim, told stories about him/her, kept his/her pictures, informed younger family members of what had happened, sent him/her letters and packages, idealized him/her

    (b) Did not speak of him/her, but maintained a belief in his/ her innocence, worked to obtain justice, did not keep pictures, but sent letters

    (c) Did not speak of him/her at all or attempt to send anything

    (d) Spoke negatively of him/her

    (e) I don't know

32. In the years right after the repressions of the late 1930s how did the victim's children relate to the victim? (*Check the answer which is closest to the children's behavior in relation to the victim.*)

    (a) Spoke of him/her regularly with pride and love, learned stories about him/her, kept his/her pictures, wanted to learn all the details of what had happened, sent him/her letters and packages, idealized him/her

    (b) Did not speak of him/her, no pictures, but sent letters

    (c) Did not speak of him/her at all or attempt to send anything

    (d) Spoke negatively of him/her

    (e) I don't know

33. What kinds of family stories or myths developed over the years about the family members who were repressed in the late 1930s?

    (a) Idealized heroes, with visible pictures and memorabilia

    (b) Talked about them as normal family members with struggles and weaknesses

    (c) Reviled them

    (d) Never mentioned them, no pictures or memorabilia

    (e) Other (please describe)

34. When did private family conversations about these lost family members begin? (Check the decade.)

    ____ 1930s

    ____ 1940s

    ____ 1950s

    ____ 1960s

    ____ 1970s

    ____ 1980s

    ____ 1990

    ____ Never

35. Did your parents mention the lost family members as positive or negative examples for you?

    (a) Positive

    (b) Negative

    (c) Did not mention them as examples

    (d) Did not mention them at all

36. Did your grandparents have any special talents or interests which you have continued? (*Circle one*)   YES   NO   I DON'T KNOW

37. Do you personally have any photographs, mementos, or objects made by the family members who were repressed in the late 1930s? (*Circle one*)   YES   NO

38. Have children or grandchildren been named after the family members who were victims of the repressions of the late 1930s? (*Circle one*)   YES   NO

39. Does anyone in your generation look like the family members who were repressed in the late 1930s? (*Circle one*)   YES   NO

40. Did you lose any relatives in World War II? (*Circle one*)   YES/NO
    I DON'T KNOW MUCH ABOUT IT   I DON'T KNOW ANYTHING ABOUT IT

41. If you answer "yes" to question 40,
    A. How many relatives died? _____
    B. Which relatives did you lose? (List)
        (a) From your grandparents' generation _____
        (b) From your parents' generation _____

42. How did your family keep alive the memory of those relatives who were killed in the War?
    (a) Spoke of them regularly with pride and love, kept their photographs, told the younger members of the family about them
    (b) Did not speak of them frequently, but kept their photographs
    (c) I know practically nothing about them

C. COMMUNIST PARTY MEMBERSHIP

43. Were any of the following people ever Communist Party Members?
    (a) Yourself _____
    (b) Your mother _____
    (c) Your father _____
    (d) Your maternal grandmother _____
    (e) Your maternal grandfather _____
    (f) Your paternal grandmother _____
    (g) Your paternal grandfather _____

44. If you answered "yes" to question 43, were any of the following people paid functionaries of the Communist Party? (*Please list the years of Party employment*)
    (a) Yourself _____
    (b) Your mother _____
    (c) Your father _____
    (d) Your maternal grandmother _____
    (e) Your maternal grandfather _____
    (f) Your paternal grandmother _____
    (g) Your paternal grandfather _____

45. Were any of the following people ever subjected to persecution or government-imposed restrictions in the post-war period? (*Indicate the intensity of persecution: arrest = 5, expulsion from job, apartment = 4, denied promotion = 3, having your abilities ignored = 2, moral pressure = 1*)
    (a) Yourself _____
    (b) Your mother _____
    (c) Your father _____

(d) Your maternal grandmother _____

(e) Your maternal grandfather _____

(f) Your paternal grandmother _____

(g) Your paternal grandfather _____

46. Did any of your family members do anything in the postwar period for which the government might have persecuted them? (*Indicate the possibility of the following dangers: arrest = 5, expulsion from job, apartment, etc. = 4, denied promotion = 3, having your abilities ignored = 2, moral pressure = 1*)

(a) Yourself _____

(b) Your mother _____

(c) Your father _____

(d) Your maternal grandmother _____

(e) Your maternal grandfather _____

(f) Your paternal grandmother _____

(g) Your paternal grandfather _____

47. If any member of your family did something for which the government persecuted them or might have persecuted them, what do you think were their motives? (*Use the following scale: accidental or impulsive decision = 1, went along with friends = 2, disagreed with restrictions on personal rights = 3, struggled for personal rights =- 4, fought against the system = 5*)

(a) Yourself _____

(b) Your mother _____

(c) Your father _____

(d) Your maternal grandmother _____

(e) Your maternal grandfather _____

(f) Your paternal grandmother _____

(g) Your paternal grandfather _____

D. LIFE IN THE PRESENT TIME

48. Who currently lives in your household?

A. (Check all that apply)

(a) You live alone _____

(b) Marital or other adult partner _____

(c) Your children (give number) _____

(d) Your siblings (give number) _____

(e) Your mother _____

(f) Your father _____

(g) Your maternal grandmother _____

(h) Your maternal grandfather _____

(i) Your paternal grandmother _____

(j) Your paternal grandfather _____

(k) Other (specify) _____

B. Give the total number of people living in your household _____

49. How does your present adult household (those living with you) function in present-day Russia? (*List excellent = 5, good = 4, fair = 3, badly = 2, very badly = 1*)

(a) Financial stability _____

(b) Survival issues (food ___ shelter ___, clothing ___)

(c) Health of adults _____

(d) Health of children _____

(e) Adult attitude toward education _____

(f) How are the children doing in school? _____

(g) Satisfaction with professional work _____

(h) General satisfaction with life _____

(i) Attitude toward the future _____

50. How would you describe the following relationships in your present adult life?

(a) With your parents _____

(b) With your spouse _____

(c) With your children _____

(d) With your grandparents _____

(*Choose one of the following in characterizing your relationships*)

(a) Very close and dependent, can't get along without each other

(b) Friendly-close

(c) Conflicted-close

(d) Friendly-distant

(e) Conflicted-distant

(f) Cut off, no contact

51. Have you maintained religious traditions in your adult household which come from one of the following families? (Write   YES   SOMEWHAT   NO)

(a) Your parents _____

(b) Your maternal grandparents _____

(c) Your paternal grandparents _____

52. If you answered "yes" or "somewhat" to the previous question, what form do religious traditions take in your household" (*Circle all that apply*)

(a) We have religious objects at home

(b) We celebrate religious holidays

(c) We attend church

53. Have you had a new baby since August 1991 or do you plan additional children? (*Answer YES or NO to the following*)

(a) New baby _____

(b) Planning additional children _____

54. What is your reaction to the new processes in Russia since August 1991? (*Circle one*)

(a) Wholeheartedly welcome the changes

(b) Basically support the changes, although with some reservations

(c) Indifferent

(d) Don't support the changes

(e) Strongly oppose the changes

     My opinion fluctuates

55. What is your children's reaction to the new processes in Russia today? (Open-ended response.)

56. Have you been involved in the new processes in Russia since August 1991? (*Circle YES or NO*)

(a) YES   NO   Voting

(b) YES   NO   Reading newspapers
(c) YES   NO   Participation in demonstrations/on the barricades
(d) YES   NO   Personal connections with Western cultures
(e) YES   NO   Travel abroad
(f) YES   NO   Membership in a new political party
(g) YES   NO   Directly involved in political process as a leader
(h) YES   NO   Involved in social initiatives
(i) YES   NO   Organized/involved in business initiatives
(j) YES   NO   Passive disinterest
(k) YES   NO   Actively opposed
        Other?

57. Do you think there are any connections between the events your family experienced in the period of repression at the end of the 1930s and the way your life developed for you? (*Open-ended response*)

58. Have you been actively involved in collecting information about your family members who were victims of repression? (Investigation, reading documents, collecting historical information, etc.) (*Open-ended response*)

26

The Social Process and the Transgenerational Transmission of Trauma in Chile

DAVID BECKER and MARGARITA DIAZ

INTRODUCTION

At the end of the Chilean dictatorship, one could have expected that a central political goal would be the active participation of the population in the democratization process. But this clearly did not happen. To the contrary, in the process of transition toward democracy, it became obvious that the internalization of political threats and the mechanisms of self-repression maintain themselves after the end of the dictatorship. Repressive processes that were open during the military government are being converted into less visible but even more effective authoritarian structures in the new democracy. There is no real social and political participation. People succumb and wait to see what the government will do. A society of alienated subject develops, in which participants feel distant and mistrustful toward the political process, even more so, because they wrongly supposed that they might be central to the new order.

The fact that we see processes of alienation in a modern democratic society is not in itself surprising. But that this happens in a society that only recently suffered the individual and collective consequences of political repression, where one of the main arguments in the fight against dictatorship was the defense of human rights and the necessity of truth and justice, obliges us to ask the following: How is it possible to maintain so much denial? How is it possible that one of the main issues in Chile today is not human rights but the fight against delinquency and terrorism? How can we understand the fact that the victims of persecution, with a certain amount of legitimacy, feel more marginal today than during the dictatorship?

It is in reference to this sociopolitical context that we discuss the problems of the children of the persecuted in Chile. They express, more than any other part of Chilean society, the basic conflict we are dealing with: the necessity to overcome a traumatic past, the impossibility of developing a future without a past, and the obligatory confusion within the present sociopolitical

DAVID BECKER and MARGARITA DIAZ • Instituto Latinoamericano de Salud Mental y Derechos Humanos, Nunez de Arce 3055, Nunoa, Santiago, Chile.

International Handbook of Multigenerational Legacies of Trauma, edited by Yael Danieli. Plenum Press, New York, 1998.

situation. It is difficult to label these children in terms of generation. On the one hand, it would be wrong to describe them as second generation, since most of them experienced persecution directly. On the other hand, it is also true that, officially, and in their own perception, the parents are the real victims. They, the children, have the task of overcoming and repairing the destruction their parents suffered. Very few of the children have direct memories of the Allende Government. They grew up as children of those against whom the military directed their coup. In this sense, they are second generation. At present these children are experiencing a nearly unsolvable contradiction: If they try to be typical youths of today and leave behind the world of the marginalized and the persecuted, then they lose their basic reference to their families and enter into insufferable loyalty conflicts. If they try, on the contrary, to integrate their history and consciously act as children of their parents, then they begin to form part of a social dynamic that is inevitably marginalizing and retraumatizing. Neither society nor their own families seem very interested in allowing them to understand these dynamics.

The Latin American Institute for Mental Health and Human Rights has provided medical, social, and therapeutic help to the victims for many years. Our research has not only been oriented toward detailed registering of the data of our patients and their treatment, but it has also included larger social dimensions, such as the existence of fear in the Chilean population and the existing attitudes toward human rights. The material presented in this chapter is a product of these research activities. But if the destruction we are dealing with is not only individual but also social, then our research cannot be exterior to the reality with which it deals. We are thus not neutral investigators intending to understand an alien reality, but are active participants in therapy and research, operating within the political process. Some people might consider this an unscientific attitude. We would suggest that at least within the context of man-made disasters, real science can only be nonneutral, because the choice here is not between objectivity and subjectivity, but between victims and victimizers.

A CASE HISTORY

Miriam's mother, Juana, sought family therapy at ILAS in 1992. In 1974, Juana, who was 7 months pregnant with Miriam, and her husband, Jose, were taken prisoners. Both of them were severely tortured for several weeks. Miriam was born in prison. In order to not disturb the other inmates, Juana always offered Miriam her breast when she started crying. Miriam met her father for the first time when she was 6 months old, through a fence, in the prison camp where both parents were held. In 1975, the parents were released from prison, expelled from the country, and went into exile in France. In the following years, they pursued various political activities related to Chile, changing countries of residence, and separating several times, with one of them always keeping Miriam. By 1990, when Miriam was 16 years old, they had changed countries four times, and had not lived together for more than 12 months. Deciding that it was time to go home again, they sent Miriam back to Chile to check out the situation. Miriam lived alone in Chile for 7 months, then her mother came back, and in 1991, the father. For the first time in many years, they tried to live a normal family life. Their economic situation was poor. Miriam had shown abnormal eating behavior since early childhood, stuffing herself with all the food she could get. Now, after reunification with her family in Chile, she developed openly bulimic symptoms accompanied by severe states of depression and anxiety. The parents first sent her to individual therapy. When Miriam started to develop a more trustful relationship to her therapist, the mother decided that this therapy did not help, and that there was no money to pay for it anyway. After

3 months with no treatment, they came to ILAS, where treatment costs are low, and where family treatment is available.

Both parents seem a lot older than they really are. A little overweight, Miriam gives a very bright, adult impression. She articulates well the strange way this family communicates, as well as the history of her own suffering. She complains that her parents sabotaged her therapy but also declares that she does not want to pick it up again. The father states that he does not believe in therapists. But all of them confirm that they respect the mother's decision to come to ILAS and ask for family treatment. In the following sessions, Miriam speaks more about her fears, her insecurities, and her confusion. She has stopped going to school, spending the whole day at home crying, eating, and vomiting. The parents express concern, but not to the extent of really taking care of her at home. During sessions, the mother and daughter fight and discuss a lot, while the father either keeps quiet or makes lengthy explanations, which quickly bore mother and daughter, and are even difficult for the therapist to listen to. But once he starts talking, he will not be interrupted.

Listening to the three of them is like attending a course in double-bind communication. Father and mother disagree about almost everything, but at the same time insist that they are a couple, finally reunited, whose only problem is their daughter. Miriam basically tries to confirm this opinion, but at the same time, she makes varying alliances with one or the other in order to disqualify the person outside of the alliance as pathological and guilty of the existing confusion. When the therapists try to pinpoint one of the apparent conflicts, all of them are very quick to rearrange or change the topic of discussion. Each of them convincingly explains the traumatization of the other two but denies his or her own problem. Miriam explains that her parents have suffered, but she, herself, is only ungrateful and egotistical. Juana confirms the extreme suffering of her daughter, having been born in prison, never having had a home and a trustful family atmosphere. She also describes the trauma of her husband, his frustrations, and how he encapsulated the experience of horror and never again talked about it, although he has nightmares, often feels depressed, and so on. She herself though is okay, with only minor problems. The father says that he has overcome his personal problems, but that his wife and daughter have a highly neurotic relationship, that Juana never knew how to control herself, that she is highly aggressive, and so on. In other words, all of them give quite adequate descriptions of the difficulties of the others but deny their own. During sessions, basically two scenarios seem possible: Either there is high tension and conflict, shouting, and crying or there is nothing, a strong depressive silence in which everything seems dead.

EXTREME TRAUMATIZATION

Miriam is one of many youths we have been treating these last few years. Her story is unique but also similar, even nearly identical, to many others. Many times, it is the parents (mothers) that seek treatment for their children, because they exhibit "antisocial behavior," drug addiction, impulsive behavior, aggression (often against their own family), problems at school, and family crises. Less often, the youths themselves ask for help because of difficulties with their boy- or girlfriends, separations, and difficulties in their studies or at work. Symptomatically, we find insomnia, nightmares, fear, depressive crises, and psychotic breakdown. Furthermore, psychosomatic symptoms, such as digestive difficulties, blood pressure problems, allergies, and low defenses are frequent. It is impressive how most of these patients appear to be very adult, while at the same time showing extremely regressive behavior in certain areas. Thus, for example, most use a very developed and rational language, and are able to describe their difficulties eloquently. At the same time, they are insecure and feel confused in many situations, show the typically exaggerated trustful and dependent behavior so well known in children in public homes, and have difficulties in determining adequately the demands of external reality. Many have histories of being exceptional students that at some point, to the surprise of everybody, feel completely unable to work or go to school and confront the next exam. Symptoms usually appear in connection with an external sociopolitical event that is relevant to them, such as the finding of mass graves in the north of the country, or in response to specific family occurrences such as birth of a sibling, death of a grandparent, and so on.

We define our patients as "extremely traumatized" (Becker, 1992; Becker & Castillo, 1990). The term *extreme traumatization* implies for us that the victims have had traumatizing experiences within the context of state terrorism that surpass the capacities of the psychic structure and therefore cannot be integrated. We believe that the analogous use of Keilson's concept of "sequential traumatization" (Keilson, 1992) is possible and useful in Chile. He shows that a process of cumulative traumatization can turn into chronic trauma whenever the context of the traumatic situation refers to political persecution and repression. He makes it very evident that not only can the consequences of trauma persist a long time after the actual traumatic situation is over, but also that after the end of political persecution, the trauma itself continues. Furthermore, his theories, in agreement with Bettelheim (1943) and others (Grubrich-Simitis, 1980; Mitscherlich & Mitscherlich, 1967; Parin, 1975), help us confirm that external and temporal realities can explain a traumatic (psychic) process, although this does not mean that the internal qualities of experience of the trauma were already understood. Keilson established his sequences in reference to Jewish war orphans in the Netherlands, differentiating between the beginning of persecution, the actual separation of the children and their parents when the parents were taken to concentration camps, and the time after the war, when families in some cases were reunified and others were not. In reference to other countries, the sequences will be different. Also, within the same country, for different persons, different individual sequences will apply, although the overall picture does not change. In Chile, we can differentiate the sequences.

First Traumatic Sequence

It begins with the military *coup d'état* and ends with the specific repressive experience: imprisonment, disappearance, death. The main characteristic of this sequence is the general insecurity because of the military activities, searching of houses, imprisonment, and shootings. Intrafamily tensions, fear, and insecurity occur regularly. Additionally, all kinds of trust in the surrounding world have to be given up. The individual, his or her family, and the group they belong to become suspects, and certain political convictions automatically make one belong to the "enemy." From then on, anything can happen. The family and social context have abruptly changed on September 11, 1973. What was law the day before is now outlawed. Fathers and mothers are still alive, but they could be dead tomorrow. Within the families, parents try to convince their children, husbands their wives, that they do not need to fear, that they can still believe in the traditional roles of parental and marital protection. All this, while in reality, the threat is already omnipresent, and death has become a part of everyday life.

In the case of Miriam, she has not yet been born, but her conception was during this period, perhaps a last try of the parents to go on with life as usual. While they daily risk their lives, they try to maintain the illusion of normal family development. Even before being born, Miriam is already a symbol of a life project, lost forever, or, better said, she is a tangible symbol of life for parents that are dealing with death.

Second Traumatic Sequence

The second traumatic sequence begins with the specific repressive situation and ends with the end of dictatorship, sometime between October 1988 (plebiscite) and March 1990 (first election of democratic government). During this sequence, terror is experienced directly by one or more members of the family. But also the family members not directly affected now basically deal with the political issues, with fighting against the government, looking for those that have been imprisoned. Family life itself has become secondary.

The life of the children in this period is marked by the loss and/or sudden separation from the people most important to them. This loss is not only related to different members of the family but also to the home and the social surrounding, in fact, to the whole world as it was until that time. It is also in this sequence that the affected persons have no choice but integrate into the world of the marginalized and persecuted. In order to survive, this new world of terror cannot be perceived anymore as an exception. It has to become *the* world.

For Miriam, this world of trauma begins with the first day of her life. She is born in jail. Instead of feeding to be nurtured, she is fed in order to be silenced. Her other is alive through her. But life has to be silent and secret. She really meets her father only in exile. From ages 4 to 5, she lives alone with him, then again with the mother, and in-between, a few months with both. In her memory, all of these years feel like having lived alone, occasionally sustaining adult conversations with her parents. She does not feel at home in any country. She does not remember friends or places she specially liked, not even toys. All she remembers is a small orange, made out of wool or felt, that she loved. She gave it away when once again she had to change countries. Coming back to Chile all by herself seems quite normal to her. What she does not understand is why she feels so depressed now, when everything seems to be "okay." Also, she does not know why her tendency to eat a lot has changed into the habit of eating and forced vomiting.

Third Traumatic Sequence

This last sequence begins with the end of dictatorship, and it is uncertain when it will end. Its traumatic character depends on how and if individual and social reparation occurs after the dictatorship. Keilson (1992) has shown that the consequences of this sequence for the victims are possibly more destructive than the other sequences (see also Danieli, 1992). The unfulfilled promise of reparation for the victims is potentially more traumatizing than the worst experience that happened before, because then the faith existed that once the dictatorship was over, truth and justice would occur and the terror would have an end.

We have earlier mentioned the retraumatizing effect this sequence has for the children of the victims. For a Chilean youth in 1983, it was still possible to establish a direct link between his or her personal suffering and that social process. A frequent slogan of these days was "It's okay to die fighting, but, damn no, not of hunger" (Morrir luchando—de hambre ni cagando). It expressed quite adequately part of the individual trauma and its destructive potential, but also a certain amount of hope that was shared with the majority of the Chilean people. But all of this is history in postdictatorial Chile. There is no political participation and even less a political youth movement. The children of the victims are forced to deny their past in order to appear normal. The historical truth can only appear as individual craziness.

When Miriam begins to tell her story, she laments her dependency on others, especially her parents. She is angry about her symptoms, because they forced her parents into therapy. She feels confused and different from everybody else. She had hoped that now everything would be okay, but life seems more hopeless than ever. When she prepared the homecoming of her parents, she was convinced that everything would turn out fine. And now she feels sad, wanting to be a baby, and hating herself for it. She feels guilty for doing harm to her parents. They feel that they do not know her, that she is less ill and more blackmailing them. They oscillate between ignoring her problems and trying to convince her rationally to overcome them. Miriam feels that she can talk to other youths about her eating problem but not about her past, her time in exile, or the fact that she was born in jail. It is easier to try to be a hysterical youth with severe eating problems than to confess the history of persecution and loss. Since her birth, Miriam has known that dependency is dangerous and has to be avoided. One should not be a child, and if she is, as is happening to her now, it is disastrous. Through Keilson's sequences, we can understand how she came to her strange, contradictory convictions. Her conduct makes sense. But how can we explain the extraordinary process of adaptation this girl managed from her birth day onwards?

Relying on Winnicott (1973, 1974, 1976), we can understand the traumatic situation as a failure of the holding environment (mother) in its function as mediator of the child's needs. Also, afterward, the environment is not able to provide a good enough situation to enable the child to elaborate about the traumatic experience. On the contrary, the threat within the social context is maintained, and grief processes cannot happen. The "holding environment" and/or the "primary object-relationship" (Balint, 1966, 1968) are traumatic in themselves. Individuation and identity formation happen under conditions that permit activities of adaptation but not the development of the true self. The trauma is dissociated, and during adolescence, the crisis becomes visible because this is the moment where instead of real autonomy the pseudoreality of the autonomy enacted up until then can no longer be denied. It is therefore unsurprising that so many of our patients are adolescents.

It was Ferenczi (1988) who first described the extreme division, nearly impossible to overcome, that exists between the traumatic experience and the posttraumatic structure. In his clinical diary, he describes how fragmentation, the splitting into two personalities, helps one to survive the traumatic experience. But this same defense mechanism also implies that, afterward, there is no direct access to the trauma. If in the therapeutic process the trauma is reconstructed, the dissociation is nevertheless maintained, because the split between a destroyed part of the person and a part that perceives this destruction is repeated. On the other hand, if the person "regresses" to the situation of experiencing the trauma, he or she is in a "trance," feeling but not knowing" what is happening. When the patient awakes from this "trance," once more the immediate evidence of the trauma disappears. Once again, it is only reconstructed from the outside, without a feeling of conviction. What, in Ferenczi's terms, could be understood as a mere clinical technical problem in reality describes extremely well the core problem of people that have survived trauma. The theory of sequential traumatization describes how the social context produces breakdown and the maintenance of the dissociative process. Ferenczi offers us a bridge to approach the inner psychic world of a traumatized person.

The English psychoanalysts, Kinston and Cohen (1986), quite similar to Winnicott (1974), understand psychic structure as a lifelong mediating process with the surrounding environment. They speak of trauma as "primary repression," which, in contrast to Freud's (1926) opinion on this issue, can happen at any point in life. Depending on the specific psychological development of the individual, the defense mechanisms might vary but the basic consequence of trauma is always the same: a hole in the psychic structure. The satisfaction of needs lead to psychic representations that themselves are the basis for the development of wishes, without which there can be no object relations. Trauma means that basic life needs are not satisfied. Where there is no wish, there cannot be a psychic representation or capacity of symbolizing. There can only be a hole, primary repression.

The experience of the child in these cases is not "My mother has abandoned me," but the feeling of falling endlessly. Just like Ferenczi's patients, most children survive this experience of death and develop what Winnicott (1973, 1974) calls a "false self." Children are confronted with the obligation to assume premature control over their environment instead of being able to discover it slowly. The healthy fantasies of omnipotence that children can have when they can believe that they invented the object are being replaced within the traumatic experience with an omnipotence that tries to cover up the very real failure of the environment. Instead of inventing the environment, the children have to live with the frustration of having had to assume prematurely responsibility for the world.

Our clinical experience shows that this is exactly what happened to our patients. They had to develop the capacity to understand the world very early in their lives, grow up immediately, and become protectors of their own parents. They really believe that it is their task to solve all family problems, including that of income. They justify their attitude with opinions such as "They (other family members) are still so young, have suffered so much, are so insecure." Even if they want to, they find it extremely difficult to leave behind this role. Miriam, for example, can perceive her parents only as victims that need help. Her own needs seem to appear in spite of her, causing her extreme feelings of guilt. No matter how bad she feels, she still thinks that the inability of her parents to produce a decent income is her problem. She finds a job in addition to attending school and makes more money than her father, who works all day. Just as she took care of her mother's fears in jail, nursing at any time and keeping quiet, so she continues her preoccupation with others. Her relationship to peers reflects the same model: She is the therapist, the mother to whom others tell their troubles. Children such as Miriam have had to learn very early to adapt to the demands of their surroundings. They have, therefore, developed very rigid false-self structures in order to protect their true selves, their spontaneity and, most of all, to defend against feelings of loss, destruction, and death. They have perceived dependency as limbo, as a void. They never experienced the "holding mother," never had an adequate mirroring. They had to dispose of their own need for protection in order to protect the vulnerable objects around them. They had to assume complementary ego functions for their parents. But in this process, it is important not to forget that the vulnerability of the parents was real; it was not the product of some secret illness, but of a sociopolitical process.

Because of their age, the children could not really understand this process. The only choice they had was either to attempt magically to save their parents and thereby themselves, or together with their parents be a victim of primitive fears, feelings of void, and loss of body, all of which were not psychotic feelings but a reflection of a very concrete exterior world.

Paradoxically, the premature recognition of the environment leads to the incapacity to really perceive this environment and construct real object relationships. While a true self permits a person to feel real, a false self always implies a feeling of inexistence, of nothingness, of not being. Miriam often reported this feeling of not being, of being outside herself. She ascribed the same meaning to her bulimic activities: She feels hollow and wants to fill herself up. After eating a lot, she feel stuffed but equally void. So she vomits. In this process, she feels herself a little more, basically as pure pain.

For a true self to develop, the object has to be recognized as a real object outside of the self. Following Winnicott (1974), this is only possible if the child can destroy the object and find out that the object survives. If the child experiences that the object cannot be destroyed, then his or her omnipotence has limits. And because of that, it is possible to believe in the object, to permit its protection. Concern becomes possible in the form of gestures of reparation, while internally the child can go on fantasizing the destruction of the object. Thus, the child learns to use the object and to develop object constancy.

Our patients never had this experience. Aggression as a central element of healthy development had to be repressed. The perceived and very real destructibility of the parents forced the children to succumb to the parents' needs. Instead of being mirrored, they had to mirror. The mirroring of the parents often takes the form of idealization and also copying behavior, beliefs, and social relationships. Miriam and her mother reflect this kind of magical closeness, of artificial symbiosis. They understand each other without talking; they feel the same about everything. Obvious differences are denied. Aggression has to be dissociated. Miriam is bulimic, but she does not feel hate against her mother. When Miriam makes her first tentative steps toward autonomy when relating to her therapist, her mother intervenes and breaks off this *liason dangereuse*. Miriam suffers, but she knows her mother is right.

We believe that children and youths who, together with their parents, have had direct experience with death through torture and persecution, generally tend to understand aggression as an equivalent of destruction. Aggressive feelings within a relationship are experienced as the very real death of oneself and the other. To attack somebody means to be the torturer, the executioner, and there is no experience that would permit a belief in the possible survival of the object. In this manner, aggression as a normal part of human development is being inhibited, while the illusory object relationship that is supposed to cover up the nothingness and represents the subjective object is maintained. The sickening omnipotence is reinforced while feelings of unreality and rupture dominate the internal world and the perception of external reality.

FAMILY AND SOCIAL IDENTITY

It is important to look at the processes of traumatization of the youths that up to now we have been discussing in terms of true and false self, and also in terms of identity development. We have seen that identity development has been severely hindered, if not impossible, because the youths have never been able to experience themselves as persons within a continuity in time and space. As Grinberg and Grinberg (1980) point out, central tasks of the crisis of adolescence are the elaboration and integration of the losses of the childhood object relationships that have invariably changed during psychosocial development. A healthy grief process in these terms is the core of adult identity. Extremely traumatized youths cannot experience this process. Instead of remembering and grieving "holding," fear and experience of destruction reappear. Instead of finding basic elements of identity in the past, they only find pieces of multiple losses of self. Instead of grief, they reexperience death. The only identity that promises some continuity is the identity of discontinuity and rupture. The denial of reality on an individual and social level, the repetition of destruction, rupture, and insecurity thus appear as possibly the most authentic expression of identity in these youths.

These vulnerable identities are not only the inevitable answers of the youths to the destruction they experienced but are also the product and the expression of a sociopolitical process that had implied a series of specific intrafamily delegations and demands in the second traumatic sequence, and confirm the social process of alienation and the maintenance and continuity of authoritarian structures within the third traumatic sequence.

Within the families, the experience of repression and persecution has produced a series of delegations and demands only seemingly independent of the social process:

1. The children are supposed to maintain themselves as closely connected to their families throughout their lives. Any intention of separation, implied by the normal growth

process, is seen as a disloyal act, since separation is seen as identical to the involuntary losses during the original traumatic experiences.

2. The children have to replace the lost or damaged and always idealized objects. Wishes and needs directed toward these objects have to be satisfied by the children, and they have to represent the idealized object in their behavior.

3. The children must help the parents to diminish their feelings of guilt and extreme humiliation. They have to overcome the total powerlessness of their parents. They also have to overcome and right the social stigma that defined them as criminals during dictatorship. They can do this by assuming a scapegoat role, or by hating and seeking vengeance.

4. They must overcome the trauma itself to make the past disappear; they must start living when the parents have stopped doing so. They have to finish the story and live the lives their parents would have lived if disaster had not struck. In accordance with the posttraumatic idealization of the past, they have to be good students, learn an important profession, and build good and lasting partner and family relationships.

It is not difficult to recognize the contradictions, the mutual exclusiveness in these demands. At the same time, it is obvious how these demands seek to solve and overcome within the family the sociopolitical experience of impotence and destruction. Therefore, the children have to accept these delegations but are also condemned to fail. They will fail because a social problem cannot be solved within the family, and also because only in failure can they be completely loyal to their parents.

The political process after dictatorship, for a short time, suggested to the victims that there was a real possibility of ending the madness, of facilitating collective elaboration. But rather quickly, it became evident that this is an illusion, the maintenance of which not only denies the reality of the victims but also reinforces their collective impotence. As Mitscherlich and Mitscherlich (1967), Parin (1975), and, most importantly, Adorno (1982) have pointed out, the negligence of postdictatorial society in dealing with its victims, with the collective past, is a way of pretending that democracy has come, while in reality, authoritarian structures are being retained. We can thus speak of a double victimization where, first during dictatorship, the victims were repressed and persecuted in order to establish a new order. Afterward, these same victims were denied, pushed into the fragile existence of sick people with a private problem.

We can see how the intrafamily delegations and the social process unfortunately complement each other. While the general social process facilitates the development of false-self psychic structures, those structures make it more difficult to recognize the social basis for the individual suffering. The youths are trapped. If they recognize the destructiveness of the social process, they are even more dependent on the family delegations. If they rebel against these delegations and try to integrate normally into society, they can only do so by covering up their personal false selves with social false selves.

TREATING MIRIAM

Therapy cannot solve social dilemmas, but it must be conscious of them if some kind of help is to be offered to the victims. More precisely, if the social context is as we described it earlier, then sometimes therapy loses its connotation of basically being something private and becomes a relevant social space where personal and social reparation can begin. The therapeutic process is the endeavor to begin a relationship, to facilitate a bond, to invent a transitional space

(Winnicott, 1973) in which the patients can play. Basically, the idea is to bring together the bits and pieces of a life history that is full of terror and fear, losses and black holes. The fundamental problem in these therapies is less to establish a relationship than to facilitate a process where symbolization can occur. We have learned that a perspective of life can only be developed if we are ready to recognize the death our patients have experienced as such, and integrate it into a living relationship.

The treatment of Miriam and her parents was long and complicated, and cannot be reproduced here in detail. But some information on the work with her seems helpful. After 6 months in family therapy, as well as individual sessions for Miriam, we had established some kind of trust. While Miriam was getting more and more depressed, in sessions, she was more able to confront her parents. The parents, on the other hand, began reconstructing their own history, facilitating a slow, differentiating process. Miriam stopped vomiting but continued to eat excessively. One afternoon, when her parents were not home and she knew they would be late, she took a considerable amount of sleeping pills and went to bed. Late that night, her father found her. She was unconscious for 2 days and nearly died. After this event, things began to change dramatically. While the parents assumed a real parental attitude for the first time, not only giving love, but also setting limits, Miriam accepted dependency, being a child. Within the following months, she grew rapidly. When a year later we finished therapy, Miriam summed up the experience as follows: "When I tried to commit suicide, a part of me wanted to die, but another part of me wanted to live more than ever. Waking up afterward was painful but intensely gratifying. It was like being born again. In these last months, I feel I have won myself parents. Life is still difficult, but I don't feel lost anymore."

The parents said, "What happened was terrible. But we feel we got a second chance. For the first time, there was no other issue than fighting for her survival. We feel we are a family now. We are sad for the lost time, sad because our child is grown up now. But we are happy to be a family who has had to mourn many losses but survived."

These comments perhaps sound like the typical happy ending reported after so many therapeutic processes. There can be no doubt that, in many cases, we cannot help. But for us, Miriam's case quite dramatically shows the road one youth had to take to begin the process of symbolization. She could have died. But through luck, this suicide attempt could be worked through as the beginning of a healthy grief process, as the end of death as it had been up to now, and the beginning of life.

REFERENCES

Adorno, T. W. (1982). Was bedeutet Aufarbeitung der Vergangenheit. In G. Kadelbach (Ed.), *Erziehung zur Mündigkeit* (pp. 10–28). Frankfurt: Suhrkamp Verlag.

Balint, M. (1966). *Die Urformen der Liebe und die Technik der Psychoanalyse*. Stuttgart: Klett Verlag.

Balint, M. (1968). *Therapeutische Aspekte der Regression*. Stuttgart: Klett Verlag.

Becker, D. (1992). *Ohne Hass keine Versöhnung: Das Trauma der Verfolgten*. Freiburg: Kore Verlag.

Becker, D., & Castillo, M. I. (1990). *Procesos de Traumatización Extremas y Posibilidades de Reparción*. Santiago: ILAS.

Bettelheim, B. (1943). Individual and mass behavior in extreme situations. *Journal of Abnormal and Social Psychology, 38,* 417–452.

Danieli, Y. (1992). Preliminary reflections from a psychological perspective. In T. C. van Boven, C. Flinterman, F. Grunfeld, & I. Westendrop (Eds.), *The right to restitution, compensation and rehabilitation for victims of gross violations of human rights and fundamental freedoms* (pp. 196–213). *Netherlands Institute of Human Rights [Studie- en Informatiecentrum Mensenrechten]. Special issue* No. 12.

Ferenczi, S. (1988). *Ohne Sympathie keine Heilung: Das klinische Tagebuch von 1932*. Frankfurt: S. Fischer Verlag.

Freud, S. (1926). *Hemmung, Symptom und Angst.* G. W., Bd. XIV. London: Imago.

Grinberg, R., & Grinberg, L. (1980). *Identidad y Cambio.* Madrid: Paidós.

Grubrich-Simitis, I. (1980). Vom Konkretismus zur Metaphorik. Gedanken zur psychoanalytischen Arbeit mit Nachkommen der Holocaust-Generation—anlässlich einer Neuerscheinung. *Psyche, 38*(1), 1–28.

Keilson, H. (1992). *Sequential traumatization in children (English Ed.).* Jerusalem: Magnes Press, Hebrew University.

Kinston, W., & Cohen, J. (1986). Primal repression: Clinical and theoretical aspects. *International Journal of Psychoanalysis, 67,* 337–355.

Mitscherlich, A., & Mitscherlich, M. (1967). *Die Unfähigkeit zu trauern.* München: Piper Verlag.

Parin, P. (1975). Geselschaftskritik im Deutungsprozess. *Psyche, 29,* 97–117.

Winnicott, D. W. (1973). *Vom Spiel zur Kreativität.* Stuttgart: Klett Verlag.

Winnicott, D. W. (1974). *Reifungsprozesse und fördernde Umwelt.* München: Kindler Verlag.

Winnicott, D. W. (1976). *Von der Kinderheikunde zur Psychoanalyse.* München: Kindler Verlag.

27

Transmission of Trauma

The Argentine Case

LUCILA EDELMAN, DIANA KORDON, and DARÍO LAGOS

THE SITUATION IN THE DICTATORSHIP PERIOD
IN ARGENTINA, 1976–1983

Between 1976 and 1983, a military dictatorship overthrew the Argentine government and installed itself by means of state terrorism. During this period, the worst form of political repression in Argentina's entire history was carried out. It was characterized by the illegal detention of many people in clandestine prisons and the "disappearance" of about 30,000 people, the majority of whom were killed after having endured terrible tortures; the illegal detention in known prisons of more than 10,000 people over a long period of time (more than 2 years), who also underwent torture and inhuman conditions of detention; murders, many of which were carried out to set an "example" (for instance, a few bodies were dynamited together); the kidnapping of children and the changing of their identity (more than 400 are still missing); and hundreds of thousands of people who went to other countries as refugees.[1]

After the military coup, the Executive Power was destituted and Parliament was dissolved. A large number of judges were removed from their positions, and those that remained took oaths in the name of what was then called the Statute of National Reorganization Process, whose postulates were placed higher than those of the National Constitution. This statute was, in turn, violated by the dictatorship itself. The Judicial Power was subordinated to the decisions of the new Executive Power.

All the crimes committed during the period of dictatorship were protected by the impunity that the military power granted itself. There were no trials. In 1983, shortly before the first summons to free elections, the dictatorship sanctioned a self-amnesty law.

---

[1]The conditions of terror that were present and the events are detailed in the report on the situation of Human Rights in Argentina—CIDH (OAS) Chapter 3, 1979—and in the book *Nunca Más* (*Never Again*) that was edited by the National Commission of Missing People (CONADEP), Ed. EUDEBA.

LUCILA EDELMAN, DIANA KORDON, and DARÍO LAGOS • Equipo Argentino de Trabajo e Investigacion Psicosocial, Rodriquez Peña 279 "A" (102o), Buenos Aires, Argentina.

International Handbook of Multigenerational Legacies of Trauma, edited by Yael Danieli. Plenum Press, New York, 1998.

During the later constitutional period, pushed by a massive popular movement that clamored for justice, trials against the first three military juntas and some officers who had acted in the repression were started. Not long after the sentences of the highest-ranking officials were pronounced, the laws of Final Point and Due Obedience were passed, which excused all those who had been found responsible, with the exception of the highest-ranking officers.

The Law of Final Point, which is particularly abhorrent at the fundamental level, proposes the following:

1. The torturers of low military rank would not be held responsible for their actions.
2. The torturers could not decline against any order that was given to them, due to the state of war under which they supposedly were acting.
3. A serious alteration in the system of ethical values, since it excused kidnapping, torture, and murder, but not the robbing of tangible private property. This law placed private property above life itself.

Under the second constitutional government, the Executive Power sanctioned two pardons that granted freedom to the members of the juntas of the military government that had been put on trial and condemned. These "pardons," although constitutional, gave the president the unique power to pardon, exclusive and independent of all social consensus. Before the pardons to those most responsible for the genocide in Argentina were actually granted, a large number of protest marches took place. The decree of this pardon installed a system of exceptions and privileges that questioned legal and ethical norms and values.

The massiveness of the phenomenon of the "missing detainees" made it paradigmatic of the type of political repression that was used by the military juntas. Taking its characteristics into account, we can consider it as a particular form of torture in itself, a torture that the missing detainees suffered but that was also suffered by the relatives and friends of the victims.

The pyschosocial status of the missing detainees was similar to that of someone who was living in a "no-man's land," or who was "beyond life and death." He or she had no legal help and was at the mercy of his or her captors. On a family level, this presence–absence brought about a high degree of psychic suffering and a profound alteration in the everyday events of the affected groups, both in intrafamily and extrafamily relationships.

To assure complete social control, the dictatorship created not only terror but also an intense propaganda campaign, the characteristics of which would have to be analyzed in detail to be able to understand the complex psychological phenomena that not only were produced in the relatives of the missing detainees but also in the whole social body.

A silence regarding the repressive events that occurred was induced. Even though there were events and information that proved the existence of missing detainees, any public mention of them was forbidden. The effect on a person is particularly sinister if he or she has been a witness to the kidnapping of a son or daughter, a friend or a neighbor, and is continually told by outsiders that it is not true, or the outsiders do not want to accept the truth, or simply deny the perception.

The situation is frankly psychotic (Galli, 1984; Macci, 1985), especially if added to this there is a total absence of information about what happened, and about the fate of the person in question, that lasts for many years on the part of those who must answer these questions. On the other hand, the society could not believe that a person could be kidnapped and turn out to be a missing detainee. Though political repression used to be common, Argentinians had never lived through events of such horrendous characteristics and magnitude.

Many parents whose sons and daughters had been missing detainees never thought that being detained, no matter how violent, would result in the disappearance and/or murder of their loved ones.

After a long period of unsuccessful efforts to determine the whereabouts of their children, the relatives, under threat by the authorities that nothing would be made known about what was happening, under the pretext that this could increase the risks for the persons they were looking for, began to suspect that something sinister was happening. They still did not contemplate the possibility that their children would never return home, but they began to understand that, beyond what they had ever imagined possible, a system of political repression had been established in which the victims were "swallowed up by the earth." Not believing in the possibility of these events was also based on the efficiency of the historical silence concerning the indigenous genocide that had been carried out over a century earlier by the Argentine oligarchy using quite similar methods.

During the first three years of the dictatorship, there did not even exist a term for the status of the kidnapped people. Although the violence of the kidnapping was not expressed, and because the word *kidnapped* had a terrifying connotation, in time, a new word, *disappeared* (or *missing detainee*), was coined as a social representation that defined the fate of the people who had been the victims of these actions.

In some cases, some missing detainees were released. Under threats to their lives, these people also accepted or went along with the mandate of silence regarding the events that they had lived, witnessed, or heard from their repressors. In many cases, they were forced to collaborate with the forces of repression upon release from the concentration camps.

Little by little, reconstructed from the few testimonies that could be obtained, the truth of the terrible physical and psychological suffering of those missing detainees became known: the existence of clandestine prisons; brutal and sophisticated torture methods systematically applied to all prisoners; the so-called "transfers," which usually meant assassination and disappearance of the bodies of the victims; the number of people that were drugged and thrown into the Rio de La Plata or into the sea in an attempt to cover up all traces of them; and, finally, the atrocities that were implemented by the fascist repression of the dictatorship.[2]

Different human rights organizations began the difficult task of collecting information and making the corresponding denouncements. At the same time, from the start of the repression, the relatives of those who disappeared attempted to search systematically for their loved ones. In particular, the mothers began to gather and meet, and occupied the public squares in an attempt to break the walls of silence imposed by the dictatorship, Thus, the movement of the Mothers of Plaza de Mayo was formed.

Children were also a target of repression. Hundreds disappeared while they were preadolescent or adolescent. One of the most dramatic and significant episodes was the "Night of the Pencils," in which a group of secondary students from the city of La Plata, who had been calling for the continuation of a student bus fare, were kidnapped, tortured, and finally disappeared. Many adolescents and students involved in student centers also disappeared, especially those from secondary schools connected with the University of Buenos Aires.

On the other hand, the dictatorship implemented the practice of delivering, under false identities, very small children or babies born in captivity to families who registered them as their own children. These families were often couples who could not have children, who were associated with groups carrying out the repression. A notorious case is that of a sheriff of the Federal Police, Miara, married to a woman who was also a member of the Police Force, who appropriated the Reggiardo-Tolosa twins.

The pregnant women who gave birth in captivity to children underwent horrendous treatment. The majority of the women were violently separated from their children before being

[2]In 1995, an ex-officer of the Navy, Adolfo Scilingo, publicly acknowledged that, in a systematic way, prisoners were thrown out alive from airplanes into the river or the sea.

assassinated. Eloquent testimony of one of these cases was given by Ms. Adriana Calvo de Laborde, who, after giving birth to her son in captivity, was released.

Inés Ortega de Fossati, a girl of 17, was one month more advanced in her pregnancy than me and more or less a month before her due date; at the end of February, she started to have contractions. It was her first childbirth so we called the guards to help. After a long time of calling for someone, Berges appeared with his usual brutal gang, with cars entering at high speed, doors opening, and the slamming of car doors (you had to be there to be able to imagine all this). This made us get further into our cells and crouch in a corner because we knew that those noises were the signs of what was to come. Just as we had imagined, "the gang" entered our cell; it was something that was felt rather than seen. But this time, besides the "gang," Berges also came. He asked who had been complaining and a guard pointed to Inés Ortega. They dragged her by her arm and took her away. And, unfortunately for me, when they were leaving, a guard saw me and remembered that I was there and said, "This one is also pregnant." I felt them grab me by an arm and then start to drag me. Inés was ahead and I went behind. They made us go up a very steep cement staircase because I banged my feet trying to go up. With our eyes blindfolded and our hands tied behind us, they pushed us on our backs and we hit ourselves against those cement stairs. We went up a flight of stairs, and when I reached the top, I felt them start to push my chest. They pushed us backward and we both fell to the floor, and then I realized with horror that they were taking off my panties and examining me manually. This examination did not last more than 30 seconds. It was horrible. There was Berges; he was a medical doctor, a gynecologist, an obstetrician. He rapidly announced that we were both in very good condition, and in the same fashion that they had taken us up to that room, they dragged us down the stairs and threw us into the cell again.

A short time later, Inés went into labor. She was more than 12 hours in labor, alone with us in the cell, which in reality was the best situation she could have been in. I remember that not many of us there had already had children. There were women that were much younger and, with Patricia Huchansky, we took turns helping Inés. We tried to teach her how to breathe, how to push the air into her abdomen. And we tried to calm her. All of the others were at the gate shouting "guards, guards" for 12 hours nonstop. Then Berges arrived again and we all felt terrified by the shouts of the "gang." The shouts were also directed to the guards, who were also terrified. At last they were coming to take Inés. They took her to the kitchen, which was very close to our cell, so we all knew what was going on, partly from what we heard, partly from what we imagined, and partly from what she told us afterward. They put her on top of the kitchen table and tied her legs and hands; in this situation, she gave birth to her son, surrounded by the guards. We heard the laughter, the insults: It was horrible, the screams of the doctor, until we finally heard the baby crying. Leonardo had been born. This was March 12, 1977. We all breathed a bit. He had been born, he was crying, he was alive. It was our first experience. Imagine what it meant to me, because I knew what was going to happen to me. They then took her to a small cell that was next to ours but which was not connected to ours, but we could hear what was going on. Inés stayed there 24 hours with her baby. We heard her talking to the guards. The guards told her that the Colonel wanted to see the baby, that it was a beautiful baby. She told them that she had named him Leonardo after his grandfather. Twenty-four hours later, they came and took the baby away. They took Inés out of her cell and threw her into the common cell in which we were all together. We never heard anything more about the baby or of her either. . . .

Inés Ortega and her baby are still missing. Elena de la Cuadra gave birth to her daughter in the Fifth Precinct Police Station; both mother and daughter are still missing. When I arrived at the pit at Banfield, they told me that a few days earlier Eloisa Castellini had given birth to her daughter there and that she had been the most affected by the presence of Teresa because she had just had a daughter. In her case, they didn't even take her to another room. After a lot of shouting, Patricia was allowed to go out into the corridor with Eloisa, who gave birth to her daughter with Patricia's help. They were given a kitchen knife with which the umbilical cord was cut and immediately afterward, the baby was taken away. Nothing more was heard of either Eloisa or her baby. The fourth case is the one of Silvia Isabella Valenzi, whom I also met at the Banfield Pit. She "disappeared" at the Quilmes Pits and she was also pregnant. Silvia was a really beautiful girl, with blonde hair and green eyes. She was so beautiful that they called her "the cat." She realized that they were waiting for her baby. Her baby had been reserved. They took care of her, they gave her special food, and they even took her to the Quilmes Hospital to have her baby. Berges himself took her there. Silvia managed to ask the nurse and midwife to tell her family; the midwife did indeed tell the family and then disappeared. Immediately after having the baby, they took Silvia to the Banfield Pit and she disappeared. The baby had been left in the Quilmes Hospital.

Among other repressors, General Camps, the Chief of Police of the Province of Buenos Aires during the dictatorship, explicitly stated that children who were educated by the same families that had brought up their parents would also be opposers or "subversives."

And even though the kidnapping of children was expressly excluded from the laws that guaranteed impunity, it has been extremely difficult to obtain the return of those children, who were located by the untiring work of human rights organizations, to their legitimate families. It is calculated that there are approximately 400 children in this situation. To date, only 54 have been found; 7 were killed, 13 continue with their adopted families, and the rest, 34, have been returned to their families of origin.

INCIDENCE OF IMPUNITY

Until today, impunity has been maintained. We consider impunity to be a new traumatic factor (Edelman & Kordon, 1955a; see also Danieli, 1992; Danieli, Rodley, & Weisaeth, 1996). Not only has nothing been done to achieve the symbolic reparation offered by justice, but in an inexorable manner, impunity has been accompanied by a periodic reappearance in the mass media of the same psychological campaigns of the dictatorship, repeating the same arguments of those times, or presenting denouncements of the period of terror as "fantasies" of those who resisted the military dictatorship.

These campaigns have been particularly notorious in the case of the return of kidnapped children and to justify, though different arguments, not giving back these children to their biological families. The most common argument used to defend this way of thinking is stating that these children will lose the love of those who appropriated them.

They tried to cover up the crimes committed against these children's parents. They proposed a concept of family love in which assassination did not produce any mark in the constitution of the identity or in the new family ties that the children established (Edelman, 1995). There was a tendency to suggest that the appropriators of those children, who had themselves participated in the kidnapping and assassination of the parents as well as in the abduction of the children, could function as excellent "parents." Some cases that became publicly known showed evidence of the level of perversion and psychopathy of these appropriators and the appearance of these traits in their relationship with these appropriated children.

Thus, in an attempt to generate a favorable social consensus toward these appropriators as part of impunity, the true story of the parents of the children was kept secret while the families of origin were continually degraded and blamed.

On May 11, 1994, Law No. 24321 was passed, Article 2 of which states:

> In accordance with this Law, let it be understood that forced disappearance of a person means that a person's personal liberty has been taken away and that this event is followed by the disappearance of the victim, or if the person has been detained in clandestine places or deprived, under any other form, of the right of jurisdiction. The same must be justified

through a denouncement which has already been presented to the competent legal authority, the ex-National Commission on the Disappearance of Persons (decree 158/83) or to the Sub-secretariat of Human and Social Rights of the Interior Ministry or the ex-National Board of Human Rights. (*Boletin Oficial de la República Argentina,* 1994, p. 2).

This law is the first acknowledgment of responsibility on the part of the state in connection with the missing detainees. It also makes it possible for the families to determine the status of the disappeared person.

PSYCHOLOGICAL CONSEQUENCES

The effects were multigenerational in the sense that various generations were affected simultaneously.

In this chapter, we analyze some of the problems observed in the generation that was born and grew up during the dictatorship, in particular, the problems of those children of missing detainees. We also examine some problems appearing in the next generation. Our ideas are the result of clinical observations based upon having assisted many people affected by repression, either individually or in group therapy, from the start of the military dictatorship to the present. From 1977 to 1990, we worked in the Psychological Team of Assistance to the Mothers of Plaza de Mayo, and from 1990, until today, in the Argentine Team of Psychosocial Work and Investigation.

As an example, and before going in depth into some of the problems, we would like to describe a mother's narration of what has been happening to her 7-year-old son, whose father had been kidnapped when the child was 11 months old.

When my husband was kidnapped, Facundo abruptly moved from an organized family to a situation in which he was handed from one relative to another in different places where he could be hidden. He first showed inbalances in his sleep and in his appetite: in one day he shift[ed] from serious constipation to a severe diarrhea. I had to abandon my house because the police took possession of it, and I left my job as if I were a fugitive. My child continued to grow up in this situation.

Almost 2 years later, I managed to reconstruct what had happened to my husband. He had been kidnapped on the street. At that moment, he screamed his name, denouncing that he was being abducted, and asked for help. Someone who happened to be passing by went to a police car nearby and asked for help. They told him: "You haven't seen anything." Some time later, I managed to meet this person.

I never lied to Facundo about the situation. From the beginning, I talked quite a bit about it but he didn't seem to understand because he was a baby. One day when he was 3 years old and we were traveling toward Buenos Aires along the Avenida de la O.E.A. he asked me: "OK, Mom, what happened to Daddy?" My answers, although true, were rather confusing. At his age, they were not something that could be logical, but they were logical in the sense that he was frightened that this might be repeated. At this stage, his constipation problems were quite serious. And I had been able to reconstruct my life with some stability.

This was the period of "I don't know if Daddy is going to come home." The father's coming home implied that the child's liberation could also become a reality.

When the dictatorship was over, Facundo was 7 years old. At that time, he narrated a dream he had to a reporter during an interview: A big bird is attacking and killing all the people who are within eyesight except for the children. Then, the bird tries to enter Facundo's room to go after him. His mother closes the window just in time, cutting off one of the toes of the bird. Facundo constantly has nightmares. The reporter asked Facundo if the bird had died and he answered, "No, Mummy just cut off his toes." At this point Facundo started to ask me if he also could have been taken away.

THE QUESTION OF INFORMATION AND TRUTH

Many families, particularly during the first years of the dictatorship, had great difficulty in informing the children about what had happened to their parents (Kordon & Edelman, 1988b). Some of the reasons were as follows:

- The widespread nature of the mandate of silence.
- The fear that what had occurred could also happen to the children or to their families if the children spoke about it to their classmates or friends.
- The difficulty of the adults in accepting the suffering caused by the disappearance of a loved one. This difficulty was projected to the children in the fear that the information could cause harm or suffering.

That is why, in many cases, the absence of the parents was explained as a trip or work, or some other similar lie. In fact, these explanations could be interpreted to suggest a voluntary abandonment of the children by the parents (Kordon & Edelman, 1988b).

As we have proven in the majority of the cases, children, especially those who were already going to school, knew that the information they had been given was false and, in some cases, were aware of the fate of their parents. Nevertheless, they supported the family "secret" by agreeing with the prohibition of talking about what happened to the family. The lack of support from natural groups often included the extended family. In fact, the breaking up of families due to situations of fear, or differences in reasons about whether to keep silent about what had happened, led to important emotional losses.

In the majority of the cases, this silence was also maintained outside of the family, even in relation to their peers. This denied them the possibility of support from their natural groups. In other cases, the situation was told on a confidential basis to some friend of the same age.

Experience has shown (Danieli, 1995) that it was essential for children to have detailed information about what had happened, since the pathological effects of silence and secrecy could become even more important than the situation of loss, especially in situations where the substitute parental figures were adequate. Children want to know the truth. It was essential to clarify this to relatives, since the return of the person who had disappeared was not an option. On the other hand, it was possible, through a careful process of comprehension within the family, to withdraw, even if only partially, from the induced silence and social distance and to manage the truth in relation to the children.

In contrast, the children of the families who were committed to the public search for those who had disappeared, and who did not keep silent, avoided talking about the subject, especially in times of latency. This brought about feelings of anguish to the relatives, who viewed it as a sign of negation of the real events. A frequent consequence was the adults' compulsive insistence and children's rejection or hostility. In other cases, where the families had informed the children of the truth of what had happened, they were subjected to the mandates of silence and were quite relieved to avoid the subject.

Especially during the first years of the dictatorship, an important aspect of our clinical work was to collaborate in different ways with the transmission of information to the children of those who had disappeared.[3] In some cases, it was in group reflection that these conflicts were especially discussed; in other cases, it was through individual interviews with relatives in

---

[3]The purpose of the first groups of reflection with the relatives of the disappeared was the discussion of this problem that generated anguish and conflict within the families.

charge of the children; in still others, it was through individual interviews with us present at the precise moment when the information was being given.

The access to the truth produced, in all the cases to which we have been linked, a very important feeling of relief (Palento & Braun, 1985).

Some children explained that they did not insist on asking questions because they did not want to increase the anguish of their relatives. A similar situation is described in children of survivors of the Nazi Holocaust (Danieli, 1993). In these cases, the two parties had a pact to sustain a situation that both knew was false but which was intended to allow each to take care of the other. This pact was based on a misunderstanding about the possibility of not increasing the suffering of the other. It was quite inadequate for both.

THE STATUS OF THE DISAPPEARED

One of the pressures that was most frequently put on relatives was that they themselves should admit that the disappeared were really dead.

This was a particularly traumatic and complicated situation. On one side, the dictatorship that denied the existence of the missing detainees simultaneously induced their relatives to admit that they were dead. This was accomplished through "well-intentioned advice" given by public officials, people in the armed forces, or Church members who were a part of the police or armed forces when the relatives went to them in search of information about their loved ones.

Another frequent struggle between family members occurred when the parents of a disappeared person insisted that their son or daughter had been kidnapped and that it was necessary to continue the search for them, while the husband or wife of the disappeared person preferred to believe that he or she was dead and to transmit this information to their children. This preference was linked to the possibility of forming a new couple. As observed later on, many couples who were rapidly formed during that period seemed under the illusion that they were avoiding abandonment and blocking the difficult process of mourning. Many of them split up immediately after the dictatorship ended.

Simultaneously, many therapists who were consulted about how to manage the situation of the children, and who were also alienated by the inducements of the dictatorship and/or contratransferentially needed to give answers that could solve the psychotic ambiguity of the presence–absence situation of those who had disappeared, advised that it was better to believe that the disappeared person was dead and to inform the children, so that the family and the children could work through their mourning accordingly.

THE PROBLEM OF ABANDONMENT

As mentioned earlier, many explanations that were used as substitutes for the truth left the impression of voluntary abandonment. It is for this reason that we did not agree with therapists who, during the constitutional period, proposed to characterize the situation that the children had lived through as a "forced abandonment," as though the second word characterized the whole term.

From the children's point of view, both in clinical contacts and in groups of reflection for them, we found a conflict between the conscious acceptance of their parents' disappearance as an involuntary event and feelings of hostility and reproach for having been "abandoned" by them. The children tended to hide the latter because it was unacceptable to them, but it was nonetheless expressed many times in their aggressive attitude toward the other members of the family who were taking care of them, especially if these relatives were of the same generation as their own parents, at the therapists, and at the coordinators of the groups.

In the transference, explosions of anger were numerous, evidently motivated by the displacement of the original hostile feelings toward parents.

TRAUMATIC EFFECTS

We have found differences among children both according to the way each family faced the circumstances and the meaning each child gave the traumatic situation that he or she had lived through. In many cases, the children of disappeared people did not show disturbing psychological effects during early childhood that drew the attention of relatives, teachers, or themselves. But they did occur upon entering adolescence, a particularly critical period of their lives. Obviously, these effects did not necessarily spring forth in a direct manner from the early traumatic situations to which these children had been subjected. During their treatment, the interior articulation of both situations was established with clarity.

Contingency

In some cases, the principal clinical problem was related to the lack of adequate contingency for the development and growth of the children. In each case, this is expressed in different ways, from the impossibility of adopting adequately the integration of the ego to the most circumspect problems.

For example, a 6-year-old had been $1^{1}/_{2}$ months old when placed in the care of some neighbors for approximately a week after his parents had been kidnapped. He was later found by his grandparents and brought up by them. There was frequent contact with his aunts, uncles, and cousins. This child presented a single symptom, encopresis, each time his grandparents left him, even if only for a short period of time, or when his teachers were changed at kindergarten or school. This symptom was repeated at the beginning of his treatment, before going on vacation or during a short illness of his therapist. Luckily, it was solved during psychotherapeutic treatment.

In other cases, children assumed, at stages too early in their lives, the roles of adults. They occasionally occupied the place of their mother or father who had disappeared and structured a personality with features that were overadapted.

Gustavo was referred to our team by his mother's therapist. He was 17 years old when he started treatment. His father had disappeared when his mother had been pregnant with his younger brother, Julian. His mother, from then on, had never had a stable partner, and they could not count on relatives for any kind of help. They moved from one city to another and could not settle down anywhere.

During our first interviews with him, we were struck by the way Gustavo accepted things: He showed an understanding attitude toward all the difficult situations he had been through and did not manifest any aggressive feelings. He was studying and working to help to support the household. He also supported his mother and brother emotionally. When we interviewed his mother, she indeed expressed guilt toward Gustavo because she constantly overburdened him with her own anguish.

Gustavo seemed to be a man but had an adolescent aspect. A compensation for narcissistic self-esteem is evidenced in the role he had assumed in the family. After a year of treatment, when the mother finally achieved a greater degree of autonomy and personal stability, had a stable partner, and the general conditions of the family were more favorable, Gustavao, who, up to that moment, had shown high intellectual achievement, decided to leave his studies and entered a period of tumultuous adolescence characterized by the systematic abandonment of all situations that characterized personal achievement. This was followed by a period of narcissistic retraction in which apathy and abulia were the fundamental clinical expressions.

The pathology of overadaptation appears to be more frequent in boys, especially at the beginning of adolescence. Also, boys more frequently show a "defensive" attitude by avoiding talk about the traumatic situation. The phenomenon of overadaptation is probably linked to the social role of men regarding the functions of protection. When boys find themselves alone with their mothers or grandmothers, that is to say, in a relationship with a female figure, they develop their protective function at an earlier stage. When boys had the presence of a substitute father figure during adolescence, the pathological effects were more linked to infantile and/or impulsive behaviors.

We also noticed a family situation in which symbiotic and endogamous situations predominated and outside circumstances were considered as dangerous or persecutorial.

> Since Alicia was 10 years old, she had to change homes frequently because her mother participated in a political organization opposed to the government and tried to elude repression by constantly moving. Her parents had separated some time earlier, and she and her brother (2 years older than Alicia) lived with the mother. The father did not share the mother's political activities. When she was 12, while staying at her maternal grandmother's house, her mother and her 14-year-old brother were kidnapped, and, since then, nothing has been heard from either of them. Alicia continued to live with this grandmother, economically sustained by a father who remarried and formed a new family in which she did not find a place. She finished secondary school with some difficulty. From then on, Alicia found it very difficult to continue any activity. When she turned 19, she sought refuge in all the places whose activities were related to human rights. She moved from one human rights group to another, entering into conflict with each of them as soon as there were differences or signs that the institution was not going to take total and absolute care of her. In this case, it is evident that different human rights organizations are sought as maternal substitutes, because they simultaneously give identity and perform containing functions.

Identity Problems

Acknowledging that being "the son–daughter of a disappeared person" was an important traumatic social situation during the first years of dictatorship (Nicoletti, Bozzolo, & Siacky, 1988), we wondered what weight it would bear on the child's personal identity. How much of the personal identity would be shaped by it? How much capacity for full development of persona ego potentials would remain?

To this day, years later, many children of disappeared people still search for different groups. The objectives of these groups vary from participating in social and political activities whose purpose is to ensure that those responsible for crimes during the dictatorship are punished, to the support of the historical memory, to carrying out entertainment activities that are suitable for adolescents.

Some groups are created to accomplish an activity, such as making a film, or organizing homages, such as those that are held at the University of La Plata, where students and teachers that disappeared during the military dictatorship are remembered. In other cases, they are long-lasting groups that sometimes become associations.

These groups have simultaneously sprung up all over the country. Clearly, aspects of identity exist that necessitate being processed in peer groups that have undergone the same problems. These are those aspects of personal identity that are related to the origin, to the traumatic situation, that had been socially silenced.

The silence, the social denial of the existence of disappeared persons, and the tendency to blame those who disappeared and the families characterized the context in which the children grew up to such an extent that the young men and women of today tend to gather together. All these events seem to have deeply marked the aspect of personal identity that corresponds to social belonging and that, in many cases, is required for the elaboration of the construction of a group matrix, that of a group of peers with the same problems. Probably these peer groups, like those of the mothers who went out in search of their disappeared children, operate simultaneously as groups of belonging (with aspects of a primary group in the sense of a giver of identity), and as groups of reference that provide social representations capable of identifying support even for those young people who do not directly participate in them. The peer group thus functions as an intermediate space in the identifying process.

These groups have begun to develop practically one generation later, that is to say, 18 years after the beginning of the dictatorship.[4]

Like a historical paradox, the appearance of these groups within the social scene coincides with the reactivation of the problem of the repressors' impunity, but more particularly with the appearance of the "speakers," those who repressed and tortured, and who are protected by the framework of impunity and go to the mass media to "confess" the crimes in which they participated.

Each time they meet people who had something to do with their parents, most children of the disappeared ask what their parents were like in every aspect, from the expression on their faces to their ideas. They maintain an important identification with them, which is expressed in different types of interests, careers, and so on. They try to reconstruct an image of the family, identifying both the parents and themselves simultaneously. The identifying process covers everything from attempts to imitate to trying to find common traits, physical features (such as the way of smiling), how they dealt with matters, how they had communicated with them, if they had changed their diapers or not, everyday habits, and so on. They ask if certain personality traits that they possess could have been inherited from their parents. In some cases, there may even be character traits that they consider to be negative but would have the value of somehow assuring the genealogy.

For many years, we chose not to hold long-term therapy groups with children or adolescent children of people who had disappeared, so as not to encourage an identity that was ascribed to the traumatic situation as a fundamental and distinctive aspect of personal identity. Moreover, we tried not to favor the tendency to stigmatize or to marginalize, which was encouraged in relation to the people who had been affected in a direct manner by repression (Danieli, 1995).

During treatment, adolescents tend quickly to link their conflicts to the trauma that they have lived through. In therapy, they find an adequate space to face these problems, because in many families, it is still conflictual to talk about this. The males maintain a more pronounced defensive disassociative level.

On the Generation Gap

One of the situations that has produced an important effect on the level of personal identity is that of the "crossing out" of a whole generation. We are referring in this case to the situation that was brought forth in young grandparents (those of about age 40) who were left in

---

[4]In Argentina, 18 marks the legal coming of age.

charge of their grandchildren (if both parents had disappeared), and who established an almost direct parent–child relationship with them. Concretely, their grandchildren called them Father and Mother. They claimed that it was better for the child so that he or she did not feel different from other children. What it hid was the attempt to deny the death of their own children and/or the substitution of that grandchild who occupied the place of the lost child. Serious disturbances in behavior and refusal to accept any kinds of limits were observed in these cases. Worse, these children, whether they had detailed information concerning the fate of their parents or not, were enormously confused, unconsciously, about the parent images and the structure of family roles. They were greatly different from children who lived with their grandparents but fully understood the generation gap that existed between them.

Younger Brothers and Sisters of People Who Disappeared

A special comment should be made about the situation of younger brothers and sisters of people who disappeared, and who lived through a situation of repression during their childhood. These children had to elaborate a situation of loss simultaneously with the destructuring and melancholic effects that were brought about in the midst of the family.

In the cases where the parents, and most especially the mother, participated in some group movement in search of the disappeared child, profound recriminations linked to feelings of abandonment existed. In other words, the children who suffered the loss of an older brother or sister felt they needed more protection from their parents. The parents, on the other hand, were in the middle of the process of mourning for their loss. At the same time, there was an abrupt modification in the structure of family roles due to the activities demanded by the search for this child. The sense of abandonment that these children lived through was very important. The parents spent less time with them at precisely the moment when they needed their parents more. They also had feelings of devaluation in reference to the narcissistic acknowledgment on the part of their parents, since the disappeared child became more idealized with the passing of time. At the same time, somewhat contradictory and overprotective attitudes of parents were quite frequent due to the fear of the risk implied by the child's development of independence. (This referred not only to the political posture, but also to normal events in the process of growing up such as traveling alone at night or leaving the house to go and study elsewhere, and so on).

All these elements created a highly conflictual situation that was complicated by the resulting feelings of hostility, which were subjected to self-censure.

Many of these younger brothers and sisters maintained dependent relationships toward the family that lasted too long (reinforcing the family symbiosis), or broke away from the family at a too early an age (demonstrating a type of pseudoindependent behavior such as marrying while still in adolescence).

During the last years, the problems that arose in connection with the sale and traffic of children have become public. Although beyond the scope of this chapter, it is worth mentioning that since the state was responsible for the kidnapping and appropriation of children, a situation of anomaly is produced in the organization and social normalization of the family structure and in the generational transmission that is much more general, and that transcends those who were affected by the repression of the dictatorship.

The subject of child trafficking, a problem that undoubtedly existed prior to the dictatorship, today has a different meaning and has been broadened in view of the crisis in the social delimitation of what is licit and what is illicit. This problem has been extended to the question of the traffic of children's organs. Myth or reality, once again this is a symptomatic consequence of impunity.

The institution of adoption, in general terms, is one of the most affected by the kidnapping of children and impunity. In Argentina, the subject of adoption is in itself conflictual, since it recognizes social and class roots. But the persistence of the undetermined status of disappeared people and of the majority of kidnapped children and the situation of impunity have cast a great suspicion over all adopted children, especially those born between 1976 and 1980.

Many parents do not tell their children that they are adopted, so as not to cause them pain. In reality, it is they themselves who cannot bear this information. The absence of truth always bring about symptoms by occluding areas of the child's psychic development behind that which must not be known. If what leads to the concealment has something to do with the impossibility of elaborating mourning for the biological maternity–paternity, this is curable with treatment. But if what is concealed has something to do with the social environment, then the elaboration of this situation is much more complex. It must be noted that we are not referring here to situations of direct or indirect complicity in the appropriation of children by the repressors.

Many families blame themselves when they think of the possibility that their adopted children might be children of disappeared people. This doubt fills the adopting father/mother–adopted son/daughter relationship with anguish and reproach.

In opposition to the generalized suspicion, many adopted adolescents wish that they had been children of disappeared people.

Susana was adopted[5] and her parents have not given her a clear version of her origin. Years before, she had undergone a histocompatibility test, with negative results, to see if there existed the possibility that she were the child of some person who had been registered as disappeared by the Mothers of Plaza de Mayo. She presented a serious abandonment pathology.

Susana wished to be the daughter of a disappeared couple. Under her true situation of abandonment, if she were the daughter of a disappeared person, it would mean, at least to her subjectivity, a place of acknowledgment and external desire, which she feels she is lacking. In the face of the possibility of not having been a child desired by her biological parents and having been abandoned voluntarily, and also in the face of a destructured family with scare resources for her care, the desire to be the daughter of disappeared parents implies that she was desired by her real parents, from whom she was separated by force.

Although this chapter focuses on problems related to the disappearance of persons, the traumatic situation that was lived, from the transgenerational point of view, also takes into account children of people who had disappeared and then reappeared, of people who had been in prison for a long time, as well as children whose parents had gone into exile and then returned, and who have suffered identity or behavior disturbances as a result of the different processes of transculturation that, in the majority of cases, came about in an abrupt manner and in unfavorable conditions.

Conceptualization

We are analyzing the psychological consequences over a long period of time that were produced in children who today are adolescents and young men and women, and who suffered the conditions of secrecy that they had to live in, as their parents had been political opponents of the dictatorship. If we take into account the number of consulations that we have today, we are only beginning the analysis of these types of problems.

The nature of the traumatic situation affects the family structure and the individual subjects at the multi- and transgenerational levels (Puget, 1991). We characterize the traumatic

---

[5]*Adopted* in Argentina means that a nonbiological son or daughter is declared a son or a daughter by a legal procedure or a false inscription pretending to be a biological son or daughter. The latter is very common in Argentina.

situation as that which is constituted by events of political repression (disappearance, torture, etc.) and by the social inducements produced by the state and implemented through the mass media.

Impunity, as well as silence and the induced guilt, are decisive components of this traumatic situation. The longer they persist, the greater is the iatrogenic effect that they produce and the greater the possibility of the production of pathologies over a long period of time and in the plane of transgenerational transmission.

The psychopathological incidence of impunity varies according to the containing capacity of the families, the possibility that these families have of adequately managing the information and sustaining the truth, the previous levels of symbiotic functioning, the depth of the depression after the loss, and the degree of the endogamous return that is produced as a result of the repressive event.

It can be affirmed that a personal elaboration of the trauma isolated from the conditions of social elaboration does not exist. In this social elaboration, various factors must be taken into account. One of the most important of these is the collective answer produced by the same people who had been affected (either direct victims or their relatives). This solution helps the personal preservation of those who participated in those actions and functions as a reference even for those who were affected but did not have direct participation.

On the other hand, this socially organized solution allows the members of the next generation to find a starting point from which to resignify their own history. Experience has indicated that this historicization in the next generation constitutes a necessary step in the passage from adolescence to adulthood.

In the context of the reconstruction of this history, adolescents search for the narration of the history of their parents. They also want to know about identifying features such as personality traits and even habits or gestures that make them recognize themselves more intimately as the children of those people who, many times, they have never met.

In the Argentine experience, from the beginning of the social trauma produced by the kidnapping of children, many social and legal mechanisms were affected, apparently without connection to the repressive situation, as was the case of the institution of adoption that affected the transgenerational level.

In this regard, the analysis will be centered on one of the situations that produced the most controversy in Argentina, which is the return of the kidnapped children or children born in captivity to their families, in which the two levels that were mentioned earlier are manifested.

Even though the return of these kidnapped children to their families is a very complex matter, where ethical, legal, and political factors play an important role, mental health professionals were asked to give expert opinions on this subject. Indeed, many times, we went beyond our professional intervention when faced with concrete cases.

A few months ago, a baby girl was stolen by a woman, perhaps psychotic, from the maternity ward of the Spanish Hospital. After a few days, the baby was taken to a church. In this case, nobody doubted that she should be returned to her parents. This is an act of justice, of reparation. This is basically an ethical position based on not validating, not excusing and leaving unpunished one of the most terrible crimes of the dictatorship.

We think that the return of children consists of giving back of the *patria potestad* to the legitimate family. But what has happened to this view?

When the film *La Historia Oficial* (*The Official Story*) was shown in Argentina, it aroused an enormous popular reaction. The people identified themselves with the character portrayed by Norma Aleandro. The character's decision to search for the true story of her adopted daughter was in reality the true story of the country. That was a hushed-up story, whose existence the dictators, from their positions of power, tried to deny. In that search, the woman portrayed by Norma Aleandro was willing to give the little girl back to her legitimate family.

This story was probably not different from another official story, which unfolded in the context of the human rights politics of the constitutional government—not so much for what it said but, rather, for what it omitted. And it encouraged, from this point of view, the expectation of personal reparation without full justice, which would also include punishment of the perpetrators.

Some years later, during several procedures of return of the children, but most especially in the case of Juliana Sandoval Fontana, a very intense propaganda campaign was waged on two principal arguments:

- One was psychological: not to inflict damage or even further damage on the children, separating them from the false parents.
- The other was legal: Abandonment automatically legitimates adoption. Returning a child violates the legal order.

A part of the population identified with the position of not giving back the small girl. Others felt extremely torn internally upon facing the conflict.

What has happened in the time that elapsed? What are the factors that determine this change?

Elsewhere (Kordon & Edelman, 1998a, 1998b; Macci, 1985; Nicoletti *et al.,* 1988; Pelento & Braun, 1985; Puget, 1991; Viñar, 1992), we have analyzed how the state has intervened in creating the social systems of representation. During the dictatorship, a series of statements that tried to establish its necessity and inevitability was produced. The dictatorship, through the manipulation of the mass media, and through self-justifying statements and a set of inducements, the most important of which was the inducement to silence, tried to make people believe that the violence they were using was both necessary and natural. A situation of terror favored identification with the dominating discourse. In the face of these proposals, there were different answers between the poles of discrimination–resistance and heeding–submission.

Since the film was first shown, the laws of Final Point and Due Obedience were enacted. This not only deprocessed and guaranteed the impunity of the great majority of those responsible for the crimes committed during the dictatorship, but it also excused them. Only the kidnapping of children and the theft of property were not included in this law of Due Obedience. But to think that the question of the kidnapped children could be solved, isolated from the global situation, within a framework in which justice was lacking and impunity existed was merely an illusion, or, in any case, an illusion for those who made these laws. The case of Juliana shows quite plainly how totally illusory it is. And it goes beyond the desire of many to cling to this to be able to sustain a fictitious personal calmness. From this point of view, it works in the same manner as what was instructed in *Nunca Más* (*Never Again*), besides the concrete conditions of punishment of those who were guilty so as to guarantee that "Never Again."

The kidnapping of children during the dictatorship was not simply another atrocious act. It showed explicitly or implicitly that certain families were determined by the state as not fit for creating new subjects, as long as these subjects were not a part of the dominating sociocultural model.

This campaign again tried to show the victims as guilty of harming the girl because they seek her return.

The subsistence of these proposed models of the state and the implacable logic that intertwines them induce a certain identification with the power in such a way that it is possible to begin collaborating in the search for kidnapped children and to end up in the position of the "creators of public opinion" in favor of the dictatorship.

By omitting everything that happened until Juliana's arrival at Casa Cuna (Hospital), an attempt was made to reduce her case to the equivalent of a struggle between, for example, separated parents, and to make the people decide among options that pertain to this type of problem, thus creating a situation of internal schism between the desire for justice and the desire to keep the children.

This is what has happened to us. But what has happened to the children?

We know that every person is constituted through a process of identification that is developed at an early age in the nucleus in which he or she lives. This process of identification implies an internalization of the bonds with these people.

Do these children have the kidnapping, the violent separation from their mother, the conditions of their birth, and the violent basis of their identity registered inside of them? We think they do through a double mechanism: on the one hand, the register of what is archaic in the psyche; on the other, because all conflicting family situations are present in the relationships that are internalized in each subject.

The social discourse, the social marks, operate as an internal factor in the family structure and in the relationships. There will be present, for example, an attempt to hide the assassination of the parents or the fear of revenge that the child may take upon him- or herself to pay for what happened to his or her parents, in the case of children who are living with repressors, or when the suspicion of the true origin of the child exists. But can we believe that the suspicion of the origin of the child in this case is a strictly personal situation? We think that in every case, but more especially in the situations generated by the social violence of state terrorism, the suspicion is more of a social nature than a personal one. And this social suspicion inexorably impregnates the personal relationship.

Can this child become, for those who are bringing him or her up, a persecutory object that must be controlled?

How does one answer these children's questions about their origin?

If the fantasy of having robbed a child from his or her mother is present in parents who adopted a child under legal conditions and this has its effects, then is this not present in these families where the theft of the child is not a mere fantasy but a reality?

We think that without a change in the existing conditions, it is not possible to open any possibility of psychic health and productivity (Galli, 1984). By no means do we believe that the return of these children, who many times have been years within another family, will function as a miraculous cure. Since they were separated from their mothers, they have been submitted to psychic situations that border on the catastrophic.

But the child's return does open the way for the integration of his or her subjectivity with what is genealogical, historical, transgenerational, and social that may give the necessary support for his or her personal identity.

REFERENCES

Boletín Oficial de la República Argentina, No. 27.910, 1st Section, June 12, 1994.

Danieli, Y. (1992). Preliminary reflections from a psychological perspective. In T. C. van Boven, C. Flinterman, F. Grunfeld, & I. Westendrop (Eds.), The Rights to Restitution, Compensation and Rehabilitation for Victims of Gross Violations of Human Rights and Fundamental Freedoms. *Netherlands Institute of Human Rights [Studie-*

en Informatieecentrum Mensenrechten]. Special issue No. 12 (pp. 196–213). Also published in N. Kritz (Ed.), *Readings on the transitional justice: How emerging democracies reckon with former regimes.* Washington, DC: U.S. Institute of Peace.

Danieli, Y. (1993). Diagnostic and therapeutic use of the multigenerational family tree in working with survivors and children of survivors of the Nazi Holocaust. In J. P. Wilson & B. Raphael (Eds.), *International handbook of traumatic stress syndromes* (pp. 889–898). New York: Plenum Press.

Danieli, Y. (1995). Who takes care of the caretakers? The emotional consequences of working with children traumatized by war and communal violence. In R. J. Apfel & B. Simon (Eds.), *Minefields in their hearts: The mental health of children in war and communal violence.* New Haven, CT: Yale University Press.

Danieli, Y., Rodley, N., & Weisaeth, L. (Eds.) (1996). *International responses to traumatic stress.* Amityville, NY: Baywood.

Edelman, L., & Kordon, D. (1995a). Efectos psicosociales de la impunidad. In B. Kordon, L. Edelman, D. Lagos, D. Kersner, V. Bird, M. Lagos, C. Quintana, G. Taquela, *La Impunidad. Una perspectiva psicosocial y clinica.* Buenos Aires: Sudamericana Publishing Company.

Edelman, L. & Kordon, D. (1995b). Trauma y Duelo. Conflicto y elaboración. In D. Kordon, L. Edelman, D. Lagos, D. Kersner, V. Bird, M. Lagos, C. Quintana, G. Taquela. *La Impunidad. Una perspectiva psicosocial y clinica.* Buenos Aires: Sudamerican Publishing Company.

Freud, S., (1912). Totem y Tabú. *O. C.* Amorrotu editores. Tomo XIV.

Galli, V. (1984). Terror, silencio y enajenación. *Jornadas de Salud Mental: Efectos de la Represión, la Dimensión de lo Psíquico.* November.

Kaes, R., H. Faimberg, M. Enríquez, & J. J. Baranes (1993). *Transmission de la vie psychique entre generations.* Paris: Dunod.

Kordon, D. & Edelman, L. (1988a). Psychological effects of political repression I. In D. Kordon, L. Edelman, D. Lagos, E. Nicoletti, R. Bozzolo, O. Bonano, & S. Siacky (Eds.), *Psychological effects of political repression.* Buenos Aires: Sudamericana Planeta.

Kordon, D. & Edelman, L. (1988b). Psychological effects of political repression II. In D. Kordon, L. Edelman, D. Lagos, E. Nicoletti, R. Bozzolo, O. Bonano, & S. Siacky (Eds.), Buenos Aires: Sudamerican Planeta.

Nicoletti, E., Bozzolo, R., & Siacky D. (1988). Childhood and political repression. In D. Kordon, L. Edelman, L. Lagos, E. Nicoletti, R. Bozzolo, O. Bonano, & S. Siacky (Eds.) *Psychological effects of political repression.* Buenos Aires: Sudamerican Planeta.

Pelanto, M., & Braun, J. (1985). *Las vicistudes de la pulsión de saber en ciertos duelos especiales.* XV Congreso Interno and XXV Symposium "El malestar en nuestra cultura," organized by Asociación Psicoanalítica Argentina, Buenos Aires.

Pujet, J. (1991). Violencia y Espacios Psìquicos. *Jornadas de Asociación Argentina de Psicologia y Psicoterapia de Grupo.*

Viñar, M. (1992). Una historia clínica: El hijo de un desaparecido en el exilio. *Ficha Cátedra de Psicología, Etica y Derechos Humanos, Facultad de Psicología,* University of Buenos Aires.

28

The Impact of Culture on the Transmission of Trauma

Refugees' Stories and Silence Embodied in Their Children's Lives

CÉCILE ROUSSEAU and ALINE DRAPEAU

INTRODUCTION

Studies of intergenerational transmission of trauma have reported complex, even contradictory, findings (Kaufman & Zigler, 1989; Solkoff, 1992) and have taken many different views of what can be transmitted from one generation to the next, independent of context. Moreover, the wide variety of traumatic settings observed introduces the concept of specificity of transmission, which may fragment our understanding of the phenomena of transmission to such an extent that generalization becomes totally impossible. This attention to context usually tends to focus on the characteristics of the traumatic settings, paying scant heed to those of the groups that experience the traumatic events.

Some main trends are evident, however. One group of writings tends to consider the individual, usually a parent, and the family as bearers and potential transmitters of trauma-related psychopathology that either translates into specific behaviors or modifies intrapsychical representations. Other, more anthropological and sociological writings instead consider society as a whole to be the bearer of social trauma, which, by effecting profound changes in the webs of human relationships and collective representations, has a direct influence on future generations (Lykes & Farina, 1992; Martín-Baró, 1994; Vinar, 1993).

From both perspectives, the question that cannot be avoided, although it is rarely tackled directly, is the degree to which culture influences the transmission of trauma. Behaviors and representations of families and individuals, as well as collective representations, are shaded, even shaped, by culture. Obeyesekere (1985) suggests that culture provides the tools for grieving. When it comes to trauma, culture, which is obviously involved in the reparative process, may be equally involved in determining how, and how intensely, trauma is relived.

CÉCILE ROUSSEAU and ALINE DRAPEAU • Department of Psychiatry, Montreal Children's Hospital 4018, Montreal, Quebec, Canada.

International Handbook of Multigenerational Legacies of Trauma, edited by Yael Danieli. Plenum Press, New York, 1998.

If the specific time and place of a culture and trauma are taken into account, the question becomes even more complex.

With regard to the concept of place, there has been much debate over whether the particular problems observed in second- and third-generation Holocaust survivors are the result of the trauma itself or of the displacement it entailed (Weiss, O'Connell, & Siites, 1986). In the case of refugee children, a number of authors have stressed that exile and uprooting play a major role in the persistence of the impact of trauma, but there is no consensus in this area.

Time is of special importance in considering the transmission of trauma to children. There is a great deal of literature showing that the child's age at the time of a direct trauma influences the symptoms that develop later in life (Green *et al.*, 1991; Pynoos & Eth, 1985), but not much attention has been paid to the impact of the child's stage of development on the consequences of various ways trauma is transmitted.

This study compares two populations of refugee children from contrasting cultures (Southeast Asian and Central American) at two stages of development (8–12 years and 12–16 years) by examining the relationship between family trauma and mental health problems.

The influence of the culture of origin and the child's stage of development on the transmission of family trauma is discussed in light of our data on the impact of family trauma on the two groups of young refugees studied.

First, we briefly review the literature on the interactions among culture, context, and transmission of trauma, focusing on what is known about the two groups under study. We then explain the methodology of the two surveys, present the quantitative and qualitative data obtained, and discuss the results.

CULTURE AND INTERGENERATIONAL TRANSMISSION OF TRAUMA

The influence of culture on intergenerational transmission of trauma cannot be reduced to a single variable having an influence parallel to that of other determining factors.

Culture imbues and shapes what the person, the family, and the community construct around a disease that becomes illness (Kleinman, 1988). We therefore do not go into all the ways that culture influences the transmission of trauma, but by concentrating on some factors known to be important in intergenerational transmission, we attempt to show the importance of culture and propose some hypotheses concerning the mechanisms involved.

Four areas are especially relevant to a consideration of the influence of culture: posttraumatic signs and symptoms, changes in family dynamics, individual and collective meanings associated with trauma, and reparative processes.

Influence of Culture on Parental Symptomatology Associated with War Trauma

As a result of war, adults, who are likely to become parents, may display a wide variety of symptoms, ranging from posttraumatic disorders to depression and anxiety-related problems. Much of the work on war-related psychopathology has taken a diagnostic approach, concentrating in particular on what is defined as posttraumatic stress disorder (PTSD) (Kinzie *et al.*, 1990; Mollica *et al.*, 1990). Some authors, however, have rightly pointed out that the psychological effects of war cannot be reduced solely to posttraumatic symptoms (Danieli, 1985; Kestenberg, 1993), while others question the cross-cultural validity of PTSD as a category, which was established to deal with the specific problems that Vietnam veterans presented for American society (Richman, 1993).

It is well known that anxiety and depressive disorders take different forms in different cultures, whether in terms of the dominant clinical symptoms (somatization, depressive affect, dissociative reaction, etc.) or the importance attributed to the symptoms. Obeyesekere (1985) points out that among Buddhists, for example, anhedonia and low self-esteem are not considered to be symptoms but rather the end results of an internal progression.

In the case of posttraumatic disorders, cultural variability is just starting to be investigated. Many authors tend to assume that the symptoms of PTSD are universal (Kinzie, Sack, Angell, Manson, & Roth, 1986; Kinzie *et al.*, 1990), but some object to jumping to such conclusions. According to Eisenbruch (1991), in Cambodian refugees, nightmares and reliving experiences, for example, cannot be interpreted outside the framework of their traditional cultural significance, that is, a normal part of grieving for their Cambodian homeland. Rechtman (1992) points out that among survivors of the Pol Pot regime, the return of "ghosts" is not regarded as being pathological the way nightmares are in the West but is actually a normal occurrence when the dead have not been laid to rest with proper funeral rites.

Based on an ethnopsychological analysis of manifestations of distress in Salvadoran refugee women, Jenkins (1991) suggests that the political context mediates the way emotions associated with a traumatic situation are expressed. She shows how the culture of origin provides modes of expression of these emotions, called *calor* (heat) or *nervios* (nerves) in El Salvador. These categories are the main concern of trauma victims and their families, even if symptoms do actually fit DSM-IV–type diagnoses. Allodi (1989) notes that the Latin American refugee children in his study seemed to be fairly well protected against the effects of the trauma despite their parents' serious posttraumatic symptoms and raises the question of how the social context of the symptoms might potentially attenuate their impact.

Without going into too much detail about culturally determined variations in trauma symptomatology, it is interesting to consider which aspect of parental symptomatology is more likely to affect children: the symptoms identified using a classification from outside the group, or those that the group considers to be a problem. The impact of the parents' symptoms on the children should perhaps be examined as a function of the significance assigned to them: the difference between major depression and normal grieving, between dissociation and possession, between reliving traumatic experiences and the return of ghosts not properly laid to rest.

In looking at the possible impact of parental symptomatology on intergenerational transmission of trauma, the relationship between parents' symptoms and their ability to function must also be considered (Sack *et al.*, 1995). In both cases, the community's cultural definitions of what is normal and abnormal are certainly a crucial factor.

Influence of Culture on Changes in Family Dynamics Associated with War Trauma

The impact of trauma on families has been studied in many different contexts. The transmission of war trauma through changes in family dynamics is a central theme of research on the families of Vietnam veterans (Rosenheck & Nathan, 1985; see also Chapter 14, this volume). In her review of the question, Harkness (1993) points out the high rates of divorce, conjugal discord, and domestic violence in this population. After systemic analysis of the families, she classified them according to three characteristics: enmeshment, disengagement, and impulsivity and violence. Various family profiles have also been identified in work with Holocaust survivors (Danieli, 1985), but they are quite different from those of veterans' families, largely owing to the differences between the analytic and systemic models used. It seems clear, however, that contextual factors also play a central role in shaping family reactions. For instance, genocide driven by ethnic and religious motives does not have the same impact on the family as a lost war that nobody wants to talk about.

Yet even if fairly similar, prolonged armed conflicts are compared, there are still differences in the ways family dynamics change. In the case of Southeast Asia, for example, Tsoi, Gabriel, and Felice (1986) report that very high family cohesion seems to be the reason why few problems are observed in children whose families have been through many traumatic experiences in the Hong Kong refugee camps. This perception of a tightening of family ties, which are already very close in Southeast Asian cultures, is shared by several authors (Kinzie et al., 1986). Others, such as Ima and Hohm (1991), however, mention an increase in child abuse in Cambodian and Vietnamese families, the groups most affected by armed conflicts in Southeast Asia, and hypothesize that there may be an association between family violence and the social violence in their background. These disparities may partially reflect a discrepancy between what families say and what they actually do. Thus, as Sack et al. (1995) observe, Cambodian families tend not to report conflicts within the family or community, but this does not necessarily mean that they are not a problem.

Looking at Central America, several authors (Bottinelli, Maldonado, Troya, Herrera, & Rodriguez, 1990; Farias, 1991; Walter & Riedesser, 1993) clearly emphasize the possible link between family violence and conflict on the one hand, and armed violence on the other. Jenkins (1991, 1995) suggests that what she calls a "political ethos of violence" structures large areas of personal and social experience, particularly interpersonal and family relations. In her opinion, forms of domestic terror, such as the fear of being a victim of witchcraft, occur in parallel with forms of state-sanctioned terror. The repercussions of state-sanctioned violence within the family are different depending on the primary victim; in men, they take the form of physical violence against their wives and children, whereas in women, a tendency to overprotect the children is more often seen, although they also sometimes abuse them physically.

Traumatic phenomena associated with war therefore affect the degree of family cohesion and conflict, among other things. More specifically, cultural factors seem to have a direct influence on family conflicts or violence that may develop in the wake of traumatic events, and on the types of situations or times when the family closes ranks and becomes more cohesive.

Influence of Culture on Personal, Family, and Collective Meanings Associated with Trauma

Beyond the feeling of horror, inhumanity or, on the contrary, too much humanity (Girard, 1977) associated with the violence of war and armed conflict, individuals, families, and communities attach special meanings to trauma. These meanings make it easier, or sometimes more difficult, to situate a trauma within a community's common universe of meanings.

As Mollica (1988) says, these specific characteristics are reflected linguistically in the etymology of the words for torture, rape, and so on. Outside a context of war, Lefley, Scott, Llabre, and Hicks (1993) have shown how cultural beliefs associated with rape vary with the ethnic group concerned and influence the degree of acceptability and suitability of different types of intervention.

Although several interwoven etiological layers are usually involved in construing the meanings of trauma, more often than not, a single explanatory system predominates. For example, in the case of a traumatized person of Khmer origin, the healer looks for the source of a problem in one of three worlds: the world of ancestors, the world of humans, or the world of demons (Eisenbruch, 1992). But this does not exclude the possibility that both the person and the group may come up with sociopolitical explanations, complementary to the meaning–attribution systems and usually of secondary importance. Eisenbruch stresses the idea that the structure assigned to the social space in which the meaning of traumatic events is construed must be understood from an emic point of view,[1] rather than on the basis of categories corresponding to a Western vision that might lead to a misinterpretation of the relationships between the social, the political, and the religious.

From this perspective, it is interesting to consider how the discourse on trauma resulting from war or armed conflict in Central and South America is structured. In the last few decades, a Marxist sociopolitical language has clearly been dominant in the way people in general, and therapists in particular, talk about the meaning of trauma, but some groups have introduced issues of ethnic and racial identity, referring to the continuity and reenactment of the traumatic event since the conquest and colonization (Lebot, 1992).

More recently, with the collapse of traditional political models and oppositions, it appears that religious meanings that used to be very much of secondary importance are now regaining prominence in explicit discourse. It is highly likely, however, that, implicitly, religion has always been very important in assigning meaning in Latin America, although this has been partly denied (Lebot, 1992).

The complex way that various levels of meaning—collective, family, and personal—fit together, and their implicit or explicit nature, play a key role in the transmission of traumatic events as bearers of meaning and of a possible historical context for future generations. Much has been said and written, both by clinicians and researchers, on the subject of denial, taboo, secrecy, and avoidance in discourse on traumatic events of human origin (Bar-On, 1993; Danieli, 1982). The basic assumption of most of this theoretical and clinical work has been psychodynamic: that shedding light on reality could counteract the potentially harmful effects of the implicit transmission of trauma.

Cross-cultural comparisons may well make it necessary to call into question, at least in part, two aspects of this statement. First, it seems increasingly clear that in the case of trauma, we cannot speak of one reality, but must acknowledge that several meaningful realities may coexist. In writing about his own personal experience, Semprun (1994) clearly explains the impossibility of giving an objective account of the trauma of the concentration camps, and suggests that only through symbolization can the experience be transmitted and understood in all its complexity. Second, the ability to make the various meaningful realities coherent may have a greater impact on the child than whether what is transmitted is implicit or explicit (Antonovsky, 1986). The construction of this coherence, which is based both on what is said and left unsaid, no doubt differs with the equilibrium that each culture establishes between various means of expression and the extent of the group or family's desire to unify discourse around one meaningful reality or another.

Influence of Culture on the Reparative Process

As with most physical or mental problems, therapeutic responses and avenues offered by a community or society depend on how the problem is identified and the meanings assigned to it (Corin, Uchoa, Bibeau, & Koumare, 1992). The posttraumatic reparative process may therefore be individualized and medical, as it is in most Western countries, or it may be more group

[1]An emic perspective is the perception a community or a culture has of itself, in contrast with an etic perspective, which is the perception of a cultural group by an external person or group.

oriented and based on social issues. Work with Holocaust survivors, which has generated the most literature on the reparative process, provides a good illustration of both the development of psychoanalytical and therapeutic trends, and the centrality of religious and identity issues, among others.

In the case of Latin America, reparative processes are part of the universe of sociopolitical meanings attached to trauma. Bearing witness is viewed as therapeutic (Lira & Weinstein, 1984), and the collective strength of the protests of trauma victims as a lever for political change. A typical example is the downfall of the dictatorship in Argentina, partly as a result of pressure from the movement of mothers of the "disappeared," the *madres de la plaza de Mayo* (Kordon & Edelman, 1992).

In Southeast Asia, reparative processes involve more of a return to tradition: reestablishing links with ancestors, appeasing the spirits of the dead, and so on (Eisenbruch, 1988; Williams, 1991).

These processes, whether individual or collective, are ongoing, frequently lasting longer than the traumatic events themselves. The children and grandchildren of trauma victims have direct or indirect contact with these processes, or lack of them, and this may also have a structuring or destructuring effect on their lives.

METHOD

Context of Studies and Sampling Method

The first study involved 156 children aged 8–12, enrolled in Montreal elementary schools, and the second involved 158 adolescents in Montreal high schools.

Subjects were selected by systemic cluster sampling in seven elementary schools and six secondary schools with a high concentration of students of different ethnic backgrounds. Due to their minority status, such children in schools with a low ethnic concentration adapt differently than they would in schools with a high ethnic density; this could have introduced unwanted diversity in our samples. The schools chosen were all French-language public schools belonging to the two main school boards in Montreal. They are situated in parts of the city where housing is cheaper and newly arrived immigrants and refugees tend to concentrate, in other words, in relatively deprived socioeconomic areas. The schools were chosen according to two criteria: whether children born outside Canada made up more than 25% of enrollment (in some schools this figure reached 85%), and whether they had children from both the communities under study (Central Americans and Southeast Asians). Almost all schools contacted agreed to participate in the study.

Student enrollment records served as the basis for sampling, and the children were selected on the basis of the following four criteria:

1. Children must be from Southeast Asia (Cambodia or Vietnam in primary schools, Cambodia only in secondary schools) or Central America (Honduras, Guatemala, or El Salvador). Both these regions have endured prolonged armed conflicts, which makes them at least somewhat comparable in terms of premigration conditions; while there is no denying the significant national and local differences within these regions, each presents a certain cultural homogeneity. Given the differences between the characteristics of traumata of the Vietnamese and Cambodians, however, and the fact that the high-school sample was composed of only Cambodians, here, we will be discussing the quantitative data on the Cambodians alone ($n = 67$ elementary students, and $n = 76$ high-school students). It is important to note that all the

Central American families in the sample identified their culture as being Hispanic, or *Ladina* (non-Indian). There are very few refugees of Mayan origin in Canada for two reasons: the cost of migrating such a long distance, and their traditional attachment to the land, which means that they are more likely to choose a place of exile close to the land of their ancestors.

2. Children must be born outside Canada. Defining refugees on the basis of birth outside Canada served two purposes: first, it allowed the inclusion of children who arrived in Canada under a family reunification program but who were not themselves necessarily granted refugee status; second, it allowed the exclusion of children who did not directly suffer the tribulations of the premigration and migration processes, although their parents may themselves have been refugees.

3. For elementary schools, children must be in the third, fourth, fifth, or sixth grade in a regular or special class in one of the elementary schools chosen, that is, children between the ages of 8 and 12, approximately. For high schools, children must be in first or second year (seventh or eighth grade), that is, between the ages of 12 and 16, approximately.

Variables

The two studies gathered quantitative and qualitative data on variables characterizing the premigration period (traumata and separations) and postmigration period (family variables, immigration status, socioeconomic conditions, social network, and acculturation). In this chapter, we will be considering only a few of these variables, which can be divided into three categories:

- Those describing the children's emotional problems as perceived by the parents.
- Those describing the family history of traumata connected with the sociopolitical situation.
- Those that can mediate the effect of the family trauma on the children (intermediate variables).

Emotional Problems of Children and Adolescents. Emotional problems of children and adolescents were assessed using the version of the Child Behavior Checklist (CBCL) completed by parents. The psychometric features of this instrument have been described elsewhere (Achenbach & Edelbrock, 1983).

The CBCL has often been used in a multicultural context. Spanish translations have been validated in Chile and Puerto Rico (Bird, 1987). The CBCL is also available in Vietnamese and Cambodian. These translations enabled us to have the subjects' parents answer the questions in their native tongue, thus reducing any bias that might be due to a limited understanding of English or French.

In a transcultural context, the norms of North American instruments such as the CBCL may prove inadequate. Bird, Canino, Bould, and Ribera (1987) concluded that the CBCL is capable of effectively detecting the presence or absence of psychopathologies in Latin American children. It should be noted, however, that although the critical scores based on North American norms are sensitive enough in the case of Hispanic children, they do not seem to be specific enough. This may be due to differences between Hispanic and American children in type and severity of symptoms. Using the CBCL on an Asian Buddhist population, Weisz, Suwanlert, Chaiysit, Weiss, and Walter (1987; Weisz *et al.*, 1989) suggested that the problem posed by norms with Hispanic children also applies to Southeast Asian children, albeit in a different manner. For the purposes of our study, we followed the procedure used by Weisz *et al.* to compare the global mean internalizing and externalizing scores obtained by different groups. This procedure avoids the problem of the possible invalidity of norms based on other populations. We used the global scores to compare the general symptom profiles of the children in the two cultural groups being studied.

Family History of Trauma.   In order to assess the history of war traumata suffered in connection with an armed conflict, we used the same instrument as in an earlier study (Rousseau, Corin, & Renaud, 1989), that is, a trauma scale based on the Breslau and Davis (1987) model that takes into account the severity and number of traumata experienced by the family and by the child. The scale examines traumatic events arising within a context of war or armed conflict, as reported by key informants from the country or region concerned. The Latin American version of the instrument had been developed for use in a preliminary study (Rousseau *et al.,* 1989). The Cambodian version was constructed along the same lines. Rape was not studied directly since, after consultation with our key informants, we realized that a direct question on such a taboo subject would be too invasive in this type of interview. None of the respondents brought up rape spontaneously in relating the traumata experienced by the nuclear or extended family, which shows how much the topic is avoided, but this says nothing about how widespread rape is, although there is ample literature confirming its frequency (Khuong, 1988).

This history of traumata was assessed in terms of two raw scores that correspond to the number of traumata reported by the child and by his or her family before and after the birth of the child. This instrument can also weigh traumata according to severity, as established by key informants from the same culture with a good knowledge of the context of war or armed conflict. The various aspects of trauma that we examined are intensity of the familial trauma, the bond between the traumatized person and the child, and the child's age at the time of the trauma.

Analysis of our findings shows that for the Central Americans, there is a strong association between the severity of emotional problems and the total number of traumata reported (raw scores). At first glance, these findings seem to call into question the literature associating intensity of trauma and risk to mental health, and confirm, rather, the importance of the multiplicity of traumata on the development of psychiatric trauma (Terr, 1991). It should be noted, however, that the children and adolescents in our sample who have experienced many traumata either directly or indirectly have also, on the whole, experienced more severe traumata. We preferred to use only the raw scores, since they did not significantly change the results obtained, and we were not attempting to conduct an in-depth study of trauma measurement.

The emotional burden associated with events experienced during the premigration period was sometimes revealed by a vagueness in responding to questions about traumata, which could be seen as an avoidance strategy. Concern over retraumatizing the respondents forced the interviewers to respect this vagueness, which may reflect a difficulty inherent in trauma research (Danieli, 1982).

Intermediate Variables: Parental and Family Characteristics.   The literature on children in general, and refugee children in particular, mentions two salient indicators of family dynamics that can be influenced by contextual stress: family cohesion, which stands out as a protective factor (Tsoi *et al.,* 1986; Wolkind & Rutter, 1985), and conflict, which is a risk factor (Garmezy, 1983).

The selection of an appropriate instrument for measuring family dynamics was based on three criteria: potential for clearly assessing the dimensions of conflict and cohesion, respondent acceptance of the instrument, and cross-cultural suitability.

The Family Environment Scale (FES) developed by Moos and Moos (1986), which is used to evaluate global family behaviors without identifying specific actors (children or parents), is better suited than others to contexts where the rules governing interactions among family members do not correspond to the Western model. Moos and Moos note that the psychometric characteristics of the cross-cultural versions of the FES are highly comparable to those of the English version; the norms, however, may vary across ethnic groups. For this reason, we avoided using any cutoff point and considered the scale as a continuous measure. The Spanish version of the FES, which was developed and validated by Szapocznik, Kurtines, and Foote (1983), was used on our Central American sample, For the Cambodian sample, key informants from this ethnic group were recruited to translate the FES. The accuracy of this version was checked through back-translation.

Among the parental characteristics suggested as likely to transmit the impact of trauma from parents to children and adolescents, the level of parental depression stands out as particularly significant, owing to its direct repercussions on the emotional availability of parents (Barankin, Kostantaveas, & Bosset, 1989; Sigal, Silver, Rakoff, & Ellen, 1973). The Self-Rating Depression Scale developed by Zung (1969) was used to measure depression in our subjects' parents. The advantage of this scale is that the range of symptoms it measures does not focus on the more cognitive aspects of depression. This consideration is of particular interest in a cross-cultural context, where the cognitive/affective dimension may vary considerably. The Spanish version used was validated by Zung. The Cambodian translation was validated in the same way as the FES.

The following sociodemographic characteristics were documented: time in Canada, sponsorship (or lack of it), immigration status, income level, and employment status and command of host-country languages (French and English). Table 1 gives some of the sociodemographic characteristics of the sample.

We performed t tests and correlational analyses to investigate the relationships between CBCL scores, trauma scores, and family variables.

Qualitative Method

We gathered qualitative data on several aspects of the experiences of refugee families from the two communities under study in two ways. First, we did an ethnographic survey of parents and adolescents from the two communities. Second, we devised a semistructured interview covering key aspects of experiences: trauma suffered in their homeland and separations resulting from their exile, the acculturation process in different social spheres, and personal and family ideas of what the future held. For this part of the study, all elementary and high-school subjects were interviewed. The two sets of data were analyzed for content by comparing the Central American and Southeast Asian respondents, as well as the parents and the children. The following presents only the qualitative material most relevant to the question of intergenerational transmission, concentrating the analysis on two issues:

1. What the children, adolescents, and parents say and do not say about the trauma: Have the parents talked to their children about what happened? If now, why not? If so, what have they said? What do the children and adolescents know? What have they guessed? Would they like to know more about it or less? Does the family refer to the trauma in other, inexplicit ways?

2. The subjective desire to transmit the past: What do the parents wish or not wish to transmit about their origins and their past? What do the children and adolescents wish or not wish to hold on to?

Table 1. Sociodemographic Characteristics of Cambodian and
Central American Refugee Children and Adolescents

Sociodemographic characteristics	Children		Adolescents	
	Cambodian ($n = 67$)	Central American ($n = 56$)	Cambodian ($n = 76$)	Central American ($n = 82$)
Sex (%)				
Male	52.2	57.1	60.5	57.3
Female	47.8	42.9	39.5	42.7
Mean age (years)	10.3	10.7	13.7	14.4
Mean length of stay in Quebec (years)	5.2	5	9.8	6.6
Household income (%)				
Moderate	56.7	17.9	18.4	34.1
Low	43.3	82.1	81.6	65.9
Employment status of parents (%)				
Employed	38.8	71.4	40.8	46.3
Unemployed (both)	61.2	28.6	59.2	53.7
Mean size of household (people)	5.6	3.9	5	4.8
Type of household (%)				
Two-parent	91.0	71.4	72.4	64.6
Single-parent	9.0	28.6	27.6	35.4
Parents' educational level (%)				
Elementary	53.7	33.9	61.8	30.5
High school	46.3	58.1	35.5	59.8
University	—	7.1	2.6	9.8
Parents' French or English proficiency (%)				
Nil	10.4	8.9	14.5	8.5
Poor	89.6	64.3	75.0	63.4
Good	—	26.8	10.5	28.0

RESULTS

Nature and Intensity of Family Traumata

The trauma profile reported by the families varied according to geographic context. The greatest traumata in both number and severity, reported by Cambodian respondents for both the children and adolescents, were suffered before the birth of the child; for the Central Americans, trauma was worse after the birth (Tables 2 and 3). The traumata most frequently reported by the Cambodian respondents (Table 2) that occurred in the child's lifetime were confinement in a refugee camp (98.5% for children, 98.7% for adolescents) and fleeing their homeland on foot (43.3% for children, 30.3% for adolescents). The journey out of the homeland was fraught with peril. Some parents even reported leaving their older children with peasants met along the way, for fear they would die if they stayed with them. Forced labor

Table 2. Percentage of Families of Cambodian and Central American Refugee Children and Adolescents Having Experienced Trauma, by Type of Trauma and Time of Trauma

| | Children | | | | Adolescents | | | |
| | Cambodian (n = 67) | | Central American (n = 56) | | Cambodian (n = 76) | | Central American (n = 82) | |
Type of trauma	Before	After	Before	After	Before	After	Before	After
In homeland								
Persecution	1.5	1.5	7.1	46.4	10.5	6.6	6.1	51.2
Threats	11.9	4.5	1.8	39.3	34.2	10.5	6.1	63.4
Imprisonment	1.5	—	1.8	14.3	2.6	—	3.7	20.7
Execution	68.7	—	8.9	25.0	32.9	3.9	4.9	35.4
Torture	3.0	6.0	5.4	21.4	3.9	1.3	7.3	32.9
Disappearance	32.8	3.0	10.7	19.6	15.8	2.6	9.8	25.6
Forced labor	86.6	—	—	—	77.6	10.5	—	4.9
Violence witnessed by child	—	—	—	12.5	—	—	—	30.5
Other	3.0	4.5	7.1	39.3	47.4	36.8	1.2	62.2
During migration								
Crossing borders illegally	44.8	43.3	1.8	16.1	35.5	30.3	—	30.5
Attack by soldiers	13.4	9.0	—	—	19.7	18.4	—	9.8
Flight from country by boat	—	1.5	—	—	1.3	5.3	—	1.2
Other	46.3	37.3	1.8	28.6	38.2	35.5	1.2	50.0
Stay in refugee camp	—	98.5	—	—	—	98.7	—	1.2
Birth in refugee camp	—	53.7	—	—	—	52.6	—	—

(86.6% for children and 77.6% for adolescents) and the execution of a relative (68.7% for children and 32.9% for adolescents) were the most often reported family traumata that occurred before the birth of the child.

The main traumata in the child's lifetime, as reported by the Central American respondents, were persecution and threats for both the children and adolescents; execution and assassination (25.0% for children, 35.4% for adolescents), and torture (21.4% for children, 32.9% for adolescents) were also frequent. In addition, 19.6% of the children and 25.6% of the adolescents had a relative disappear. Fewer traumata were suffered before the birth of the child, and most of them in the adolescent sample involved difficulties in leaving the country, especially crossing national borders on foot.

If we consider traumata reported for the entire family, the respondents in the samples of both children and adolescents reported a greater number of traumata suffered by the nuclear family than by the extended family (Table 4). The Cambodian respondents in the children's sample were especially vague in identifying the members of the nuclear family who suffered traumata; 10.4% reported a trauma suffered specifically by the father of the child, 6.0% by the mother, and 1.5% by a sibling of the child, for a total of only 17%. The figure 95.5% is explained by the fact that respondents often reported that the entire family had suffered a trauma, particularly in connection with life in a refugee camp and crossing borders. The type of trauma reported by the Cambodian parents of this sample (i.e., associated with life in a refugee camp

Table 3. Means and Standard Deviation of CBCL Internalizing and Externalizing Scores, Trauma Scores, and Family Scores

	Children		Adolescents	
	Cambodian	Central American ($n = 56$)	Cambodian	Central American ($n = 82$)
CBCL scores				
Internalizing				
M	6.6	19.2	5.4	12.4
SD	4.2	13.9	3.7	8.1
Externalizing				
M	7.3	18.5	4.3	8.6
SD	4.6	13.5	4.3	8.6
Trauma index				
Before birth				
M	3.7	0.5	4.2	0.5
SD	1.8	1.3	2.8	1.3
After birth				
M	2.9	3.1	2.1	4.9
SD	1.5	2.9	2.9	3.3
Family scores				
Cohesion				
M	8.3	7.5	8.1	7.8
SD	1.0	1.2	(1.3)	(1.4)
Conflict				
M	1.4	1.8	0.8	1.6
SD	1.3	1.9	(1.1)	(1.6)
Parental depression				
M	38.2	31.6	36.1	32.9
SD	5.0	8.0	(6.0)	(8.7)

Table 4. Percentage of Families of Cambodian and Central American Refugee Children and Adolescents Having Suffered Trauma, by Relationship between the Trauma Victim and the Child

	Children		Adolescents	
	Cambodian ($n = 67$)	Central American ($n = 56$)	Cambodian ($n = 76$)	Central American ($n = 82$)
Trauma victim				
Nuclear family				
Father	10.4	55.4	42.1	46.3
Mother	6.0	25.0	32.9	19.5
Sibling	1.5	5.4	11.3	2.4
Entire nuclear family	95.5	64.3	80.3	48.8
Extended family				
Grandparent	20.9	7.1	9.2	13.4
Other family member	40.3	57.1	19.7	46.3
Entire extended family	52.2	14.3	67.1	41.5

and crossing borders on foot) would appear to be at the root of this discrepancy. Interestingly, however, the rates of trauma reported by the parents of Cambodian adolescents involving the father (42%) or mother (33%) are much higher than in the families of children.

In the case of Central American respondents, the profile of traumata suffered directly by parents is similar for both children and adolescents. As in the case of parents of Cambodian adolescents, more direct traumata involving the father than the mother were reported (Table 4).

Characteristics of Family Variables

According to the FES, from the parents' point of view, Cambodian families were more cohesive than Central American ones in both samples, while the conflict level did not vary significantly between the groups in the children's sample but was significantly higher in the Central American adolescent sample (Table 3). The level of parental depression was significantly higher among the Cambodians than among their Central American counterparts.

Association between Emotional Problems, Traumata, and Intermediate Variables

The association between the scores for traumata experienced before and after the birth of the child and the emotional symptoms reported by parents varied with the cultural group and stage of development (Table 5). For the Cambodians, there appears to be a significant association between the number of traumata experienced by the family after the birth of the child and internalizing problems only among adolescents. Further analysis reveals that the effect is sex-linked, and that it is adolescent Cambodian girls ($r = .47$; $p = .008$), for whom an increase in the number of family traumata is associated with an increase in internalized symptoms.

Among the Central Americans, there is a strong association between the number of traumata experienced by the family after the birth of the child and internalized and externalized symptoms in the children. The number of traumata before the child's birth is also significantly correlated to externalized symptoms in the children. For Central American adolescents, only the number of traumata after their birth is associated with internalized symptoms. The relationship between the number of traumata and emotional symptoms does not vary with sex for either Central American children or adolescents.

Table 5. Pearson's Correlation Coefficients between CBCL Internalizing and Externalizing Scores in Refugee Children and Adolescents and Trauma Occurring before and after the Birth of the Child

Timing of trauma	Children				Adolescents			
	Internalizing		Externalizing		Internalizing		Externalizing	
Cambodia								
Before birth	−.0577	(.643)	−.0315	(.800)	.0711	(.542)	.0297	(.799)
After birth	−.0594	(.633)	.1302	(.294)	.2433	(.034)	.1259	(.278)
Central America								
Before birth	.1825	(.178)	.2870	(.031)	.0690	(.538)	−.0380	(.735)
After birth	.5017	(<.000)	.4146	(.001)	−.0138	(.902)	.2279	(.039)

Note: Numbers in parentheses indicate two-tailed levels of significance.

Table 6. Pearson's Correlation Coefficients between Intermediate Family Variables and Trauma Occurring before and after the Birth of the Child

	Children			Adolescents		
Timing of trauma	Cohesion	Conflict	Parental depression	Cohesion	Conflict	Parental depression
Cambodia						
Before birth	−.2522	.0627	.0702	−.0566	.0610	.0062
	(.040)	(.614)	(.572)	(.627)	(.601)	(.958)
After birth	.1308	.0626	−.0105	−.0825	.0318	.3173
	(.291)	(.615)	(.933)	(.479)	(.785)	(.005)
Central America						
Before birth	.0226	.1026	.1039	−.0979	.0806	−.1555
	(.869)	(.452)	(.446)	(.382)	(.472)	(.163)
After birth	−.0900	.4406	.3379	.1362	−.1283	.1445
	(.510)	(.001)	(.011)	(.222)	(.250)	(.195)

Note: Numbers in parentheses indicate two-tailed levels of significance.

As in the case of emotional symptoms, the association between trauma scores and family variables that may modify the effect on the children varies with the ethnic group and the sample (Table 6).

In the Cambodian samples, there is a significant association between the number of traumata experienced before the birth of the child and low family cohesion in families of children, while the number of traumata after the birth is linked to the level of parental depression in the families of adolescents. For the families of Central American children, the number of traumata after the birth is associated with the degree of family conflict and parental depression. A similar association is not found in the families of adolescents, however (Table 6).

The three variables that describe the family—cohesion, conflict, and parental depression—are also associated in various ways with the emotional symptoms of the children and adolescents of both cultural groups (Table 7). Overall, in the case of Cambodian children and adolescents, a higher degree of family cohesion is associated with a decrease in emotional symptoms. Depression in Cambodian parents is also strongly associated with emotional problems, but only among adolescents. In Central American families, family conflict and parental depression are associated with emotional symptoms in children and adolescents, whereas the lack of family cohesion seems to play an insignificant role.

After controlling for significant intermediate family variables (conflict, cohesion, and parental depression) and length of time in Canada, partial correlations between traumata before and after the child's birth and emotional problems in Central American children and adolescents do not change in any meaningful way. For Cambodian adolescents, on the other hand, the correlation between traumata after the birth and internalized symptoms shrinks to insignificance when family cohesion, parental depression, and time in Canada are controlled for ($r = .24$; $p = .034$ before; $r = .14$; $p = .215$ after).

Further analysis shows that the relationship between trauma after the birth and internalized symptoms among Cambodian girls is still significant, even after controlling for family variables and length of time in Canada ($r = .47$; $p = .008$ before; $r = .38$; $p = .04$ after). Parental depression and length of time in Canada are partially responsible for the variation in the strength of the correlation.

Table 7. Pearson's Correlation Coefficients between Intermediate Family Variables and CBCL Internalizing and Externalizing Scores in Refugee Children and Adolescents

	Children			Adolescents		
CBCL scores	Cohesion	Conflict	Parental depression	Cohesion	Conflict	Parental depression
Cambodia						
Internalizing	−0.1993	0.1875	0.0946	−0.2182	0.1288	0.4383
	(.053)	(.064)	(.223)	(.058)	(.268)	(<.000)
Externalizing	−0.0668	0.2242	−0.1663	−0.4626	0.1515	0.4431
	(.296)	(.034)	(.089)	(<.000)	(.191)	(<.000)
Central America						
Internalizing	−0.1144	0.3456	0.3488	−0.2883	0.3978	0.3599
	(.200)	(.005)	(.004)	(.009)	(<.000)	(.001)
Externalizing	−0.1637	0.3295	0.1971	−0.0842	0.2297	0.2768
	(.114)	(.007)	(.073)	(.452)	(0.038)	(.012)

Note: Numbers in parentheses indicate two-tailed levels of significance.

RESULTS OF QUALITATIVE ANALYSIS

Implicit and Explicit Family Discourse on Trauma

Before going into the specific question of how the family refers to trauma, let us take a brief look at the major differences that have traditionally existed, independent of traumatic events, in parent–child communications in these two cultural groups.

The concept of respect is central to the parent–child relationship in both groups. For Southeast Asian families, respect is part of the code of conduct that governs all family and social relationships, and is embedded in a complex hierarchical structure. Relationships are fundamentally unequal, and the language reflects the fact that a person does not exist alone, but only as a function of all these relationships (Atlani, 1994). The Southeast Asian parents we met in the course of our research were very often puzzled by questions regarding what they had said to the child, or what was important to the child. The Southeast Asian interviewers also found it difficult to understand these questions that treated the child as an independent individual. The parents' answers reestablished the proper relationship: They were the ones who knew what was important for their children, or what they should think, and there was no point talking directly to their children about it.

In Central American families, respect is a type of consideration among family members that implies emotional closeness more than obedience. Dialogue, mutual understanding, and love are the signs of this respect.

In both communities, the way a family talks about trauma depends on preexisting patterns of intrafamily communications; it may reinforce them, or change them subtly, or even break them.

Southeast Asian Families. On the whole, the Southeast Asian parents rarely spoke to their children, of any age, about their traumatic past and the war. When they did, they tended to talk about family members who had not been "properly laid to rest" and whose spirits might still affect the living, or about their past poverty and hunger, so that the children would appreciate the gains they had made in the host country.

· The parents offered the following justifications for the fact that they had not told the children what was happening: They were too young, it would have been dangerous, they might have talked, it would have been pointless. Even now, they still speak only occasionally and anecdotally about the past, saying that there is no point, that the children/adolescents cannot understand, that the children/adolescents do not speak their native language well enough to talk about anything but day-to-day matters. Last, some parents say that their children are not interested, while others acknowledge that the children sometimes talk about it, but that they do not answer: "I let her talk and then that's the end of it."

Many Southeast Asian adolescents express a desire to know more about the family's past and the war. They mention that they feel left alone with their sketchy memories or vague impressions about things that might be secret. "There's nobody I can talk to" and "I think about it all the time" were comments often heard. Some ask their parents questions, but often get no reply: The television is on, their parents say they haven't the time or simply remain silent. Often, the adolescents accept this state of affairs as unchangeable, although they wish it were not.

Some adolescents acknowledged that they did not like "those stories," or said that their memories mixed with snatches of stories seemed unreal: "It's almost as if it never happened." They also seemed to have trouble talking to their friends about the past. One adolescent reported that his friends "don't believe it; they say it isn't true," or could not imagine that it could be true. He mentioned that some teachers at school were "curious," however.

More implicitly, parents acknowledged being afraid for their adolescents. Rape was frequently mentioned in adult conversation as a very real threat. A mother quoted this proverb: "Girls are like cotton: Once it falls in the mud, it's no good anymore. Boys are like gold: If it gets dirty, you just wash it off and it shines." The world outside the community was seen as threatening and violent, especially for girls. Unlike their parents, the adolescents did not see the source of the danger of violence as lying exclusively outside the community. A number of them admitted to being members of gangs from the community and committing violent acts within the community—facts that the parents seemed to be unaware of or denied. Although they did not explicitly mention the danger of rape, some adolescent girls expressed a need for male "protectors" against other men, and they sometimes chose gang members for this role.

Central American Families.   The Central American families spoke more of the past and history in their homeland than did the Asian families. Questions about the traumatic events and the war were often treated generally as *la politica,* or, in the case of El Salvador, *la situación.* Some parents expressed a desire to distance themselves from this history and *la politica,* whereas others had a desire to share their past political commitment and continue it through their children.

Many parents said that they had already explained to the children their departure and the misfortunes they had suffered as a result of the traumatic events. A fairly large number of these parents gave explanations that either skirted around the traumatic events ("I told him that we were going to visit his aunt," "We were going to Canada because her father was there") or were even false ("I told him we were going on vacation"), with the implicit goal of protecting either the child or the family's safety. A large number of parents said nothing to the children because they felt they were too young, because they did not want them to worry, or because they themselves were not psychologically up to it: "I went crazy." Some parents explained that they had said nothing because they had the impression that the children already knew what was going on.

After many years in the host country, parents were more willing to talk about what had happened in their homeland, although the desire to avoid painful memories and frequent political opposition within the family may limit what is actually said. The Central American adolescents often placed themselves at what they felt as a necessary distance from the past. They said that they remembered "enough," that they "know nothing about politics," even though they knew that their parents did. Some adolescents said that their parents had spoken to the older children and were waiting for the right time to tell them. They showed no impatience or desire to know more, and on the contrary, seemed much more comfortable at this relative distance.

Implicitly, despite the distance the families put between themselves and politics, which is strongly associated with armed violence, some concepts traditionally associated with the language of Central American political activism emerged very frequently. The concepts of equality and inequality, of discrimination and dominance, for example, partially structured family members' observations regarding relationships both within the community and outside it. Similarly, while material prosperity was generally viewed in a positive light, *el materialismo* was seen as one of the evils undermining family and community relations.

Subjective Desire to Transmit or Not Transmit the Past

Southeast Asian Families.   Southeast Asian parents wanted to pass on to their children the aspects of their culture of origin that define the code of acceptable conduct in the community, mostly emphasizing respect and obedience. Some parents defined the code of conduct in more detail: Specifically, their main concerns were the importance of not living together until after marriage, and behavior with respect to the opposite sex. Parents sometimes mentioned customs and religion, but they had little or no desire to pass on their native language. Religion was seen as protecting against the risks of future violence: "It preaches nonviolence and gratitude toward parents; it distinguishes between good and evil." Parents did not say that there were some aspects of their culture of origin that they did not wish to pass on to their children. Rather, anything negative (violence, extreme liberty, abandonment of parents) was attributed to the host community.

Southeast Asian adolescents appreciated and wished to hold on to the reserve, politeness, and respect that they felt characterized their culture of origin. Several questioned the lack of freedom and the frequent physical violence that they reported in parent–child relationships in their community. They had a less dichotomized view of the positive and negative aspects of their own culture, and of that of the host country, than did their parents.

Central American Families.   The main things Central American parents wanted to pass on to their children were their language and customs. Intrafamilial communication, love, and respect for parents were also seen as fundamental values that characterize the culture of origin and should be transmitted to the children. Central American parents named some aspects of their cultural heritage that they did not want to pass on: *machismo*, irresponsibility, laziness, submissiveness, and armed violence.

The Central American adolescents identified themselves as *Latinos*, and this identity is built up largely around language, birthplace, and, for some, a certain way of relating to others: "warmth . . . consideration." *Machismo* was mentioned as one of the negative aspects of the culture of origin. Many adolescents expressed contempt for and felt betrayed by those young people of their community who identify "too much" with Quebeckers.

Interestingly, in both cultural groups under study, there is a definite convergence of what parents wish to pass on to their children and what the adolescents value and consider to be the key aspects of their culture of origin. The numerous conflicts between refugee parents and adolescents seem to leave these spheres untouched for the most part, at least, as they are defined in theory. The two groups of parents take different approaches to the transmission of violence, with the Asians emphasizing the aspects of their own culture (e.g., religion) that protect them against violence and perceiving the risk of violence as coming from outside the community, while the Central Americans see the transmission of the violent social environment in which they used to live as a possible risk. One of the preventive strategies they have adopted seems to be to promote a distancing from politics and a new appreciation of religion. This importance of religion is not mentioned in most of the Latino-American studies of trauma. This may be explained in part by the fact that the majority of these consider population from the southern part of Latin America, where the religious phenomena may be less important than in Central American countries (Jenkins, 1991).

DISCUSSION

For a number of reasons, the quantitative and qualitative results of the two studies presented here must be interpreted with caution when it comes to understanding intergenerational transmission of trauma.

First, despite similarities in the sociodemographic and traumatic profiles of the samples of children and adolescents, this was not a longitudinal study, and differences between the patterns of associations between variables in the two samples may be caused, accentuated, or reduced by facts other than the child's stage of development. In particular, the differences in the traumata suffered directly by fathers or mothers of the Cambodian children and adolescents may be evidence of different degrees of direct exposure to war.

Moreover, for the two samples, there is an overlap between the traumata experienced before the birth of the child and those experienced afterward, often when the child was quite young. Although, in the case of very young children with no direct experience of the traumatic event, for whom transmission of trauma may well be very close to purely intergenerational, the fact remains that the association with other events, such as separations, makes these traumata different.

It should also be noted that the two groups display marked differences in exposure to family trauma before and after the child's birth. These differences may be due to a different degree of geographic proximity to the armed conflict and introduce some confusion as to whether cultural origin or contextual differences are more significant.

Other limitations have to do with the characteristics of the family variables examined: Only depression was studied; thus, parental symptomatology was not considered globally and other aspects of family dynamics could also have been studied.

Despite all these limitations, the observations made in these two studies raise some interesting questions about possible interactions between child development, cultural origin, and context of trauma in the family transmission of the impact of trauma.

The first question has to do with the possibility that family transmission of the impact of trauma is not a linear function of time elapsed since the trauma occurred, but that the culture of origin and different stages of the child's development play roles in mediating the relationship.

This hypothesis, which is backed up by observations on fluctuations in the relative importance of risk and protective factors at different stages of development (Werner, 1989), challenges the common assumption found in the literature that refugee children eventually become just like any other immigrants (Rumbaut, 1991), and that the impact of trauma decreases linearly with the passage of time. The relationship between family trauma and emotional problems seen in Central American youngsters remains constant if we control for time spent in the host country. Furthermore, in the case of the Cambodians, the appearance of emotional problems associated with the family trauma observed in adolescent girls can be attributed only partially to a variation in family dynamics (cohesion, conflict, parental depression) or to length of time in Canada. These variations could be partially due to the way the families of the two cultural groups talk about their traumatic past. The Central Americans talk more explicitly about the trauma, and in the younger children, this seems to be associated with a greater invasion of the child's emotional world. The Central American adolescent distanced themselves, which could be a protective avoidance mechanism. Among the Southeast Asians, the silence surrounding the past seems to protect the children at first, but indirect references to the past through allusions to rape seem to have an impact on anxiety and depression levels in pubescent girls. This indirect reference, which could also be termed a return of the repressed, seems to breach the relative protection provided by silence, which also served as an avoidance mechanism.

Another question has to do with the patterns in which family variables such as parental symptomatology or family dynamics are involved in transmission. The results of our two studies of Central American children and adolescents suggest that trauma may sometimes affect the family climate, which in turn had a major impact on the symptoms displayed by children and adolescents. The impact of trauma on children, both before and after birth, seems to be relatively independent of these family conditions, however. What is more, the association between family climate and trauma does not appear to be immutable, even for two samples of the same ethnic origin having fairly comparable trauma profiles. This underscores the need to try to understand the relationship between trauma, conflict, and family cohesion in all its complexity.

A third and final question concerns the establishment of continuity between past and present, between children and parents, beyond the ruptures caused by traumata and migration.

The literature on adolescent immigrants and refugees has greatly emphasized the importance of intergenerational conflict and the gap created by the fact that young people are acculturated much more quickly than their parents. The convergence seen in the qualitative data between what parents wish to pass on of their culture and what adolescents value highlights another dimension: the means of establishing continuity based on cultural anchors that help them cope with rupture. This continuity, which should be investigated to determine whether it is only paid lip service or actually influences behavior, may develop in parallel to many conflicts about everyday matters. Given the many losses these populations have to come to terms with, it is possible that continuity may play a protective role and facilitate the inevitable grieving process that Eisenbruch (1988) calls "cultural bereavement."

In the way they talk about the transmission of trauma to their children, both cultural groups studied seem to employ strategies that could be described as "preventive neutralization," although the two groups differ radically in where they feel this violence is rooted. The Central Americans see violence as existing within the community, and they talk openly about the risk of transmission and the need to avoid it. The Southeast Asians, on the other hand, see violence as chiefly coming from the outside world and being transmitted to children and adolescents through bad influences when they breach the code of conduct.

Although the two communities' strategies to counter the spread of violence differ in form—a code of conduct as opposed to respect and mutual understanding—they are similar when it comes to refocusing on values considered to be characteristic of the culture of origin that subjectively underlie family cohesion and strength.

CONCLUSION

Research into the interactions of culture and context in the intergenerational transmission of trauma is only just beginning, and a great deal remains to be done to develop a better idea of their specific roles.

An understanding of intergenerational transmission of trauma in light of the strategies devised by various cultures may not only enhance our prevention and intervention efforts for those suffering the consequences of direct or indirect trauma but may also open up avenues for understanding how the hate and hostility that underlie many modern conflicts as much as, if not more than, immediate economic interests, have been passed on from time immemorial.

REFERENCES

Achenbach, T. M., & Edelbrock, C. (1983). *Manual for the Child Behavior Checklist and Revised Child Behavior Profile*. Burlington, VT: University of Vermont Department of Psychiatry.

Allodi, F. (1989). The children of victims of political persecution and torture: A psychological study of a Latin American refugee community. *International Journal of Mental Heath, 18*(2), 3–15.

Antonovsky, A. (1986). Intergenerational networks and transmitting the sense of coherence. In N. Data, A. L. Greene, & H. W. Reese (Eds.), *Life-span developmental psychology: Intergenerational relations*. Hillsdale, NJ: Erlbaum.

Atlani, L. (1994). *Les adolescents d'origine Vietnamienne réfugiés à Montréal: Acculturation et événements traumatiques*. Thèse de maitrise. Paris: Université de Paris IV.

Bar-On, D. (1993). Children as unintentional transmitters of undiscussable traumatic life events. Paper presentedat the Conference on Children: War and Persecution. Hamburg, Germany.

Barnakin, T., Konstantaveas, M., & Bosset, F. (1989). Adaptation of recent Soviet Jewish immigrants and their children to Toronto. *Canadian Journal of Psychiatry, 34*(6), 512–518.

Bird, H. R., Canino, G., Bould, M. S., & Ribera, J. (1987). Use of the behavior checklists as a screening instrument for epidemiological research in child psychiatry: Results of a pilot study. *Journal of the American Academy of Child and Adolescent Psychiatry, 26*(2), 207–213.

Bottinelli, M. C., Maldonado, I., Troya, E., Herrera, P., & Rodriguez, C. (1990). *Psychological impacts of exile: Salvadoran and Guatemalan families in Mexico*. Washington, DC: Center for Immigration Policy and Refugee Assistance, Georgetown University.

Breslau, N., & Davis, G. C. (1987). Post-traumatic stress disorder: The etiologic specificity of wartime stressors. *American Journal of Psychiatry, 144*(5), 578–583.

Corin, E., Uchoa, E., Bibeau, G., & Koumare, B. (1992). Articulation et variations des systèmes de signes, de sens et d'action. *Psychopathologie Africaine, 24*(2), 183–204.

Danieli, Y. (1982). *Therapists' difficulties in treating survivors of the Nazi Holocaust and their children* (Doctoral dissertation, New York University, 1981). *University Microfilms International*, No. 949–904.

Danieli, Y. (1985). The treatment and prevention of long-term effects and intergenerational transmission of victimization: A lesson from Holocaust survivors and their children. In C. R. Figley (Ed.,), *Trauma and its wake* (pp. 295–313). New York: Brunner/Mazel.

Eisenbruch, M. (1988). The mental health of refugee children and their cultural development. *International Migration Review, 22*(2), 282–300.

Eisenbruch, M. (1991). From post-traumatic stress disorder to cultural bereavement: Diagnosis of Southeast Asian refugees. *Social Science and Medicine, 33*, 673–680.

Eisenbruch, M. (1992). The ritual space of patients and traditional healers in Cambodia. *BEFEO, 79*(2), 283–316.

Farias, P. J. (1991). Emotional distress and its socio-political correlates in Salvadoran refugees: Analysis of a clinical sample. *Culture, Medicine and Psychiatry, 15*, 167–192.

Garmezy, N. (1983). Stressors of childhood. In N. Garmezy & M. Rutter (Eds.), *Stress, coping and development* (pp. 43–84). New York: McGraw-Hill.

Girard, R. (1977). *Violence and the sacred*. Baltimore: Johns Hopkins University Press.

Green, B. L., Korol, M., Grace, M. C., Vary, M. G., Leonard, A. C., Gleser, G. C., & Smitson-Cohen, S. (1991). Children and disaster: Age, gender, and parental effects on PTSD symptoms. *Journal of the American Academy of Child and Adolescent Psychiatry, 30*(6), 945–951.

Ima, K., & Hohm, C. F. (1991). Child maltreatment among Asian and Pacific Islander refugees and immigrants. *Journal of Interpersonal Violence, 6*(3), 267–285.

Jenkins, J. H. (1991). The state construction of affect: Political ethos and mental health among Salvadoran refugees. *Culture, Medicine and Psychiatry, 15,* 139–165.

Jenkins, J. H. (1995). An anatomy of cruelty locating violence in civil and domestic war. Paper presented at the Canadian Anthropological Association meeting.

Kaufman, J., & Zigler, E. (1989). The intergenerational transmission of child abuse. In D. Cicchetti & V. Carlson (Eds.), *Child maltreatment: Theory and research on the causes and consequences of child abuse and neglect* (pp. 129–150). Cambridge, UK: Cambridge University Press.

Kestenberg, J. S. (1993). The diversity of child survivors of the Holocaust. Paper presented at the Conference on Children: War and Persecution. Hamburg, Germany.

Khuong, D. T. (1988). Victims of violence in the South China Sea. In D. Miserez (Ed.), *Refugees: The trauma of exile: The humanitarian role of Red Cross and Red Crescent* (pp. 18–38). Dordrecht, The Netherlands: Martinus Nijhoff.

Kinzie, D., Sack, H. W., Angell, H. R., Manson, S., & Roth, B. (1986). The psychiatric effects of massive trauma on Cambodian children: I. The children. *Journal of the American Academy of Child and Adolescent Psychiatry, 25*(3), 370–376.

Kinzie, J. D., Boehnlein, J. K., Leung, P. K., Moore, L. J., Riley, C., & Smith, D. (1990). The prevalence of posttraumatic stress disorder and its clinical significance among Southeast Asian refugees. *American Journal of Psychiatry, 147*(7), 913–917.

Kleinman, A. (1988). *Rethinking psychiatry.* New York: Free Press.

Kordon, D., Edelman, L. I., Lagos, D. M., Nicoletti, E., & Bozzolo, R. C. (1988). *Psychological effects of political repression.* Buenos Aires: Sudamericana/Planeta Publishing Company.

Lebot, Y. (1992). *La guerre en terre Maya. Communauté: Violence et modernité au Guatemala.* Paris: Karthala.

Lefly, H. P., Scott, C. S., Llabre, M., & Hicks, D. (1993). Cultural beliefs about rape and victims' response in three ethnic groups. *American Journal of Orthopsychiatry, 63*(4), 623–632.

Harkness, L. (1993). Transgenerational transmission of war-related trauma. In J. P. Wilson & B. Raphael (Eds.), *International handbook of traumatic stress syndromes* (pp. 635–643). New York: Plenum Press.

Lira, E., & Weinstein, E. (1984). *Psicoterapía y represión politica.* Mexico City: Siglo Veintiuno.

Lykes, M. B., & Farina, J. J. (1992). *Niños y violencia política. Dossiers bibliograficos en salud mental y derechos humanos.* Buenos Aires: Editado por Centró de Documentación.

Martín-Baró, I. (1994). War and the psychosocial trauma of Salvadoran children. In A. Aron & S. Corne (Eds.), *Writings for a liberation psychology* (pp. 122–135). Cambridge, MA: Harvard University Press.

Mollica, R. F. (1988). The trauma story: The psychiatric care of refugee survivors of violence and torture. In F. M. Ochberg (Ed.), *Post-traumatic therapy and victims of violence* (pp. 295–314). New York: Brunner/Mazel.

Mollica, R. F., Wyshak, G. Lavelle, J., Truong, T., Tor, S., & Yang, T. (1990). Assessing symptom change in Southeast Asian refugee survivors of mass violence and torture. *American Journal of Psychiatry, 147*(1), 83–88.

Moos, H. R., & Moos, S. B. (1986). *Family environment scale manual* (2nd ed.). Palo Alto, CA: Consulting Psychologists Press.

Obeyesekere, G. (1985). Depression, Buddhism, and the work of culture in Sri Lanka. In A. Kleinman & B. Good (Eds.), *Culture and depression: Studies in the anthropology and cross-cultural psychiatry of affect and disorder* Berkeley: University of California Press.

Pynoos, R. S., & Eth, S. (1985). Children traumatized by witnessing acts of personal violence: Homicide, rape or suicide behavior. In R. S. Pynoos & S. Eth (Eds.), *Post-traumatic stress disorder in children* (pp. 168–186). Washington, DC: American Psychiatric Press.

Rechtman, R. (1992). L'apparition des ancêtres et des défunts dans les expériences traumatiques: introduction à une ethnographie clinique chez les réfugiés cambodgiens de Paris. *Cahiers d'Anthropologie et Biométrie Humaine, 10*(1–2), 1–19.

Richman, N. (1993). Annotation: Children in situations of political violence. *Journal of Child Psychology and Psychiatry, 34*(8), 1286–1302.

Rosenheck, R., & Nathan, P. (1985). Secondary traumatization in children of Vietnam veterans. *Hospital and Community Psychiatry, 36*(5), 538–539.

Rousseau, C., Corin, E., & Renaud, C. (1989). Conflit armé et trauma: Une étude clinique chez des enfants réfugiés Latino-Américains. *Canadian Review of Psychiatry, 34,* 376–385.

Rumbaut, R. G. (1991). The agony of exile: A study of the migration and adaptation of Indochinese refugee adults and children. In F. L. Ahearn, Jr. & J. L. Athey (Eds.), *Refugee children: Theory, research, and services* (pp. 53–91). Baltimore: Johns Hopkins University Press.

Sack, W. H., Clarke, G. N., Kinney, R., Belestos, G., Chanrithy, H., & Seeley, J. (1995). The Khmer adolescent project: II. Functional capacities in two generations of Cambodian refugees. *Journal of Nervous and Mental Disease, 183*(3), 177–181.

Semprun, J. (1994). *L'écriture ou la vie.* Paris: Gallimard.

Sigal, J. J., Silver, D., Rakoff, V., & Ellen, J. (1973). Some second generation effects of survival of the Nazi persecution. *American Journal of Orthopsychiatry, 43*(3), 320–327.

Solkoff, N. (1992). Children of survivors of the Nazi Holocaust: A critical review of the literature. *American Journal of Orthopsychiatry, 62*(3), 342–358.

Szapocznik, J., Kurtines, M. W., & Foote, H. F. (1983). Some evidence for the effectiveness of conducting family therapy through one person. *Journal of Consulting and Clinical Psychology, 51*(6), 889–899.

Terr, L. C. (1991). Childhood traumas: An outline and overview. *American Journal of Psychiatry, 148,* 10–21.

Tsoi, M. M. Y., Gabriel, K. K., & Felice, L. M. (1986). Vietnamese refugee children in camps in Hong Kong. *Social Science and Medicine, 23*(11), 1147–1150.

Vinar, M. U. (1993). Children affected by organized violence in South America. Paper presented at the Conference on Children: War and Persecution. Hamburg, Germany.

Walter, J., & Riedesser, P. (1993). Why has my father changed? Children, fathers, persecution and exile. Paper presented at the Conference on Children: War and Persecution. Hamburg, Germany.

Weiss, E., O'Connell, A. N., & Siites, R. (1986). Comparisons of second generation Holocaust survivors, immigrants, and non-immigrants on measures of mental health. *Journal of Personality and Social Psychology, 50,* 828–831.

Weisz, J. R., Suwanlert, S., Chaiyasit, W., Weiss, B., Achenback, T. M., & Trevathan, D. (1989). Epidemiology of behavioral and emotional problems among Thai and American children: Teacher reports for ages 6–11. *Journal of Child Psychology and Psychiatry, 30*(3), 471–484.

Weisz, J. R., Suwanlert, S., Chaiyasit, W., Weiss, B., & Walter, B. R. (1987). Over- and undercontrolled referral problems among children and adolescents from Thailand and the United States: The Wat and Wai of cultural differences. *Journal of Consulting and Clinical Psychology, 55*(5), 719–726.

Werner, E. E. (1989). High-risk children in young adulthood: A longitudinal study from birth to 32 years. *American Journal of Orthopsychiatry, 59*(1), 72–81.

Williams, C. L. (1991). Toward the development of preventive intervention for youth traumatized by war and refugee flight. In F. L. Ahearn, Jr. & J. L. Athey (Eds.), *Refugee children: Theory, research, and services* (pp. 201–217). Baltimore: Johns Hopkins University Press.

Wolkind, S., & Rutter, M. (1985). Separation, loss and family relationships. In M. Rutter & L. Hersov (Eds.), *Child and adolescent psychiatry.* Oxford, UK: Blackwell Scientific Publications.

Zung, W. W. K. (1969). A cross-cultural study of symptoms in depression. *American Journal of Psychiatry, 126,* 154–159.

29

The Second Bullet

Transgenerational Impacts of the Trauma of Conflict within a South African and World Context

MICHAEL A. SIMPSON

And death is no longer a chance event. To be sure, it still seems a matter of chance whether a bullet hits this man or that, *but a second bullet may well hit the survivor,* and the accumulation of death puts an end to the impression of chance.

SIGMUND FREUD (1915, pp. 291–292)

The only way to stop feeling so bad is a new kill.

—SOUTH AFRICAN PERPETRATORS AND THEIR CHILDREN

Few people have had access to Southern Africa's most feared perpetrators, members of the notorious killing team called Koevoet, an "antiguerrilla" group of the South African army, which fought in Namibia. Members wore T-shirts inscribed "Murder is our business: And business is good!" "Sometimes we killed them quickly, sometimes we killed them slowly. . . . We felt fantastic. We drank a beer and said a short prayer: 'Thank you, Lord.' " The group killed large numbers of black guerrillas representing the Namibian forces that now govern that country. These former killers speak of the satisfaction it gave them, commenting, "After a day, you must have another *kill,* to feel the adrenaline in your blood."

Braam (1994), with the assistance of myself and others, conducted one of the very few studies of these perpetrators. They describe routine atrocities, which give a thrill they liken to that of drugs: "You get addicted to it, you can't do without it." They speak nostalgically of the kick of describing the latest kill at the bar with your mates, and of knowing they had survived he episode. After each kill, they talk of standing in silent prayer: "Thank you, Lord, for taking this life." They talk of experiencing withdrawal symptoms when they inadvertently went

---

Note: This chapter is dedicated to Hlalanathi Sibankulu, Legai Pitje, and other friends who were assassinated, and were thus not allowed to join us in solving today's problems of freedom.

MICHAEL A. SIMPSON • National Centre for Psychosocial and Traumatic Stress, P.O. Box 51, Pretoria 0001, South Africa

International Handbook of Multigenerational Legacies of Trauma, edited by Yael Danieli. Plenum Press, New York, 1998.

a week without a "kill." Between deaths, they describe feeling a depression, and "the only way to stop feeling so bad is a new kill. But as that becomes more normal, more usual, you need still more, it must be more gruesome" (e.g., Braam, 1994, p. 42). "Maybe I became mad. . . . I have photos in which I drag the brains out of someone's head. I would so much like you to see that. You must see the photos." No one teaches them to stop killing. They describe classic symptoms of posttraumatic stress disorders (PTSD). Some burned their trophies and photographs; some still treasure them. They watch war—the Gulf War, Bosnia—endlessly on television, watching CNN all night during the active phases of such warfare, though it brings back the nightmares.

One showed his albums of color pictures: holidays, a wedding—and kills. His 5-year-old son was watching and obviously thoroughly familiar with them as he showed the pictures, six per page, page after page, of bodies with huge gaping wounds. He described with expert relish which weapons caused which wounds. Then another album, and another. Bodies split open, spilling their contents. "I sometimes wonder if there's something wrong in my head." The boy is undisturbed: "Show my favourite video, Papa!" This video shows the orgiastic final days of killing: prisoners walk miserably between Koevoet soldiers. "Kaffirs!" exclaims the boy. "Terrorists," corrects the father. Now, the prisoners are on the ground, twitching, bleeding, dead. Hundreds of bodies, now being pulled together and posed in weird postures. When the video is completed, he sends the boy to bed, and continues talking about his experiences.

In 1989, toward the end of the 23-year-war, there was a United Nations-overseen ceasefire. When young Southwest African People's Organization (SWAPO) soldiers (members of the liberation forces) crossed into the territory to give themselves up to UNTAG (United Nations) forces, Koevoet soldiers killed over 300, mostly by close-quarter shots in the head. The bodies were dumped into massed graves. Soon afterward, the group was officially disbanded, and millions of rands were spent on "golden handshakes" (tax-free retirement gratuities) to the 613 members. They had earlier kept a scoreboard of "kills," and were paid Kopgeld (literally, head-cash) bonuses per body, dead or alive: R 1,000 for a SWAPO fighter, R 500 for his gun, and so on: killing on commission. It was easier to kill and bring back the body for the bonus than to try to bring back a live "Terr." The bodies would be tied to the vehicle bumper or to the spare wheel, like hunters returning with deer, except that they had been hunting humans. But live captives were also valued by their "security force" bosses. According to one source, these were used to test torture and interrogation techniques, as well as to get information. The prisoners, kept in solitary confinement, were formally paid R 20 per month, so that they could be accounted for as in the service of the South African forces, and thus not be available for Red Cross access. "Koevoet took no prisoners of war: only new recruits," says one.

Suicide is quite common in Koevoet veterans. The survivors complain of hearing of the suicide of old comrades: "To Hell with this world." They have been candid, and feel relieved to speak of things they have done, what they describe as things you can't talk of, even with your own wife. They feel there is no place for them in the "new South Africa," having seen their former enemies form the governments of Namibia and South Africa, and they resent the lack of recognition and gratitude for their deeds. "No one understands us," they complain. More recently, we have been consulted by members of the radical black "Self-Defense Units" (see below), wholly on the other side of the political spectrum in Koevoet. They have no photo albums but describe the same symptoms, and complain in the same way, of a high suicide rate.

INTRODUCTION

Myth and legend have a reliable record of revealing insights that scientists have taken centuries to rediscover laboriously. In Africa, traditional beliefs have always emphasized the continuing and active relevance of the ancestors in current life affairs and the lasting contamination caused by violence and trauma. Similarly, as Goodwin (1993) and especially Robbins (1993) have shown, gross intergenerational cycles of violence were a consistent and basic feature of the ancient Greek legends. Robbins impressively retells the case of Oedipus, for example, as "part of a pattern of continuing multigenerational familial dysfunction in a violent lineage noted for breaching norms, biological as well as societal" A long litany of matricide, parricide, filicide, incest, rape, bestiality, war, and assassination, with children abused, abandoned, and killed, is a central thread in these complex tales of human and social misery. We vary in what we learned from myths such as the story of Oedipus. Freud and others emphasized the enduring intrapersonal and intergenerational reverberations of such trauma; more recently, we have accepted the long-lasting interpersonal and multigenerational effects among family members. Albeck (1994), himself a second-generation survivor, who has provided a usefully critical review of the concept of intergenerational consequences of trauma and agrees with this point of view, says, "Until very recently, psychological explanations for trauma's effects have tended to focus on intrapsychic factors at the expense of the interactive social, political, and historical aspects" (p. 109).

This understanding of the individual principally within the full context of family, community, and nation, is basic to our African worldview. Figley (1995) admits that much of the traumatology literature "is dominated by Western-oriented conceptions" and focused "almost exclusively on individual functioning" But he then enlarges this viewpoint only so far as to include individual families, calling this "systemic PTSD." However, this is a similarly Western limitation, which still ignores the larger systems of community and nation, within which such traumatic reactions are always contextually embedded. Similarly, Westermeyer (1995), though discussing cross-cultural aspects of trauma care, fails to grasp the issues from anything but a profoundly Western and Eurocentric viewpoint.

In this chapter, I wish not only to explore those aspects of the traumatic experiences of South Africa, but also to emphasize the remaining, and even more widely ignored, dimension (so clearly represented in so many early myths): the abiding effects of unresolved conflict on communities and nations. The continuing sociopolitical fallout of individual and larger social forms of violence and trauma, generating lasting multigenerational cycles of trauma, are a significant historical force deserving study by clinical and psychological experts, as well as historical and political commentators. I explore the fact that there are clear societal changes in the wake of major traumatic historical events that are highly analogous to the individual symptoms of posttraumatic disorders. Our growing understanding of PTSD and trauma reactions can advance our understanding of history, and an understanding of history can assist us in comprehending individual and community responses to trauma.

THE TRAUMA OF CHANGE

Since 1987, researchers have concentrated greatly on PTSD, which has proved such a fruitful concept, but have too often overlooked the fact that there are a variety of other posttraumatic syndromes. There is what has been called "complex PTSD" (Herman, 1992), and "partial PTSD" [in patients who persistently suffer from severe PTSD symptoms without fully meeting the diagnostic criteria of the DSM-IV (American Psychiatric Association, 1994) at one point in time]. Even more neglected, there are posttraumatic dissociation disorders, and posttraumatic somatization disorders, identity problems, repetition compulsions, reexposure problems, and others. For years, I have emphasized (e.g., Simpson, 1993c) that there are broader and consistent patterns of communal response to trauma, in-group and community posttraumatic pathologies, which often contribute significantly to continuing social unrest and violence.

Just as Danieli (1984) emphasized countertransference reactions among therapists in individual psychotherapy with Holocaust survivors, so I have described (Simpson 1993c, and elsewhere) similar patterns of denial in social and professional responses to the facts and victims of repression. Disguised by a pretense of neutrality, most world health workers and general citizens ignore widespread abuses of human rights, fail to take even those actions readily open to them that would discourage such abuses, and maintain friendly and profitable relationships with perpetrators and collaborators while avoiding victims. In the face of evil events, doing nothing, or ignoring the facts, is not being neutral: It is giving essential support to the perpetrators. There are not two sides to every issue. No one feels bound to be neutral toward cancer or to balance evenly the needs of the patient and the cancer, or to be neutral toward child abuse, or earthquakes: Why should repression and torture be more privileged? Even the most rabid eco-fanatics, who have argued that the preservation of every species (however obscure) is a higher priority than regular human needs, have not mounted a "Save the Smallpox" campaign.

Innovation and transition are stressful, even when voluntary, planned, desired, and occurring in safe settings. How much more is the pathological impact when they are involuntary, unplanned, ambivalently welcomed, and in situations of long-lasting instability. The prospect (Simpson, 1993c) of giving up the relative predictability of a familiar repression for the uncertainty of an unpredictable future, which may certainly be different but may not necessarily be better, is daunting. Getting what you have struggled and suffered for, for decades, and discovering that it is not as sweet and satisfying as you dreamed it would be, magnifies the effect.

Marris (1974), in an often overlooked book, described "anxieties of change" in situations that are individually or communally traumatic. Relevant to the situations in South Africa and in former Yugoslavia, he discussed tribalism as a response of those who lose their bearings in a heterogenously changing society. They cling to natural or invented "national" group identities, which they relate to a past that is only partly realistic (but usually irrelevant to current needs) and largely mythological. One sees the invention of "instant traditions": new practices, designed to resemble ancient historic forms and claimed as evidence of archaic status. Retreating within such tribal boundaries enables them to project their ambivalence, fears, and internal conflicts on the rest of society at large and especially upon close neighbors. They become organized around an ideology of inevitable conflict in which they see themselves as brave and innocent martyrs, valiantly withstanding an onslaught from barbarian hordes external to themselves and unable to comprehend the mystic centrality of their ethnic purity. At the social level, this variation of the typical process of "blaming the victim" is even more malignant. Those people who are the prime and continuing cause of conflict and its exacerbation, often the actual perpetrators of human rights abuses, are able to portray themselves as victims of those they are in fact victimizing.

SOCIAL RESPONSES TO CONFLICT AND WAR

There is a German term *vergangenheitsbewältigung,* referring to the attempt to come to terms with the past, a necessary exercise for nations and communities, as well as individuals. In 1994–1995, the popular literature was full of articles about the strong and persistent memories, including vivid negative emotions, evoked by anniversaries of World War II. It seemed widely agreed, as Jackson (1994a) wrote, that "50 years is not long enough to dissipate the bitterness of Allied soldiers who suffered" (p. 37). There were demonstrations and protests, and demands for apologies and other acts demonstrating repentance and regret by representatives of the perpetrators of past trauma. This provided a poignant backdrop to the very opposite situation in South Africa, where the millions of victims of a much longer, as well as more recent, period of severe suffering were being lectured by their new rulers to forget promptly and to stop referring to their pain. In the dubious name of "national reconciliation" (no one has yet explained how you can achieve reconciliation of groups that have never before been conciliated), they were told to "forgive and forget." No one in power, neither the representatives of the old regime still sharing government, nor the new figures who were once leaders of the liberation movement, showed any sign of recognizing the impossibility of commanding such complex emotional responses or of requiring such intricate sociocultural processes.

Similarly, while there was also broadly expressed consensus that, as Jackson (1994b) wrote, applying to the Balkan tragedy the lessons of World War II, the war-crimes trials held in Germany and Japan after World War II set the standards for such proceedings, establishing the principle that leaders may be held responsible for atrocities committed during the conflict. In contrast, in South Africa, politicians of all parties, with striking and unusual unanimity, announced that "of course" nothing resembling the Nuremberg Trials was conceivable in the South African situation. Recent studies of the lasting effects of national as well as individual guilt (e.g., Buruma, 1995; Heimannsberg & Schmidt, 1993) are highly relevant to the South African situation. Rarely has such a widespread and deliberate failure to learn from history been so obvious. Some may fondly imagine that this was a noble response, springing entirely from virtuous motives. This would have been easier to believe if those who waxed so eloquent about "forgiveness" had anything they personally needed to forgive, and if none of the politicians who reached this rogues' accord were in any way at risk of appearing before such Tribunals. Perhaps it was more cynical realism: Who, after all, were or will be tried or punished for the atrocities in Cambodia, El Salvador, Lebanon, Tibet, Somalia, and the many other killing fields of this century? Perhaps a Nuremberg resolution requires that the victims are on the side that wins a decisive ultimate victory, a rare situation.

CULTURAL ASPECTS OF RESPONSES TO TRAUMA IN AN AFRICAN SETTING

There are broad similarities in relevant cultural beliefs about how the dead influence the living, surely the primal instance of transgenerational impacts of trauma. The comparative anthropological studies of Fraser (e.g., 1933/1934/1936/1937) illustrate this. There has been widespread belief that those who have died traumatically can and do return to wreak vengeance on those living who were responsible, and mutilation of the dead to seek to prevent knowledge that this has been a common practice (see, e.g., Fraser 1934, Vol. 2, pp. 75–96, citing examples in Europe). There is a curious echo of the mutilations reported to have occurred in Vietnam, in the ancient Greek practice (Fraser, Volume 2, 1934, p. 81) whereby murderers would cut off the ears and noses of their victims to weaken the ghost's potential for returning, bent on vengeance. Apart from the general fear of the dead, which is Fraser's main theme, there are numerous examples of the belief that the traumatically killed are more likely to haunt and damage the survivors. This is best exemplified in Chapter 3 of Fraser's third volume (1936, pp. 103–303). He concluded that there are almost always consistent and major distinctions in relation to the cause of death. The most dangerous ghosts are widely recognized to be those of those slain, those who have died a premature and violent death, or those who have been murdered, or suicides, or those who died in battle or were killed by wild animals.

In Zulu thought, for example, Death is associated with pollution (*umnyama*), which diminishes one's resistance to disease and creates a situation predisposing to misfortune (*amashwa*) (see Ngubane, 1977). In a manner reminiscent of the A criterion in the *Diagnostic and Statistical Manuals* DSM-III and DSM-III-R, these traditional beliefs specify that death from an accident or from unusual misfortune, war, accident, or crime leads to a special and more severe type of *umnyama* called *umkhoka*. There is, of course, also a central belief that the ancestors continue to be powerful influences on their descendants. They can bring health and good luck when pleased, and if displeased, the withdrawal of their protection leaves their descendants vulnerable to disease and misfortune. Thus, it is obvious that transgenerational effects of trauma are recognized in the traditional African way of thinking.

THE CHANGING NATURE OF WAR TRAUMA AND ITS IMPACT AS EXEMPLIFIED IN SOUTH AFRICA

Evolving strategies conflict have led to varying patterns of trauma, so far largely ignored by most specialists in this field. World War I, and especially World War II, explicitly blurred the distinction, often previously kept clear, between soldier and civilian. It has since almost wholly disappeared. Civilians became absolutely explicit targets, whether in the bureaucratically vicious concentration camps or the indiscriminate bombing of large cities. More like the earlier instances of siege, the degree of suffering and privation inflicted was deliberately sought as a means to place pressure on the enemy politicians and their military complex.

In the recent South African conflict, while the regime victimized the population at large, the African National Congress (ANC) and liberation movement took this trend still further, using large masses of the civilian population as an instrument of conflict. This included the organization of large marches and mass stay-aways from work, which are traditionally nonviolent means of protest *when used in democratic and nonrepressive societies,* but which otherwise usually lead to violent confrontation. To some extent, this encompasses the tactic expressed in the student confrontations in Europe and American in the 1960s, that by provoking acts of violence against oneself, one can force a regime to reveal its true nature, converting covert repression into explicit and well-publicized violent acts. One convincing view of the basic nature of terrorism is the use of violence by one party against another (preferably symbolically significant and innocent) in order to produce an impact on a third party. This tactic is related to the hunger strikes used earlier by the Irish Republican Army in Britain and later in South Africa as a special form of terrorism in which the person causing or inciting the violence and the person receiving and suffering its direct effects is conflated into the same individual. The intention is still to disturb and affect the behavior of an audience of others not party to the direct conflict. But such tactics are effective only against a government with scruples, or at least capable of shame, or more realistically, one that is acting covertly at variance with its public self-image and declared ideals, and is thus open to embarrassment. Gandhi could be effective against the British in India by revealing to them that they were acting in ways their ideals would declare them incapable of doing. But Gandhi was ineffective against the Boers in South Africa, because it never occurred to them that they should not be beastly to non-Boers.

More damaging in its lasting effects was the ANC policy of rendering large areas "ungovernable" by encouraging civil unrest and damage to social and community structures and organization. Such methods were perhaps inevitable results of the creativity of a resistance movement faced with a world that provided much verbal support but little real logistical support for conventional warfare. But the risk, demonstrated in South Africa, is that large areas become not merely ungovernable by the unpopular regime but by all forms of governance. This has had a severe, lasting, and damaging impact on South African society, which seems likely to last for many generations.

Hansson and van Zyl Smit (1990), among others, have reviewed relevant aspects of the old regime's evolving attempts to destroy the opposition to apartheid. Earlier, in the P. W. Botha presidency, there was the "total strategy," conceived as a response to the "total onslaught" of an international communist conspiracy (all opposition to apartheid was automatically seen as communist) against capitalism (epitomized, bizarrely, by the twisted socialism of South African racism). Any and all means were seen as justifiable in responding to such a wholly evil offensive. It was argued that intense, widespread, and violent oppression was essential to produce "law and order" as a prerequisite to any reform. This view prescribed more of the brutal force, which had caused the unrest in the first place, as necessary to end it, while the policies that engendered it would be changed only after the violence they were causing had ended. Not surprisingly, this approach caused massive misery and steady escalation of trauma. As ex-President de Klerk was once quoted as saying, in using such counterinsurgency methods, "it may be that the enemy is the majority of the population" (de Klerk, 1989, in Hansson & van Zyl Smit, 1990).

Later, around mid-1986, there was increased use of "low-intensity conflict or low-intensity warfare," a post-Vietnam counterinsurgency stratagem (see, e.g., Hippler, 1987). Among its tenets were strenuous efforts to separate guerrilla forces from the general population, such as by disinformation (using the huge resources of the State) and by staging atrocities that could be blamed on the guerrillas, a tactic used by the regime at least up to the April 1994 first elections, in the opinion of many experts. The traumatogenic potential of such methods has been little studied. Other methods include population resettlement (traumatic in itself and reducing access to the normally strong community support mechanisms) and a more deliberate and focused rather than indiscriminate use of violence directed at civilians. By this means, a State causes massive damage to its own citizens, but covertly, disguising the author of the trauma. It is, as Hippler wrote, a fight without appearing to fight. Military objectives are sought by social manipulation, while overtly courting social popularity. There are superficial reforms, with much attention given to providing and publicizing the simulation of modification and a veneer of program, while ensuring as little substantial reform as possible. There is careful targeting of activists and of political and community leadership, further damaging the community and its ability to heal itself. The State acted to achieve its aims, but so far as possible by surrogates, such as vigilante groups like the Witdoeke, (Theological Exchange Program, 1987). The WHAM policy (Winning the Hearts and Minds) actually damaged both. Like a deliberate induction of DESNOS or complex PTSD, there is premeditated promotion of distrust and disillusionment.

Overt and covert violence became official and formal state policy from 1976 on, while among the resistance movements, violent reaction was seen as legitimate and even popular. In a sort of privatization of conflict, they declared a "people's war." After the regime had made all civilians targets of discrimination, and of indirect and direct violence, the resistance declared all civilians to be combatants. Tactics, successful to a degree in the short term, have proved to have long-lasting damaging effects showing a significant variety of the transmission of trauma via enduring harm to social structures. A government that refuses to allow any nonviolent means of achieving change (as the South African government did so assiduously) creates a crucible of violence. Violence may, in such a situation, become the only effective means of promoting desirable reforms. Even if inefficient, it can at least convincingly simulate change. A government that forbids other means of resolving conflict will inevitably promote violence. Criminalizing politics politicizes crime.

THE ROLE OF CHILDREN IN THE SOUTH AFRICAN STRUGGLE FOR FREEDOM

Youth played a leading part in the struggle for democracy from early times. The ANC Youth League was founded in the late forties out of the feeling that the established leadership of the time was not vigorous enough in opposing the regime. The youth leaders prominent at that time included Nelson Mandela and Walter Sisulu, now elder statesmen, themselves facing a restless and unsatisfied youth. Once again, in the late 1960s, new groups arose, such as the Black Consciousness movement of Steve Biko and others dissatisfied with the failure of older activists to achieve meaningful changes. Saths Cooper (1994) has suggested a progressive development: the "young Turks" of South African politics in the 1940s were in their thirties; Biko and his peers were in their early twenties. In the 1970s and 1980s, leaders in community activism were in their teens, and in early teenage years at that. Successive older generations were seen as having compromised the cause. The major traumatic events that shaped the course of political developments (such as the Sharpeville massacre of March 21, 1960, and the Soweto uprising of June 16, 1976) were youth-led acts of resistance, leading to the deaths and suffering of youth in government counterresistance. The successive waves of political activists moving into exile became younger, leaving still younger groups of activists, with few or no significant older leaders. As the society of the oppressed majority produced successive crops of leadership, these were regularly depleted by voluntary or involuntary exile, or by government-orchestrated deaths and imprisonments, driving the locus of leadership younger and younger. Youth, precisely became of its lack of experience of previous attempts and of failure, is more easily able to adopt a single-minded and simplistic optimism and zealousness, unhampered by awareness of the complexities of the situation.

In any society, old activists are rare. The longer the succession of life experiences in which the individual has been unable to influence the course of events, the less likely it is that anyone will seriously question the inevitability of the status quo. In the case of apartheid, an entire social structure was designed with the active participation of social and behavioral scientists (Breyten Breytenbach called them "spychologists") to magnify that effect and to induce a substantial degree of learned helplessness (Seligman, 1975) on its citizens. Only by such means, by convincing the majority that resistance cannot succeed, can any minority regime maintain power. Only the young, not yet fully subdued by this, retained the capacity to act and to resist.

Facing a common and rather undiscriminating menace, enhanced peer socialization and the induction of a "struggle mentality," which has proved hard to give up, apartheid deliberately (see, e.g., Simpson, 1995) provided black youth with poor education designed to maintain a menial status. In response, the youth boycotted such "education," inducing large-scale disruption of family structures. Cooper (1994) reports finding that 6 out of 10 youths involved in the struggle could not identify with one parent, usually male, because he was not around or they did not know who he was. In some areas, 75% were born in single-parent homes. Completely contrary to the traditional black society, their socialization came from their peers, not their unavailable elders.

Black children were often in the forefront of the organized resistance to the regime. This may have mitigated, to some extent, the damage caused to them, by promoting self-esteem, pride, dignity, and self-respect, and reducing the sense of powerlessness. Indeed, at times, it promoted an unrealistic and exhilarating sense of power. In practice, it was difficult to render a community ungoverned and ungovernable. It is far more difficult to regain civic governance and social cohesion. In the same way, any idiot with a hammer can stop a clock: Very few can mend one, and very different tools are needed. These youth often led their elders. White South African children often grew up with a black "nanny": a woman, often forced to neglect her own children in order to provide prolonged and intimate care of "the young master." There have been no adequate studies of the impact of the long-term effects of such child-rearing practices. White children almost totally ignored participation in the struggle, concentrating instead on enjoying and entrenching their unearned privileges. There were white participants in the struggle, but only on a very small scale, and usually aged from the twenties up. Ironically, one of the most politicizing and radicalizing forces for white youth was the enforcement of compulsory military conscription. Many of the richer youths avoided the draft, usually by emigrating, under rather comfortable circumstances, then enjoying the claim of having opposed a system they had in truth done nothing whatever to oppose other than merely to escape its tedious inconveniences. Poorer and lower class white youths did not have this option. While the Army used conscription very deliberately as a means of political indoctrination, the gradually increasing racial integration of the army and its facilities (born of necessity, and against the wishes of the ideology) brought white and black youths together, sharing risks and scarce comforts, and making the discovery (monumentally huge for some of them) of how much they had in common, and how little they differed. Apartheid had successfully hidden this fundamental fact from them and from their elders.

Black youth became a specific target of State terrorism, trying to destroy their resistance. Youths took on the task of protecting their communities, and many were killed or exiled. Evidence is only now becoming available that proves beyond reasonable doubt the reality of the previous allegations of so-called "Third Force" terrorism that became rampant as the nation moved toward a negotiated settlement. The State "security" forces sponsored, trained, and armed black vigilantes to conduct acts of extreme violence and terrorism that could then be blamed on the liberation forces. To those denied any role whatever in positive social ascendancy, the only source of power was violence. Thus, repressive regimes create the resistance they claim to be responding to. They became desensitized to violence. It was still feared but no longer really shocking, thus lowering the threshold to ordinary social and domestic violence.

Despite the world's applause, the bulk of the people were in fact even more marginalized by the negotiations, which were strictly limited to the politicians, who met their own needs rather than those of the people and never consulted those most affected by their decisions. Youth was especially ignored. As one young Soweto activist complained, "We were the lions you asked to roar: now the only ones who listen to us are the drug dealers." As Cooper (1994) comments, "Their usefulness expended, they are being infantilized by the new compact between erstwhile oppressor and erstwhile oppressed." Not just superfluous, they were seen to threaten the cosy, mutual back-scratching of the politicians who were demonstrating the essential identity of the species, offering the chronically dispossessed further alienation, not affirmation.

CHILDREN AS AGGRESSORS

Recent African experience has also revealed the increasing role played by child soldiers. Children were recruited or conscripted into partisan armies as young "comrades" seeking confrontation. Showing aggressive responses to trauma or its threat can be adaptive for some individuals, though damaging for the community. Once, random violent acts that disrupted society were praised by some as "crippling apartheid" but were later criticized as lawless, confusing their authors. "Self-defense units," set up to defend communities from State and factional violence, themselves grew to become heavily armed, powerful, and feared. Never mind *quis custodiet custodies:* Who defends us from our defenders? Who will liberate us from our liberators? To the ill-educated or uneducated, unemployed or never employed, in bleak, arid, and boring environments, crime and violence can become the main means of entertainment and stimulation, the sole source of any sense of self-worth, the *raison d'etre* for the only groups within which many individuals can feel a sense of belonging and mutual respect. As adults were seen as unable to protect the young, they were no longer seen as valid authorities or sources of norms of conduct.

Prior exposure to trauma can sensitize or "steel" the individual to later incidents. Ideology explained and led to an expectation of state violence. Intracommunity violence was less explicable, less comprehensible, and often more traumatizing. The longer the duration of exposure to violence, the less the protective effect of mediating factors such as available caretakers. The effects of apartheid, other than direct trauma, were such as to be adjuvant factors, enhancing the pathogenicity of traumatic events. There were no safe places: family violence, dangerous streets and schools, rebounding trauma. We have also found that children are more likely to show symptoms of stress disorders when their caregivers have PTSD or other significant stress symptoms themselves. Similarly, Famularo *et al.* (1994), in their study of mothers and children following earlier occurrence of severe maltreatment of the child, found a relationship between the mothers' responses and those of the children, with PTSD "significantly overrepresented in the children of mothers diagnosed with PTSD"

In 1994, a hasty, unrepresentative, and self-appointed Commission of Inquiry (Duncan & Rock, 1994) studied other people's work in South Africa on the effects of political and social violence on children, drawing heavily on the present author's work (Simpson, 1993a, 1993b, 1993c, 1993d, 1993e). Studies have suggested that the more often children encounter violence, the more likely they may be later to perpetrate violence (Aysen & Nieuwoudt, 1992; Dawes & Tredoux, 1990; Hirschowitz, Milner, & Everatt, 1992; Klassen, 1990; Malepa, 1990). Straker, Moosa, Becker, and Nkwale (1992) emphasized the relatively recently recognized issue of children as aggressors involved in hideous acts of cruelty (like "necklacing," in which the victims, hands tied, have a car tire filled with petrol placed around their neck, which is then set on fire) and other murders of perceived political opponents.

THE INFANTILIZING OF BLACK ADULTS

Apartheid had the concept of *baasskap:* of boss-ness, or master-ness, a worldview that saw whites as an *ubermensch* and blacks as children needing the paternalistic and firm guidance of the white "boss." The cross-culturally dominant image of adult blacks as children persisted. To this day, adult black men and women are often called "boys" or "girls": "Just give it to the Boy, and ask the Girl to bring in the tea!" At best, they might be called by their first name, or, more insultingly, by a generic first name: "Jim", or "Mary", irrespective of their true name. Even the autonomous political act of resistance to tyranny was persistently and insistently misrepresented by the regime as entirely due to the actions of outsiders: "agitators" or "intimidators"—as if any sensible person subjected to the treatment prescribed by apartheid would fail to be agitated by it, without someone else fomenting ill-feeling. Blackness was equated with the rampaging and lurking id, controlled only by the presence of a white superego.

These old practices meant that today's young blacks grew up in a world where their parents were treated as children. There was a clear inversion of traditional leadership structures, with the young involved actively in liberation political action and their parents often discouraging this as dangerous. Cycles of loss and trauma were apparent. As the freedom to hold public gatherings was severely curtailed as politically perilous, funerals, especially of those who were seen as victims of government action, became the focus of community solidarity and mobilization, and thus were politicized. They were then, in their turn, controlled by the State. Criminalizing ordinary political activity led to a concomitant politicization of ordinary criminality. Now, we see criminals who claim that they rob banks—not, as the famous crook once said, because that's where the money is—but because they were representatives of the underprivileged nonparticipants in capitalism, or some such political guff. They were not stealing bankrolls, they were "redistributing wealth." The fact that it was being redistributed rather exclusively to themselves, and with even less benefit to the community at large than before, largely escaped attention. The regime had been in so many aspects a kleptocracy. Theft, graft, and corruption have become endemic in all sectors of the community and especially in the "public service." Vast amounts of scarce funds were wasted and stolen, as new administration officials now admit. A veteran of the liberation movements, Dr. Siphiwe Stamper, is quoted, referring to an honored old liberation slogan that meant "The struggle continues", as now saying, "A *luta continua* was given a new meaning here . . . "the looting continues" (van der Linde, 1995). As Bulhan (1985) remarked, "Violence breeds more violence . . . and a community of victims, unaware of its history and unable to control its destiny, engages in much autodestructive behavior" (p. 174).

THE EFFECTS OF CHILD TRAUMA ON PARENTS

In the existing world literature, the main concern seems to have been with the effects of traumatized parents on their children. But also important is the effect of traumatized children on the parents and the interactions when both are traumatized, as well as the impact of adult trauma on those who were traumatized, similarly or differently, as children. Elsewhere (Simpson, 1993b), I have reviewed in much greater detail the effects of political violence and repression on children and adolescents, and the effects of torture and coercive interrogation (Simpson, 1993a, 1996). In the latter study, I emphasized the frequency with which we have seen in South Africa the reverse of the effects often described in regard to Holocaust survivors. In our setting, "the younger generation has been, preponderantly, the victims, and it is the older, parental generation that shows the secondary effects. Not infrequently, the effect of the martyrdom or victimization of the child has been a radicalization of the parents (often very conservative people originally) and a move toward the parents' sharing their child's ideals and joining the struggle" (p. 681).

THE EFFECT OF PARENTAL TRAUMA ON CHILDREN

Most of the studies one sees in the literature on multigenerational effects of the Holocaust seem to be of parents who experienced the Holocaust and children born after it, rather than of instances where both parents and children shared the experience of the Holocaust. Parents are described as absorbed in their own pain, leaving the children to "separate development"; we have found this to be a frequent response in South African. Parents, themselves trapped in intolerable life situations, often act out their frustration in verbal and physical abuse of their small children. A desperate mother is quoted (Duncan & Rock, 1994) as saying of her obviously malnourished child: "I hit him because he is naughty. He is always crying for bread." The children learn that they are regarded as bad, without having done anything to deserve this label, and may later feel justified in undertaking any self-serving actions, however bad, as appropriate to the identification that was forced upon them. They also express no confidence in their own ability, in due course, to be parents.

Harkness (1993) writes of transgenerational or intergenerational trauma from father to children. She says that even in the comparatively peaceful United States, 50% of the population have a first-degree relative who is a veteran. Effects described include numbed responsiveness and social withdrawal. Quality research needs the advantages American researchers had: a period of trauma to an identifiable and significant group, followed by peace with sufficient prosperity and access to psychiatric/psychological care to enable studies to take place. In the developing world, we lack all those advantages. Harkness says Vietnam veterans with PTSD have a high incidence of divorce, marital discord and domestic violence, high unemployment, drug and alcohol abuse, and suicide. *So does the South African population as a whole.*

The effect may depend on the degree and nature of the child's identification with the parents. In South Africa, many were conflicted. Children rejected their parents' passivity in the face of apartheid and their failure to take effective action to end it (Simpson, 1993a, 1993b). Apartheid severely damaged families. In contrast to the small and schismatic modern nuclear (or postnuclear) North American families, African families (more like European Jewish and Romany families before the Holocaust) were especially vulnerable, as adherents of the concept of *ubuntu,* experiencing the large community as an enlarged, extended family. Harkness writes of Vietnam veterans having disengaged relationships with spouses and families, and of families with a relative absence of structure, order, and authority. Apartheid all too often enforced that. Migratory labor and other pressures forced families to break up, weakened the ties between family members, and greatly reduced opportunities for mutual support and joint problem solving of the traditional sort. Harkness also writes of Vietnam veteran families that "it is not unusual to find a child elevated to a parental-functioning role" (p. 636). We have seen exactly the same situation in South Africa: Young children, in the absence of the parents as breadwinners, away in distant towns, having to become active in the raising of still younger children. This was compounded by what became a growing tendency for the young to take leadership in political activism from their passive elders whose learned helplessness so frustrated the young.

Dawes and Tredoux (1989) reported briefly on children exposed to political violence in a South African squatter community in which, within 3 months, 53 people were killed and 20,000 were made homeless by vigilante attacks. They concentrated on acute effects, but still noted such effects as changed attitudes to the police and effects on socialization. They noted an association between more serious disturbances in children and maternal PTSD. Methodological weaknesses, including very limited measures of other factors, limit the generalizability of these specific findings, but their conclusion that "maternal stress increases the risk of child problems" matches general experience in this country.

MULTIGENERATIONAL TRAUMA AND THE GENESIS OF TERRORISM

A field that has been very largely neglected is the role of prior trauma in the genesis of terrorism and in the motivation of those known as terrorists. Garr (1970) wrote, "Some of the most general explanations of the origins of revolution and other forms of collective violence attribute it to the loss of ideational coherence: men's loss of faith in, or lack of consensus about, the beliefs and norms that govern social interaction." Taylor and Quayle (1994) have made an interesting contribution on this issue, though wholly outside the traditional boundaries of psychotraumatology. For example, they report a finding that is intriguing when considered in the light of our knowledge of complex PTSD and of damage to the "just-world hypothesis." They write, "The sense of a 'just world' seems to lie at the very heart of the social and psychological response to political violence of both terrorists and their victims" (p. 8). As they recognize, these viewpoints are somehow primarily opposed yet similar in nature. "The sense of remedying injustice which might lead to terrorism *creates* the injustice to the innocent bystander"; and it can thus become the basis for a responsive terrorism of retaliation, immediate or historic. "Often the injustice which initiates terrorism . . . becomes lost under layers and layers of later affronts and perceived injustice, such that the starting point no longer has relevance other than through mythology. But whatever might be the starting point of terrorism, its central quality seems to be that it creates a self-sustaining cycle of injustice which once established, experience suggests is very difficult to break." Terrorists are acting out an unjust-world hypothesis; in a very real sense, they are acting out the characteristics of their trauma experience.

As Taylor and Quayle (1994) emphasize (see also Simpson, 1988), a central element in the terrorist act is the lack of any direct relationship between the victims and the specific political agenda of the organization taking such action. We protest loudly, as we are meant to, at the "innocence" of the victims. Our outrage is precisely the response sought: guilty victims would not be functional. In a sense, they may be acting out the random malignity of the trauma they experienced, and the chord they so deliberately touch in all of us is strictly based on that vulnerability that our "just-world" beliefs create. It illustrates vividly the extent to which society at large holds most trauma victims as somehow to blame for their fate, that when the terrorist skillfully selects dramatically innocent victims, we are especially deeply disturbed. We feel that victims *ought* to deserve their fate, and when it is made too difficult for us to construct some sense of responsibility for them, it is acutely uncomfortable. State or insurgent terrorism uses acts of violence perpetrated against certain targets in order to produce desired effects on quite other people for political purposes. I have previously (e.g., Simpson, 1993a) shown how torture and coercive interrogation in fact represent the careful and deliberate use of trauma in order to induce desired posttraumatic syndromes in the direct targets of such violence. Terrorism deliberately (if usually unwittingly or without fully understanding) uses indirect or secondary traumatization for similarly political ends. That is why terrorism is so intimately concerned with the means of communication (as is excellently discussed by Schmidt & de Graaf, 1982). Where it is unable to attain media access so as to influence the secondary trauma targets, it is ineffective. Although it has been insurgent terrorism used by relatively small and unofficial structures that has attracted the most attention, one must remember that these methods were originally developed and systematically used by the State, notably in the Reign of Terror under Robespierre in France. Only later was the technique privatized.

The victims may be indiscriminate but not arbitrary. It is surely significant that the terrorist act—its timing, methods, and targets—is precisely planned to be incalculable, unpredictable, unexpected, unfathomable, and uncontrollable. Like deliberate disasters, these are acts of man planned to have the impact of Acts of God. Before those components of traumatic stress were formally recognized in DSM-IV (American Psychiatric Association, 1994) they had been embodied in all successful acts of terror. Such deeds always force the larger audience to confront the experience or witness events that cause, or threaten to cause, death or serious injury to others, and in such a way as to induce fear, horror, and especially a sense of help-lessness in those of us who are forced to be bystanders.

Although Taylor and Quayle (1994) are clear that "there seems to be no discernible patho-logical qualities of terrorists that can identify them in any clinical sense as different from oth-ers in the community from which they come," they were looking for obvious psychopathology and not the area I consider most relevant, that of responses to prior loss and trauma. In my forensic work in the last decade, I have had the opportunity to examine closely numerous men who were considered by the State to be terrorists (and by others to be freedom fighters), and have found such experiential themes to be common among them. The unusually detailed in-terviews with members of Irish and other terrorist groups reported by Taylor and Quayle ex-emplify themes I found commonplace in South Africa freedom fighters: a sense of community support for long-term involvement in "the troubles," of special comradeship within the struc-ture, of being part of an ongoing response to previous and bitterly remembered acts of the op-posite side, and "in an almost intuitive way he [the terrorist] could recognize the continuity of his present behavior with the past" (p. 28). What others see as acts of offense are seen as de-fenses of the community against external threats and as responses to past acts of violence against that community by the State.

> This appears to have its primary origins in the past through family, cultural, historical and religious traditions. . . . Many terrorist families can give a litany of past events . . . where in-dividual family members have been injured, killed or imprisoned. The present therefore has continuity with the past, and the young person growing in this environment absorbs the ethos of terrorism as part of his early socialisation. (p. 29)

Actions that others see as immoral are seen as morally required responses to the past and fu-ture violence of others. They describe a "point of no return," a form of critical psychological boundary of involvement in such a process, which is usually either a personal experience of re-pression or violence, the death of a friend or acquaintance in a political action or demonstra-tion, or an analogous incident, such as an atrocity, that damaged the community.

The cyclical and intergenerational nature of such community political violence must not be underestimated. Most attempts to stop such violence become pretexts for its continu-ance. And to South African insurgents, as with the Irish that Taylor and Quayle interviewed, prison is a powerful learning environment for ideological growth. The major prison island used for South African political prisoners is still commonly referred to as "the University of Robben Island."

Fields's studies (1986), among others, suggest that children who grow up in violent so-cieties may show a degree of moral and social retardation, but it is hard to isolate the effects of violence per se and those of the closely related poor social circumstances (see Heskin [1980], referring to Northern Ireland in particular). There are possible differences between the effects of witnessing violence to others, whether strangers or intimates, personally expe-riencing violence, and participating in violent acts. Some authors predicted that the latter would surely lead to moral breakdown (e.g., Fraser, 1974; Lyons, 1979). Torture is addictive. Any government or security force that gets a good chance to enjoy it rarely gives it up volun-tarily. In North America and Europe, there has been a privatization of bestial violence. Those people who truly enjoy maiming and killing others must stick to fantasy or become serial killers. In repressive regimes, they can look forward to a secure government job and pension. As the South African novelist, André Brink, writes (1992), "Once you start using violence to change the world to your liking, you're stuck with violence to keep it going. And there's no way out again" (p. 157).

THE "LOST GENERATION": WHO LOST THEM?
WHERE CAN THEY BE FOUND?

Many generations of children have been proclaimed a "lost generation" (see, e.g., McWhirter & Trew, 1982, on children in Northern Ireland), generally by self-proclaimed experts who propose to find them. Someone should undertake a follow-up study on all the reputedly lost generations. The degree of damage and the implications of irreparable damage seem to have been exaggerated. The Khmer Rouge and the children of Belfast, Beirut, and South Africa have all been labeled as "lost."

A number of rather minor and impressionist surveys have attracted publicity but often contradict each other. Everatt and Orkin (1993) announced that their analysis of South African youth, across all races, showed 5% to be "lost", 27% as "marginalized" (seen as most needing urgent intervention), 43% as "at risk" ("functioning, but showing signs of alienation on a few dimensions of concern") and 25% as "fine" (fully engaged with society, with the authors recommending they be trained "in peer education and leadership"). The report has serious sampling and methodological concerns, and an artificial appearance of accuracy.

Verhulst, Althaus, and Versluis den Bieman (1992) reported a study of 2,148 international adoptees and found that early neglect, abuse, and the number of changes of caretaking environment increased the risk of later maladjustment, but also that the majority of the adoptees—even those with potentially damaging backgrounds—seemed to be functioning well. What, then, are the long-term effects of early exposure to trauma and persecution? Krell (1993) points out the relatively recent recognition of distinct effects of such experiences on children in comparison with adult exposure. In the early literature on child survivors of the Holocaust, there are challenging observations. Friedman (1949), for example, expressed astonishment at "the shallowness of their emotions" after the experience of continuous danger, and Minkowski (1946) spoke of "affective anaesthesia." Krell (1993) reported on 25 child survivors, "the majority of whom were not patients" (which is important, as so many studies are limited both by small numbers and by an exclusive focus on people already in therapy), and he emphasizes that the majority of child survivors lead normal and creative lives. Lasting damage is not inevitable.

Feenstra (1995) reported the results of a 10-year study of the psychological health of post-war children of war victims, concluding emphatically that "a review of the literature compels [one] to make the tentative conclusion that, as yet, no support has been found for the assumption that post-war children of war victims, solely on the basis of the fact that their parents were traumatized in the war, are at higher risk for mental problems." He agrees that the methodologies used so far leave much to be desired and that more research is justified, but the contrast to "lost generation" claims is clear.

POLITICAL CORRECTNESS, DENYING APARTHEID,
AND REQUIRING AMNESIA

Lipstadt (1993), in her notable book *Denying the Holocaust,* has ably reviewed the meretricious and phony propaganda that promotes the obscene myth that the Holocaust never occurred or seeks to minimize its awful realities. She addresses, for instance, the fake scholarly argument used by those who advance this fable by pretending that they are merely presenting "the two sides" of the issue. About the reality of the Holocaust, like the reality of winter and death, there are no "sides": It happened. While there are legitimate differences in one's responses to or explanations of such events, denial of reality is not a "side" in an argument: It is the refusal to argue, the disguising of facts by those too cowardly to respond to the realities. Lipstadt sees the Holocaust denial phenomenon as part of a neofascist agenda. Frank discussion of such grim events and their consequences is disgustingly misrepresented by some as "hate material" (Lipstadt, p. 15) or as "threatening national healing and reconciliation" (in today's South Africa). In a disguised reversal of truth, the hateful suppression of frank discussion of the results of hatred and conflict is misrepresented as if it somehow *caused* the events it is simply describing. Lipstadt (e.g., pp. 21–22) also discusses how the Holocaust deniers not only deny or minimize grim historic realities, but also argue passionately against the assignment of any blame to any of the participants: Victors and vanquished, perpetrators and victims, are all regarded as equal; essentially (though they usually avoid revealing this logical consequence of their arguments), they would hold that there was no useful moral or other distinction between Hitler and Churchill, between the Gestapo and the Royal Air Force. She discusses the *Historikerstreit* in Germany in the 1980s, in which conservative historians sought to "normalize and relativize" the Nazi period of history.

But, at least, it took decades, some 50 years, before the Holocaust deniers grew strong enough to have any noticeable influence on the understanding of some of those who lacked firsthand knowledge of the denied events. In South Africa, apartheid denial was an extensive official government policy for decades to facilitate the continuation of those crimes against humanity. It has continued unabated and has been adopted by the new "democratic" government. South African history, written as denial propaganda for the decades of official apartheid, is still dishonest. A coercive "political correctness" enforces strong pressure against frank discussion of what has so recently happened. A mother demanding to know who killed her son a year ago is told that she is "raking up the past" and preventing a necessary process of "reconciliation."

Pross (1991) very relevantly reviewed the postwar cover-up of Nazi doctors in Germany, confirming how, after the collapse of a repressive regime, most perpetrators, helpers, and collaborators "manage to survive quite agreeably." Speaking at a Norwegian conference from which South African doctors had been excluded, he appealed to the world medical community not to be fooled again, and to "break the complicity of silence towards contemporary abuses." In fact, none of the South African doctors who behaved dishonorably during the apartheid era have been censured in any way by the South African Medical Association, or by the South African Medical Council, whose own unethical conduct during the bad years was so widely condemned. The Council is still run by appointees of the old regime and has, amazingly, been given the task of reforming itself, free from any participation by its victims.

CONTINUING EFFECTS OF SOCIAL TRAUMA: CONTRASTING EUROPEAN AND AFRICAN EXPERIENCE

We find strong echoes between the Dutch experience after World War II, and our South African experience after Apartheid. Jaffer (1995), acting on my proposal, reviewed how the Dutch dealt with the trauma of the last war, and how South Africa might learn from this. Sachs (1995), in his foreword to Jaffer's booklet, writes,

> The eagerness of the Dutch people to enter a phase of forgetfulness and happiness after the long years of conflict and suffering was understandable. Yet it is quite clear that attempts simply to bury the past because of its unpleasantness had at best temporary success. In the medium and long-term they turned out to be strongly counterproductive. . . . Reconciliation

is far more than a gesture of kindness or courtesy to those who have wronged us. True reconciliation is a deep process that deals with pain through handling the emotions of pain. It is
sufficiently confident of the endeavour to allow genuine memory to express itself. (pp. v–vi)

He reminds us of how the pain of the Anglo–Boer War was kept alive by survivors. At the
Vrouemonument (Women's Monument) is a large inscribed motto in Dutch: WE SHALL NOT FOR-
GET and WE SHALL NOT FORGIVE. As he comments, "The oppressed became the oppressors. When
will the cycle be ended? Only our generation can do it, if we have the courage to face the past
with honesty but without vindictiveness. If pain is unrecorded and unacknowledged, it surfaces
in the most bitter ways and at the most inconvenient moments. The story will never end if it is
suppressed, but finalises itself if it is properly told."

To seek understanding or comprehension of a traumatic past is seen by glib politicians as
standing in the way of economic reconstruction and development, while ignoring the needs of
psychological reconstruction and development. As in Europe in the late 1940s, there is a steadfast determination to ignore the extent of the active collaboration of many and the fact that the
resistance was only a small group. In fact, in our situation, although former resistance members still suffer, collaborators now enjoy the fruits of the international status the resistance
earned. Just as Germany was suddenly devoid of Nazis, South Africa has hardly anyone who
acknowledges having played any part in apartheid. Jaffer (1995, p. 3) describes the "let's forget the past" syndrome. Political opportunism usually dominates. But the Dutch allowed out-
of-court settlements for petty collaborators, with surveillance of the STDP (Stichting Toezicht
Politieke Delinquenten), while thousands more were tried by Special Courts and Tribunals, and
there was dishonorable discharge of thousands of civil servants (with loss of pension). In South
Africa, in strong contrast, all collaborators were guaranteed vastly generous pensions and generous lump-sum payments. Far more was spent on such rewards for the unworthy than on care
for their victims. The Dutch set up University Purge Boards that inquired into the conduct of
students and professors, and other, similar boards examined the roles played by journalists,
doctors, and lawyers. In South Africa, medical collaborators have been richly rewarded, and
the lawyers who played such an active role in the repression remain at work (if government
employees) and still get the majority of government legal work (if in private practice). Those
who made great sacrifices to fight for human rights during the repressive era have received no
government appointments, contracts, or work. The Dutch provided adequate pensions for the
survivors of repression; South Africa has ensured that no pensions whatsoever will be available
to our survivors.

As Jaffer (1995) has written,

The initial over-emphasis on economic reconstruction and "forgetting the past" only submerged serious problems which then had to be attended to years later—at great human cost
to families. The collective blacking-out of memory did little to help heal the victims. . . . Allowing people to speak about their experiences; recording their experiences for posterity;
publicly acknowledging that damage has been done and wrongs committed is an essential
part of the healing process.

Most reviews of the South African experience (e.g., Levett, 1989) tend to ignore intergenerational aspects and are largely obsessed with political correctness and doctrinaire political interpretations of the trauma experience in terms of dated neo-Marxist political themes, not
so as to understand better the micropolitics and sociopolitical context of the survivor's experience, but to support standpoints in the internecine warfare of ideologies.

After the 1967 classic, *The Inability to Mourn* (Mitscherlich & Mitscherlich, 1967),
Mitscherlich-Nielson (1993) recently revisited the topic. She describes the "pull of silence" in

postwar Germany concerning Nazi atrocities, by which "guilt and shame were negated," enabling public avoidance of remembrance of (let alone the needed active memory for) the millions of German and non-German war victims. She sees a parallel in the current German situation with hostility toward foreigners, asylum seekers, Jews, and Gypsies also "mutely condoned by a silent majority" She sees this as showing the same denial of shame and guilt, and the same lack of empathy for the poor and underprivileged.

THE SOUTH AFRICAN EXPERIENCE OF LASTING EFFECTS OF SOCIAL VIOLENCE COMPARED TO OTHER COUNTRIES

Curran (1988) expertly discussed the impact of 18 years of terrorist violence in Northern Ireland and the difficulties involved in competently studying such issues. Despite gloomy predictions that society would be "broken down" under such stresses, he emphasizes that, so far as can be judged from the results of community surveys, hospital admission and referral data, psychotropic drug usage, suicide rates, and assessment of victims, the impact, in his careful phrase "has (not) been judged considerable" This is unlike the situation in South Africa, where every index of social pathology scores high. Among the reasons he discusses for such findings, apart from the underestimated resilience and adaptivity of human beings, are underreporting, migration of the most afflicted and vulnerable, denial and habituation to violence, a possible latency period (as described by Porot, 1957, after the unrest in Algeria), and a possibly cathartic effect of the disinhibition and direct expression of violence. Casper (1995), studying the legacies of authoritarian rule following the Marcos and Aquino eras in the Philippines, as well as examples in Latin America, explored the long impact on society of authoritarianism: the damage to social institutions, for instance, caused by the intervention in politics of the church and/or the military, and the fragility of redemocratization.

It has been commonly observed that neurotic patients often seem to cope better when faced with external stress. Mira (1939), for instance, recorded this during the Spanish Civil War, as did Ierodiakonou (1970) during the civil war in Cyprus, whereas psychotic patients are generally little affected, as Solomon (1995) reported in Israel during the Gulf War. No such effect has been described in South Africa, where mental health services have been so primitively developed that sufficiently sensitive observations, especially of those most exposed to the threat, were not possible. The work of Curran (1989) and others (e.g., Kee *et al.,* 1987) has suggested a limited duration of the impact of civil violence in many cases, at least as regards the duration of formal psychiatric illness. Also intriguing in its implications is the study of Greenley, Gillespie, and Lindenthal (1975) in their study of the impact in New Haven of a period of severe urban rioting, arson, vandalism, and assault. They found that suburban male whites felt significantly psychologically better both during and 2 years after the riot; white females felt no different during the rioting and significantly better later. Neither black men nor black women felt worse during or after the riots. Fogelson (1970), commenting on the American riots of the 1960s, noted "the outpouring of fellow-feeling, of mutual respect and common concern . . . exhilaration so intense as to border on jubilation . . . a sense of pride, purpose and accomplishment. . . . Their common predicament revealed in the rioting, blacks looked again at one another and saw only brothers" We saw a similar sense of cohesion and positive sense of brotherhood and community during the struggle against apartheid, and as that has been replaced by a general era of greed and self-seeking, many greatly miss the positive aspects of the days of struggle.

THE NATURE OF APARTHEID AND ITS TRAUMATIC IMPACT

Other political conflicts have led to wars and similar periods of violence that had secondary effects of damaging family and community structures. Apartheid had the primary effect of damaging those structures: The overt acts of violence were in many senses secondary to that. The Holocaust had as a primary aim the annihilation of the Jews and others deemed unworthy to find a place in the Aryan society. It was prepared to make use of their labor in the service of that primary ideal. Apartheid may have caused the deaths of very large numbers of people, but its principal purpose, though hardly less chilling, was even more ambitious: It was the deliberate creation of an eternal underclass of subservient peoples, providing a docile and cheap workforce for the master race. I call it a more ambitious project in the sense that, at least, people once dead stay dead. Apartheid aimed at keeping them alive and perpetually submissive, tractable and adapted to the needs of others. Verwoerd was very explicit that the function of education of the black majority was precisely that. While human physiology makes it relatively easy to kill large numbers of people, the Afrikaners were to discover that human psychology and sociology makes it far more difficult to transform independent people into happy slaves.

Also, the Afrikaner, in creating apartheid, had to live in a very different world to that which enabled the Nazis to act out their ignoble aims: an international environment changed by the experience of the horrors of the Holocaust, such as to make it somewhat more difficult to get away with genocide and similarly gross aims (difficult, but far from impossible, as experience has shown, in Cambodia, and Rwanda). But the Afrikaner enterprise was in no way limited by scruples or tenderheartedness, nor any moral considerations, nor by any cautions imposed by their endlessly compliant churches and academics. Rather, as economists talk of maximal sustainable output or profit, the Afrikaners, with great skill and the use of warped scientific knowledge and the deliberate induction of trauma, achieved maximal sustainable repression, the greatest degree of repression they could get away with in the modern world. And their hegemony lasted much longer than the Third Reich.

The ability of black families and communities to cope with the violence and to provide a functionally nurturing ambience for child development was greatly impaired by the requirements of apartheid. Communities were uprooted and displaced (ethnic cleansing long before Bosnian Serbs adopted the technique), and their homes were bulldozed flat. Social norms were damaged by economic conditions enforcing migrant labor. Forced to live in very poor-quality housing, usually in "locations" distant from the place of work, parents often had to leave home at 3:00 or 4:00 A.M. in order to reach their workplace by 7:00 A.M., getting home well after dark. Thus, even in theoretically intact families, there could be very limited contact. Overcrowding, poor services, crime-ridden neighborhoods—all these are well-known in every country. But rarely are such conditions deliberately planned and forcibly executed by acts of government, and seldom are people confined to such circumstances by the force of law rather than economic pressure. Unable to rebel effectively against the tyranny experienced, many frustrations inflamed internecine violence. As Emily Brontë (1847) wrote in *Wuthering Heights:* "The tyrant grinds down his slaves and they don't turn against him, they crush those beneath them"

PARALLELS WITH THE ANGLO–BOER WAR IN SOUTH AFRICA

Even at the time of the Anglo–Boer War in South Africa at the turn of the century, the potential for multigenerational effects was recognized. Joseph Chamberlain (1896), not long before the war, warned in the British Parliament that such a war "would leave behind it the embers of a strife which I believe generations would hardly be long enough to extinguish" Kruger (1958) remarked that the Jameson Raid, which helped precipitate that war, "injected into race relations more poison than the past sixty years have been able to eliminate, especially as the Boer has an Irishman's memory" (p. 35). It is widely forgotten that the British Army in South Africa faced the first modern war, with many new features later to become routine, especially guerrilla warfare. It devised responses also due to be widely imitated, such as a scorched earth policy and the invention of the concentration camp. Commenting on the lasting effects of such methods, Kruger says that "if some of his Boer descendants are reproached for remembering bitterness too long . . . to the Boer the war was not over . . . it refined a consciousness of their national identity previously less coherent or passionate" (p. 376).

The concentration camps were intended to concentrate Boer women and children in specific places, to provide care for them while preventing them from providing support to their menfolk who were fighting. They were, at first, ineptly run, with a high death rate from disease: One in five inhabitants died within a year, especially children. Lloyd George, the British opposition politician prophesied that "a barrier of dead children's bodies will pile up between the British and Boer races in South Africa" There was much exaggerated propaganda about the camps, perhaps later influencing the disastrous minimizing of reports of the awful truth about German concentration camps in World War II. In fact, living conditions were so precarious, and the incidence of disease so rife among those attempting to stay at home, that, eventually, Boer leaders actually encouraged their families to move into the British camps (General Botha said, "We are only too glad to know that our women and children are under British protection" [p. 462]). The death rate in the camps dropped greatly with reorganization, and conditions became sufficiently favorable that British leadership was worried that this provision helped the guerrillas significantly. It is too easily forgotten that some two-thirds of the enormous number of British Army fatalities in the Boer War were also due to infectious disease. There was often deliberate encouragement of lasting enmity. Lord Kitchener (e.g., Kruger, 1958, p. 438), suggested whipping up hatred between those Boers who had surrendered and those still fighting, "so that they would in future hate each other more than the British."

The parallels are intriguing. Corruption was rife in the government of President Kruger, as it was in the Afrikaner governments of the apartheid era. The Boer War also ended by negotiation, and inconclusively, without a conclusive defeat of the Boers, although they were wholly unable to win. Then, too, the Boers achieved all they needed in the generous terms allowed after their defeat. The Boer War was also followed by a highly controversial amnesty, but that amnesty was expressly limited to those who had not broken the rules of civilized war, unlike the current South African amnesty, which is expressly designed to benefit those who broke such rules and committed war crimes.

It is unfortunate that there are so few recorded observations of the direct psychological impact of this war, as it offers a good opportunity to contrast the effects of two very different military systems facing the same highly traumatic war events. The British had an extremely rigid system, allowing very little autonomy to the men actually at risk, giving great power to some of the most barmy military commanders of recent history, such as Buller, while the Boers, with great advantage, encouraged individual initiative. The British system led to appalling troop losses due to their obtuse leaders persistently snatching defeat from the jaws of victory; to the consternation of their leadership as well as their opponents, the Boer system led to unpredictability.

THE POSSIBLE RELATIONSHIP BETWEEN EXPERIENCING TRAUMA AND CAUSING IT

The issue of whether individuals who have been traumatized later become perpetrators of violence toward others is still controversial, but it seems that whereas most victims of trauma do not later become prime causes of violence toward others, some do, and trauma victims are overrepresented in numerous studies of perpetrators of various kinds. There is little clarity as to what determines what happens to individual victims. On the broader social scale of responses to trauma, the cycle of recursive violence is clearer though less remarked upon. One might naively imagine that after the experience of severe victimization, a people would say, in effect, "Never again! After our experience, we will try to ensure that this will never happen again to anybody. We won't do such things to anyone."

But, sadly, the more common response is "To Hell with anyone else: We are prepared to become perpetrators in our turn, to inflict on others what we suffered earlier, to protect our own sense of security." Perhaps political processes are all too often more adept at compounding and reflecting the more ignoble elements of our individual personalities.

In the South African example in earlier centuries, the Boers had cheerfully killed large numbers of black people (even observing the date of one of their greatest massacres as a holy holiday until 1994), displacing populations and destroying societies. Then, in their wars with Britain, the Boers themselves suffered defeat and humiliation, and damage to their fledgling, crude, and fragile culture. Devouring their own propaganda, the Boers passionately embraced the identity of victim, gathering international support for their cause. They discovered the potential power provided by exploiting the status of victim, and the role, since profitably elaborated by others, of professional victims who feel perpetually entitled and empowered to do anything, at whatever cost to others, to promote their own sectional interests. Abu-Lughod (1990) demonstrates relevant parallels between the responses of the British Colonial administration in Palestine and the more recent Israeli responses to the Intifada.

THE PLIGHT OF THE SURVIVOR IN THE "NEW" SOUTH AFRICA

Like the "flight into health" so psychoanalytically familiar, South Africans' current "flight into reconciliation" is also phony, flimsy, and avoidant of reality rather than healthy. Survivors feel a strong sense of betrayal, loss, and abandonment as their experience and histories are ignored, and feel even more hopeless than during the worse years of apartheid. Now that the world has decided, whatever the facts of the situation, that there is no problem remaining in South Africa, they have no audience for any complaints, and no support is available. Danieli (1993 and elsewhere) wrote of the *conspiracy of silence:* In South Africa, this is not merely a psychological mechanism, it has been imposed. As Bettelheim (1984, p. 166) wrote, "What cannot be talked about can also not be put to rest; and if it is not, the wounds continue to fester from generation to generation." Danieli (1984, and elsewhere) eloquently described the countertransference problems of therapists who were themselves not involved in the Holocaust, when confronted with survivors. In South Africa, there are no such therapists: Most played an active role in our national tragedy, mostly on the side of the perpetrators or, at least, as very helpful bystanders whose passivity was a necessary precondition for the success of apartheid. They are unlikely to be able to appreciate the problems of the survivors, and survivors will not trust them as therapists. Vietnam veterans experienced difficulty at times in trusting the Veterans Administration as a source of help. This problem is far greater in South Africa.

It must be remembered that the worst period of apartheid lasted for over 50 years, with many of its nastiest features being nearly a century old. This has been a very long conflict. Although in America there are studies of the multigenerational ripples of a single, comparatively brief episode of trauma, however awful, on succeeding generations living in peace and prosperity and with abundant therapy available, we are looking at multigenerational effects in which the trauma has lasted through three or four generations. We have yet to have any postwar generations.

AMNESTY OR AMNESIA?

Truth Commissions, set up to investigate periods of human rights abuses, are often lauded as if they were a form of therapy for multigenerational trauma. But many have failed (Hayner, 1994), and the South African Truth and Reconciliation Commission is showing consistent flaws, including conspicuous lack of expertise. While making generous provision for privacy and protection for perpetrators (whose pensions are guaranteed), and making pathetically limited provision for any form or care or restitution for survivors (only temporarily at best, and only if funds can be found), it carefully removes the victims' rights to all forms of redress against admitted and known perpetrators, even preventing any form of civil action against them. The law establishing it explicitly breaches international law in the extreme care it takes to provide for comprehensive exoneration of those found responsible for crimes against humanity. After a period when the whole system of laws served to protect the strong from the weak, and, rather than serving justice and morality, often required injustice and immorality, the proposed Bill of Rights was preceded by this Bill of Wrongs.

Although most states and people deplore "crimes against humanity" as the worst of human crimes, these are the most rarely punished of all. Of all categories of criminal, none is so likely to be zealously protected and rewarded or to retire on a fat pension. This fact, which makes a mockery of all Human Rights charters, compounds the continuing damage suffered by the victims of such abuses.

Helplessness and powerlessness are the essential insults of trauma, and amnesty imposes perpetual helplessness and powerlessness on the victims. It demands that the unspeakable shall remain unspoken. The conflict between denial and testimony is the central dialectic of psychological and social trauma. But as the folklore of all peoples insists, such ghosts will not rest in premature and hasty graves until their story has been told. Healing of individuals and of societies requires remembrances, truth, revelation, repentance, recognition, and mourning for what has been lost. Even divine forgiveness, in most traditions, is not unconditional and must be earned by confession, repentance, and atonement. In South Africa, identification with the aggressor is now official State policy, enforcing a compulsory happy ending.

EPILOGUE: THE SECOND BULLET ... TO KILL A SECOND TIME?

Yet there are transcendent moments. I recall a young black cleric (Anonymous, personal communication, 1988) with whom I was working on a project in Soweto. Late one night, he began recalling his experiences in detention. After a particularly brutal session, his chief interrogator began to jeer at him and to promise an endless misery. "Don't forget," he gloated, "not only will I interrogate you forever, but my children will interrogate your children, and my grandchildren will interrogate your grandchildren." After a brief pause, the young man replied, "I am so sorry to hear that you have so very little ambition in life."

Survival imposes a heavy burden. We are now closer relatives of the dead, and we are obligated to speak for them. We are their true memorials; for many, we are their only memorials. "Do not forget us when we are gone: The only place where we can still live in peace is in your memories" (Simpson, 1993c). As Wiesel (1993) wrote, we are duty-bound to try to communicate what we know of such events, because "not to do so would mean to forget. To forget would mean to kill the victims a second time. We could not prevent their first death; we must not allow them to vanish again. Memory is not only a victory over time, it is also a triumph over injustice" (p. 14).

REFERENCES

Abu-Lughod, I. (1990). Introduction: Achieving independence. In J. R. Nassar & R. Hencock. (Eds.), *Intifada: Palestine at the crossroads* (pp. 1–11). New York: Praeger.

Albeck, J. H. (1994). Intergenerational consequences of trauma: Reframing traps in treatment theory: A second-generation perspective. In M. B. Williams & J. F. Sommer (Eds.), *Handbook of post-traumatic therapy* (pp. 106–125). Westport, CT: Greenwood Press.

American Psychiatric Association. (1994). *Diagnostic and statistical manual of mental disorders* (4th ed.). Washington, DC: Author.

Aysen, N. B., & Nieuwoudt, J. (1992). Attitudes of black senior primary school pupils to the 1991 Soweto township violence and unrest. *UNISA Psychologist, 19*(1) 24–29.

Bettelheim, B. (1984). Afterword. In C. Vogh (Ed.), R. Schwartz, trans. *I didn't say goodbye.* New York: Dutton.

Braam, C. (1994, September 24). De killers van Koevoet. *Vrij Nederland, 38,* 38–45.

Brink, A. (1992). *An act of terror.* London: Minerva.

Brontë, E. (1847). *Wuthering heights,*

Bulhan, H. (1985). *Frantz Fanon and the psychology of oppression.* New York: Plenum Press.

Buruma, I. (1995). *The wages of guilt: Memories of war in Germany and Japan.* New York: Meridian.

Casper, G. (1995). *Fragile democracies: Legacies of authoritarian rule.* Pittsburgh: University of Pittsburgh Press.

Chamberlain, J. (1896). *Hansard, 8 May.* Fourth Series. Vol. XI, columns 914–915. Cited in Kruger, 1958, p. 36.

Cooper, S. (1994). Political violence in South Africa: The role of youth. *Issues: A Journal of Opinion, 22*(2), 27–29.

Curran, P. S. (1988). Psychiatric aspects of terrorist violence: Northern Ireland 1969–1987. *British Journal of Psychiatry, 153,* 470–475.

Danieli, Y. (1984). Psychotherapists' participation in the conspiracy of silence about the Holocaust. *Psychoanalytic Psychology, 1*(1), 23–42.

Danieli, Y. (1993). Diagnostic and therapeutic use of the multigenerational family tree in working with survivors and children of survivors of the Nazi Holocaust. In J. P. Wilson & B. Raphael (Eds.), *International handbook of traumatic stress syndromes* (pp. 889–897). New York: Plenum Press.

Dawes, A., & Tredoux, C. (1989). Emotional status of children exposed to political violence in the Crossroads Squatter areas during 1986–87. *Psychology in Society, 12,* 33–47.

Dawes, A., & Tredoux C. (1990). Impact of political violence on the children of K.T.C. In Centre for Intergroup Studies (Ed.), *The influence of violence on children* Cape Town: Centre for Intergroup Studies.

de Klerk, F. W. (1989). Quoted in Hansson, & van Zyl Smit, 1990 (op cit); and in the *Weekly Mail*, December 1, 1989.

Duncan N., & Rock, B. (1994). *Inquiry into the effects of public violence on children: Preliminary report. Commission of Inquiry Regarding the Prevention of Public Violence and Intimidation.* Johannesburg: Goldstone Commission.

Everatt, D., Orkin, M. (1993, March). *Growing up tough: A national survey of South African youth.* Paper presented to the National Youth Development Conference, Broederstroom, South Africa.

Famularo, R., Fenton, T., Kinscherff, R., *et al.* (1994). Maternal and child post-traumatic stress disorder in cases of child maltreatment. *Child Abuse and Neglect, 18*(1), 27–36.

Feenstra, W. (1995). De psychische gezondheid van naoorlogse kinderen van oorlogsgetroffenen: Resultaten van tien jaar onderzoek [The psychological health of post-war children of war victims: Results of ten years of research]. *Maandblad Geestelijke Volksgezondheid, 49*(5), 541–553.

Fields, R. (1986, August 25). *The psychological profile of a terrorist.* Paper presented at the American Psychiatric Association Annual Meeting, Washington, DC.

Figley, C. R. (1995). Systemic PTSD: Family treatment experiences and implications. In G. S. Everly & J. M. Lating (Eds.), *Psychotraumatology: Key papers and core concepts in post-traumatic stress* (pp. 341–358). New York: Plenum Press.

Fogelson, R. M. (1970). Violence and grievances: Reflections on the 1960's riots. *Journal of Social Issues, 26,* 141–163.

Fraser, J. G. (1933/1934/1936/1977). *The fear of the dead in primitive religion* (Reprint of 3 volumes in 1 volume). G. Geddes, G. J. Gruman, & M. A. Simpson (Eds.). New York: Arno Press.

Fraser, M. (1974). *Children in conflict.* Harmondsworth, UK: Penguin.

Freud, S. (1957). Thoughts for the times on war and death: II. Our attitudes towards death. In J. Strachey (Ed.), *The Standard Edition of the Complete Works of Sigmund Freud,* Vol. XIV (14), pp. 291–292. London: Hogarth Press. (Original published 1915)

Friedman, P. (1949). Some aspects of concentration camp psychology. *American Journal of Psychiatry, 105,* 601–605.

Goodwin, J. M. (Ed.). (1993). *Rediscovering childhood trauma: Historical casebook and clinical applications.* Washington, DC: American Psychiatric Association Press.

Green, A. (1993). Childhood sexual and physical abuse. In J. P. Wilson & B. Raphael (Eds.), *International handbook of traumatic stress syndromes* (pp. 577–592). New York: Plenum Press.

Greenley, J. R., Gillespie, D. P., & Lindenthal, J. J. (1975). A race riot's effects on psychological symptoms. *Archives of General Psychiatry, 32,* 1189–1195.

Gurr, T. R. (1970). *Why men rebel.* Princeton, NJ: Princeton University Press.

Hansson, D., & van Zyl Smith, D. (Eds.). (1990). *Toward justice? Crime and state control in South Africa.* Cape Town: Oxford University Press.

Harkness, L. L. (1993). Transgenerational transmission of war-related trauma. In J. P. Wilson & B. Raphael (Eds.), *International handbook of traumatic stress syndromes* (pp. 635–644). New York: Plenum Press.

Hayner, P. B. (1994). Fifteen Truth Commissions—1974 to 1994: A comparative study. *Human Rights Quarterly, 16*(4), 597–615.

Heimannsberg, B., & Schmidt, C. J. (Eds.). (1993). *The collective silence: German identity and the legacy of shame.* San Francisco: Jossey-Bass.

Herman, J. L. (1992). Complex PTSD: A syndrome in survivors of prolonged and repeated trauma. *Journal of Traumatic Stress, 5,* 377–390.

Heskin, K. (1980). *Northern Ireland: A psychological analysis.* Dublin: Gill & Macmillan.

Hippler, J. (1987, January–February). Low-intensity warfare: Key strategy for the Third World Theatre. *Middle East Report,* pp. 32–38.

Hirshowitz, R., Milner, S., & Everatt, D. (1992). *Growing up in a divided society.* Braamfontein, Johannesburg: CASE.

Ierodiakonou, C. S. (1970). The effect of a threat of war on neurotic patients in psychotherapy. *American Journal of Psychotherapy, 24,* 643–651.

Jackson, J. O. (1994a, June 6). Coming to terms with the past. *Time,* p. 37.

Jackson, J. O. (1994b, June 20). The Balkans: Unfinished business. *Time,* pp. 23–27.

Jaffer, Z. A. (1995). *How the Dutch dealt with the traumas of the Second World War: Some lessons for South Africa.* Cape Town: Justice in Transition.

Kee, M., Bell, P., Loughrey, G. C., *et al.* (1987). Victims of violence: A demographic and clinical study. *Medicine, Science and the Law, 27,* 241–247.

Klaasen, E. (1990). The impact of violence on children. In Centre for Intergroup Studies (Ed.), *The influence of violence on children.* Cape Town: Centre for Intergroup Studies.

Krell, R. (1993). Child survivors of the Holocaust: Strategies of adaptation. *Canadian Journal of Psychiatry, 38*(8), 384–389.

Kruger, R. (1958). *Goodbye dolly gray: The story of the Boer War.* London: Cassell.

Levett, A. (1989). Psychological trauma and childhood. *Psychology in Society, 12,* 19–32.

Lipstadt, D. E. (1993). *Denying the Holocaust: The growing assault on truth and memory.* New York: Free Press.

Lyons, H. A. (1979). Civil violence: The psychological aspects. *Journal of Psychosomatic Research, 23,* 373.

Malepa, M. (1990). The effects of violence on the development of children in Soweto. In Centre for Intergroup Studies (Ed.), *The influence of violence on children.* Cape Town: Centre for Intergroup Studies.

Marris, P. (1974). *Loss and change.* New York: Pantheon Books.

McWhirter, L., & Trew, K. (1982). Children in Northern Ireland: A lost generation. In E. Anthony & C. Chiland (Eds.), *The child in his family* (Vol. 7, *Children in Turmoil: Tomorrow's Parents*). New York: Wiley.

Minkowski, E. (1946). L'anesthesie affective. *Anales Medico-Psychologiques, 104,* 80–88.

Mira, E. (1939). Psychiatric experience in the Spanish war. *British Medical Journal, 1,* 1217–1220.

Mitscherlich, A., & Mitscherlich, M. (1967). *Die Unfahigkeit zu trauern: Grundlagen kollektiven verhaltens.* Munchen: Piper.

Mitscherlich-Nielson, M. (1993). Was konnen wir aus der vergangenheit lernen? *Psyche, 47*(8), 743–751.

Ngubane, H. (1977). *Body and mind in Zulu medicine: An ethnography of health and disease in Nyuswa-Zulu thought and practice.* London: Academic Press.

Porot, M. (1957). Les retentissements psychopathologiques des evenments d'Algerie. *Press Medicale, 65,* 801–803.

Pross, C. (1991). Breaking through the postwar coverup of Nazi doctors in Germany. *Journal of Medical Ethics, 17*(Suppl.), 13–16.

Robbins, K. X. (1993). Oedipus: Uncovering intergenerational cycles of violence. In J. M. Goodwin (Ed.), *Rediscovering childhood trauma: Historical casebook and clinical applications* (pp. 7–26) Washington, DC: American Psychiatric Press.

Rosenheck, R. (1986). Impact of post-traumatic stress disorder of World War II on the next generation. *Journal of Nervous and Mental Disease, 174*(6), 319–327.

Sachs, A. (1995). Preface. In Z. Jaffer (Ed.), *How the Dutch dealt with the traumas of the Second World War: Some lessons for South Africa* (pp. v–vii). Cape Town: Justice in Transition.

Schmidt, A. P., & de Graaf, J. (1982). *Violence as communication: Insurgent terrorism and the Western news media.* London: Sage.

Seligman, M. (1975). *Helplessness: On depression, development and death.* San Francisco: W. H. Freeman.

Simpson, M. A. (1988). *The nature of terrorism and psychiatric findings in the case of three patients alleging torture and coercive interrogation.* Report to the Court in the case of State v. Tshika and others. Supreme Court of South Africa, Natal Region, Pietermaritzburg, South Africa.

Simpson, M. A. (1993a). Traumatic stress and the bruising of the Soul: The effects of torture and coercive interrogation. In J. P. Wilson & B. Raphael (Eds.), *The international handbook of traumatic stress syndromes* (pp. 667–685). New York: Plenum Press.

Simpson, M. A. (1993b). Bitter waters: The effects on children of the stresses of unrest and oppression. In J. P. Wilson & B. Raphael (Eds.), *The international handbook of traumatic stress syndromes* (pp. 601–624). New York: Plenum Press.

Simpson, M. A. (1993c, June 6–10). *Change as trauma: Challenges in the transition to democracy in South Africa.* Closing Plenary address, Third European Conference on Traumatic Stress, Bergen, Norway.

Simpson, M. A. (1993d, June 6–10). *The heavy-hearted joy of my survival . . . on surviving assassination attempts.* Paper presented on the Third European Conference on Traumatic Stress, Bergen, Norway.

Simpson, M. A. (1993e, June 6–10). *"Curl up the small soul . . ." : The effects of traumatic repression on children in South Africa.* Paper presented to the Third European Conference on Traumatic Stress, Bergen, Norway.

Simpson, M. A. (1995). Reforming health care in South Africa. In D. Seedhouse (Ed.), *Reforming health care: The philosophy and practice of international health reform* (pp. 101–126). Chichester, UK: Wiley.

Simpson, M. A. (1996). What went wrong? Diagnostic and ethical problems in dealing with the effects of torture and repression in South Africa. In R. J. Kleber, C. R. F. Figley, & B. P. R. Gersons (Eds.), *Beyond trauma: Cultural and societal dynamics* (pp. 187–212). New York: Plenum Press.

Solomon, Z. 1995. Coping with war-induced stress: The Gulf War and the Israeli response. New York: Plenum Press.

Straker, G., Moosa, F., Becker, R., & Nkwale, M. (1992). *Faces in the revolution: The psychological effects of violence on township youth in South Africa.* Cape Town: David Philip.

Taylor, M., & Quayle, E. (1994). *Terrorist lives.* London: Brassey's.

Theological Exchange Program. (1987). *Low intensity conflict: South Africa under threat* (Pamphlet). Cape Town: Author.

van der Linde, I. (1995). Eastern Cape chaos. *South African Medical Journal, 85*(9), 815–816.

Verhulst, F. C., Althaus, M., & Versluis den Bieman, H. J. (1992). Damaging backgrounds: Later adjustment of international adoptees. *Journal of the American Academy of Child and Adolescent Psychiatry, 31*(3), 518–524.

Weisel, E. (1993, May 17–31). For the dead and the living. *New Leader,* pp. 13–14.

Westermeyer, J. (1995). Cross-cultural care for PTSD. In G. S. Everly & J. M. Lating (Eds.), *Psychotraumatology: Key papers and core concepts in post-traumatic stress* (pp. 375–395). New York: Plenum Press.

30

Intergenerational Responses to the Persecution of the Baha'is of Iran

ABDU'L-MISSAGH GHADIRIAN

Persecution and torture in physical and psychological forms have been associated with religious and societal movements throughout history. In view of the fact that this chapter examines the psychological and spiritual dimensions of persecution based on the Baha'i teachings, and in particular explores the impact of persecution and atrocities on the Baha'is of Iran, it is necessary to briefly acquaint the readers with the Baha'i faith.

Founded in 1844, the Baha'i faith is the youngest and among the fastest growing of the world's independent religions. With followers in over 233 countries and dependent territories, it has become the second most widespread faith, surpassing every religion but Christianity around the globe (Barrett, 1992, p. 269). Its founder, Baha'u'llah (1817–1892), who was born in Iran, was persecuted and banished from His native land and is regarded by Baha'is as the most recent of God's chosen Messengers, including Abraham, Moses, Buddha, Krishna, Zoroaster, Christ, and Mohammed. Baha'u'llah appointed His eldest son, 'Abdu'l-Baha (1844–1921), as His successor and interpreter of His teachings. 'Abdu'l-Baha in His will and testament appointed His grandson Shoghi Effendi as his interpreter and successor.

> The Revelation proclaimed by Baha'u'llah, His followers believe, is divine in origin, all embracing in scope, broad in its outlook, scientific in its method, humanitarian in its principles and dynamic in the influence it exerts on the hearts and minds of men. . . . The Baha'i Faith recognizes the unity of God and of His Prophets, upholds the principle of an unfettered search after truth, condemns all forms of superstition and prejudice, teaches that the fundamental purpose of religion is to promote concord and harmony, that it must go hand-in-hand with science, and that it constitutes the sole and ultimate basis of a peaceful, an ordered and progressive society. It inculcates the principle of equal opportunity, rights and privileges for both sexes, advocates compulsory education, abolishes extremes of poverty and wealth, exalts work performed in the spirit of service to the rank of worship, recommends the adoption of an auxiliary international language and provides the

Part of this chapter is based on an article previously published by the author in 1994 in the *Journal of Baha'i Studies* 6(3): 1–26.

ABDU'L-MISSAGH GHADIRIAN • Faculty of Medicine, McGill University, Montreal, Quebec, Canada H3A 1A1.
International Handbook of Multigenerational Legacies of Trauma, edited by Yael Danieli. Plenum Press, New York, 1998.

necessary agencies for the establishment and safeguarding of a permanent and universal peace. (Shoghi Effendi, 1938, pp. 44–46)

With the advancement of science and technology, humankind has acquired new skills for inflicting physical and psychological pain and suffering. Torture has been used in different forms and in many countries of the world. According to Amnesty International, the use of "brutal torture and ill-treatment" was practiced in more than ninety countries in 1980 (Turner & Gorst-Unsworth, 1990). The figure has risen considerably in recent years. The 1995 Amnesty International annual report reveals that, despite the extraordinary global political changes since 1989, violations of human rights increased in virtually every category (Wright, 1995). Accordingly, in 1994, torture was documented in at least 120 countries, which is almost two-thirds of the countries of the world. The report indicates that opposition groups and governments no longer try to hide evidence of their atrocities, because they do not believe that the international community will make them pay the price. Sadly, some countries even legislate freedom from prosecution. The human atrocities are not limited to ethnic cleansing, religious persecutions, or political strife. They extend to the family, the basic unit of society, and, more specifically, to women. The Amnesty International report shows that "countless women are battered to death by their husbands, burned alive for bringing 'disgrace' on the family, killed for non-payment of dowries, bought and sold in unacknowledged slave markets" (Wright, 1995, p. B1). The report includes the following conclusions:

- At least 54 governments or their agents have carried out extrajudicial executions.
- At least 78 countries have detained or imprisoned prisoners of conscience.
- In 34 countries, prisoners died of poor treatment.
- In 29 countries, people "disappeared" under suspicious circumstances.
- In 36 countries, torture, hostage taking, and deliberate or arbitrary killings were undertaken by armed opposition groups (Wright, 1995).

The Report of the Task Force on Human Rights of the American Psychiatric Association (1985) outlines the techniques of torture used in certain countries, including some in South America, consisting of "beatings; electric shocks; sexual abuse; drugs; underwater submersion; deprivation of food, water and/or sleep; various forms of personal humiliation; confinement to very small spaces; sham executions and death threats against family members" (p. 1393). The Task Force concluded that the impact of these tortures was felt both psychologically and physically. However, the physical effect disappeared earlier, while the psychological impact lasted longer.

The purpose of this chapter is threefold: (1) to examine the nature and characteristics of persecution and suffering in the light of current knowledge and the Baha'i teachings as well as to elaborate on tests and trials in personal development and the role of empowerment in overcoming personal adversities; (2) to explore the psychological as well as spiritual dimensions of adversity and martyrdom and to dispel myths and misconceptions about them; and (3) to elaborate on the recent persecution of the Baha'is of Iran as an example of human rights violations in the land where the religion was born. With these objectives in mind, I set out a general outline of the physical and psychological aspects of persecution and suffering. Then, I examine the concept of suffering and martyrdom by bringing individual cases from the lives of persecuted Baha'is of Iran as tangible examples of human atrocities.

TRAUMA OF PERSECUTION: DEFINITION AND CHARACTERISTICS

Torture is defined as a willful act of infliction of severe pain or suffering (physical or psychological) on a human subject for the purpose of obtaining information, exerting discrimination and punishment, and creating intimidation or coercion against the will of the victim (Turner & Gorst-Unsworth, 1990).

One of the common features of torture is subjugation of the will of the victim by the perpetrator (Turner & Gorst-Unsworth, 1990). For each person who suffers torture and persecution, there are many more who also suffer with them, particularly family and friends. Federico Allodi (1993) refers to one study in which 500 victims of eight hostage-taking episodes were followed up in The Netherlands. In an examination 9 years after the incident, it was reported that 50% of the victims and 29% of the families showed symptoms of posttraumatic stress disorder (PTSD), anxiety, phobias, and psychosomatic symptoms. According to Allodi, victims of persecution experienced the following symptoms:

- Denial is the most common and first defense to appear. Its variants are avoidance, forgetfulness, shifting themes, silences, confusion, and so on.
- Fearfulness and anxiety.
- Feelings of vulnerability, aberration, distress, helplessness, and apocalyptic fear.
- Depression and inability to experience other emotions, particularly love or pleasure.
- Acting out in the form of alcohol or drug abuse.

Traumatized individuals have low tolerance for psychological and physical irritation (van Kolk, 1987). Their reaction to a stressor is either physical aggression toward self or others, or passivity and withdrawal. They may experience emotional excitement or emotional numbing, depending on their personality and their coping defense mechanisms.

Dehumanization of victims is another phenomenon often observed in persecuted subjects. A closer look and deeper reflection on the plight of those who suffered in the Nazi concentration camps during World War II and in the refugee camps in Asia after the Vietnam War or, in more recent times, the tragic events of genocide in Bosnia and Rwanda show that victims of violence were treated as less-than-human objects. They could be entirely innocent, but innocence did not count, because the perpetrators saw virtually everyone else as a real or potential enemy.

Pain and Suffering

Although pain and suffering are often used interchangeably, a distinction between them is necessary. Cassell (1983) states that suffering is usually perceived as a psychological experience, whereas pain is quite often referred to as a physical experience. Patients may tolerate severe pain and not consider it as suffering if they know that the pain is controllable and will end. In contrast, a minor pain may become the source of suffering if that pain stems from a dire and uncontrollable cause such as cancer. In such circumstances, the feelings of helplessness and hopelessness may intensify suffering.

Cassell defines suffering as "the state of severe distress associated with events that threaten the intactness and wholeness (or integrity) of the person. Suffering continues until the threat is gone or the integrity of the person can be restored in some other fashion" (p. 522).

Suffering, Masochism, and Fanaticism

Masochism has been described as "pleasure derived from physical or psychological pain inflicted either by oneself or by others" (Stone, 1988, p. 97). Today, it is very tempting and even fashionable to think of contentment in personal suffering as a masochistic response to life crises. Very often, such a judgment is not only inspired by the materialistic orientation of contemporary psychology but also indicates an inability to see beyond the limitations of the present "state-of-the-art" psychology and discover the spiritual dimension of human reality. The power of faith and its effect in the transformation of human character, as noted in each religious epoch, have baffled many behavioral scientists.

I believe that acceptance of pain and suffering for persevering in one's belief in truth, whether spiritual or scientific, should not be confused with masochism. Scientists who make new discoveries often face the challenge of resistance, rejection, or opposition until the new thesis is proven to be true. Likewise, a person who chooses to tread the path of a new spiritual truth may have to be content with adversities for having dared to be different from those who oppose his or her views. Neither the former nor the latter person intentionally seeks pain and torment for personal satisfaction in the pursuit of perfection. In masochistic pursuit, however, the individual seeks or incites situations where pain or punishment becomes a means of gratification for certain emotional or instinctual needs.

Fanaticism is defined as an excessive and unreasonable enthusiasm or zeal, often involving blind religious fervor and superstitions. When a religious belief departs from logic and proven scientific knowledge, it may very easily lend itself to superstition and fanaticism. However, the Baha'i concept of proclaiming truth is compatible with neither masochism nor fanaticism: It rejects asceticism and intentional infliction of pain upon one's physical or psychological self. The human body is viewed as a temple of the soul, to be cared for and protected. Moreover, the Baha'i faith teaches harmony between science and religion, and repudiates superstition, fanaticism, and any form of prejudice.

The Baha'i view of suffering differs from that of some other religions in that suffering is not seen as a means for personal salvation or to attain the reward of paradise. Nor is it believed that an individual is born sinful and therefore should suffer. The Baha'i faith teaches nobility of the human being and sees in inevitable suffering a challenge for personal growth. The human soul is believed to be unaffected by physical pain and afflictions (Baha'u'llah & 'Abdu'l-Baha, 1971). An example of this can be seen in the life of persecuted Baha'is of Iran and early believers of other religions of the world. In spite of every conceivable type of torture and inhuman adversity, they remained calm and content, reflecting many noble attributes. Indeed, undergoing suffering may have transformed their lower and material qualities into higher and spiritual attributes.

In many of these circumstances, the faith and certitude of the victim may empower him or her to endure pain and suffering. But the victim can also become an embodiment of fanatical emotions and prejudices within a certain movement. The question is, then, what is the prime motive and nature of the movement that has led to this struggle? Does it promote an altruistic, mature, and peace-loving attitude toward humanity, or does it encourage a power struggle for personal or political gain? What is the difference between the gentle disciples of Christ, who suffered brutal persecution, and devout followers of Hitler, many of whom also suffered in their plight? The message of the former was a message of true love and fellowship, whereas the dictum of the latter was hate and power. At the root of suffering and adversity, one can find prejudices of many kinds. From Auschwitz to Hiroshima, from Vietnam to Bosnia, from Kampuchea to Lebanon and Rwanda, one can discern the impact of various forms of prejudice disguised in struggles for ethnic cleansing, religious intolerance, or political dominance.

ON MARTYRDOM

The term *martyrdom* has also been misused by various groups for political reasons to exploit opportunities for enhancement of certain objectives toward which a group or society is striving. Thus, the meaning of slaying has been modified and controlled by the societies of the slayer and the slain in order to convey to the world a desired perception of martyrdom or a judicial retribution depending on the suitability of the one that can serve them best (Eliade, 1987). As a result, an IRA (Irish Republican Army) soldier who died of self-imposed starvation in a British jail, or a Muslim suicide bomber who attacked an Israeli military post or public place in the name of Allah, or a self-immolating Buddhist monk in Vietnam can all be declared "martyrs" alongside disciples of Christ or other prophets who were subjected to violent persecution and death. In the former, the "martyrdom" becomes a means to break through the ideological and social boundaries between conflicting groups, which often have a politically or religiously based power, whereas in the latter, it is a form of submission to a higher spiritual power and unifying divine force for which the prophets themselves suffered grievously.

It has been said that "the martyr dies convinced of his or her legitimate authority, an authority challenging that of executioners. . . . Such charismatic authority discards an older order in a breakthrough to a new social and cultural order, often conceived as a spiritual order" (Eliade, 1987, Vol. 11, p. 231). It has furthermore been stated that

> with martyrdom, the culture of the minority, its ideology and law, is sanctified, a covenant established, stamped with blood. It is written in Mekhilta, a Jewish interpretative work, that every commandment that the Israelites have not died for is not really established, and every commandment that they have died for will be established among them. (p. 233)

Baha'u'llah advised His believers to act with prudence and care and not volunteer to give their lives. Martyrdom in the path of God is the greatest bounty, provided that it takes place through circumstances beyond one's control (Taherzadeh, 1987). Indeed, in response to a believer who asked Baha'u'llah whether it was more meritorious to give one's life for the love of God or to teach the faith with wisdom and the power of utterance, Baha'u'llah replied that the latter was preferable. This view stands in contrast to some of the fundamentalists' indoctrinations to engage willfully in violent suicide attacks and "martyrdom" to promote their cause. Fundamentalism by itself may be an expression of certain mental attitudes rather than a religious belief per se: "There is a difference between the spiritual message at the core of a religion and the blind expression of that faith grounded in fear" (Nakhjavani, 1990, p. 59). This mental attitude of fanatics is charged with emotions such as hate and rage, culminating in a self-imposed "martyrdom." In contrast, the pages of history of the persecution and martyrdom of Baha'is show that these individuals, even in the moments before their death, were submissive and prayed that their tormentors and executioners be guided and forgiven (Nabil-i-Azam, 1932).

Table 1 illustrates reflections on the differing features of true (natural) martyrdom and self-imposed "martyrdom." It is to be noted, however, that the boundaries separating these two can be extremely elusive and subjective, shrouded in mystery, with many unknown areas yet to explored.

For example, Bhatia (1995) reports of a 15-year-old Muslim teenager in Gaza City, who planned to strap 8 kilograms of TNT to his body and to blow himself up in Israel. His plan was foiled by his parents a few nights before it was to be carried out. He later admitted to having been indoctrinated by fundamentalist mentors with the notion of "martyrdom" and "special privileges enjoyed by a Muslim who is willing to sacrifice himself for the sake of his homeland

Table 1. Differing Features of True and Self-Imposed Martyrdom

Natural martyrs	Self-imposed "martyrs"
Condemned to death due to their refusal to recant their belief.	Not condemned to death. Suicide wilfully planned and often intended to cause death and destruction to others to promote a cause.
Empowered with a universal love and compassion.	Often inspired by hate and instigated to punish or kill those perceived as enemies.
Death is imposed by external forces beyond one's control; true martyrdom is preordained.	Death is chosen by free will to serve dogmatic ideology and is avoidable.
Victim prays for forgiveness and guidance of tormentors.	Victim may pray for victory of self against the evil of those who are wrong.
Faithfulness to covenant rather than the desire to attain paradise is the primary goal.	The reward of paradise is often the motivating force to choose death.
Self-abnegation, detachment, and utter submission to the Will of God are the hallmarks of final hours with martyrs seeking no material power.	Self-righteousness and seeking entitlement with passion to destroy in the name of God or an ideology and search for power as a driving force for the action.
Accepts suffering and sacrifice with altruism and freedom from prejudices toward others.	Accepts suffering and sacrifice for specific religious or political reward and is motivated by prejudices.
Death becomes the ultimate witness to the truth of one's belief when all other alternatives are refused.	Death intended to arouse emotional support for a religious or political ambition.
Acknowledges absolute nothingness and seeks no name or fame save the good pleasure of the Lord.	Seeks power and sympathy in name of "martyrdom" when other attempts to that effect fail.

and Allah" (p. B1). He was so strongly brainwashed by the promise of paradise and a face-to-face encounter with Allah that he could hardly wait. His training included daily learning of the Qur'an by rote. He was instructed to carry a dummy pack of explosives around his waist or his shoulders. In his will, addressed to his parents, he expressed his clear expectation of dying a martyr and consoled them with these words: "Oh parents, rejoice. For by becoming a martyr I have opened the gates of Paradise for you and all other members of our family. Farewell with my hopes of meeting you all soon in Paradise" (p. B1). He later confessed to the Palestinian police in Gaza that he had indeed been serious about blowing himself up, with the aim of killing "as many Jews as possible" (p. B1).

SUFFERING AND HUMAN VALUES

Human values are the highest expression of a person's conviction, integrity, and character. They are the fruits of acquired and innate knowledge and personal development. To defend one's spiritual values in the face of adversity is an act of faith and fulfillment. It has been said the sign of a civilized individual is his or her ability to stand unflinchingly for his or her convictions while recognizing their relativity (Berlin, 1969).

In this connection, Shoghi Effendi (1988) stated:

It is only through suffering that the nobility of character can make itself manifest. The energy we expend in enduring the intolerance of some individuals . . . is not lost. It is transformed into fortitude, steadfastness and magnanimity. . . . Sacrifices in the path of one's religion produces always immortal results, "Out of the ashes rises the phoenix." (p. 603)

RESILIENCE TO ADVERSITY

Although severe life stressors and adversities may increase the risk of emotional disturbances (i.e., depression in the face of personal losses), most people do not succumb to these diseases (i.e., most of those who suffer personal losses do not necessarily become clinically depressed and incapacitated, although they are affected by them). According to Rutter (1985), "Resistance to stress is relative, not absolute; the bases of the resistance are both environmental and constitutional; and the degree of resistance is not a fixed quality—rather it varies over time and according to circumstances" (p. 599). Resistance can also have a spiritual dimension, which has not yet been fully explored in modern psychology. This dimension is based on spiritual education, belief, and insight into the nature of human beings and the purpose of their creation.

Exposure to adversities as they come about in the course of life may improve our adaptational capability in facing life events. Indeed, on the one hand, hardship and difficult experiences of an earlier period of life may serve as a form of psychological vaccination and personal preparation that would strengthen the individual to cope better in the future. On the other hand, unresolved traumatic conflicts of childhood may create a psychological climate that would complicate personal development in later life. These kinds of traumatic experiences requiring treatment should not be confused with hardship and difficulties due to, for example, socioeconomic deprivations that many have had to face at some point in life.

Shoghi Effendi (1988), states that through overcoming hardship and tribulation, an essential characteristic of this world, we achieve moral and spiritual development. Using an analogy from Abdu'l-Baha, he compares sorrow to a ploughman's furrow—the deeper the furrow, the greater the harvest.

Recent research studies on the survivors of torture show that repeated exposure to stress may immunize some survivors against subsequent traumatic stress experiences. Social and emotional support by the family and friends plays an important role in protecting against or overcoming traumatic experiences (Basoglu, Paker, & Paker, 1994). Researchers have debated about the impact of stress on individuals and development of PTSD. Although some believe that a person develops a form of neurosis if the stress is strong enough, others maintain that although the stressor is a necessary element, it is not sufficient to cause PTSD in every person exposed to a stressor (Choy & de Bosset, 1992). This shows the complex and multidimensional nature of human vulnerability and resilience to stressful events.

In addition to psychological coping mechanisms, one also needs to come to terms with the reality of the stressful life events and their meaning. This is a process of making an internal adjustment to a difficult problem of an external nature. Depending on educational and cultural attitudes, the coping mechanisms may vary greatly from person to person. In a life crisis of serious proportion, such as a death in the family, the following phases of mourning may take place: shock, denial, despair, recognition, and acceptance. An individual's attitude toward death and belief in life after death will have an important bearing on the ability to cope.

Tolerance and magnanimity have been observed among the early believers of each religion and even among certain pioneers of science who defied opposition with peaceful tolerance and raised questions concerning the validity of stress response theory in the face of life crises. One explanation could be that when the life threat, whether psychological or physical, can be explained and made sense of in the light of scientific or spiritual conviction, that insight will arouse considerable courage that will, in turn, abate the fear and anxiety created by the threat. Moreover, faith itself is a potent force in which human beings find their "ultimate fulfillment" (Tillich, 1957). With true faith, one sees in an inevitable death a fulfillment of one's spiritual convictions. Thus, faith gives a new meaning to suffering, which can transform fear into joy and despair into hope. The heroic lives of the martyrs, their determination and perseverance for their cause in spite of torture and torments inflicted upon them, testify to the strength of their faith and loftiness of their belief, for which they give their most precious possession: life itself.

The history of religions shows that human tolerance to suffering goes far beyond the psychological formulation of defenses and stress adaptation. In such cases, I think, suffering is neither perceived as a traumatic state of despair, nor as a grievous blow to human defenses. Rather, it is welcomed with faith and contentment. This does not imply that victims of religious persecution are free from pain and sorrow; rather, it suggests that their spiritual conviction and faith have changed their perception and attitude toward suffering, and have empowered them to gain greater tolerance. No one knows with scientific certainty at present how a profound spiritual conviction can raise the physiological threshold to pain and suffering, as neither spirituality nor suffering is an experience that can be measured and quantified biochemically or physiologically.

THE TRIAD OF OPPRESSION—RESILIENCE

On the basis of this analysis, the impact of a stressor such as oppression may depend on the following three factors:

- Intensity of oppression.
- Personal endurance and resilience.
- Spiritual or ideological perception and attitude toward oppression (personal interpretation of the event).

Based on this model, the severity of oppression (e.g., trauma, torment, persecution) may not significantly disturb the subject if he or she is prepared to endure for a cause and finds a meaning in it that would give a purpose to his or her life. Although the severity of oppression directed toward an individual is usually beyond his or her control, resilience and behavioral attitude are important factors within his or her power, and both resilience and attitude are influenced by spiritual or sociocultural beliefs. In this process, the attitude will strengthen the will to endure and to resist the oppression. In concentration camps, those who maintained a hopeful and positive attitude or displayed active resistance are reported to have fared and survived better than those who were passive victims, because the resistance activated self-esteem and contact with the outside world (Berger, 1985). One of the most common forms of resistance in the persecution of the Baha'is of Iran was the refusal of the believers to recant their faith and, instead, actively to proclaim their belief. This refusal angered the authorities, who intensified their repression.

TRANSFORMATION OF HATE INTO LOVE

The mystic transformation of hate into love is the result of a spiritual education free from prejudices, which empowers a person to change. It would be very difficult, if not impossible, for one to develop such a capacity for personal transformation without the aid of spiritual insight and faith. This insight and faith can be acquired through the knowledge of and love for God.

Prejudices, whether religious or political, play a powerful role in the perception and suffering of the victim in the mind of the persecutor. Under the influence of political ideology or religious fanaticism, the mind can dissociate the knowledge of pain and suffering from its real feeling and experience. When feeling is dissociated from the reality of perception, and when the conscience is no longer in contact with the mind, the behavioral consequences can be tragic (MacLeish, 1959). A distinguishing feature of responses elicited by the brutal persecution of the Baha'is of Iran is the nonviolent and peaceful attitude of this people in the face of adversity. They reacted with patience and tolerance to aggression and hatred.

The process of transformation of attributes is illustrated by the example of iron, which ordinarily has the qualities of being solid, black, and cold. However, when the same metal absorbs heat from fire, its natural attributes will be sacrificed and transformed into new qualities: its solidity to fluidity, its darkness to light, and its cold to heat. Thus, as the original qualities of iron disappear, the qualities of the fire appear in their place. Likewise, in the fire of ordeals, one sacrifices one's material desires and qualities for spiritual attributes (Baha'u'llah and 'Abdu'l-Baha, 1971).

SPIRITUAL PERCEPTION OF SUFFERING

In the Baha'i writings, trials and tribulations are "preordained" (Baha'u'llah & 'Abdu'l-Baha, 1955). According to Shoghhi Effendi (1968) sufferings and privations are blessings in disguise, for they stimulate, purify, and ennoble our inner spiritual forces. Moreover, there is a great wisdom in their occurrence: "Whatsoever comes to pass in the Cause of God, however disquieting in its immediate effects, is fraught with infinite Wisdom and tends ultimately to promote its interests in the world" (p. 27). Submission to the Will of God is an essential attitude of Baha'is who are faced with adversities beyond their control.

In materialistic societies, self-centeredness and material attachment become impediments to one's submission to the greater Will, and therefore discontentment is prevalent. In such an environment, personal contentment is often sought through material qualifications and success rather than through spiritual fulfillment. "Were it not for tests, pure gold could not be distinguished from the impure. Were it not for tests, the courageous could not be separated from the cowardly. Were it not for tests, the people of faithfulness could not be known from the disloyal" (Baha'u'llah & Abdu'l-Baha, 1986, p. 87). He (Baha'u'llah, 1985) emphatically adds, "O Son of Man! If adversity befall thee not in My path, how canst thou walk in the ways of them that are content with My pleasure? If trials afflict thee not in thy longing to meet Me, how wilt thou attain the light in thy love for my beauty?" (p. 20). It is interesting to note that our interpretation of tests and trials can be very different from the wisdom inherent in the occurrence of these events. Our judgment is finite and limited, while the divine purpose of these calamities is limitless and infinite.

SUFFERING AND RELIGION

The major religions of the world, at the height of their development, were the source of the renewal of civilization and progress in the material and spiritual affairs of humankind (Hofman, 1960).

The birth of every religion has been marked by fierce opposition to, and oppression of, its followers. Throughout history, we have seen this pattern repeat itself. As the Baha'i Faith is a new religion, the persecution of its followers in Iran is a human experience closer to our time, making it possible to analyze objectively the tragic events following its inception. Having discussed the nature and characteristics of persecution and adversity in general, the following focuses on the psychological and spiritual responses of persecuted Baha'is of Iran. The manner of response of these individuals and their attitude toward religious atrocities reflects human response to suffering in light of the Baha'i teachings.

Targeted Victims of Persecution

In recent times, various forms of psychological intimidation and torture of the mind have become potent instruments for aggressors in the religious and political arena to crush human will and defenses. Among different psychological methods used to torment, subjugate, intimidate and oppress innocent Baha'is in Iran, the following are but a few.

Torture the Victims

- Mock executions and other acts of terror as an attempt to force Baha'is to recant their faith or admit to false accusations.
- Forced exposure of the Baha'is to the torture of their family members and friends, or to witness the horrifying scene of the lacerated and injured bodies of these victims in order to arouse fear.
- Total solitary confinement in isolated cells (i.e., 1.72×2 meters) without verbal contact with anyone, including prison guards, for weeks or even months (Universal House of Justice, 1984). Such sensory deprivation and human isolation for a long period of time usually leads to serious psychological consequences.

Psychological and physical intimidation, threats, and torture of victims were common. Kidnapping prominent Baha'is and leveling false accusations to humiliate the victims and incite the mob were carried out to extend repression.

Terrorizing the Families and Community

- In some cases, after issuing the death sentence of a group of Baha'i prisoners, the government withheld the identity of those condemned, causing enormous psychological stress and anguish among relatives and friends. The relatives were left to speculate constantly and painfully about the fate of their loved ones and possible reunion with them (*The Baha'i Question*, 1993).
- Often, after the execution of Baha'is, family members were not informed, and when the death was eventually discovered, the authorities would refuse them any access to the body, thus increasing the sorrow of the grieving survivors. Many of the martyrs whose bodies were not delivered to the family most likely were subjected to cruel physical torture and injuries prior to death.
- After the victim was executed, his or her house and belongings were confiscated, leaving the surviving spouse and children homeless. To add insult to injury, the survivors of those who were executed by firing squad were ordered to pay for the cost of the bullets that took the lives of their loved ones. Family members in some areas were asked to make regular monthly payments for the expenses of the inmates, another example of contempt for the Baha'is (*The Baha'i Question*, 1993).
- Mobs in some towns or cities attacked Baha'i cemeteries and desecrated graves. This reflects the extent of out-of-control violence. Attacks were also directed toward the Baha'i sacred writings.

Assault on Children

- Baha'i children have also experienced psychological pressure in their neighborhoods by being labeled as the offspring of heretics. Young girls were abducted to be converted to Islam.
- Many Baha'i women or girls were victims of rape and assaults. Some were forced to marry Muslims under Islamic law and were deprived of the right to rear children as Baha'is.
- Hundreds of children were expelled from primary and secondary schools because they refused to recant their faith. This caused significant hardship, and although they were later permitted to return to school, they suffered discrimination and insult. University students were also expelled, some in their final year, and even just prior to their final examination. They continued to be denied admission into Iranian universities.

THE ATTACK OF PERSECUTORS—A PROFILE

Persecution is very often the consequence of racial, economic, political, or religious strife. The primary aims of persecution arising from these sources are twofold: (1) rejection of the belief to invalidate, discredit, or undermine the basic beliefs and precepts of the victim; and (2) rejection of the believer, characterized by physical assaults, torture, imprisonment, starvation, and death, or psychological insults and abuses by means of false accusations, humiliation, threats, and deprivation from personal and social rights and privileges.

In 1981, Professor Manuchihr Hakim, an outstanding, gentle, and much-loved physician, was murdered in his office while caring for patients in Tehran. His assailant posed as a patient who needed medical advice after office hours. Professor Hakim's only "crime" was to be a member of the Baha'i Faith. Five years earlier, he had been decorated by the French government with the Legion of Honor for his humanitarian services. Well known for his scientific endeavors, he graduated from the Medial College of Paris and was cited in the prestigious *Le Rouviere,* the French medical encyclopedia, for his anatomical discoveries (Hakim-Samandari, 1985). As a physician and academician, he served thousands of his sick and suffering fellow citizens with the highest degree of dedication and professional integrity, but even his profile of service to humanity did not spare his life from those who could not come to terms with his belief as a Baha'i. This is more evidence of the terrible influence of blind prejudices that dissociate human virtue and noble accomplishment from personal belief in another religion or ideology.

Steadfastness by the believer can evoke an even greater hatred in the persecutors, as this is seen as a sign of the latter's failure. Distortion of truth and manipulation of public conscience as a means of discrediting the subject and justifying the hatred against the victim is quite common. In such circumstances, the public's ignorance creates an ideal climate for accomplishing fanatical objectives. As an example, in the persecution of the Baha'is in Iran, the principle of equality of the rights of men and women in the Baha'i community, and the fact that there is no segregation of sexes in the Baha'i gatherings, have been attacked by the Muslim clergy as immoral deviation in a society where male domination has been the rule for centuries (*The Baha'i Question,* 1993).

MOTIVES FOR ACCUSATION

Accusations against Baha'is have taken different forms at various stages of the history of this religion in Iran. At one point, Baha'is were accused of being connected to the Russian tsars; at another time they were labeled as servants of British or American imperialism. In recent times, they have been accused of being agents of Israel and Zionism. The Baha'is were declared to be *mahdur-addamm* ("those whose blood may be shed") (Martin, 1984), or involved in the "corruption of the earth," "warring against God," and so on. Faced with mounting negative world opinion and pressured by the criticism of human rights violations, the Islamic Republic of Iran denied that the Baha'is were being killed because of their religious beliefs. Rather, they stated, they were being punished for the crime of serving as spies of foreign powers. This was a clear concealment of the earlier actions of their revolutionary courts, which sentenced Baha'is to death on religious grounds. Baha'is were viewed as pagans and heretics who were not people of the Book (Muslims, Jews, Christians, Zoroastrians) and thus must be eliminated. Hence, acts of violence toward Baha'is were sanctioned with the promise of paradise for the perpetrator. The condemned Baha'is reacted with forbearance and compassion, and transcended their physical sorrow and suffering by relying on the Will of God. They embraced their ultimate destiny, an imposed death, and refused to recant their belief. This noble response to the brutal punishment of perpetrators further enraged and frustrated the clergy and government officials, as it was a clear affirmation of faith and reliance on an inner truth that no exterior power could eradicate. Ironically, if the victims had recanted their faith, their "sins" would have been washed away, and they would have been freed with publicity and fanfare. This clearly unmasked the real intention of total extinction of a minority the Islamic regime would neither tolerate nor recognize.

RESPONSE TO PERSECUTION

According to the Baha'i teachings, the creative words of a divine revelation can empower the soul, transform the heart of individuals, and create a new race of people as a result of their unique vision of life. This transformation gives a new meaning and purpose to life that dissipates existential fears and anxieties, replacing them with tolerance and contentment. When the vision of the true purpose of life and its ultimate destiny is blurred with doubts and superstitions, these individuals are no longer able to maintain that sense of security and forbearance at the time of trials and tribulations.

Baha'u'llah (1955) reveals that the suffering his followers experience is preordained to proclaim the Cause of God in this new dispensation and, therefore, empathizes with his followers in their suffering. Moreover, He elucidates that one's love of God will enable one to resist the powers arising against him or her and to overcome any fear. The result is courage and confidence, as observed in the multitude of Baha'is who have experienced torture and atrocity.

He also described a significant association between true love and pain in *The Seven Valleys and the Four Valleys:*

> The steed of this Valley (Love) is pain; and if there be no pain this journey will never end. In this station the lover hath no thought save the Beloved, and seeketh no refuge save the Friend. At every moment he offereth a hundred lives in the path of the Loved One, at every step he throweth a thousand heads at the feet of the Beloved. (pp. 8–9)

IMPACT OF PERSECUTION AND MARTYRDOM
ON SURVIVING FAMILY MEMBERS

In view of the fact that intergenerational impact of persecution and martyrdom has not been systematically studied among first-degree relatives of Baha'is who were persecuted and executed in Iran, the following survey was designed and carried out on a sample of population affected by the recent persecution of Baha'is of Iran. The survey was not intended, however, to be a large-scale study with exhaustive statistical data and detailed analysis. Such an endeavor would require greater freedom of contact with family members, who are still largely in Iran, than the present sociopolitical climate of oppression toward the Baha'i religious minority permits. In fact, it renders that goal dangerous and unattainable. Thus, the present study is confined to those children and grandchildren, as well as spouses of the Baha'i martyrs, who, during the past two decades, have left Iran and settled in different parts of the world. The author was able to contact some of them who reside in North America in order to accomplish this objective as is outlined later.

The Sample Description

The sample consisted of 27 Persian members of families of victims who were killed by the Islamic Revolutionary Government of Iran from 1979 to 1989. The participants, all of whom were contacted by mail, consisted of 19 children and grandchildren (only 2), and 8 spouses (all wives). The mean age of children and of grandchildren was 33 years, whereas the mean age of wives was 60.12 years. The mean age of the entire sample was 41.03 years. Gender distribution was 19 females and 8 males. The objects of these responses were 17 adult Baha'is who were killed: All but one were men.

Each participant received by mail a structured and uniform questionnaire, and their participation in this survey was entirely voluntary. Only those who agreed to respond through the initial telephone call received the questionnaire and the explanatory letter by mail. Out of 31 survivors who were contacted, 4 declined and 27 responded. One of those who declined, a daughter, indicated that the memories of her father's suffering and execution were too painful to relive. Another, a wife of North American origin, indicated that she did not wish to respond, but no reason was given. The remaining 2 simply did not respond. One of these was a son who had been in Iran at the time of his father's imprisonment and execution and was deeply affected emotionally. All of the respondents were living outside of Iran at the time of contact.

Identification of individuals to participate in this program was through informal contact in the Baha'i Community of Canada. All but 7 respondents were residents of Canada at the time of responding to the questionnaire. The questionnaire consisted of a brief demographic section, followed by five questions, as follows:

1. What do you know or remember about the martyred person in your family before he or she was killed?
2. What are your thoughts and impressions (imagined or perceived) of the moments when he or she was being martyred? (Please answer even if you were not there.)
3. What impression do you have in your mind about him or her after the martyrdom?
4. Do you think that you were affected in any way by his or her martyrdom? Yes __ No __ If the answer is yes, please explain how.
5. What are your thoughts and feelings about those who were responsible for the execution of your martyred family member?

Data Analysis.   Study of the responses was conducted on the basis of careful content analysis. There were five variables in this study: four of them were independent variables (questions 1, 2, 3, and 5) and the other (question 4) was a dependent variable. Descriptive findings and analysis are outlined. In the following results, the responses to each question are treated separately.

Results

Knowledge and Memory of the Martyr before Execution.   Question 1: What do you know or remember about the martyred person in your family before he or she was killed?

Respondents pointed out attributes and defenses of the deceased person. These attributes, without exception, were positive in nature. Some noted the deceased person's emotional strength and will to persevere. Others described positive affect such as happiness and joy in life. But these are the views of those who lived for years, or most of their lives, with the martyrs, and the impression imprinted upon them is reflected in their statement. Knowledge and memory of survivors of their loved ones who were executed were all positive. Among the positive emotions they recalled of these individuals were a sense of happiness and calmness that prevailed in the days prior to the execution of some of the martyrs. With regard to the will to face the tragic ending of life, the survivors sensed a remarkable courage in their loved ones before their death. This courage has special significance given the fact that each one of the executed persons was offered release from prison should they repudiate their belief in Baha'u'llah, the Prophet–Founder of the Baha'i Faith. Despite this enticing option, the martyrs chose not to recant and remained faithful and submissive to the will of God. This submission is part of the Baha'i teachings to accept suffering in the path of God.

Among the personal attributes of the martyrs, there were a number of noble characteristics reported, such as their eagerness to serve humanity with altruism, their kindliness, detachment, devotion to their family, resilience in the face of adversity, love for their Faith, love for life and nature, and deep literary interest. A son whose father was killed wrote that "he taught us from an early age to be useful and serve society to the best of our capability." A young boy depicted the tender memory of his grandfather, who was executed in the city of Tabriz, with these words: "He taught me to love and value nature and everything in creation." Another person described his father as "the best father anybody could ask for . . . kind and full of love for his family and everybody around him."

Thoughts and Images of Execution.   Question 2: What are your thoughts and impressions (imagined or perceived) of the moments when he or she was being martyred?

Answers to this question had to be subjective and impressionistic, as no one was allowed to be present at the sites of execution which were mostly done in secret and in some cases after brutal torture (*The Baha'i Question,* 1993).

Several family members experienced emotional pain and agony in the days before or just after the execution. Some described a period of serenity before the storm as they were waiting for the news of the fate of their loved ones. A daughter wrote, "Prior to his martyrdom, emotionally I was in a turmoil. For 3 years, I grieved and had a lot of anxiety. . . . Fortunately his imprisonment was only 2 weeks. Toward the end of his imprisonment, one day, when I was getting home, I suddenly experienced a change in my heart. . . . That change was my surrender to the will of Baha'u'llah. So the next day [when] I was informed about his martyrdom, I easily accepted and did not grieve the way I thought that I would."

A wife, whose husband was arrested and imprisoned, wrote about a deep feeling of calm and serenity she had before the execution, the like of which she had never experienced before. "This was the quiet period before the coming of a violent storm and the silence preceding the fury. I felt the coming of a tempestuous occurrence, an unprecedented event which would change the destiny of mankind. . . . The images of opposing forces of oppression, destruction and calamities on the one hand, and the divine light of glory and majesty on the other, like two theatrical scenes, flashed before my eyes."

Another spouse described her impression of the moments of her husband's execution with these words: "I knew that at the time of his martyrdom, my husband, with full submission and detachment, stepped into the arena of sacrifice. . . . Therefore, we have to accept it whole-heartedly. We have to be thankful that a lover has attained the presence of his Beloved." This reflects a mystic perception of death in the path of God, the outcome of which is leading the lover to his Beloved, God.

Another woman praised her husband's steadfastness and prayerful attitude at the final moments of his life. "It is related that at the very moment my husband faced the bullets of the enemies, he had lifted up his face for prayers and communication with his Beloved (God), for the autopsy showed that the first bullet had struck him in the throat. Such was his joy to offer up his life in the path of his Lord." And as to how she, herself, felt about her husband and his dire fate, she wrote, "I yearned for his life to be spared, and yet I prayed for his steadfastness in the path of Baha'u'llah."

A woman, who was 10 years old at the time of her father's execution, reacted to the news of his death with these words: "I felt such a wave of heat, it was as if I was being scorched in a fire." Another daughter described her reaction by saying, "I felt lost thinking how life without my dad could exist and how it would be. I had and still have many questions about the last days of his life in prison, his thoughts and feelings, his trial, how he faced his firing squad and so on. Although these questions are partly answered, I don't feel the need to know the rest. I believe these questions are born out of human curiosity and mean very little in the great scheme of things."

Not all were comforted with faith and serenity. One daughter noted that after she heard the news of the killing of her father, she went into "shock" and could not believe what had happened. She feared that he felt abandoned in those final hours of his life in prison.

Many expressed their impressions in terms of certain attributes that they assumed characterized their martyr's final hours of life, such as being calm, detached, happy, steadfast, and brave. No adversarial expressions, such as aggression, vengeance, and violence, were noted throughout the responses. One person reported that eyewitnesses (Baha'i and non-Baha'i) reported that the martyr went to his death while chanting prayers. Even an Islamic court authority responsible for his execution admitted to his bravery.

Psychological and Spiritual Imagery of the Victim after Execution.   Question 3: What impression do you have in your mind about him or her after the martyrdom?

The immediate response was a sense of loss. "I miss him terribly as 'my dad,'" one said. One woman, now 47 years old, mentioned that although on the logical level she accepted the martyrdom of her father, on the emotional level, even after 14 years, she had not come to grips with it. However, because it was in the path of God, this separation caused less agony than it otherwise would have. Many viewed the martyrdom of their loved one as an honor of which they were proud and felt closer to the martyr after his or her death. They also felt that the principle of obedience to the will of God, enshrined in the Baha'i teachings, enabled them to accept and endure this suffering. As for the victim,, they felt that he or she was spiritually elevated to a new rank and was probably beaming with joy in the world beyond.

Several family members indicated their images of the martyr being happy and peaceful after his or her death and endowed with courage, steadfastness, dignity, and honor.

The Impact of Martyrdom on the Families.   Question 4: Do you think that you were affected in any way by his or her martyrdom?

Of 27 respondents, 24 stated that the death of their father, mother, husband, or grandfather affected their lives. Two said it had no effect, and one said he had no response. Of those who were affected, 10 experienced a negative effect such as being deprived of the person, being abandoned by him or her, missing him or her and feeling sad about his or her absence. Fourteen felt it had a positive effect on them. It caused them to become more mature, more dedicated; it created a spiritual atmosphere, strengthened the person, and empowered the family with unprecedented courage.

The family members reacted to the death of their loved one in both positive and negative ways. For example, one widow said it was a shock for her to learn that her husband had been killed, but on the other hand, it led her to develop patience and forbearance in the face of afflictions. Others felt that the loss inspired them to greater devotion, courage, and steadfastness in their faith. One person who witnessed the mutilated corpses of her husband and companions was inspired by an unprecedented courage and bravery. "For days it seemed as if I moved in a different realm, and to this day, I remember those moments with great joy and longing." She felt this change of her weakness into strength was through the assistance of Providence. The event "changed me into a volcano possessed of such driving power that, fearless and oblivious of all the dangers which surrounded me, I cried out to the truth of this revelation and to the innocence of the martyrs against the onslaught of the oppressors," she remarked.

Another widow, a 67-year-old woman and a mother, described the effect of the martyrdom of her husband in two ways. On the one hand, it created a more spiritual and unifying climate within their family and fostered a strong spirit of faith in her older children. On the other hand, the loss of her husband created a vacuum in their lives:

> Deprived of his presence, we felt despondent and abandoned. My youngest son, who was 13 years old at that time and very attached to his father, missed him dearly and remained affected for a long time. It took him a great deal of time to come to understand the significance of the event and the station of those souls who sacrificed their lives in the path of God. I remember very well the day when we had to sell the car which belonged to my husband. On that day (my son) was so unhappy that he wept and did not want us to hand over the car key to the new owner. You can well imagine the depth of our agony and the anguish of our souls.

This human dimension of suffering underlines the other side of the impact of loss of a parental figure and the daily struggle of the spouse and offspring to cope with the brutal consequences of persecution and death.

Reaction toward the Persecutors.   Question 5: What are your thoughts and feelings about those who were responsible for the execution of your martyred family member?

Some of the respondents reacted by saying that although initially they had a feeling of hatred and anger, later on, they developed a sense of forgiveness. Others felt that the persecution was part of a greater plan of God to promote His Cause: "He doeth what He willeth." In this plan, the protagonists on the scene of persecution played their role, while submission and acceptance became the lot of those who suffered. One person blamed the cleric system and not the individuals for the tragedy. As a whole, there was no sense of revenge. This is not a denial of underlying anger as much as it is an expression of belief based on tolerance and forgiveness. It also reflects a broader vision of calamity, which is viewed as a disguised blessing that ultimately leads to the expansion of the Faith. For example, a daughter grieving the death of her executed father commented that because of the Divine Plan, "I do not feel any hatred toward those who contaminated their hand with the blood of my father. . . . May God forgive their transgressions. I pray fervently for them."

What is interesting is that several of the respondents reacted initially with anger and hate, but soon these feelings yielded to more positive effects as compassion and forgiveness prevailed. This is a transformation of hate into love. Some left the aggressors to be judged and dealt with by God. Others pitied them for their ignorance.

Of the 27 first-degree family members, 3 declined to forgive and hoped that justice would be done, but felt pity for the perpetrators. There were 2 siblings who lost both of their parents. One stated that she had "absolutely no feeling, since any feeling is too good for anyone who can kill my wonderful parents." Here is a repressed rage and anger that is not allowed any expression, as the tragedy of oppression is too hideous to be confronted with words. Yet her brother, on the same question, spoke of his feeling openly saying, "I have no hate for those responsible for my parents' martyrdom. I feel pity towards these individuals."

One person whose father was executed believed that the perpetrators would experience their own punishment through realization of the truth of the Baha'i faith in this world or in the worlds to come. "Revelation of truth," she pronounced, "to these people will pain their conscience to a degree that death may be an easier choice." The perception of this young woman conveys a profound sense of maturity and vision on the basis of which human conscience will stand on trial at the moment of its awakening to a reality that it refused to acknowledge at the moment of committing the hideous act. Such an enlightened concept releases the persecutee or the relatives from the rage of revenge or hatred.

INTERGENERATIONAL PERCEPTION OF MARTYRDOM: RESPONSES OF GRANDCHILDREN

Among the respondents were 2 grandchildren, 1 male and 1 female, from two different families, who lived or were associated closely with the martyred person during their childhood in Iran. Their responses are analyzed and compared with the reactions of their mothers, who also participated in this study. The grandchildren were less emotionally distraught than their parents and more able to recall fond childhood memories. Both idealized their grandfathers, stating that they wished to strive to attain their nobility of character. With regard to question 4, in one case, the mother denied having been affected by the arrest and execution of her father, while her son stated that he had been deeply affected, wishing to emulate his grandfather. In the second case, both daughter and mother were greatly affected in a very positive way, stating that the experience had caused them to become more peaceful and mature.

Regarding the last question, concerning the attitude toward the persecutors, one grandchild stated that he felt neither anger nor empathy toward the persecutors, while his mother denied hatred and expressed prayerful forgiveness toward them. In the second case, the grandchild felt great anger at first toward her grandfather's executioners for taking him away from her, but later she forgave them. Her mother also had an initial feeling of anger toward her father's executioners, but she, too, decided to leave them to God and to pray for them.

A comparison of the responses of children and grandchildren of the martyrs reflects a difference in perception of and attitude toward forces beyond their control, which may be related to age and personal development. Although the number of grandchildren in this study was limited, their responses, like those of their parents, were guided by their Baha'i belief in the importance of maintaining a peace-loving and forgiving attitude. One might ask, if the grandchildren had not been Baha'is, would their reaction have been the same? It is my hope to repeat this study 5 or 10 years from now, expanding it to a larger number of respondents to see if, with the passage of time, changes in perception occur.

Discussion

This brief survey reflects certain reactions and defenses of wives and children of Baha'is of Iran who were recently executed. For the most part, these defenses included idealization of martyrs and transformation of anger and rage into submission to the Will of God, leading to acceptance. Nevertheless, several respondents admitted experiencing emotional turmoil and agony in the perplexing days and hours prior to execution. Two referred to this period as one of "serenity before the storm." And when the storm struck (announcement of execution), the sudden stroke of grief ultimately yielded to tolerance and contentment, to a greater Will. Indeed, some rejoiced at the victory of the soul over the violent and fatal attack to their loved ones. They praised the martyrs for their courage, steadfastness, and their unfailing determination to remain constant in their faith. But the "storm" was not a messenger of joy for everyone. Some suffered bitterly and, as one person stated, it was like being "scorched in a fire." Particularly intense was the pain of despair affecting the younger children who could not make sense out of the loss of their fathers in the fire of ordeal and fanatic persecution. (It is to be noted that the execution occurred 10–15 years ago and some of the respondents were quite young at the time.)

After the killing, a sense of loss was felt by all, and yet many felt this event was an honor bestowed upon their family. Had the martyrs denied their faith, for which they and their families were being persecuted, and survived, the impact may have been more devastating, as it would have been a rejection of truth.

As a whole, the death of the martyrs in defense of truth enhanced and augmented the affiliation of family members to the Baha'i faith and had a unifying effect on the lives of the survivors. They discovered that love more than hatred could become an instrument to awaken the souls and bind together hearts, allowing the healing process to take place. No doubt Baha'i teachings played a crucial role in bringing about such a peaceful attitude. These positive defenses were ego-syntonic and not ego-alien in this population.

Sigal (1995), in his study of Holocaust survivors, pointed out that "endowment, temperament, or familial environmental factors that preceded the persecution can be advanced to explain these resilience producing traits" (p. 8). This can explain the steadfastness and resilience of the family members prior, during, and after the execution, owing to the educational influences of the teachings of Baha'u'llah. As Viktor Frankl (1963) stated, "Suffering ceases to be suffering in some way at the moment it finds a meaning, such as the meaning of sacrifice" (p. 179).

Conclusion

Persecution, suffering, and martyrdom characterize the evolution of world religions, particularly in their early stage of development and expansion. Although there is a general pattern of tolerance and submission to the Will of God in the persecution of the early believers of each religion, it is only recently that we have been able to explore the psychological dimension of these atrocities in relation to their spiritual aspects. The persecution of the adherents of the Baha'i faith, which is the most recent divine religion, allows us to study more closely the attitude of the persecuted individuals, more notably the martyrs close to our time, as well as the reaction of their family members, and to discover the uniqueness of their psychological and spiritual perceptivity and submission to the Will of God and dedication of their lives to humanity. The chapter also outlines the differential features between militant and self-imposed "martyrdom" and real martyrdom. It furthermore delineates different aspects of human values, resilience, and responses to various forms of human suffering and adversity. It is hoped that more research will be done in the future to illuminate further this dark side of human suffering in order to appreciate the true spiritual destiny of humankind on this planet.

REFERENCES

Allodi, F. A. (1993). Terrorism and torture. In A.-M. Ghadirian & H. E. Lehmann (Eds.), *Environment and psychopathology* (pp. 141–157). New York: Springer.

American Psychiatric Association. (1985). Report of the Task Force on Human Rights. *American Journal of Psychiatry, 142*(11), 1393–1394.

The Baha'i Question: Iran's secret blueprint for the destruction of a religious community. New York: Baha'i International Community.

Barrett, D. (1992). Religion: World's religious statistics. In *Britannica Book of the Year* (p. 269). Chicago: Encyclopaedia Britannica.

Baha'u'llah. (1985). *The Hidden Words of Baha'u'llah.* Kuala Lumpur, Malaysia: Baha'i Publishing Trust.

Baha'u'llah. (1955). *The seven valleys and the four valleys* (3rd ed.). Marzieh Gail with A. K. Khan, Trans. Wilmette, IL: Baha'i Publishing Trust.

Baha'u'llah & 'Abdu'l-Baha. (1955). *The Baha'i revelation: A selection from the Baha'i holy writings.* London: Baha'i Publishing Trust.

Baha'u'llah & 'Abdu'l-Baha. (1986). *Divine art of living.* M. H. Paine (Ed.). Wilmette, IL: Baha'i Publishing Trust.

Baha'u'llah & 'Abdu'l-Baha. (1971). *Reality of man.* New Delhi: Baha'i Publishing Trust.

Basoglu, M., Paker, M., Paker, O., *et al.* (1994). Psychological effects of torture: A comparison of tortured with non-tortured political activists in Turkey. *American Journal of Psychiatry, 151*, 76–81.

Berger, D. M. (1985). Recovery and regression in concentration camp survivors: A psychodynamic re-evaluation. *Canadian Journal of Psychiatry, 30*, 54–59.

Berlin, I. (1969). Two concepts of liberty. In *Four essays on liberty.* New York: Oxford University Press.

Bhatia, S. (1995, May 2). Luring children to death with visions of paradise. *The Gazette* (Montreal), pp. B1, B8.

Cassell, E. J. (1983). The relief of suffering. *Archives of Internal Medicine, 143*, 522–523.

Choy, T., & de Bosset, F. (1992). Post-traumatic stress disorder: An overview. *Canadian Journal of Psychiatry, 37*, 578–583.

The Encyclopedia of religion (1987). Eliade (Editor-in-Chief). New York: Macmillan.

Frankl, V. E. (1963). *Man's search for meaning.* New York: Simon & Schuster.

Gollwitzer, H. (Ed.) (1965). *Dying we live.* (R. Kuhn, Trans.). London: Macmillan.

Hakim-Samandari, C. (1985, Fall). A victory over violence: A personal testimony. *World Order, 20*(1), pp. 9–29.

Hofman, D. (1960). *The renewal of civilization.* London: George Ronald.

MacLeish, A. (1959, March). The poet and the press. *Atlantic Monthly,* pp. 44–46.

Martin, D. (1984). Persecution of the Baha'is of Iran, 1844–1984. *Baha'i Studies, 12/13.* Ottawa: Association for Baha'i Studies.

Nabil-i-Azam. (1932). *The dawnbreakers: Nabil's narrative of the early days of the Baha'i revelation.* Shoghi Effendi (Trans. & Ed.). Wilmette, IL: Baha'i Publishing Trust.

Nakhjavani, B. (1990). *Asking questions: A challenge to fundamentalism.* Oxford, UK: George Ronald.

International—Iran. *Newsweek,* June 18, 1994, p. 57.

Rutter, M. (1985). Resilience in the face of adversity. *British Journal of Psychiatry, 147*, 598–611.

Sigal, J. J. (1995, August). *Long-term effect of the Holocaust: Resilience in the first, second, and third generation.* Summary of studies using representative sample, presented at the 103rd Annual Convention of the American Psychiatric Association, New York, NY.

Shoghi Effendi. (1938). *World order of Baha'u'llah.* Wilmette, IL: Baha'i Publishing Committee.

Shoghi Effendi. (1968). *Baha'i administration: Selected letters 1922–1932* (5th ed.). Wilmette, IL: Baha'i Publishing Trust.

Shoghi Effendi (1988). Quoted in *The lights of guidance* (Comp. Helen Hornby. 3rd ed.). New Delhi: National Spiritual Assembly of the Baha'is of India.

Stone, E. M. (1988). *American psychiatric glossary* (6th ed.). Washington, DC: American Psychiatric Press.

Taherzadeh, A. (1987). *The revelation of Baha'u'llah* (Vol. 4). Oxford, UK: George Ronald.

Tillich, P. (1957). *Dynamics of the faith.* New York: Harper & Row.

Turner, S., & Gorst-Unsworth, C. (1990). Psychological sequelae of torture: A descriptive model. *British Journal of Psychiatry, 157,* 467–480.

Universal House of Justice. Letter of May 13, 1984.

van Kolk, B. A. (1987). The psychological consequences of overwhelming life experiences. In B. A. van Kolk (Ed.), *Psychological trauma* (pp. 2–3). Washington, DC: American Psychiatric Association.

Wright, R. (1995, July 6). Governments ignoring rights abuses, Amnesty International says in report. *The Gazette* (Montreal), p. B1.

VIII

Domestic Violence and Crime

31

Intergenerational Child Maltreatment

ANN BUCHANAN

INTRODUCTION

It is now more than 30 years since Henry Kempe was credited with "rediscovering" child abuse (Kempe, Silverman, Steele, Droegemueller, & Silver, 1962). Since then, there has been a sustained international effort to afford effective protection to children. Yet, today, a large number of children continue to suffer. What is worse, when these children themselves become parents, many are unable to protect their offspring or may actually inflict the suffering they themselves endured. This intergenerational legacy of trauma has become known as the "cycle of abuse."

The purpose of this chapter is to reexamine current world literature emanating from psychiatry, psychology, anthropology, sociology, social policy and social work, and related disciplines in order to elicit new insights into our understanding of the phenomenon. Although it is recognized that there are inextricable links between family violence and child maltreatment, the main focus of the review is on maltreatment of children, and there is only limited material on sexual abuse of children.

For the purposes of this review, a broad definition of child maltreatment has been used: "Abuse of children is human-originated acts of commission or omission and human-created or tolerated conditions that inhibit or preclude unfolding and development of inherent potential of children" (Gil, 1981, p. 295).

The Intergenerational Hypothesis

Since the first studies by Steele and Pollock in 1968, the cycle of abuse has been one of the most enduring yet controversial theories of child maltreatment. Much of the early evidence supporting this theory came from psychiatric studies that noted pathological features in abusing families and, in particular, among these families in their own histories of abuse.

In the United States, there was a strong reaction to the "cycle of abuse hypothesis." Courts could unfairly judge parents as more likely to abuse their child on the evidence that they had been abused themselves (Cicchetti & Aber, 1980).

ANN BUCHANAN • University of Oxford, Department of Applied Social Studies, Oxford OX1 2ER, United Kingdom.

International Handbook of Multigenerational Legacies of Trauma, edited by Yael Danieli. Plenum Press, New York, 1998.

This "inevitability" was not supported by studies that looked at large samples of parents from the general population who had experienced abuse in their childhood. These studies found a much weaker correlation between early abuse and later abusive parenting. The findings shown in Table 1 demonstrate the apparent contradiction.

The studies, however, were not as contradictory as they appeared. First, the methodological approaches determined what results were found. Retrospective clinical studies of abusing parents, particularly severely abusing parents, often found nearly a 100% correlation. Prospective studies found that the association between past and present abuse was much weaker. Second, there was also evidence that in self-report studies of past abuse, findings may have been biased by the tendency for abused parents to idealize their childhoods (Oliver, 1993). Third, those studies that viewed the wider social context found poverty and structural inequalities significantly correlated with later abuse (Gil, 1970). The hypothesis was that intergenerational patterns of maltreatment related to a cycle of disadvantage rather than a cycle of abuse. Despite the controversies, there is now some consensus among researchers studying family violence in the United States and United Kingdom that around 30% of those who have been abused will go on to abuse their own children (Gelles & Loseke, 1993; Kaufman & Zigler, 1989). This figure constitutes a significant risk factor, being approximately six times the base rate for abuse in the general population (5%) (Kaufman & Zigler, 1989).

There was a further dilemma. As most of the studies originated in the United States and United Kingdom, it was initially felt that child abuse and the cycle of child maltreatment was

Table 1. Rates of Intergenerational Child Abuse

Study	Year	Rate IGT	Type of study
Oliver & Taylor	1971	100%	Retrospective agency record linkage of severely abusive families.
Steele & Pollock	1968	100%	Retrospective study of abusive parents. No controls. Wide definition of abuse.
Hunter & Kilstrom (Retrospective)	1979	90%	Retrospective: Agency record/self-report/controlled.
Egeland & Jacobvitz	1984	70%	Prospective multiple interviews of high-risk parents. Comparison: abusive versus non-abusive group/various rating scales. Wide definition of abuse.
Herrenkohl et al.	1983	47%	Retrospective self-report clinical study with comparison subjects.
Egeland et al.	1988	40%	As 1984 study above, but minus "borderline" abuse categories.
Straus	1979	18%	Retrospective self-report, nationally representative sample.
Hunter & Kilstrom (Prospective)	1979	18%	Prospective self-report, controlled.
Gil	1970	7–14%	Nationwide survey, self-report.
Altemeier et al.	1986	2–5%	Prospective self-report, controlled.
Widom	1989	1%	Prospective agency records for validated child abuse, controlled.

a specific feature of life in advanced economies (Korbin, 1987). However, studies in other cultures have confirmed that this is not so.

Kaufman and Zigler (1989) feel that the time has come for researchers to cease arguing over the precise percentages of how many abused children will become abusing parents. Instead, there is a need to focus efforts on the conditions under which the transmission of abuse is most likely to occur. This review moves in this direction.

THE FOUR CYCLES

The literature can broadly be grouped into four major cycles that directly or indirectly lead to intergenerational child maltreatment. These cycles are cultural, sociopolitical, psychological, and biological. The first two are extrafamilial, with factors in societies as the focus, whereas the last two are predominately intrafamilial and personal. The separate divisions are, of course, artificial, as the four cycles interrelate, but it is the thesis of this review that the separate mechanisms need to be unwound in order to target appropriate interventions.

Cultural Factors in Intergenerational Child Maltreatment

Cross-cultural studies demonstrate that parents around the world are faced with a similar task when rearing children. In all societies, the helpless infant must be protected from the risks threatening survival and turned into a responsible adult obeying the rules of his or her community.

Whiting and Edwards (1988) have shown that as both elicitors and actors, children share panhuman characteristics that equip them for survival. However, cultural forces modulate social development and lead to increasing differences in the kinds of behavior adults expect. Although the needs and environment of different societies play an important role in developing different parenting styles, how parents parent is largely passed from generation to generation.

Although no society condones child maltreatment, what is, and is not, defined as abusive is culturally constructed (Finkelhor & Korbin, 1988). Children the world over are at risk from a wide variety of violence that is generally carried out by their parents or with their parents' tacit approval (Levinson, 1989). In extreme circumstances such as infanticide, abuse of children can be seen as consistent with the drive for survival. Most types of culturally condoned violence only occur in a few societies. The major exception is the use of physical punishment in child rearing (Radda Barnen Organisation, 1993). The problem is that there is a relationship between severe chastisement and serious injury to children.

Levinson (1989) has shown that there is also a relationship between different forms of violence, in particular wife beating, and child physical chastisement. Physical punishment is not, however, a prerequisite for successful rearing. In his study of 90 societies, he found 16 in which there was no physical chastisement of children, or indeed any other form of family violence. These 16 societies were found in all geographical regions of the world. Family violence was less common in societies that were characterized by cooperation, commitment, sharing, and equality.

These findings are supported by other researchers. Mejiuni, for example, in Nigeria, demonstrated that within cultures, there can be a support system that permits and encourages forms of child maltreatment (Mejiuni, 1991).

Korbin has shown that there is considerable resistance to the fact that appropriate parenting is not an infallible and innate attribute of all parents. This inhibits the recognition of child maltreatment (Korbin, 1991). The media in many countries have played an important role in identifying abuse and raising social awareness (Ikeda, 1982; Kokkevi & Agathonos, 1987; Mejiuni, 1991).

Studies from around the world demonstrate that there are wide cultural variations in defining what is abuse. In Nigeria, for example, Obikeze (1984) discovered that economic exploitation of children was felt by the local population to be the number one form of child maltreatment. Other forms regarded as abusive, such as child pawning may be unknown in other areas. Korbin suggests that in coming to internationally accepted definitions of child abuse, there is a need for both an EMIC approach—where the local community makes the definitions—and an ETIC approach—where there is an international consensus on types of behavior toward children that are deemed abusive (Korbin, 1980, 1987).

Finkelhor and Korbin (1988) have also shown that cross-culturally, particular categories of children are vulnerable to maltreatment. These children are those with inferior health status, malnourished children, deformed or handicapped children, excess or unwanted children, and stigmatized children (such as illegitimate children). Children are also at particular risk in different societies at different developmental stages. In addition, in many countries, gender can compromise the health and survival of the girl child, while in Greece, higher expectations of the male child can place him at risk (Agathonos-Georgopoulou, 1992). Children with socially diminished supports, such as stepchildren, are a particularly vulnerable group.

Studies, mainly from the United States, have shown that children and families moving into areas with different lifestyles or living in changing socioeconomic situations can find their traditional child-rearing patterns are no longer protective to children (Gray & Cosgrove, 1985; Reid, 1984; Spearly & Lauderdale, 1983). Urban environments, in particular, can have an inhibiting and even destructive effect on the supportive functions of the family. However, where effective support networks can be maintained, these serve a protective role for family functioning and child welfare.

Sociopolitical Factors in Intergenerational Child Maltreatment

Most families, even in the most extreme conditions, do not maltreat their young, but small changes in social conditions have important effects on lowering the thresholds in which many parents can parent effectively. Although child abuse cuts across social and economic groups, it does so unevenly. The poor are always most at risk (Gelles, 1973; Gil, 1970; Straus, Gelles, & Steinmetz, 1988). This is related not only to poverty but also to the correlates of poverty, such as poor nutrition and health, and lack of access to effective health care, education, housing, and employment opportunities. In the industrialized countries, drug abuse and criminality may also correlate with poverty. Minority and ethnic groups may be particularly disadvantaged, and this is a feature of both developed and developing countries. Single parents can be the most disadvantaged of all. Rutter, Quinton, and Liddle (1983) in the United Kingdom have shown although there are discontinuities from disadvantage, there are also considerable continuities. Parents need what Rutter has called "permitting circumstances" (Department of Health and Social Security, 1974) in order to parent. These relate not only to the adequacy of basic needs such as food, housing, health, and financial well-being but also to support from family and friends, and the community. When the "permitting circumstance" thresholds are lowered, more families are at risk and more children are abused.

Fostering Human Security.   State policies have an important role in increasing or decreasing these thresholds. For example, state policies, directly or indirectly, can lead to a lack of human security. Human security (United Nations Development Program, 1994) refers to cataclysmic events such as war and national disasters, as well as to job, income, health, access to education, environmental security, security from crime and violence, and social integration.

Definitions of Human Security

If a country is at war how are people supposed to feel secure? (Child in Iraq)

I feel secure when I know that I can walk the streets at night without being raped. (Child in Ghana)

When we have enough for the children to eat, we are happy and feel secure. (Father from Thailand)

Robberies make me feel insecure. I sometimes feel as though even my life will be stolen. (Man in Namibia)

Human security indicates faith in tomorrow, not so much as having to do with food and clothing, as with stability of the political and economic situation. (Man in Ecuador, United Nations, 1994, p. 23)

In countries undergoing rapid socioeconomic change, traditional family support systems can be disrupted. State policies have an important role in managing socioeconomic change in such a way that it maintains, as far as possible, effective family functioning. The lack of human security has intergenerational continuities, and there is a growing realization that even after the original threat has diminished, there can be an emotional cost that affects the parenting abilities of future generations (Schwebel, 1992).

Every Child a Wanted Child. In Romania, Professor Radulian (1992), President of the Romanian National Committee for UNICEF, spoke of the savagely espoused policy of a forced birthrate legislated by the previous totalitarian system in his country that changed the very spirituality of Romania. *"Paradoxically instead of growing and educating children, families have come to the stage of not wanting their children . . . leading to an increasing number of abandoned and handicapped children, of orphaned and vagrant children, the very destruction of the family"* (Radulian, 1992, p. 1).

Dytrych (1992), in a study in the Czech Republic spanning more than 20 years, has also shown that when women were denied abortion and when this was upheld on appeal, "unwanted" children had considerably more difficulties than a comparison group of "wanted" children, and there were intergenerational continuities.

Both pronatalist policies in industrialized countries and family limitation policies in developing countries can have profound and sometimes unexpected repercussions on the well-being of children. There is concern that the mandatory limits on family size in China may have led to a generation of overindulged and overweight young men. On the other hand, population forecasts in particular areas indicate considerable urgency in assisting families to limit the number of children they have. Some economists argue that development is the best contraceptive. As the World Congress on Population (Cairo 1995) highlighted, children's well-being cannot be separated from women's well-being.

Policies to Protect Women. Women cannot effectively rear healthy babies if they themselves are ill, malnourished, overworked, insecure within their families, and treated by society as a disadvantaged group. The patterns are particularly strong in developing countries, although in the developed world a similar pattern can be seen among inner-city groups. The double disadvantage of being born poor and female is vividly illustrated by UNICEF in their booklet *The Girl Child* (1991). Ill health and low quality of life for girl children lead to ill health and low status when they become women. This may be linked to lack of education, poverty, malnutrition, and an unhealthy environment. There may be harmful traditional practices such as female circumcision (Bruce-Chwatt, 1976) and child marriage, as well as lack of family planning and lack of health care, especially during labor. Such intergenerational patterns may be compounded by violence, abuse, and insecurity within the family and within society (El-Mouelhy, 1992). The irony is that the health and well-being of *both* male and female children are affected by the disadvantages experienced by their mothers.

Policies That Promote the Family.   The rapid rise in the number of parents who divorce and the increase in single parenthood is a disturbing phenomenon in industrialized countries (United Nations, 1994). Single parenthood is largely accounted for by those who are separated or divorced, but there has also been a rise in unmarried parenthood. There is considerable evidence on a range of indicators that many children of single parents do less well than children of two-parent families (Essen & Wedge, 1983; Brubaker, 1993). In the United Kingdom, there is a powerful relationship between poverty and lone parent status, most of whom are women (Bradshaw & Millar, 1991). Policies in the United Kingdom have placed many single mothers in a welfare poverty trap, and there are considerable intergenerational continuities (Rutter, 1989). The controversial Child Support Act of 1990 in England and Wales is intended to combat lone-parent poverty but it remains to be seen how effective this will be. Polices have also not encouraged the reliable day care that enables mothers to go out to work. The United Kingdom has some of the lowest levels of day care in Europe.

Effective Policies to Protect Children.   For many children in the world today, protection is manifestly inadequate. Munir (1993) suggests this is because children have no political power. The voice of the child is not easily heard. Specific groups of children live in what the United Nations describes as particularly "difficult circumstances." Among these groups are street children, child prostitutes, child refugees, and children with AIDS. The countries with the highest number of street children are paradoxically not the poorest. According to Moorehead (1989), 20,000 children are said to roam the streets of New York. Child prostitution exists because it answers a demand. Sex tours are advertised in Western travel guides for pedophiles.

AIDS is a major threat to the well-being of children and to the abilities of their parents, if they survive, to care for them. Denial, shame, and lack of education, which hindered preventive efforts in the United States and Europe 10 years ago, are still crippling effective measures to limit the disease in Asia and Africa. AIDS does not respect national boundaries (*Time*, 1994).

Child refugees are the result of conflicts, but 80% of all military expenditures and 90% of all arms exports are provided by industrialized countries. These difficult problems suggest both an international responsibility and the need for global strategies.

Protection That Protects.   There is growing evidence in the West that child rescue policies, far from rescuing children, have in some circumstances led to further abuse (Department of Health, 1995). In the United Kingdom, there has been a run of scandals among children placed in the residential sector. A recurring feature of the many inquiries into such scandals has been that the voice of the child was not heard (Buchanan, Wheal, Walder, MacDonald, & Coker, 1993). Children who have been in the public care are a high-risk group for suicidal behavior (Buchanan *et al.*, 1993) and the risk of depression in adulthood among such children and young people is much higher than those, even from disadvantaged backgrounds, who have not been in care (Cheung & Buchanan, 1997). It is a paradox that many of these children were originally separated from their parents in order to protect them and to improve their well-being. Gurry (1993) has noted that sending a child to a welfare home in a developing country represents further abuse. In the United Kingdom, the situation may be different, but when decisions are taken about a child's future, the likely harm to the child of remaining in the family situation is rarely balanced against the possibility of harm in the long term to the child from the care setting.

Further evidence is accumulating that the very process of investigation in child protection may be abusive for the child. Sharland, Seal, Croucher, Aldgate, and Jones (1993) have found that children going through a child sexual abuse investigations are often as depressed or more depressed after the investigations than before, especially if nothing has changed. Ongoing research from the University of East Anglia in the United Kingdom (Audit Commission, 1994) implies many child abuse investigations may be unnecessary.

These issues are not easily remedied because children have to be protected, and in order to be protected, their situation needs to be assessed. The challenge is to make greater efforts to foster family preservation in the first place, to limit investigative procedures through better initial indicators of high-risk situations, and, if children need to be separated, to ensure that child protection interventions do in fact protect.

In England and Wales, the Children Act of 1989 has tried to encourage practitioners to develop family support approaches. Central to these approaches is working in partnership with families, identifying their strengths, and using these to meet needs. How successful these approaches are remains to be seen, but the indications are that fewer children are now compulsorily separated from their families (Department of Health, 1993).

Psychological Research Supporting the Cycle of Abuse

Theories to support the cycle of abuse have come from different psychological traditions. The early psychiatric studies, which were largely based on the psychodynamic model, related child abuse to the damaged "ego" of parents who had themselves been abused as children. Aggression was related to a subconscious "inner drive." Social learning theorists rejected this idea. They argued that aggression was both learned and that it took place within a social context. According to the behaviorist perspective, the child came into the world as a *tabula rasa* and was molded by the treatment he or she received from the parents. Children not only learned that violence paid, but they also learned the moral justifications for their behavior (Gelles & Cornell, 1990). Developments from social learning theory include the cognitive behavioral approaches, among which are Newberger and White's (1989) work on parental cognitions. Parents with troubled relationships with their children were frequently unable to perceive their children as having needs and rights of their own, separate from the parent. An important finding from this work was that parental awareness was a developmental process that unfolded during childhood and continued to develop with parental experience. Parental reasoning was responsive to intervention efforts. Attachment theory, although based on the psychodynamic tradition, in fact links with social learning ideas, in that early attachment relationships between the caregiver and the child are felt to be a prototype for later relationships (Ainsworth, 1973; Egeland & Sroufe, 1981). Crittenden and Ainsworth (1989) have shown that the maternal style of child rearing begins to influence the child at a very young age and that most children are influenced to be similar to their parents. Zeanah and Anders (1987) add that these early working models compel individuals to recreate their relationship experiences in their own lives. Not violence per se but the ongoing theme of the caregiving relationship was passed on.

Work from Straus (1979), Garbarino (1977), Bronfenbrenner (1977, 1979), and Belsky (1980) has demonstrated the limitation of single linear models. Intergenerational child maltreatment can better be understood if it is seen as a product of the interaction of social systems operating at individual, family, and societal levels. The ecological model developed from Belsky highlights risk and protective factors operating in four domains: (1) The *ontogenic level* includes individual factors; (2) family factors are considered in the *microsystem level;* (3) community factors exist at the *exosystem level;* and (4) cultural factors operate at the *macrosystem level.*

According to the ecological model, having a high IQ, resolve not to repeat the abuse, positive attachments, healthy children, a supportive partner, good social support, economic security, few stressful life events, and living in a supportive culture opposed to violence were protective. In contrast, a history of abuse in the parent, low self-esteem, low IQ and poor interpersonal skills, marital discord, single parenthood, having children with behavior and/or health problems, poverty, unemployment, isolation, poor social supports, and living in a culture that accepts violence and views children as possessions were risk factors (Kaufman & Zigler, 1989). Intergenerational child maltreatment was best understood by the transmission of risk factors. Cross-generational transmission was operated by increasing vulnerability or decreasing protective factors.

There are a number of dilemmas in using psychological theories as a basis for intervention. First, the intervention depends on the theory espoused (Gelles & Loseke, 1993). Second, many approaches involve high-cost, postabuse individual programs that may not be cost-effective in large populations. The value of these studies is that they have elicited a range of risk and *protective* factors that can assist in identifying vulnerable families. There are considerable problems in risk lists (Kaufman & Zigler, 1989). Such lists still only predict *potential* rather than *actual* risks. Further work is necessary before abusing families can be predicted with more certainty. Straus's (1979) extensive model of the characteristics associated with abuse only identified one-third of all the abusing families, which was little more than the single indicator of a history of abuse in the parent.

In the long term, further work on identifying *protective* factors and/or *strengths* in abusing families may be more helpful than an unrelenting pursuit of pathological features.

Biological Factors in Intergenerational Child Maltreatment

However, having said this, the biological cycle of child maltreatment relates to two realities. Some parents *are* biologically more vulnerable to the risk of abusing their children, and some children *are* biologically more vulnerable to be being abused (Rutter, 1989). First, biological factors may relate to intergenerational patterns of disease and poor health care; for example, more children are born damaged, and more mothers have poor health. Second, they may relate to inherited characteristics that lower the ability of the parent to parent and the child to be reared effectively. Third, they may relate to factors present in the environment such as pollution and drug and alcohol abuse, which bring about biological changes in the mother and/or child.

Intergenerational Patterns of Disease and Poor Health.   Intergenerational child maltreatment cannot be separated from patterns of disease and poor health in mothers and children (Blaxter, 1982; Blaxter & Paterson, 1981). The infant death rate is a good indicator not only of the numbers of children who die at birth, but also the numbers of children who will be born damaged and, as a result, be more difficult to rear (United Nations, 1994). Similarly, the maternal death rate will predict not only mothers who die but also mothers who find child rearing more difficult because they are in poor health. Diseases such as AIDS and tuberculosis, if they do not kill, may leave both mothers and children vulnerable to the experience of difficulties in child rearing. A disturbance of the cognitive processes due to injury or disease in early childhood may lead to a greater risk of psychiatric disorder, and the effects of this may persist and impede the child's long-term adjustment in many important areas (Robins & Rutter, 1990). Neurological factors have also been implicated in abusive behavior (Elliott, 1988). Iodine deficiency can lead to both a reduced capacity to parent and mental retardation (UNICEF, 1993). Programs that improve the health of parents and children and limit disease will have the secondary effect of improving parenting.

Inherited Disorders That Affect Parenting. For many practitioners, heredity was simply something that you could do nothing about. Rutter *et al.* (1990a, 1990b) suggest these views are no longer tenable. As knowledge increases, genetic disorder may increasingly be treatable by environmental manipulation. One of the most striking examples of this is phenylketonuria. Even when environmental manipulation is not possible, some genetic disorders may be limited by effective genetic counseling. There is also ample evidence that even if a child or parent is at definite risk due to biological deficits, in many cases, positive features of the environment can "buffer" the child and parent (Robins & Rutter, 1990).

Some inherited mental disorders, such as Huntington's chorea, in which a parent in middle age develops dementia, directly affect parenting ability (Oliver & Dewhurst, 1969). Similarly, inherited learning difficulties (mental handicap), inherited mental disorders, and neurological handicaps can affect both the child and parent, and their relationship. Such a child may be more vulnerable to abuse than a child without a disorder (Buchanan & Oliver, 1977).

With many of these disorders, current research is illustrating important links between both nature and nurture (Plomin, 1994). Evidence suggests the operation of synergistic interactions between biological predisposition and subsequent environmental stress. A vulnerability to schizophrenia, for example, may not become apparent in less stressful environments (Tienari *et al.,* 1990).

The current interest in behavioral genetics (Loehlin, 1992) has given rise to the idea that genetics will unlock the secrets of behavior. The situation is infinitely more complex. It is felt unlikely that a single gene will be identified that will predict particular forms of behavior, for example, aggression, but it is felt that genes play a part in the inheritance of broad temperamental traits (Loehlin, 1992). These traits may make parenting more or less difficult (Caspi, Elder, & Herbener, 1990). Some character traits, such as high reactivity in the parent or difficult temperamental characteristics in the child, may be associated with abuse (Casanova, Dominic, McCanne, & Milner, 1992; Crowe & Zeskind, 1992). However, these may be offset in positive environmental conditions. Rutter *et al.* (1990b) suggest that higher-order interactions are also important. Early stress on a vulnerable child can both *sensitize* children to extreme reactions in later life or *steel* them to become less vulnerable. Wachs (1992) has shown that what is an optimal environment may vary depending on the age of the child and individual characteristics.

Research by Plomin (1994) illustrates another important issue. Basically, people choose the environment that suits their genetic makeup best. Children in schools seek out preferred "niches'" and perform better in preferred environments. Correlates of parenting emphasize the importance of parental personality, life events, and social support. Genetic factors influence these domains and thus create a relationship with parenting. The issue is, however, that many parents do not have the opportunity to find their preferred "niches."

Environmental Factors Leading to Biological Changes in Parents and Children. The health of both parents and children can be affected by factors in the environment. Lead poisoning, for example, can lead to a range of difficulties in the parent–child relationship. Maternal alcoholism may lead to fetal alcohol syndrome. Similarly, the fetus may be damaged by substance abuse in the pregnant mother.

Although a genetic link has not yet been identified that predicts alcoholism or drug abuse, it is widely recognized that some people are more vulnerable to alcoholism than others (Ackerman, 1988). But as Rutter points out, to become an alcoholic requires the availability of alcohol (Rutter *et al.,* 1990b).

Interaction between the Cycles

> If we had one preventic program we could put in place, and knew it would succeed, we would opt for a program that would ensure every baby born anywhere in the world would be a healthy, full-term infant weighing at least eight pounds and welcomed into the world by economically secure parents who wanted the child and had planned jointly for her or his conception and birth. I would add the hope that the baby would be breast-fed by an adequately nourished mother who was not on drugs. I would also ask for good health care for expectant mother and child. Such an arrival in the world would go a long way toward assuring later healthy relationships, reduced mother and child mortality, reduced retardation and reduced mental disorders. (Albee, 1992, p. 313)

Such a strategy would also go a long way toward breaking cycles of child abuse.

This quotation illustrates how the separate mechanisms interact in our four cycles. Culturally, socially, psychologically and biologically, handicapped children are at greater risk of child maltreatment. Socially and psychologically, two-parents families who are economically secure are better able to parent. Culturally and socially, "wanted" children thrive better than "unwanted" children, and there are intergenerational continuities. Socially, psychologically, and biologically, mothers on drugs present a risk both to the biological health of their children and to their own parenting effectiveness. Through all the cycles, sick children are at greater risk than healthy children of growing up to repeat the tragedy of child abuse. The certainty of repeating the pattern is multiplied by the mechanisms operating in each cycle.

INTERVENTIONS IN THE FOUR CYCLES

The challenges in breaking cycles of intergenerational transmission are immense. So interwoven are the mechanisms, it is often hard to disentangle the constituent parts and find appropriate strategies to effect change. So vast is the task, many may feel overwhelmed. Research, however, indicates that progress can be made by the pooling of international, national, and local knowledge and resources. Research also indicates that to encourage us on our way, we need simple indicators at every level to demonstrate that we are moving toward our target.

The strategies suggested here come from a range of sources. In this short chapter, it is only possible to touch on a few of these ideas. Some of the most interesting ideas come from individual projects around the world that found solutions to the particular problems they faced. Sadly, it is not possible to list all their achievements here. However, a central finding from this review is that change is most likely to come when the expertise within communities is built upon and the strengths within communities mobilized to combat the forces that lead to child abuse.

Interventions in the Cultural Cycle

Cross-cultural research indicates that both an EMIC (coming from within), and an ETIC (coming from without) perspective, are necessary when defining what is, and what is not, abuse (Finkelhor & Korbin, 1988; Korbin, 1980, 1981, 1987; Levinson, 1989).

Central to the EMIC strategy is working with local communities. Communities are the experts both in knowing the concerns of their area, and in devising possible solutions to them. In mobilizing public opinion against child maltreatment, the local media have played a role. Communities around the world that have to come to their own decisions in defining what they feel is abusive parental behavior, and that have decided priorities and targets for intervention, have proved effective in limiting child maltreatment. Practical considerations suggest these efforts are more effective when there is at least one named person in each community who belongs to that community and has specific responsibilities for promoting the well-being of children.

In the United Kingdom, many local authorities are developing Children's Rights Officers. Save the Children has also been developing child advocates in Romania. The theory is that children are experts, both in the maltreatment they experience and possible solutions to limit their suffering. Sometimes their perspective is different from that of adults. Research with groups of young people in public care, for example, found that young people were more concerned about bullying from their peers than other forms of maltreatment (Buchanan et al., 1993). Some areas are now developing young people's forums to monitor the effectiveness of child protection. A good measure of the effectiveness of child protection in a particular area is to ask a group of children from that area "To whom can you go for help if you are being seriously maltreated, and is that person able to help you?"

Cross-cultural research demonstrates that we need to combat isolation in families and promote supportive networks among families, especially in areas where families are moving into new social environments. Community liaison workers can be particularly effective in such areas. The extent of community participation in each area can indicate the value of such work. It may need to be asked whether all groups within the community, particularly minority or ethnic groups, are equally represented (Buchanan, 1994).

International associations such as the International Society for the Prevention of Child Abuse and Neglect (ISPCAN) and, it is hoped, UNICEF have a role in establishing ETIC definitions and targets of specific types of child maltreatment that are internationally unacceptable. Acceptance of these standards needs to be promoted in all societies. For example, international support for the girl child, in particular, will pay dividends. An international data bank monitoring particular types of abuse is necessary. This will give a baseline against which changes can be measured.

Interventions in the Sociopolitical Cycle

The challenge here is to develop programs that combat factors that lower parenting thresholds. State policies have an important role in fostering human security in all its manifestations; for example, the health and well-being of children, education, freedom from violence, economic security, and promoting social integration. Greater human security will significantly raise the thresholds above which many families abuse their children. Human security indicators (United Nations, 1994) therefore will also indicate, to some degree, the rise and fall in levels of intergenerational child maltreatment.

State fiscal and family policies need to promote the well-being of the family (Brubaker, 1993). The dilemma is that policies do not always have the intended outcomes. They need to be monitored to ascertain if they are indeed having the intended effects. Although there are many other factors involved, in industrialized countries, it could be argued that lower rates of divorce and youthful single parenthood, as well as increased economic status of lone parents, could be among the indicators of the effectiveness of family policies.

The urgency for, and the current controversies around, population control in some developing countries indicate there are no easy answers. What is certain is that "wanted" children fare better than "unwanted" children, and, therefore, effective family planning has an important role in breaking intergenerational patterns of child maltreatment. It may be that state policies need to ensure that communities have access to *acceptable* forms of family-planning knowledge and practices. Local communities may need to decide what type of family planning is acceptable in their community and develop appropriate services. Increased levels of economic security, particularly among women, may be better indicators of the success of such policies than specific targets and numbers using family planning.

The recent concerns in the United Kingdom surrounding state care of children and the effects of investigations further emphasize that state policies need to develop child protection procedures that foster family preservation and limit formal investigative procedures to the few at high risk. If children have to be separated from their families, it is important they are not further abused. It may not be enough to monitor the numbers who come to protective agencies. It is appropriate to monitor the numbers of children in state care and the outcomes for such children. In the United Kingdom, the Looking after Project (Department of Health, 1994) is developing assessment and action records for use with children who are in state care. These records both monitor the progress of the children and act as useful management tools in planning services (Department of Health, 1994).

Some intergenerational patterns of child maltreatment call for international strategies. In particular, global strategies, together with state and local initiatives, may be necessary to tackle the problems of children in especially difficult circumstances, for example, child refugees, child prostitutes, and street children. We need to learn from each other. More accurate number counts will demonstrate how successful our strategies have been.

The Psychological Cycle

The overall challenge is to promote a climate of positive parenting. The international research community has the task of developing further lists that not only identify risk but also potential protective factors in families. These are strengths that can be mobilized to meet needs.

In England and Wales, the current struggle is how to identify and measure the numbers of children "in need" as defined under the Children's Act of 1989. This is a wider definition than children at risk of abuse and neglect; therefore, it is less stigmatizing. The focus is on the specific needs of the child and whether the parent is able to meet these needs. It incorporates children who may be at risk because of poor health, poor development, disabilities and behavioral problems, as well as abuse and neglect. Under the legislation, local authorities have a duty to provide a range of support services in order to keep families together and to promote the well-being of such children. A positive approach to parenting encourages families with difficulties to ask for help and work in partnership with the helping agencies to overcome their difficulties.

Local communities may wish to develop their own methods to identify areas where groups of children and families may be "in need." Community profiling may be effective here (Buchanan et al., 1995). This can come, for example, from local records of children being seen at health centers or from census data. Under this model, families are encouraged to seek help voluntarily before they reach a crisis point. The HOMESTART model, where semitrained community volunteers are linked to families of children in need (Audit Commission, 1994), is now developing outside the United Kingdom. Measuring outcomes for children "in need" is another current concern of child welfare researchers in the United Kingdom. Some authorities are bringing groups of parents of such children together to ask them what needs they have, how they are currently met, how they could better be helped, and what their priorities are (Buchanan *et al.*, 1995). The dilemma is that this can measure parental satisfaction with services but does not necessarily measure positive outcomes for children. Further work is needed in this area.

Effective day care may have an important role in reducing disadvantage and levels of intergenerational child maltreatment. State policies, together with those of local communities, need to foster the development of safe day care for mothers of children at risk of abuse or in need, especially single mothers who may have to work. Audits of present-day care arrangements of such mothers might indicate their preferences and suggest cost-effective strategies for future developments.

The Biological Cycle

The recurring message from this international review of literature is that programs that improve the health of women and children, particularly around birth, will also reduce the transmission of intergenerational child maltreatment. Programs that effectively limit disease will have a similar effect. Experience in India has shown that positive health education for mothers is effective and cost-sensitive. In the United Kingdom, after 40 years of the National Health Services there is a realization that further gains in health, especially among disadvantaged groups, will not be achieved without a greater focus on preventive medicine (Audit Commission, 1994). The Healthy Cities Project initiated by the European Office of the World Health Organization (Stark, 1992) may well have wider applicability.

Early identification of children at high biological risk may facilitate targeting protective or "buffer" programs on this group. In England and Wales, the Audit Commission (1994) has recommended the mandatory development in every local authority of Children's Service Plans. These published statements are planned jointly with health, social service, and, in some cases, education. Their purpose is to develop strategies for identifying and supporting high-risk children and to avoid duplication of resources. They also effect more efficient targeting. Under the Children's Act of 1989 in England and Wales, all local authorities already keep a register of children who have identified disabilities. Although parents of such children are under no obligation to have their child's name on the list, the registers do assist in planning services for this group.

A novel approach for the United Kingdom is the use of a mobile health/playbus with a community pediatrician on board to assess hard-to-reach children and families at risk families (Buchanan, 1994). In the United Kingdom, because we have free health care, there is an assumption that those in need will make use of it. Evidence suggests, however, that those most in need are least likely to access the services they need (Power, Manor, & Fox, 1991).

Another effective strategy in the United Kingdom has been to build on the expertise of parents. In many areas, child health records are now parent-held. Parents are experts in noting day-to-day changes in their children. Parent-held records give parents basic child health and child development information, so they can initiate a referral when they feel their child may have difficulties (Buchanan, 1994).

The study by Olds and Henderson (1989) in the United States has shown the benefits of targeted home-visiting programs by paramedics for high-risk families. In other areas, trained volunteers may fulfill this role.

Indirectly, early educative programs that develop skills and resilience in children can buffer them against biological deficits. Children who are at high risk biologically should take priority over other children in compensatory programs such as HEADSTART in the United States (Wisendale, 1993). If such programs are not available, less-structured playgroups run by parents can prove compensatory.

Factors in the environment that lead to biological changes in parents and children present a great challenge. Monitoring levels of pollution and taking action to reduce such pollution will improve the health and thereby the care of children. Substance-abusing mothers present a more difficult problem. At the Dimmock Health Center in Boston, where the infant mortality rates "careened out of control for infants of color," substance abuse in pregnant mothers was noted to be a high risk factor. They launched New Life, a small inpatient detoxification program for newly pregnant substance abusing women with an aftercare program. They demonstrated that early substance-abuse treatment in pregnancy resulted in the birth of considerably more healthy infants (Dimmock Community Health Center, 1992). The costs of the program were high, but not when compared to the direct and indirect costs of a lifetime of disability.

SUMMARY

It makes sense when thinking about miltigenerational legacies of trauma that strategies to reduce intergenerational patterns of child maltreatment should be high on the list. This review of the mechanisms that lead to the transmission of abuse has suggested that we need to examine closely extrafamilial as well as intrafamilial factors. Strategies to effect change involve both an EMIC and ETIC perspective. This means working with communities, helping them to decide on their child protection priorities, facilitating community networks, and working in partnership with children and their families and other professionals, while at the same time working with international organizations such as ISPCAN and UNICEF, mobilizing public opinion against child maltreatment, developing social policies that reduce poverty and improve maternal and child health and education. Central to this strategy is ensuring that the voice of the child is heard in every community.

The conclusion is that although interventions that focus on the intrafamilial cycles are important, interventions that focus on the extrafamilial cycles will, in the long term, do more to break the patterns of child maltreatment and the legacies from such trauma.

ACKNOWLEDGMENTS: This chapter would not have been possible without the help and encouragement of Dr. J. E. Oliver (retired), previously Consultant Child Psychiatrist, Wiltshire, England, with whom the author worked during the 1970s. Tirelessly, for over 30 years, Dr. Oliver worked and researched in this field.

REFERENCES

Ackerman, R. J. (1988). Complexities of alcohol and abusive families. *Focus on Chemically Dependent Families, 11,* 3–15.

Agathonos-Georgopoulou, H. (1992). Cross-cultural perspectives in child abuse and neglect. *Child Abuse Review, 1,* 80–88.

Ainsworth, M. D. S. (1973). The development of infant–mother attachment. In B. M. Caldwell & H. N. Riccinit (Eds.), *Review of child development research* (Vol. 3). Chicago: University of Chicago Press.

Albee, G. W. (1992). Saving children means social revolution. In G. W. Albee, L. A. Bond, & T. C. Monsey (Eds.), *Improving children's lives: Global perspectives on prevention* (pp. 311–329). Newbury Park, CA: Sage.

Altemeier, W. A., O'Connor, S., Sherrod, K. B., & Tucker, B. A. (1986). Outcome of abuse during childhood among pregnant low income women. *Child Abuse and Neglect, 10,* 319–330.

Altemeier, W. A., O'Connor, S., Vietze, P., Sandler, H., & Sherrod, K. (1982). Antecedents of child abuse. *Journal of Pediatrics, 100,* 823–829.

Audit Commission. (1994). *Seen but not heard.* London: Audit Commission, H.M.S.O.

Belsky, J. (1980). Child maltreatment: An ecological integration. *American Psychologist, 35,* 320–335.

Blaxter, M. (1982). *The health of the children: A review of research on the place of health in cycles of disadvantage.* SSRC/DHSS Studies in Deprivation and Disadvantage. No. 3. London: Heinemann Educational Books.

Blaxter, M., & Paterson, E. (1981). *Mothers and daughters: A three-generational study of health attitudes and behavior.* SSRC/DHSS Studies in Deprivation and Disadvantage. No 5. Heinemann Educational Books, London.

Bradshaw, J., & Millar, J. (1991). *Lone Parent Families in the UK,* London: H.M.S.O.

Bronfenbrenner, U. (1977). Toward an experimental ecology of human development. *American Psychologist, 56,* 197–198.

Bronfenbrenner, U. (1979). *The ecology of human development: Experiments by nature and design.* Cambridge, MA: Harvard University Press.

Brubaker, T. (1993). *Family relations: Challenges for the future.* Newbury Park, CA: Sage.

Bruce-Chwatt, L. (1976). Female circumcision and politics. *World Medicine, 1,* 44–47.

Buchanan, A. (Ed.). (1994). *Partnership in practice: The Children Act 1989.* Aldershot, UK: Avebury.

Buchanan, A. (1996). Cycles of child development: *Facts: fallacies, and interventions.* Chichester, UK: Wiley.

Buchanan, A., Barlow, J., Croucher, M., Hendron, J., Seal, H., & Smith, T. (1995). *Seen AND heard: Wiltshire Family Services Study.* London: Barnardo's.

Buchanan, A., & Oliver, J. (1977). Abuse and neglect as a cause of mental retardation. *British Journal of Psychiatry, 131,* 458–467.

Buchanan, A., Wheal, A., Walder, D., MacDonald, S., & Coker, R. (1993). *Answering back: Report by young people being looked after on the Children Act 1989,* Center for Evaluation and Development Research, University of Southampton, Southampton, UK.

Casanova, G. M., Dominic, J., McCanne, T. R., & Milner, J. S. (1992). Physiological responses to non-child-related stressors in mothers at risk for child abuse. *Child Abuse and Neglect, 16,* 31–44.

Caspi, A., Elder, G., & Herbener, E. (1990). Childhood personality and the prediction of life-course patterns. In L. Robins & M. Rutter (Eds.), *Straight and devious pathways to adulthood* (pp. 13–35). Cambridge, UK: Cambridge University Press.

Cheung, S. I., & Buchanan, A. (1997). High Malaise Scores in adulthood of young people and children who have been in care. *Journal of Child Psychology and Psychiatry, 38*(5), 575–580.

Cicchetti, D., & Aber, L. A. (1980). Abused children–abusive parents: An overstated case? *Harvard Educational Review, 50,* 244–255.

Cicchetti, D., & Rizley, R. (1981). Development perspectives on the etiology of intergenerational transmission, and sequelae of child maltreatment. *New Directions for Child Development, 11,* 31–55.

Crittenden, P. M., & Ainsworth, M. D. S. (1989). Child maltreatment and attachment theory. In D. Cicchett & V. Carlson (Eds.), *Child maltreatment: Theory and research on the causes and consequences of child abuse and neglect* (pp. 437–463). Cambridge, UK: Cambridge University Press.

Crowe, H. P., & Zeskind, P. S. (1992). Psychophysiological and perceptual responses to infant cries varying in pitch: Comparison of adults with low and high scores on the Child Abuse Potential Inventory. *Child Abuse and Neglect, 16,* 19–29.

Department of Health. (1994). *Children Act Report 1993.* London: H.M.S.O.

Department of Health. (1994). *Looking After Children Project: Assessment and action records.* London: H.M.S.O.

Department of Health. (1995). *Child protection: Messages from research.* London: H.M.S.O.

Department of Health and Social Security. (1974). *The Family in society: Dimensions of parenthood.* London: H.M.S.O.

Dimmock Community Health Center. (1992). *1991/1992 Dimmock Health Centre Annual Report.* Boston: Author.

Dytrych, Z. (1992). Children born of unwanted pregnancies. In G. Albee, L. Bond, & T. Cook Monsey (Eds.), *Improving children's lives* (pp. 97–106). Newbury Park, CA: Sage Publications.

Egeland, B., & Jacobvitz, D. (1984). *Intergenerational continuity of parental abuse: Causes and consequences.* Paper presented at the Conference on Biosocial Perspectives on Abuse and Neglect, York, ME.

Egeland, B., Jocobvitz, D., & Sroufe, L. A. (1988). Breaking the cycle of abuse. *Child Development, 59,* 1080–1088.

Egeland, B., & Sroufe, L. A. (1981). Attachment and early maltreatment. *Child Development, 52,* 44–52.

Elliott, F. A. (1988). Neurological factors. In V. B. Van Hasselt, A. Morrison, S. Bellack, & M. Hersen (Eds.), *Handbook of family violence* (pp. 359–382). New York: Plenum Press.

El-Mouelhy, M. (1992). The impact of women's health and status on children's health and lives in the developing world. In G. Albee, L. Bond, & T. Cook Monsey (Eds.), *Improving children's lives* (pp. 83–96). Newbury Park, CA: Sage.

EPOCH-WORLDWIDE. (1992). *End physical punishment of children worldwide*. London: Radda Barnen Organisation.

Essen, J., & Wedge, P. (1983). *Continuities in childhood disadvantage*. SSRC/DHSS Studies in Deprivation and Disadvantage. No. 6. London: Heinemann Educational Books.

Finkelhor, D., & Korbin, J. (1988). Child abuse as an international issue. *Child Abuse and Neglect, 12,* 3–23.

Garbarino, J. (1977). The human ecology of child maltreatment: A conceptual model for research. *Journal of Marriage and the Family, 39,* 721–736.

Gelles, R. J. (1973). Child abuse as psychopathology: A sociological critique and reformation. *American Journal of Orthopsychiatry, 43,* 611–621.

Gelles, R. J., & Cornell, C. P. (1990). *Intimate violence in families* (2nd ed.). Newbury Park, CA: Sage.

Gelles, R. J., & Loseke, D. R. (Eds.). (1993). *Current controversies on family violence*. Newbury Park, CA: Sage.

Gelles, R. J., & Straus, M. A. (1988). *Intimate violence*. New York: Simon & Schuster.

Gil, D. (1970). *Violence against children: Physical child abuse in the United States*. Cambridge, MA: Harvard University Press.

Gil, D. (1981). The United States versus child abuse. In L. H. Pelton, (Ed.), *The social context of child abuse and neglect*. New York: Human Sciences Press.

Gray, E., & Cosgrove, J. (1985). Ethnocentric perception of childrearing practices in protective services. *Child Abuse and Neglect, 9,* 389–396.

Gurry, G. L. (1993). A brighter future for ASEAN children. *Child Abuse Review, 2,* 119–126.

Herrenkohl, E. C., Herrenkohl, R. C., & Toedtler, L. J. (1983). Perspectives on the intergenerational transmission of abuse. In D. Finkelhor, R. J. Gelles, G. T. Hotaling, & M. Straus (Eds.), *The dark side of families: Current family violence research* (pp. 305–316). Newbury Park, CA: Sage.

Hunter, R. S., & Kilstrom, N. (1979). Breaking the cycle in abusive families. *American Journal of Psychiatry, 136,* 1320–1322.

Ikeda, T. (1982). A short introduction to child abuse in Japan. *Child Abuse and Neglect, 5,* 487–490.

Kaufman, J., & Zigler, E. (1989). The intergenerational transmission of child abuse. In D. Cicchetti & V. Carlson (Eds.), *Child maltreatment* (pp. 129–152). New York: Cambridge University Press.

Kaufman, J., & Zigler, E. (1993). The intergenerational transmission of abuse is overstated. In R. J. Gelles & D. R. Loseke (Eds.), *Current controversies on family violence* (pp. 209–221). Newbury Park, CA: Sage.

Kaufman, K., Johnson, C., Cohn, D., & McCleery, J. (1992). Child maltreatment prevention in the health care and social service system. In J. Willis, E. Holden, & M. Rosenberg (Eds.), *Prevention of child maltreatment: Development and ecological perspectives* (pp. 193–225). New York: Wiley.

Kempe, C., Silverman, F., Steele, B., Droegemueller, W., & Silver, H. (1962). The battered child syndrome. *Journal of the American Medical Association, 181,* 17–24.

Kokkevi, A., & Agathonos, H. (1987). Intelligence and personality profile of battering parents in Greece: A comparative study. *Child Abuse and Neglect, 11,* 93–99.

Korbin, J. (1980). The cultural context of child abuse and neglect. *Child Abuse and Neglect, 4,* 3–13.

Korbin, J. (1981). *Child abuse and neglect: Cross-cultural perspectives*. Berkeley: University of California Press.

Korbin, J. (1987). Child maltreatment in cross-cultural perspective: Vulnerable children and circumstances. In R. Gelles, & J. Lancaster (Eds.), *Child abuse and neglect* (pp. 31–53). New York: Aldine de Gruyter.

Korbin, J. (1991). Cross-cultural perspectives and research directions for the 21st century. *Child Abuse and Neglect, 15* (Suppl. 1), 67–77.

Levinson, D. (1989). *Family violence in cross-cultural perspective*. Newbury Park, CA: Sage.

Loehlin, J. C. (1992). *Genes and environment in personality development*. Newbury Park, CA: Sage.

Madge, N. (1983). *Families at risk*. SSRC/DHSS Studies in Deprivation and Disadvantage. No. 8. London: Heinemann Educational Books.

Main, M., & Goldwyn, R. (1984). Predicting rejection of her infant from mother's representation of her own experience: Implications for the abused–abusing intergenerational cycle. *Child Abuse and Neglect, 8,* 203–217.

Mejiuni, C. O. (1991). Educating adults against socioculturally induced abuse and neglect of children in Nigeria. *Child Abuse and Neglect, 15,* 139–145.

Moorehead, C. (1989). *Betrayal: Child exploitation in today's world*. London: Barrie & Jenkins.

Munir, A. (1993). Child protection: Principles and applications. *Child Abuse Review, 2,* 119–126.

Newberger, C. M., & White, K. N. (1989). Cognitive foundations for parental care. In D. Cicchetti & V. Carlson (Eds.), *Child maltreatment* (pp. 302–316). New York: Cambridge University Press.

Obikeze, D. S. (1984). Perspectives on child abuse in Nigeria. *International Child Welfare Review, 63,* 25–32.

Olds, D. L., & Henderson, R. (1989). The prevention of maltreatment. In D. Cicchetti & V. Carlson (Eds.), *Child maltreatment* (pp. 722–763). New York: Cambridge University Press.

Oliver, J. E. (1993). Intergenerational child abuse: Rates, research and clinical implications. *American Journal of Psychiatry, 150*(9), 1315–1325.

Oliver, J. E., & Buchanan, A. (1979). Generations of maltreated children and multi-agency care in one kindred. *British Journal of Psychiatry, 135,* 289–303.

Oliver, J. E., & Dewhurst, K. E. (1969). Six generations of ill-used children in a Huntington's pedigree. *Postgraduate Medical Journal, 45,* 757–760.

Oliver, J. E., & Taylor, A. (1971). Five generations of ill-treated children in one family pedigree. *British Journal of Psychiatry, 119,* 552, 473–480.

Plomin, R. (1994). *Genetics and experience: The interplay between nature and nurture.* Newbury Park, CA: Sage Publications.

Power, C., Manor, O., & Fox, A. (1991). *Health and class: The early years.* London: Chapman & Hall.

Quinton, D., & Rutter, M. (1984). Parents with children in care: Current circumstances, and parenting. *Journal Child Psychology and Psychiatry, 25,* 231–250.

Quinton, D., Rutter, M., & Liddle, C. (1984). Institutional rearing, parenting difficulties and marital support. *Psychological Medicine, 14,* 107–124.

Radulian, V. (1992, May 11). *Aspects of the situation of the Romanian children in 1992.* Keynote address at the 2nd Assembly of the World Alliance of Christian Children's Fund in Bucharest, Hungary.

Reid, A. (1984). Cultural difference and child abuse intervention with undocumented Spanish-speaking families in Los Angeles. *Child Abuse and Neglect, 8,* 109–112.

Robins, L., & Rutter, M. (1990). *Straight and devious pathways from childhood to adulthood.* Cambridge, UK: Cambridge University Press.

Rutter, M. (1984). Continuities and discontinuities in socio-emotional development: Empirical and conceptual perspectives. In R. Emde & R. Harmon (Eds.), *Continuities and discontinuities in development* (pp. 41–68). New York: Plenum Press.

Rutter, M. (1989). Intergenerational continuities and discontinuities in serious parenting difficulties. In D. Cicchetti & V. Carlson (Eds.), *Child maltreatment* (pp. 317–348). New York: Cambridge University Press.

Rutter, M. Bolton, P., Harrington, R., Le Couteur, A., Macdonald, H., & Simonoff, E. (1990a). Genetic factors in child psychiatric disorders: I. A review of research strategies. *Journal of Child Psychology and Psychiatry, 31*(1), 3–37.

Rutter, M., MacDonald, H., Le Couteur, A., Harrington, R., Bolton, P., & Bailey, A. (1990b). Genetic factors in child psychiatric disorders: II. Empirical findings. *Journal of Child Psychology and Psychiatry, 31*(1), 39–83.

Rutter, M., Quinton, D., & Liddle, C. (1983). Parenting in two generations: Looking backwards and looking forwards. In N. Madge (Ed.), *Families at risk,* SSRC/DHSS Studies in Deprivation and Disadvantage. No. 8. London: Heinemann Educational Books.

Schwebel, M. (1992). Making a dangerous world more tolerable for children: Implications of research. In G. Albee, L. Bond, & T. Cook Monsey (Eds.), *Improving children's lives* (pp. 107–128). Newbury Park, CA: Sage.

Sharland, E., Jones, D., Aldgate, J., Seal, H., & Croucher, M. (1996). *Professional intervention in child sexual abuse.* London: H.M.S.O.

Social Science Research Council (SSRC) and Department of Health and Social Security. (1976–1983). *Studies in deprivation and disadvantage.* London: Heinemann Educational Books.

Speakly, J. L., & Lauderdale, M. (1983). Community characteristics and ethnicity in the prediction of child maltreatment rates. *Child Abuse and Neglect, 7,* 91–105.

Stark, E., & Flitcraft, A. (1985). Women-battering, child abuse and social heredity: What is the relationship? *Sociological Review Monograph, 31,* 147–171.

Stark, W. (1992). Empowerment and social change: Health promotion with the healthy cities project of WHO. In G. W. Albee, L. A. Bond, & T. Cook Monsey (eds.), *Improving children's lives: Global perspectives on prevention* (pp. 167–176). Newbury Park, CA: Sage Publications.

Steele, B. F., & Pollock, C. B. (1968). A psychiatric study of parents who abuse infants and small children. In R. E. Helfer & C. H. Kempe (Eds.), *The battered child.* Chicago: University of Chicago Press.

Straus, M. A. (1979). Family patterns and child abuse in a nationally representative sample. *Child Abuse and Neglect, 3,* 213–225.

Straus, M. A., Gelles, R. J., & Steinmetz, S. K. (1988). *Behind closed doors: Violence in the American family.* Newbury Park, CA: Sage. (Original published 1980)

Tiernari, P., Lahti, I., Sorri, A., Naarala, M., Moring, J., Kaleva, M., Wahlberg, K.-E., & Wynne, L. (1990). Adopted-away offspring of schizophrenics and controls: The Finnish adoptive family study of schizophrenia. In L. Robins

& M. Rutter (Eds.), *Straight and devious pathways from childhood to adulthood* (pp. 365–380). Cambridge, UK: Cambridge University Press.

Time (1994, August 22). Battle fatigue: Scant hope emerges from this year's AIDS meeting, p. 40.

UNICEF. (1989). *Report on the state of the world's children.* New York: United Nations.

UNICEF. (1990). *Children and development in the 1990s. A UNICEF sourcebook.* New York: United Nations.

UNICEF. (1991). *The girl child—an investment in the future.* United Nations.

UNICEF. (1993). *The state of the worlds children 1993.* United Nations Children's Fund.

United Nations. (1987). *Report of the Expert Group Meeting on violence in the family with special emphasis on women.* United Nations.

United Nations. (1994). *Human Development Report,* New York: United Nations Development Program/Oxford University Press.

Wachs, T. D. (1992). *The nature of nurture.* Newbury Park, CA: Sage.

Whiting, B. B., & Edwards, C. P. (1988). *Children of different worlds.* Cambridge, MA: Harvard University Press.

Widom, C. S. (1989). The cycle of violence. *Science, 244,* 160–166.

Wisendale, S. K. (1993). State and federal initiatives in family policy. In T. Brubaker (Ed.), *Family relations: Challenges for the future* (pp. 229–250). Newbury Park, CA: Sage.

World Health Organization. (1987). *Evaluation of the strategy for health for all by year 2000: Seventh report on the world health situation—global review.* Geneva: Author.

Zeanah, C. H., & Anders, T. F. (1987). Subjectivity in parent–infant relationships: A discussion of internal working models. *Infant Mental Health Journal, 8,* 237–250.

Zeanah, C. H., & Zeanah, P. D. (1989). Intergenerational transmission of maltreatment: Insights from attachment theory and research. *Psychiatry, 52,* 177–196.

32

An Examination of Competing Explanations for the Intergenerational Transmission of Domestic Violence

RONALD L. SIMONS and CHRISTINE JOHNSON

Although domestic violence has been a feature of most societies throughout human history (Levinson, 1989), only within the last 25 years have we come to view it as a serious social problem. North America and Western Europe have been the location for much of the research on this topic, but in recent years, researchers from other parts of the world have also begun to investigate this issue. Studies of domestic violence consistently find that childhood exposure to family violence significantly increases the chances that an individual will be violent toward his or her spouse or children during adulthood. This intergenerational pattern is often referred to as a "cycle of violence" (Gelles & Cornell, 1990; Steinmetz, 1987).

Although there is strong evidence that family violence tends to be transmitted across generations, there has been little investigation of the theoretical mechanisms whereby intergenerational transmission occurs. The present chapter attempts to address this void by testing the adequacy of three theories often presented as potential explanations for this phenomenon. We begin by specifying what we mean by "domestic violence." Next, we briefly review the evidence suggesting that such actions are often transmitted across generations. We then introduce three theoretical explanations for intergenerational transmission, making special note of the competing hypotheses implied by these different perspectives. Finally, structural equation modeling with a sample of approximately 350 families is used to test the hypotheses.

THE NATURE AND SOCIAL DISTRIBUTION OF DOMESTIC VIOLENCE

Domestic violence consists of physical attacks intended to hurt, intimidate, or coerce another family member. This includes actions such as slapping, punching, shoving, kicking, and striking with an object. Such acts are widely prevalent through out the world. For example, the

RONALD L. SIMONS • Department of Sociology and Center for Family Research in Mental Health, Iowa State University, Ames, Iowa 50014.   CHRISTINE JOHNSON • Postdoctoral Fellow, Center for Family Research in Mental Health, Iowa State University, Ames, Iowa 50014.

International Handbook of Multigenerational Legacies of Trauma, edited by Yael Danieli. Plenum Press, New York, 1998.

anthropologist David Levinson (1988, 1989) found that violence toward wives occurred in the majority of households in almost half of the 90 societies that he studied, and corporal punishment of children was used frequently in 34% of these societies. In the United States, it is estimated that 90% of all parents sometimes use corporal punishment to discipline their children, and that approximately 30% of all couples experience marital violence at some point in their marriage (Straus & Gelles, 1988; Straus, Gelles, & Steinmetz, 1980).

Although many parents sometimes spank their child and a substantial proportion of married persons have been struck or pushed by their spouse, in the majority of families, the violence occurs infrequently and is not very severe. Children and marital partners exposed to severe and recurring physical attack are the ones most likely to display long-term emotional and behavioral problems. Thus, public and scientific concern has focused largely upon family violence that is harsh and persistent. Violence of this type is often labeled *child* or *spousal abuse*. Child and spousal abuse are, of course, much less prevalent than family violence in general. In the United States, for example, national survey data suggest that spousal abuse takes place in about 6% of all marriages, and abusive parenting occurs in 3–11% of all families (Straus & Gelles, 1988).

Studies indicate that fathers and mothers are equally likely to engage in violence toward their children (Wauchope & Straus, 1990), whereas, in most countries, it is much more common for husbands to hit their wives than for wives to hit their husbands (Levinson, 1989). The latter finding does not appear to hold in the United States, as several studies have reported that husbands and wives are about equally likely to hit each other (Simons, Wu, Johnson, & Conger, 1995; Straus & Gelles, 1986). However, given sex differences in size and strength, husbands are much more likely than wives to inflict physical and emotional injury when such violence occurs (Stets & Straus, 1990; Straus *et al.,* 1980).

CYCLE OF VIOLENCE: THE INTERGENERATIONAL LEGACY OF FAMILY VIOLENCE

Several studies have examined the developmental consequences of growing up in a violent family. This research indicates that childhood exposure to family violence places a person at increased risk for a number of behavioral and emotional problems (see Cicchetti & Carlson, 1989; Hotaling, Finkelhor, Kirkpatrick, & Straus, 1988; Wolfe, 1987). The most consistent finding, however, relates to the cyclical nature of family violence: Adults who either witnessed or were subjected to violence in their family of origin are at an elevated risk for engaging in violent behavior toward their spouse or children (O'Leary, 1988; Simons, Whitbeck, Conger, & Wu, 1991; Straus, 1983; Straus *et al.,* 1980).

Although growing up in a violent family increases the probability that a person will engage in domestic violence as an adult, the relationship is far from absolute. Indeed, the evidence suggests that the majority of people do not repeat the family violence that they witnessed as children. For example, based on a review of several studies, Kaufman and Zigler (1987, 1989) estimated that only about 30% of abused children grow up to abuse their own offspring. However, this statistic should not be interpreted as an indication that a history of child abuse has little impact on the chances that a person will grow up to be abusive. Survey research conducted in the United States suggests that the rate of abusive parenting is approximately 3%. Thus, a person who was abused as a child is *10 times* more likely to abuse his or her own children than an individual who was not subjected to such parenting (Gelles & Straus, 1988). A similar pattern has been found for spousal abuse. Although most persons who experience family violence as children do not grow up to engage in marital violence, they are several times more likely to display this behavior than individuals who were not exposed to family violence during childhood (Straus *et al.,* 1980).

These findings indicate that the phrase "cycle of violence" is somewhat misleading. The phrase is often taken to mean that persons exposed to family violence during childhood are doomed to reproduce this pattern of behavior with their own marital partner or children. Clearly, this is not the case. Most victims of abuse are able to avoid duplicating their parents' violent behavior. However, exposure to violent parents increases severalfold the chances that a person will be abusive as an adult. Indeed, growing up in a violent family is the most potent predictor of child or spousal abuse to be identified by social scientists. It is in this sense that a cycle of violence exists. Growing up in an atmosphere of family violence dramatically increases the probability that an individual will be a violent parent or spouse.

THEORIES OF INTERGENERATIONAL TRANSMISSION

Although researchers agree that family violence is often transmitted across generations, there is little agreement concerning the mechanisms whereby this occurs. Past studies have been concerned with documenting the existence of intergenerational effects and have devoted little attention to the theoretical processes that account for the occurrence of this phenomena. The present study evaluates the adequacy of three explanations for these intergenerational patterns.

The first explanation, which we will label the *role modeling* perspective, asserts that children learn about the role of parent by observing the parenting practices of their parents, and they acquire information regarding the role of marital partner by observing the interaction between their parents. Thus, children exposed to abusive parenting or violent parental interaction assume that aggression is a normal part of parenting or marital interaction, and, as adults, are likely to engage in such behavior when interacting with their spouse or offspring. Consistent with this view, severe treatment as a child has been found to predict harsh parenting as an adult (Simons, Beaman, Conger, & Chao, 1993a; Simons *et al.,* 1991; Straus *et al.,* 1980), while studies have reported that childhood exposure to violence between parents increases the probability of adult marital violence (Pagelow, 1981; Rosenbaum & O'Leary, 1981).

The second explanation offers a somewhat broader view of the messages that are transmitted by physically aggressive parents. Childhood exposure to family violence, whether marital violence or harsh parenting, is seen as providing lessons that foster spousal as well as child abuse (O'Leary, 1988; Straus & Smith, 1990b; Straus *et al.,* 1980). Straus *et al.,* for example, have argued that both harsh physical discipline and marital violence teach children that it is legitimate, indeed, often necessary, to hit those you love (i.e., other family members). Thus, exposure to any form of family violence is seen as promoting attitudes that increase the probability that children will grow up to behave aggressively toward their spouse and offspring. For purposes of the present chapter, this viewpoint is termed the *family relationships* perspective. Consistent with this viewpoint, there is evidence that childhood exposure to harsh parenting increases the probability of adult marital violence (Rosenbaum & O'Leary, 1981; Straus *et al.,* 1980), and that children who witness their parents hitting each other often grow up to employ harsh parenting practices with their offspring (Straus *et al.,* 1980).

Finally, the criminology literature suggests a still broader view of what is learned in an atmosphere of family violence. Several studies have shown that deviant acts tend to be correlated so that individuals who engage in one type of deviant behavior tend to participate in other types as well (e.g., Donovan & Jessor, 1985; Jessor & Jessor, 1977; Osgood, Johnston, O'Malley, &

Bachman, 1988). There is also evidence that antisocial behavior is rather stable over the life course (Caspi & Moffitt, 1992; Loeber, 1982; Loeber & Le Blanc, 1990; Sampson & Laub, 1993). Those who manifest high levels of antisocial behavior at an early age are at risk for chronic delinquency during adolescence and continued reckless and irresponsible behavior during adulthood (Farrington, 1991; Loeber & Le Blanc, 1990; Patterson & Yoerger, 1993). In other words, antisocial behavior shows the characteristics of a behavior trait (i.e., a pattern of behavior that is expressed across time and situations) (Allport, 1937). This body of literature suggests that family violence is likely to be an expression of a more general antisocial pattern of behavior. It indicates that persons who engage in persistent aggression toward family members are inclined to have a history of involvement in a wide variety of other antisocial behaviors as well.

If family violence is an expression of a general antisocial orientation, how does such an orientation develop? Criminological research suggests that antisocial tendencies tend to emerge in childhood. A number of studies indicate that children are at risk for developing an antisocial pattern of behavior when they are exposed to inept parenting, of which rejection or abusive discipline is a type (Patterson, Reid, & Dishion, 1992; Sampson & Laub, 1993; Simons, Wu, Conger, & Lorenz, 1994). Furthermore, studies indicate that there is an increased probability that parents will engage in such parenting if they have antisocial tendencies (Capaldi & Patterson, 1991; Patterson *et al.,* 1992; Simons, Beaman, Conger, & Chao, 1993b). Antisocial parents are also apt to assault their marital partner (Fagan, Steward, & Hansen, 1983; Hotaling, Straus, & Lincoln, 1990; Simons *et al.,* 1995; Walker, 1979). Together, these findings suggest that aggressive antisocial parents are likely to hit each other and engage in ineffective, abusive parenting. This inept parenting, in turn, increases the probability that their children will grow up to engage in antisocial behavior of all sorts, including violence toward their spouse and children. In other words, it is a general pattern of antisocial behavior, and not specific lessons regarding domestic violence, that is transmitted across generations in violent families. For purposes of the present chapter, we label this the *antisocial orientation* perspective.

Unfortunately, there has been little effort to apply this perspective to the phenomenon of domestic violence. Indeed, both family researchers (Gelles & Straus, 1979; Hotaling & Straus, 1980) and criminologists (Megargee, 1982) have argued that domestic violence requires a special theory and should not be approached as a subset of general violent behavior. Albeit, as Hotaling *et al.* (1990) have noted, the question of whether family violence has a similar etiology to other forms of violent and deviant behavior is really an empirical question. The remainder of this chapter is devoted to testing the hypotheses implied by the antisocial orientation, role modeling, and family relationships perspectives on intergenerational transmission of family violence.

HYPOTHESES

The three theoretical perspectives provide differing accounts of the processes whereby the past behavior of the grandparent generation (G1) increases the probability that their adult children (G2) will engage in violence toward their spouse or children. The role modeling viewpoint emphasizes lessons specific to the roles of marital partner or parent; the family relationships framework focuses on messages regarding appropriate behavior in intimate relationships; and the antisocial orientation perspective stresses the consequences of a general antisocial approach to life. Table 1 summarizes the predictions that regarding the correlation of family violence across generations, each of these points of view suggests the association between marital violence and child abuse, and the relationship between family violence and other forms of deviant behavior.

Table 1. Theoretical Predictions Regarding the Family Violence of Parents (Generation 1) and Their Adult Offspring (Generation 2)

PTheoretical perspectives	Hypothesized relationships							
	Association between G1 and G2 harsh parenting	Association between G1 and G2 marital violence	Association between G1 harsh parenting and G2 marital violence	Association between G1 marital violence and G2 harsh parenting	Association between marital violence and harsh parenting (for both G1 and G2)	Association between antisocial behavior and both marital violence and harsh parenting (for both G1 and G2)	Association between G1 family violence and G2 antisocial behavior	Controlling for G2 antisocial behavior eliminates the associations between G1 and G2 family violence
Role modeling	Yes	Yes	No	No	No	No	No	No
Family relationships	Yes	Yes	Yes	Yes	Yes	No	No	No
Antisocial orientation	Yes	Yes	Yes	No	Yes	Yes	Yes	Yes

Table 1 shows that all three perspectives imply a bivariate association between harsh parenting by G1 and harsh parenting by G2. Similarly, all three would expect a correlation between marital violence by G1 and marital violence by G2. Whereas the theories agree regarding these two bivariate relationships, the remaining columns of Table 1 present points of disagreement.

G1 Harsh Parenting and G2 Marital Violence

The family relationships viewpoint assumes an association between G1 harsh parenting and G2 marital violence, as exposure to harsh parenting teaches that it is appropriate to hit those you love. The antisocial orientation perspective would also predict an association between these variables, as exposure to abusive parenting is seen as increasing the probability of aggressive behavior of all types, including marital violence. The role modeling framework, on the other hand, would not expect such an association, as harsh parenting by G1 is seen as providing information to G2 that is specific to the role of parent. These parenting lessons are seen as having little or no effect on a person's approach to the role of marital partner.

G1 Marital Violence and G2 Harsh Parenting

The family relationships perspective posits a relationship between G1 marital violence and G2 violence toward children, as exposure to aggressive conflict between parents during childhood is thought to foster the perception that it is acceptable to hit loved ones. The role modeling viewpoint does not make this prediction. It assumes that parental conflict shapes a child's view of the role of spouse, but has little impact upon his or her ideas regarding the role of parent. The antisocial orientation perspective also does not predict an association between G1 marital violence and G2 parenting, as it assumes that it is parenting practices, and not quality of marital interaction, that fosters an antisocial behavior in children.

Spouse and Children as Targets of Violence

Both the family relationships and antisocial orientation perspectives predict that aggression toward children is associated with aggression toward the spouse. The role modeling viewpoint would not assert this relationship, as there is no reason to expect that scripts specific to the role of parent influence behavior in the role of marital partner. To a large degree, research on harsh parenting represents a separate research tradition from that focusing upon violence toward spouses (Finkelhor, 1983). As a consequence, there has been little consideration of the links that exist between child and spousal abuse. However, two recent studies have investigated this issue, and both found an association between the two phenomena (Hotaling et al., 1990; Simons et al., 1995).

Family Violence and Other Forms of Antisocial Behavior

The role modeling and family relationships frameworks portray family violence as distinct from other forms of violent and deviant behavior. The antisocial orientation perspective, on the other hand, views chronic domestic violence as part of a general antisocial lifestyle. Hence, it predicts a correlation between aggression toward children or a spouse and involvement in other forms of antisocial behavior. This association would be expected for both G1 and G2.

Some studies have reported a relationship between spousal violence and having a criminal record; however, these studies are based upon clinical samples and utilize no comparison group

(Fagan *et al.,* 1983; Flynn, 1977; Gayford, 1975; Stacy & Shupe, 1983; Walker, 1979). Although a few studies have found that fathers of assaulted children often have criminal records (Gil, 1970; Skinner & Castle, 1969; Smith, Hansen, & Noble, 1973), other researchers have not found this to be the case (Steele & Pollack, 1968; Straus, 1985). Rather than focusing upon criminal records, Hotaling *et al.,* (1990) examined the relationship between domestic violence and self-reported assaults upon nonfamily members. Using data from the 1985 National Family Violence Survey, they reported that the hitting of either a spouse or child was associated with aggression toward nonfamily members. In the present study, we examine the extent to which domestic violence is related to both violent and nonviolent deviant behaviors outside of the family.

G1 Family Violence and G2 Antisocial Behavior

The antisocial orientation perspective asserts that abusive parenting is an ineffective approach to parenting that increases the chances that a child will engage in a wide variety of risky and antisocial behaviors during adolescence and adulthood. This suggests that harsh parenting by G1 will be related to G2's involvement in a broad range of deviant activities. On the other hand, the antisocial orientation perspective does not assume a relationship between G1 marital violence and G2 involvement in antisocial behavior. It is parents' parenting practices, and not their marital interaction, that is seen as the primary determinant of children's antisocial behavior. Any bivariate correlation between G1 marital violence and G2 antisocial behavior would be considered spurious and as likely to disappear once the effects of G1 harsh parenting are taken into account.

These predictions are quite different from those of the other two theoretical perspectives. The role modeling viewpoint posits that G2 will only engage in the type of antisocial behavior displayed by the parents. Thus, G1 harsh parenting increases the chances of G2 harsh parenting, and G1 marital violence places G2 at risk for marital violence. The family relationships position is somewhat broader. It posits that any type of family violence by G1 increases the odds that G2 will engage in some form of family violence. No relationship would be expected, however, between G1 family violence and G2 involvement in other categories of antisocial behavior.

The Effects of Controlling for Antisocial Behavior

The antisocial orientation viewpoint argues that childhood exposure to inept parenting, such as harsh physical discipline, fosters and antisocial lifestyle that, in turn, increases the probability of deviance in general, including violence toward family members. If this argument is valid, there should be no relationship between harsh treatment during childhood and aggression toward either children or spouse once the level of antisocial orientation is controlled. Stated differently, the impact of childhood experience upon adult family violence should be indirect through this syndrome of antisocial behavior.

In contrast, the role modeling perspective asserts that youngsters raised in violent families learn parenting and marital scripts that influence their adult performance of these roles. This would argue for a direct relationship between G1 and G2 parenting, and between G1 and G2 marital interaction, even after controlling for G2's level of antisocial orientation. The family relationships perspective contends that both harsh parenting and marital violence teach children that it is acceptable, indeed often necessary, to hit other family members. This view suggests that controlling for level of antisocial orientation should have little or no impact on the association between G1 parental or marital violence and G2 aggression toward both children and spouse.

METHODS AND PROCEDURES

Sample and Data Collection

Data from the Iowa Youth and Families Project (IYFP) were used to test the hypotheses. The IYFP is a panel study concerned with the life-course trajectories of parents and their adolescent children. The sample consists of 451 two-parent families recruited through the cohort of all seventh-grade students, male and female, in eight counties in North Central Iowa, who were enrolled in public or private schools during winter and spring 1989. An additional criterion for inclusion in the study was the presence of a sibling within 4 years of age of the seventh grader.

The families in the study lived on farms (about one-third) or in small towns. All of the families were white, and annual income ranged from zero to $135,000, with a mean income of $29,642. Fathers' education ranged from 8 to 20 years, with a mean of 13.5 years of education, while for mothers, the range was from 8 to 18 years, with a mean of 13.4 years. Additional information regarding the sample is available in Conger, Elder, Lorenz, Simons, and Whitbeck (1992).

The same data-collection procedures were employed annually with the families. Members of each family was visited twice at their home. During the first visit, each of the four family members completed a set of questionnaires focusing upon family processes, individual family member characteristics, and economic circumstances. During the second visit, which normally occurred within 2 weeks of the first, the family was videotaped while engaging in several different, structured interaction tasks. A description of the tasks is provided in Conger *et al.* (1992). The videotapes were coded by project observers using the Iowa Family Interaction Rating Scales (Melby *et al.*, 1990). These scales focus upon the quality of behavior exchanges between family members.

Families received $250 annually for their participation, which translated into about $10 per hour for each family member's time. The analyses for this chapter are based upon data collected over the first four waves of the project. Retention rates were above 90% for each wave. Complete data for the measures used in the present analyses were available for 324 families.

Measures

G1's Harsh Discipline. At Wave 1, husbands and wives completed a 4-item Harsh Discipline Scale for each of their parents. The items were adapted from the Conflict Tactics Scale (Straus, 1979; Straus *et al.*, 1980) and asked the respondents to indicate how their mother (or father) disciplined them during adolescence. The questions asked how often they were slapped, hit, or shoved by their mother (or father) when they did something wrong. Response categories ranged along a 5-point continuum with 1 = *Never,* 3 = *About half the time,* and 5 = *Always.* Note that whereas spanking or slapping may indicate discipline that is normative during early childhood, it is less typical and more indicative of harsh parenting if it continues during adolescence (Straus, 1983). Coefficient alpha was above .70 for both husband and wife reports. The harsh discipline of the grandfather tended to be highly correlated with the practices of the grandmother ($r \geq .49$). The scores for grandfathers and grandmothers were summed to form a composite measure of the amount of harsh discipline that a husband or wife had experienced during adolescence.

G2's Harsh Discipline. At Waves 2, 3, and 4, the target child and the sibling reported on the harsh discipline of their mother and father using a scale very similar to the measure of G1's harsh discipline described earlier. Coefficient alpha ranged from .75 to .85 for the three waves. The correlation between target and sibling reports was .35 at Wave 2, .31 at Wave 3, and .28 at Wave 4. Scores for the target child and sibling were summed to form a composite measure of harsh discipline by each parent.

G1 Marital Strife.   At Wave 1, husbands and wives were asked to think back to the period when they were growing up and to describe their parents' marriage using three questions. The questions focused on intensity of fighting, hostility, and dissatisfaction. Unfortunately, the questions did not focus explicitly on violence. Thus, our measure assumes that marital violence is most apt to be present among couples who frequently fight, and who display a high level of hostility and dissatisfaction toward one another. Coefficient alpha for the instrument was. 84.

G2 Violence toward Spouse.   At Waves 2, 3, and 4, husbands and wives used a single item to report on the extent to which they had been physically hit or shoved by their partner. Respondents were asked to think about times then they had interacted with their spouse during the *previous month* and to report how often he or she had "hit, pushed, grabbed, or shoved you." Response format ranged from 1 (*Never*) to 7 (*Always*), with 4 = *About half the time.*

G1 Antisocial Behavior.   Antisocial behavior involves actions that are deemed risky, inappropriate, shortsighted, or insensitive by the majority of people in the society (Patterson *et al.,* 1992; Robins, 1974). This would include acts such as fighting, substance abuse, extramarital affairs, lying, violations of the law, and the like. At Wave 1, husbands and wives completed an 8-item antisocial behavior scale for each of their parents. The items asked about issues of irresponsibility, drug and alcohol use, emotional problems, and loss of temper and conflicts with nonfamily members. Coefficient alpha was approximately .80 for reports about both grandfathers and grandmothers. There was a .32 correlation between the scores for grandmothers and those for grandfathers. The scores for grandfathers and grandmothers were summed to form a composite measure of the level of parental antisocial behavior to which a husband or wife was exposed as a child.

G2 Antisocial Behavior Trait.   Five instruments, covering a variety of deviant acts, were used to form a composite measure of G2 antisocial behavior. Confirmatory factor analysis demonstrated that the measures grouped on a single factor with reasonable factor loadings. The loadings were generally in the range of .40 to .60.

The first instrument consisted of a *deviant behavior checklist* that asked respondents how often (0 = *Never,* 4 = *4 or more times*) during the past 12 months they had engaged in each of five deviant acts. The acts focused upon fighting, traffic violations, lying, gambling, and having been arrested. Mothers and fathers completed this instrument at Waves 2 and 3.

At Waves 1 and 2, husbands and wives completed a 14-item *substance abuse scale.* They were asked to report how often during the last 12 months (1 = *Never,* 4 = *Often*) they had engaged in the behavior or experienced the phenomenon described in each question. The items involved incidents such as getting drunk, trouble at work because of alcohol, and using illicit drugs. Coefficient alpha for the scale was above .80 for both mothers and fathers.

An *observational measure* of antisocial behavior was formed through ratings of parental behavior from the first two tasks of the videotaped interaction obtained at Waves 1 and 2. Different coders were used for the two tasks in order to provide independent assessments of behavior. Using a scale ranging from 1 to 5, the coders rated the extent to which parents were antisocial in their interactions with other family members. Antisocial behavior was defined as the degree to which an individual is self-centered and resists, defies, or is inconsiderate of others by being noncompliant, insensitive, or obnoxious. For each parent, the ratings were summed across tasks and waves of data collection. Coefficient alpha was .88 for mothers and .90 for fathers.

At Wave 3, husbands and wives completed an 8-item instrument concerning the extent to which various *deviant activities were characteristic of their spouse.* The items focused upon substance use, traffic tickets, fights, trouble with the police, and reckless behavior. Response format for the items ranged from *Strongly disagree* to *Strongly agree.* Coefficient alpha for the scale was .73 for the reports by wives and .75 for the reports by husbands.

Finally, an index concerned with delinquent behavior during adolescence was included. This instrument consisted of a list of 14 *delinquent acts,* including items such as shoplifting, skipping school, drinking alcohol, and fighting. Respondents were asked to indicate which of the acts they had engaged in prior to age 15. Coefficient alpha for this instrument was .58 and .68 for husbands and wives, respectively.

The scores for the various instruments were standardized and summed to obtain a composite measure of a husband's or wife's recurrent involvement over a number of years in a wide range of antisocial behaviors. Thus, scores on this instrument represent a persistent pattern of antisocial acts that might be considered evidence of a general antisocial orientation.

RESULTS

Table 2 shows the percentage of mothers and fathers who were reported to have engaged in violence toward the target child, sibling, or their spouse at one wave, at all three waves, or who were not reported to have engaged in violence. Table 2 indicates, for example, that 14.2% of the target children reported at all three waves that they had been hit by their mother during the prior month, whereas 49.4% reported no violence at any wave. Similar percentages are reported for fathers. The percentage of wives and husbands who reported having been hit at all

Table 2. Number and Percentage of Parents Who Were Violent across Waves

	Violent in three waves	Violent in one wave	No violence in any wave
Mother's violence			
Toward target	14.2% (45)	50.6% (160)	49.4% (156)
Toward sibling	8.9% (28)	49.7% (157)	50.3% (159)
Toward spouse	3.2% (10)	21.2% (67)	78.8% (249)
Father's violence			
Toward target	13.6% (44)	46.9% (152)	53.1% (172)
Toward sibling	9.3% (30)	46.6% (151)	53.4% (173)
Toward spouse	1.5% (5)	12.3% (40)	87.7% (284)

three waves is 1.5 and 3.2, respectively. Eighty-eight percent of the wives and 79% of the husbands did not report having been hit at any of the waves.

Based upon the figures presented in Table 2, 28% of the mothers who used corporal punishment with their target child did so at all three waves. The figure for fathers is 29%. Twelve percent of the wives who were the victims of violence reported having been hit at all three waves and 27% at two or more waves. The corresponding figure for husbands is 15%.

The percentages reported in Table 2 involve dichotomies where the parent either did or did not engage in a violent act toward a particular family member. This is not a very strong test of the continuity of violence across time, as it does not take into account the level of violence perpetrated. This is important, as it is parents or spouses who engage in high levels of violence that are most likely to persist in the behavior across time. A better test for continuity of violence over time is provided by the correlations presented in Table 3, which shows, for example, that there is a .68 correlation between the target child's reports of violence by the father at Waves 2 and 3, and a correlation of .54 between reports of violence at Waves 2 and 4. The coefficients are of similar magnitude for sibling reports of aggression by father. A comparable pattern of continuity holds for mothers' harsh discipline of both the target child and the sibling.

The husband's violence toward the wife at Wave 2 correlates .54 and .60 with his violence toward her at Waves 3 and 4, respectively. The correlations are of similar magnitude for the wife's violence toward the husband. Thus, Table 3 provides rather strong support for the idea that high levels of family violence tend to be persistent across time. Tangentially, Table 3 also indicates that violence tends to run in couples. At each wave, there are strong correlations between father's and mother's violence toward a child. Similarly, husbands' reports of having been hit are correlated with wives' reports of having been hit.

Table 4 presents the bivariate associations between the various constructs included in our study. As noted in the measures section, a single indicator (often consisting of a composite measure) was used for all of the explanatory variables. The explanatory variables were used to explain persistent G2 involvement in aggression toward spouse and children. In order to form a measure of persistent aggression toward children, child reports collected at Waves 2, 3, and 4 were used as indicators to form the latent constructs Mother's Aggression toward Children and Father's Aggression toward Children. Similarly, spousal reports from Waves 2, 3, and 4 were employed as indicators of Husband's Aggression toward Spouse and Wife's Aggression toward Spouse. Log transformations were used in place of raw scores for both the child and marital aggression measures in order to correct for skewed distributions. LISREL VII (structural equation modeling) was used to calculate the correlations between the constructs.

The family relationships and antisocial orientation perspectives suggest that aggression toward children will be related to violence toward a spouse. Table 4 provides support for this idea. The association is .20 for G2 fathers and .24 for G2 mothers. There are also significant

Table 3. Pearson Correlations for Family Violence across Waves

	Toward target child			Toward sibling			Toward spouse		
	Wave 2	Wave 3	Wave 4	Wave 2	Wave 3	Wave 4	Wave 2	Wave 3	Wave 4
Wave 2	.70*	.68*	.54*	.68*	.55*	.40*	.34*	.54*	.60*
Wave 3	.58*	.60*	.57*	.58*	.69*	.49*	.56*	.40*	.56*
Wave 4	.48*	.62*	.67*	.35*	.33*	.55*	.49*	.50*	.39*

Note: For each 3 × 3 cell, the coefficients above the diagonal are for fathers, those below the diagonal are for mothers, and coefficients on the diagonal are correlations between mother–father scores.

Table 4. Bivaritae Correlations between Latent Constructs

	1	2	3	4	5	6
1. G1 antisocial behavior	1.00	.65*	.42*	.25*	.05	.04
2. G1 marital strife	.66*	1.00	.35*	.21*	.03	.04
3. G1 harsh parenting	.62*	.45*	1.00	.29*	.15*	.06
4. G2 antisocial behavior	.26*	.19*	.33*	1.00	.19*	.24*
5. G2 aggression toward children	.11*	.04	.22*	.22*	1.00	.20*
6. G2 aggression toward spouse	.07	.04	−.01	.21*	.24*	1.00

Note. Coefficients above the diagonal are for fathers, those below the diagonal are for mothers.
* $p = .05$

correlations for the G1 parents. The coefficient between G1 Harsh Parenting and G1 Marital Strife is .35 for the parents of G2 fathers and .45 for the parents of G2 mothers.

Table 4 also shows a significant bivariate association between G1 Harsh Parenting and G2 Aggression toward Children, a relationship assumed by all three theoretical frameworks. The coefficient is .22 for mothers and .15 for fathers. In addition to this relationship, the family relationships perspective posits a relationship between G1 Marital Strife and G2 Aggression toward Children. Contrary to the theory, these correlations are *not* significant for either mothers or fathers.

The family relationships and antisocial orientation perspectives both predict an association between G1 Harsh Parenting and G2 Aggression toward Spouse. Again, the correlations are *not* significant for either mothers or fathers. The latter finding is more consequential for the family relationships than the antisocial behavior perspective, as it may be that there is no significant bivariate association between these constructs, because G1 harsh parenting is linked to G2 marital violence through its impact on G2's general antisocial orientation, that is, the effect of G1 Harsh Parenting on G2 Aggression toward Spouse is indirect through G2 Antisocial Behavior. This idea is tested below using structural equation modeling.

Finally, Table 4 shows that G1 Antisocial Behavior is correlated with G1 Marital Strife and G1 Harsh Parenting. And, G2 Antisocial Behavior is related to G2 Aggression toward Children, G2 Aggression toward Spouse, and G1 Harsh Parenting. This pattern of associations is predicted by the antisocial orientation perspective, but not by the other two theoretical positions.

Figures 1 and 2 present the results of using LISREL VII to examine the extent to which a general antisocial orientation serves to mediate the effect of G1 Marital Strife and Harsh Discipline on G2 family violence. The families in the sample were largely working class and therefore represented a restricted range of socioeconomic status. Analysis showed that neither family income nor parents' level of education was related to Antisocial Behavior, Aggression toward Children, or Aggression toward Spouse. Hence, in an effort to save degrees of freedom, these variables were not included in the LISREL VII. Also, it should be noted that the models were originally run separately by gender of child and the results were virtually identical whether the target child was male or female. Therefore, in order to increase the sample size for the analyses, the models reported are based on the total sample.

The Goodness of Fit Indexes (GFIs) and X^2 values indicate that the models provide an adequate fit of the data. The pattern of findings is almost identical for husbands and wives. As an aid to the reader, statistically significant paths are depicted in boldface. Consonant with the antisocial orientation perspective, G1 Harsh Discipline is related to G2 Antisocial Behavior (ß = .22 for husbands and .27 for wives), which in turn, shows significant associations with both Aggression toward Children (ß = .16 for fathers and .17 for mothers) and Aggression toward

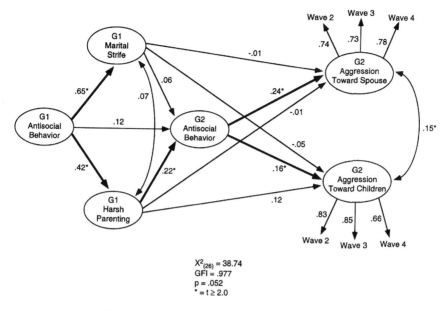

Figure 1. Structural equation model for fathers (N = 324).

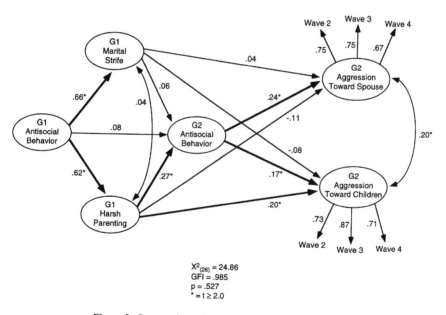

Figure 2. Structural equation model for mothers (N = 316).

Spouse (ß = .24 for both husbands and wives). There are no significant paths for G1 Antisocial Behavior or Marital Strife to G2 Antisocial Behavior, Aggression toward Spouse, or Aggression toward Children. This pattern of results suggests that antisocial parents tend to engage in marital violence and harsh parenting, and that such parenting, in turn, increases the chances that their children will grow up to engage in a wide variety of antisocial behaviors, including violence toward their spouse and children.

While the findings provide support for the antisocial orientation perspective, there is also some corroboration of the role modeling viewpoint. Figure 2 shows that after controlling for G2 Antisocial Behavior, there continues to be a significant association between G1 Harsh Parenting and G2 Aggression toward Children. It thus appears that both the antisocial orientation and the role modeling perspectives account for correlations across generations between the harsh parenting of parents and their daughters. It seems that girls exposed to harsh parenting are at risk for acquiring aggressive parenting scripts and a general antisocial orientation, and both of these consequences increase the likelihood that she will be violent toward her own children.

DISCUSSION

Studies of domestic violence have consistently found that childhood exposure to family violence significantly increases the chance that an individual will grow to be violent toward his or her own spouse and children. This tendency for domestic violence to persist across generations was also evident in our analyses. While there is strong support for the contention that family violence is often transmitted across generations, there has been little investigation of the theoretical mechanisms whereby this transmission occurs. Past studies have been concerned with documenting the existence of intergenerational effects and have devoted little attention to the theoretical processes that account for the occurrence of this phenomenon.

As noted earlier, speculation regarding the mechanisms that account for intergenerational effects generally falls into three types. The role modeling position asserts that children learn about the role of parent by observing the parenting practices of their parents, and they acquire information regarding the role of marital partner by observing the interaction between their parents. Thus, children exposed to harsh parenting grow up to hit their children, and children who witness their parents striking each other grow up to hit their spouse. The family relationships perspective posits that both harsh physical discipline and marital violence teach children that it is legitimate, indeed, often necessary, to hit those you love (i.e., other family members). Thus, exposure to any form of family violence is seen as promoting attitudes that increase the probability that children will grow up to behave aggressively toward their spouse and offspring. Finally, the antisocial orientation viewpoint contends that antisocial parents often hit each other and their children, and that such a family environment increases the probability that children will grow up to engage in antisocial behavior of all sorts, including violence toward their spouse and children.

Our analyses provided some support for the role modeling perspective, although the effect was limited to women and the role of parent. After controlling for potentially confounding factors, exposure to harsh parenting during childhood increased the chances that a mother would use harsh corporal punishment with her own children. This relationship did not hold for fathers. There was a bivariate association between a father's having been hit as a child and his use of harsh parenting practices with his own children, but this correlation disappeared once commitment to a general antisocial orientation was controlled. Also, contrary to the role modeling perspective, childhood exposure to harsh conflict between parents did *not* increase the probability that a person would grow up to hit his or her spouse. This was true for both men and women.

The finding that childhood exposure to harsh parenting influences the parenting practices of women, but not men, may be a function of the fact that the culture identifies mothers as the primary parent (LaRossa, 1986; Simons, Beaman, Conger, & Chao, 1992). Fathers are seen as playing a secondary role, which largely consists of assisting the mother in her care of the children. Given these cultural scripts, girls are more likely than boys to engage in anticipatory socialization regarding the role of parent. This concern with the role of parent might be expected to enhance their attention and awareness of the parenting practices modeled by their parents, with the result that women are more likely than men to reenact the parenting behaviors displayed in their family of origin.

Although our results provided some support for the role modeling perspective, it was the antisocial orientation viewpoint that received the strongest support. The analyses indicated that spousal and child abuse tend to be correlated. Persons who engage in persistent marital violence also tend to display aggression toward their children, and vice versa. Furthermore, we found that persons who engage in persistent family violence are also involved in other forms of deviant behavior (e.g., substance abuse, problems with the law, employment difficulties). Violence toward family members is simply one component of their general antisocial approach to life. Finally, our results indicated that it is this general antisocial orientation, rather than lessons specific to family roles, that is transmitted across generations. We found that antisocial parents tend to engage in marital violence and harsh parenting, and that such parenting, in turn, increases the chances that their children will grow up to engage in a wide variety of antisocial behaviors, including violence toward their spouse and children.

The domestic violence literature often portrays perpetrators as having few distinguishing characteristics (Pagelow, 1984). They are depicted as ordinary citizens in all respects except for their abusive behavior. This view may well be accurate for individuals who only occasionally engage in family violence. Situational factors such as economic pressure, emotional distress, and marital conflict have been linked to aggression toward children and spouse. (Conger, McCarthy, Young, Lahey, & Kropp, 1984; Simons, Lorenz, Wu, & Conger, 1993; Straus & Smith, 1990a), and one might posit that infrequent outbursts of violence toward family members are best explained by such aversive circumstances, albeit results from the present study suggest that individuals who engage in recurring family violence are often distinctive in that they participate in other forms of deviant behavior as well. Our results indicated that there is a relationship between persistent domestic violence, whether hitting of a spouse or child, and involvement in a wide variety of antisocial actions.

It is important that this finding be interpreted with proper caution. The association between domestic violence and other types of deviance did not approach unity. Therefore, while the results suggest a clear tendency for individuals who engage in family violence to participate in other forms of antisocial behavior as well, there are exceptions to this tendency. Certainly, the fact that an individual does not have a history of involvement in antisocial behavior should never be used as a reason for failing to investigate seriously accusations of child or spousal battering.

Our finding of an association between family violence and other forms of deviant behavior is consistent with recent reviews of research on spousal batterers (Hotaling & Sugarman, 1986) and child abusers (Hotaling et al., 1990) that have concluded that the demographic risk factors for these behaviors are quite similar to those for criminal violence in general. It is also consonant with the finding that adolescents and adults who engage in domestic assault often have had contact with the police for a variety of criminal behaviors (Dunford, Huizinga, & Elliott, 1990; Hotaling et al., 1990; Sherman et al., 1991). These studies have concentrated on male perpetrators, the group that represents the gravest threat to family members given the degree of injury that they often inflict upon their victims (Stets & Straus, 1990). Findings from the present study suggest that a general antisocial orientation tends to be characteristic of women, as well as men, who engage in persistent family violence.

The finding that persistent family violence tends to be part of a general antisocial orientation is important because of the treatment implications that it suggests. Effective intervention for any difficulty requires an accurate understanding of the factors that serve to foster and maintain the problem. Many programs for family violence are built on the naive assumption that such behavior is a function of distorted beliefs (learned in the family of origin) regarding the role of spouse or parent. Based on this premise, treatment programs for abusive parents usually involve teaching more constructive strategies for managing children's behavior, and interventions with men who are violent toward their wives focus on their attitudes regarding women and marriage.

While such approaches may have some value, treatment is likely to have a limited, long-term effect to the extent that it ignores the reality that in many cases, the person's behavior toward family members is indicative of a more general antisocial approach to life. The perpetrator is apt to revert back to aggressive treatment of family members if he or she continues to use substances, to get into fights, to miss work, to mismanage family finances, and so on. A truly effective treatment would be concerned with assisting the perpetrator to develop a more responsible lifestyle. Such interventions are likely to be costly in terms of both time and money. Indeed, it is not clear that current treatment technologies are able to produce such pervasive changes in a person's lifestyle, especially if he or she is resistant to change. However, results from our study, as well as those reported by others, suggest that it is only by creating such intervention programs that we will be able to help perpetrators of family violence to desist from such behavior.

REFERENCES

Allport, G. W. (1937). *Personality: A psychological interpretation.* New York: Holt, Rinehart & Winston.

Capaldi, D. M., & Patterson, G. R. (1991). Relation of parental transitions to boys' adjustment problems: I. A linear hypothesis. II. Mothers at risk for transitions and unskilled parenting. *Developmental Psychology, 27,* 489–504.

Caspi, A., & Moffitt, T. E. (1992). The continuity of maladaptive behavior: From description to understanding in the study of antisocial behavior. In D. Cicchetti & D. Cohen (Eds.), *Manual of developmental psychopathology* (pp. 472–511). New York: Wiley.

Cicchetti, D., & Carlson, V. (Eds.). (1989). *Child maltreatment: Theory and research on the causes and consequences of child abuse and neglect.* Cambridge, UK: Cambridge University Press.

Conger, R. D., Elder, G. H., Jr., Lorenz, F. O., Simons, R. L., & Whitbeck, L. B. (1992). A family process model of economic hardship and influences on adjustment of early adolescent boys. *Child Development, 63,* 526–541.

Conger, R. D., McCarthy, J. A., Young, R. K., Lahey, B. B., & Kropp, J. P. (1984). Perception of child, child-rearing values, and emotional distress as mediating links between environmental stressors and observed maternal behaviors. *Child Development, 55,* 2234–2247.

Donovan, J. E., & Jessor, R. (1985). Structure of problem behavior in adolescence and young adulthood. *Journal of Consulting and Clinical Psychology, 53,* 890–904.

Dunford, F., Huizinga, D., & Elliott, D. S. (1990). The role of arrest in domestic assault: The Omaha experiment. *Criminology, 28,* 183–206.

Fagan, J. A., Stewart, D. K., & Hansen, K. V. (1983). Violent men or violent husbands? Background factors and situational correlates. In D. Finkelhor, R. J. Gelles, G. T. Hotaling, & M. A. Straus (Eds.), *The dark side of families: Current family violence research* (pp. 49–67). Beverly Hills, CA: Sage.

Farrington, D. P. (1991). Childhood aggressive and adult violence: Early precursors and later life outcomes. In D. J. Pepler & K. H. Rubin (Eds.), *The development and treatment of childhood aggression* (pp. 5–30). Hillsdale, NJ: Erlbaum.

Finkelhor, D. (1983). Common features of family abuse. In D. Finkelhor, R. J. Gelles, G. T. Hotaling, & M. A. Straus (Eds.), *The dark side of families: Current family violence research* (pp. 1–28). Beverly Hills, CA: Sage.

Flynn, J. D. (1977). Recent findings related to wife abuse. *Social Casework, 58,* 17–18.

Gayford, J. J. (1975). Wife battering: A preliminary study of 100 cases. *British Medical Journal, 1,* 194–197.

Gelles, R. J., & Cornell, C. P. (1990). *Intimate violence in families.* Newbury Park, CA: Sage.

Gelles, R. J., & Straus, M. A. (1979). Determinants of violence in the family: Towards a theoretical integration. In W. R. Burr, R. Hill, F. I. Nye, & I. L. Reiss (Eds.), *Contemporary theories about the family* (Vol. 1, pp. 548–581). New York: Free Press.

Gelles, R. J., & Straus, M. A. (1988). *Intimate violence.* New York: Simon & Schuster.

Gil, D. G. (1970). *Violence against children: Physical child abuse in the United States.* Cambridge, MA: Harvard University Press.

Hotaling, G. T., Finkelhor, D., Kirkpatrick, J. T., & Straus, M. A. (Eds.). (1988). *Family abuse and its consequences: New directions in research.* Newbury Park, CA: Sage.

Hotaling, G. T., & Straus, M. A. (1980). Culture, social organization, and irony in the study of family violence. In M. A. Straus & G. T. Hotaling (Eds.), *The social causes of husband–wife violence* (pp. 3–22). Minneapolis: University of Minnesota Press.

Hotaling, G. T., Straus, M. A., & Lincoln, A. J. (1990). Intrafamily violence and crime and violence outside the family. In M. A. Straus & R. J. Gelles (Eds.), *Physical violence in American families* (pp. 431–470). New Brunswick, NJ: Transaction.

Hotaling, G. T., & Sugarman, D. B. (1986). An analysis of risk markers in husband to wife violence: The current state of knowledge. *Violence and Victims, 1,* 101–124.

Jessor, R. L., & Jessor, S. L. (1977). *Problem behavior and psychosocial development.* New York: Academic Press.

Kaufman, J., & Zigler, E. (1987). Do abused children become abusive parents? *American Journal of Orthopsychiatry, 57,* 186–192.

Kaufman, J., & Zigler, E. (1989). The intergenerational transmission of child abuse. In D. Cicchetti & V. Carlson (Eds.), *Child maltreatment: Theory and research on the causes and consequences of child abuse and neglect* (pp. 129–152). Cambridge, UK: Cambridge University Press.

LaRossa, R. (1986). *Becoming a parent.* Beverly Hills, CA: Sage.

Levinson, D. (1988). Family violence in cross-cultural perspective. In V. B. Van Hasselt, R. L. Morrison, A. S. Bellack, & M. Hersen (Eds.), *Handbook of family violence* (pp. 435–453). New York: Plenum Press.

Levinson, D. (1989). *Family violence in cross-cultural perspective.* Newbury Park, CA: Sage.

Loeber, R. (1982). The stability of antisocial and delinquent behavior: A review. *Child Development, 53,* 1431–1446.

Loeber, R., & Le Blanc, M. (1990). Toward a developmental criminology. In M. Tonry & N. Morris (Eds.), *Crime and justice: A review of research* (Vol. 12, pp. 375–473). Chicago: University of Chicago Press.

Megargee, E. I. (1982). Psychological determinants and correlates of criminal violence. In M. E. Wolfgang & N. A. Weiner (Eds.), *Criminal violence* (pp. 81–170). Newbury Park, CA: Sage.

Melby J., Conger, R., Book, R., Rueter, M., Lucy, L., Repinski, D., Ahrens, K., Black, D., Brown, D., Huck, S., Mutchler, L., Rogers, S., Ross, J., & Stavros, T. (1990). *The Iowa Family Interaction Coding Manual.* Ames: Iowa Youth and Families Project.

O'Leary, K. D. (1988). Physical aggression between spouses: A social learning theory perspective. In V. B. Van Hasselt, R. L. Morrison, & A. S. Bellack (Eds.), *Handbook of family violence* (pp. 31–55). New York: Plenum Press.

Osgood, D. W., Johnston, L. D., O'Malley, P. M., & Bachman, J. G. (1988). The generality of deviance in late adolescence and early adulthood. *American Sociological Review, 53,* 81–93.

Pagelow, M. D. (1981). *Wife-battering: Victims and their experiences.* Beverly Hills, CA: Sage.

Pagelow, M. D. (1984). *Family violence.* New York: Praeger.

Patterson, G. R., Reid, J. B., & Dishion, T. J. (1992). *Antisocial Boys.* Eugene, OR: Castalia.

Patterson, G. R., & Yoerger, K. (1993). Development models for delinquent behavior. In S. Hodgins (Ed.), *Mental disorder and crime* (pp. 140–172). Newbury Park, CA: Sage.

Robins, L. N. (1974). Antisocial behavior disturbances of childhood: Prevalence, prognosis, and prospects. In E. J. Anthony & C. Koupernik, (Eds.), *The child in his family: Vol. 3. Children at psychiatric risk* (pp. 447–460). New York: Wiley.

Rosenbaum, A., & O'Leary, K. D. (1981). Marital violence: Characteristics of abusive couples. *Journal of Consulting and Clinical Psychology, 49,* 63–71.

Sherman, L. W., Schmidt, J. D., Rogan, D. P., Gartin, P. R. Cohn, E. G., Dean, J. C., & Bacich, A. R. (1991). From initial deterrence to long-term escalation: Short-term custody arrest for poverty ghetto domestic violence. *Criminology, 29,* 821–850.

Sampson, R. J., & Laub, J. H. (1993). *Crime in the making: Pathways and turning points through life.* Cambridge, MA: Harvard University Press.

Simons, R. L., Beaman, J., Conger, R. D., & Chao, W. (1992). Gender differences in the intergenerational transmission of parenting beliefs. *Journal of Marriage and the Family, 54,* 823–836.

Simons, R. L., Beaman, J., Conger, R. D., & Chao, W. (1993a). Childhood experience, conceptions of parenting, and attitudes of spouse as determinants of parental behavior. *Journal of Marriage and the Family, 55,* 91–106.

Simons, R. L., Beaman, J., Conger, R. D., & Chao, W. (1993b). Stress, support, and antisocial behavior trait as determinants of emotional well-being and parenting practices among single mothers. *Journal of Marriage and the Family, 55,* 385–398.

Simons, R. L., Lorenz, F. O., Wu, C., & Conger, R. D. (1993). Marital and spouse support as mediator and moderator of the impact of economic strain upon parenting. *Developmental Psychology, 29,* 368–381.

Simons, R. L., Whitbeck, L. B., Conger, R. D., & Wu, C. (1991). Intergenerational transmission of harsh parenting. *Developmental Psychology, 27,* 159–171.

Simons, R. L., Wu, C., Conger, R. D., & Lorenz, F. O. (1994). Two routes to delinquency: Differences in the impact of parents and peers for early versus late starters. *Criminology, 32,* 247–276.

Simons, R. L., Wu, C., Johnson, C., & Conger, R. D. (1995). A test of various perspectives on the intergenerational transmission of domestic violence. *Criminology, 33,* 141–172.

Skinner, A. E., & Castle, R. L. (1969). *Seventy-eight battered children: A retrospective study.* London: National Society for the Prevention of Cruelty to Children.

Smith, S. M., Hansen, R., & Noble, S. (1973). Parents of battered children: A controlled study. *British Medical Journal, 4,* 388–391.

Stacy, W. A., & Shupe, A. (1983). *The family secret: Domestic violence in America.* Boston: Beacon Press.

Steele, B. F., & Pollack, C. B. (1968). A psychiatric study of parents who abuse infants and small children. In R. E. Helfer & C. H. Kempe (Eds.), *The battered child* (pp. 103–148). Chicago: University of Chicago Press.

Steinmetz, S. K. (1987). Family violence: Past, present, future. In M. B. Sussman & S. K. Steinmetz (Eds.), *Handbook of marriage and the family* (pp. 725–766). New York: Plenum Press.

Stets, J. E., & Straus, M. A. (1990). Gender differences in reporting marital violence and its medical and psychological consequences. In M. A. Straus & R. J. Gelles (Eds.), *Physical violence in American families* (pp. 151–180). New Brunswick, NJ: Transaction.

Straus, M. A. (1979). Measuring intrafamily conflict and violence: The Conflict Tactics (CT) Scales. *Journal of Marriage and the Family, 41,* 75–88.

Straus, M. A. (1983). Ordinary violence, child abuse, and wife-beating: What do they have in common? In D. Finkelhor, R. J. Gelles, G. T. Hotaling, & M. A. Straus (Eds.), *The dark side of families: Current family violence research* (pp. 213–234). Beverly Hills, CA: Sage.

Straus, M. A. (1985). Family training in crime and violence. In A. J. Lincoln & M. A. Straus (Eds.), *Crime and the family.* Springfield, IL: Charles C Thomas.

Straus, M. A., & Gelles, R. J. (1986). Societal change and family violence from 1975 to 1985 as revealed by two national surveys. *Journal of Marriage and the Family, 48,* 465–479.

Straus, M. A., & Gelles, R. J. (1988). How violent are American families? Estimates from the National Family Violence Resurvey and other studies. In G. T. Hotaling, D. Finkelhor, J. T. Kirkpatrick, and M. A. Straus (Eds.)., *Family abuse and its consequences: New directions in research* (pp. 14–37). Beverly Hills, CA: Sage.

Straus, M. A., Gelles, R. J., & Steinmetz, S. K. (1980). *Behind closed doors: Violence in the American family.* Beverly Hills, CA: Sage.

Straus, M. A., & Smith, C. (1990a). Family patterns and child abuse. In M. A. Straus & R. J. Gelles (Eds.), *Physical violence in American families* (pp. 245–261). New Brunswick, NJ: Transaction.

Straus, M. A., & Smith, C. (1990b). Family patterns and primary prevention of family violence. In M. A. Straus & R. J. Gelles (Eds.), *Physical violence in American families* (pp. 507–528). New Brunswick, NJ: Transaction.

Walker, L. E. (1979). *The battered woman.* New York: Harper & Row.

Wauchope, B., & Straus, M. (1990). Age, gender and class differences in physical punishment and physical abuse of American children. In M. A. Straus & R. J. Gelles (Eds.), *Physical violence in American families* (pp. 133–148). New Brunswick, NJ: Transaction.

Wolfe, D. A. (1987). *Child abuse: Implications for child development and psychopathology.* Newbury Park, CA: Sage.

33

Violence

Effects of Parent's Previous Trauma
on Currently Traumatized Children

KATHLEEN OLYMPIA NADER

> Our parental inheritance is much more than just the genes. Every cell in the body is impregnated with consciousness that is laden with the thought forms and imprints passed down from generation to generation.
>
> GRISGAM, 1988, p. 37

The belief that the actions or experiences of one family member are transmitted intergenerationally predates written history and is multicultural. It has been handed down for many centuries among Japanese cultures (Motoyama, 1992) as well as specific Native American tribes (Nahwegahbow, 1995). It can be found in both Eastern and Western religious traditions. For example, the pre-Vedic verbal tradition in India describes the transmission of positive effects (Ledgerwood, 1979). The writings, dated 15th century B.C., sacred to both the Jewish and the Christian traditions (The Holy Bible, Exodus, 34:7, Numbers 14:18) as well as Talmudic writings in the Jewish tradition from the fourth to fifth century C.E. (A.D.) (Talmud, Sota 34a) depict the transmission of negative effects. This belief has found its way into "New Age" psychological and physical healing practices that are often based upon the ancient healing and spiritual traditions of several cultures (see Grisgam, 1988, opening quotation).

The intergenerational transmission of trauma has been investigated for children of Holocaust survivors, traumatized war veterans, and previously abused parents. Investigators have disagreed about the statistically measurable existence of a *direct* effect of a parent's trauma upon the children (see Studies of Children of Traumatized Parents section). This chapter examines the association of a parent's previous trauma with trauma in children exposed to a current traumatic event. It is a clinical case examination of two groups of children, including a subsample of children exposed to a sniper attack in south-central Los Angeles, California, in 1984, and a sample of children exposed to a hostage taking and suicide in Orange County, California, in 1987.

KATHLEEN OLYMPIA NADER • Consultant on Trauma and Traumatic Grief, P.O. Box 2316, Austin, Texas, 78767.

International Handbook of Multigenerational Legacies of Trauma, edited by Yael Danieli. Plenum Press, New York, 1998.

THE TRANSMISSION OF TRAUMA

The transmission of parental trauma to a child has been explained in a variety of ways through (1) overt communications; (2) overt behaviors; (3) covert or metacommunications, subliminally; and/or (4) genetically or biochemically. Whether transmission of traumatic themes and phenomena is overt or covert may be related to the nature of traumatic memories (e.g., explicit vs. implicit memory). Explicit memory is overt, conscious, and basically factual. Implicit memory is more covert and is described as unconscious or preconscious (i.e., overt awareness of the memories is lacking). The overt transmission of trauma may include verbal prescriptions (e.g., teaching children to expect trauma, the sense of belonging to a violent community), modeling (e.g., modeling violent interactions or helplessness), or parent's posttraumatic violent behaviors (e.g., intrafamilial abuse). Other forms of transmission are also discussed.

Covert Transmission

It has been hypothesized that life experiences or their effects are covertly transmitted from one generation to subsequent generations by the nonverbal communication of intense unresolved personal conflicts, the handing down of family myths and beliefs, and the learning of life scripts. Covert transmission of trauma includes the communication of ideas, themes, and experiences without conscious awareness. This process may include issues of identification, learning, self-esteem, and mental organization. The following are a few of the theories that seek to explain the covert conveyance of repeated themes.

For children, the study of transgenerational trauma has included a discussion of intergenerationally repeated child maltreatment. Although a number of studies have observed that abusing parents report a high rate of emotional or physical maltreatment in their own childhoods (Curtis, 1963; Wasserman, 1973), the studies often do not have access to previously abused parents who are now providing adequate care for their children. Thus the maltreated–maltreating cycle may be overreported (Zeanah & Zeanah, 1989). Learning, identification, internalization, inadequate self-esteem, and impaired impulse control as a result of trauma have all been implied or discussed as explanations of the transgenerational repetition of abuse. According to Zeanah and Zeanah (1989), attachment theory (patterns of attachment to and intimately relating with others; Bowlby, 1969/1982, 1973, 1980) suggests shifting the focus to organizing themes of the parent–child relationship and their associated internal working models. In this theory, dynamic mental representations of self and others (working models), maintained largely out of awareness, guide appraisals of and responses to others. For example, mothers who are angry and punitive have toddlers who are angry and noncompliant. These toddlers have apparently internalized their parent's aggression and learned both the punitive and provocative roles of the relationship. Thus, the organizing themes of the relationship are transmitted across generations (Zeanah & Zeanah, 1989).

Szurek, in 1942, and Johnson and Szurek (1952) discussed the "superego lacunae" in relationship to adolescent delinquent behaviors. Singer (1974) summarized their theory as follows: "Specific areas of antisocial aggressive and sexual behavior coincid[ing] with the specific unconscious areas in the parents, usually the mother, that were forbidden, unacceptable and, although highly cathected, were totally unintegrated and usually unexpressed by the parent" (p. 795). These suppressed areas in the parent resulted in an unconscious dialogue between parent and child, via covert messages, characterized by an ongoing reciprocal system of message and countermessage. The unconscious sanctions for behaviors or experiences had more power than the conscious, overt messages to stop the behaviors or avoid the experiences. These metacommunications that encouraged acting out included, for example, the mother always expecting the worst. "Superego lacunae" was used to explain the behaviors of a suddenly school-phobic daughter. The family had been referred for treatment because the son had committed a minor crime; the mother also sought help for her daughter. The daughter, although unaware of her mother's childhood sexual trauma, became school-phobic when she reached the age the mother had been when first molested.

Feinstein and Krippner (1988) discuss the mythology passed down through a family, laden with the disappointments and hopes of prior generations. Genetics and cultural mythology are amalgamated into a unique "mythic" framework that shapes personal development. A personal myth is the constellation of feelings, beliefs, and images that is organized around a core theme and addresses one of the traditional functions of mythology. According to Campbell (1968), these functions, include the (1) urge to comprehend the natural world in a meaningful way; (2) search for a pathway through the succeeding epochs of life; (3) need for secure and fulfilling relationships within a community; and (4) longing to know one's part within the universe. Through these personal myths, individuals understand the present and find guidance for the future. Personal myths evolve as they are passed from one generation to the next. Similarly, Armsworth (1993) discussed the transgenerational transmission of trauma in terms of Eric Berne's "script" theory, which proposes that children learn life scripts from the opposite-sex parent and learn how to implement them from the same-sex parent.

"Self-fulfilling prophecy" is a commonly used term to denote that our strongly held beliefs often become reality (whether because of our actions or because of the actions we elicit from others). By this same process, commonly held familial or cultural beliefs may contribute to the phenomenon of transgenerational trauma as well, and thus provide a long history of anecdotal evidence that the parents' actions and experiences affect the lives of their children.

Genetic or Biochemical Transmission

Studies of both animals and humans have provided evidence that characteristics affecting life circumstances are genetically or biochemically transmitted from one generation to another. In an extensive study of mice in the 1950s, Calhoun (May, 1995) observed parent mice who, under stress, became abusive (e.g., biting the babies' necks or tails). He found that the sequence of experiences through sequential generations altered the behavior toward increasing pathology. Subsequent generations of mice became fixed at a maturation level of 21 days for males and 45 days for females, and never developed the capacity to mate or reproduce. No change was observed after they were returned to a normal situation.

In a study of Rhesus monkeys, Suomi (1995; see also chapter 36, this volume) reported that certain monkeys had higher adrenocorticotropic hormone (ACTH) and cortisol rates when placed in stress situations. These more reactive monkeys became depressed and withdrawn rather than adjusting over time to the normal parental separation during breeding seasons. Reactive male rhesus monkeys consistently produced offspring who were high reactors and had higher ACTH and cortisol levels. These patterns tended to persist from infancy to adulthood. Male monkeys who, at adolescence, must leave the troop of monkeys into which they were born and find another troop, were more successful if they were not among the high reactive group. In a comparison of female rhesus offspring placed with foster mothers during early life and maturation, Suomi observed that when monoamine metabolite levels were measured after breeding separation, daughters' monoamine metabolite rates were closer to their natural mothers' than to their foster mothers' rates. High reactors were more likely to neglect or abuse their offspring.

In a study of spine–meningeal system adaptive holding patterns, Ward (1990) suggested that psychogenetic patterns were inherited and could be traced back up to five generations (Ward, Ward, & Behan, 1993). Ward (1990) also hypothesized that every new trauma, through the fetus, becomes an inherited dysfunctional psychogenetic experience. Studying the histories of preceding generations (a history sometimes unknown to the patient), Ward related later physical traumas (e.g., debilitation from a car accident) to, for example, a murdering grandparent, the near-death abuse of mother by father during pregnancy, or a grandparent's suicide. He concluded that degenerative ailments such as muscular dystrophy, myasthenia gravis, multiple sclerosis, cystic fibrosis, and cerebral palsy could be traced back to fetal, parental, or grandparental traumatic experiences such as abandonment, suicide, or being unwanted (Ward, 1993; personal communication, June 1995).

STUDIES OF CHILDREN OF TRAUMATIZED PARENTS

A number of studies have examined the effects upon children of a parent's traumatic experience. Studies of the children of Holocaust survivors have sometimes disagreed about the etiology or existence of "effects" in children of survivors. After reviewing these studies, Solkoff (1992) concluded that clinical and anecdotal data point to psychopathology in the adjustment of children of survivors, whereas more methodologically sophisticated studies generally conclude that children of survivors are not substantially different from other children. Solkoff suggested that immigrant status may be as important as the Holocaust experience in determining differences in psychological adjustment among offspring.

Clinical studies have enumerated a variety of psychological difficulties in children of Holocaust survivors (Danieli, 1981; Freyburg, 1980; Klein & Kogan, 1986). Cited in association with these psychological effects were parenting methods characterized as overprotective, overcontrolling, and treating children like highly valued possessions (Freyburg, 1980), and parental qualities such as obsession with anxieties and fears, ambivalence, and disbelief in their children's ego strength (Klein & Kogan, 1986). In addition to issues of psychological adjustment, researchers have discussed whether or not children exhibit secondary trauma without direct exposure to their parents' traumatic experiences. Like Klein and Kogan, Barocas and Barocas (1979) reported, in a clinical sample of survivors' offspring, intrusive images and nightmares of their parents' Holocaust experiences. In order to separate the effect of a parent's posttraumatic behavior from the impact of the parent's traumatic experience, Dan (1995) examined the children (ages 12–17) of Vietnam veterans diagnosed with posttraumatic stress disorder (PTSD) and associated disorders, and children of veterans without any combat experience during the Vietnam era (with no PTSD). Both groups were substance abusing, so that differences in the children could not be attributed to any family disorganization and other effects of the substance abuse itself. Both the children of substance-abusing fathers with no PTSD and the children of substance-abusing combat-veteran fathers with PTSD had more trauma symptoms than normal children. However, most of these children had a subset of DSM-IV PTSD symptoms rather than PTSD. Children with moderate to severe PTSD levels generally had mitigating factors (e.g., high levels of violence in the home), which might explain their increased symptoms. Children of PTSD fathers had more conflict in their families.

Studies have also examined increased vulnerability during exposure to a traumatic experience as a result of a parent's previous trauma. Solomon, Moshe, and Mikulincer (1988) found that 1, 2, and 3 years after participation in the 1982 war in Lebanon, Israeli combat veterans whose parents were Holocaust survivors had higher rates of PTSD and greater numbers of

PTSD symptoms than their combat-veteran counterparts whose parents were not survivors of the Holocaust. The decrease in PTSD symptoms over time was greater for soldiers with non-survivor parents.

CHILDHOOD TRAUMATIC EVENTS
AND PARENT'S PREVIOUS TRAUMA

This chapter primarily examines the issue of vulnerability in children whose parents have had traumatic experiences. Below are the results of this examination for two groups of children who were exposed to a traumatic experience as a group.

Sniper Attack

In February 1984, a man opened fire on a crowded elementary school playground. One fifth-grade child and one passerby were killed and more than 14 others were injured, including one school staff member. Children witnessed as bullets went through one side of a fifth-grade girl, exiting the other side with lung and heart tissue. The passerby was cut open across his abdomen by the same automatic gunfire, and intestines were emerging from his abdomen. One child sustained severe intestinal and other abdominal injuries, another lost the use of his hand, and still another child had a pellet lodged in her throat. The sniper appeared to be shooting at any moving target, and many children were pinned down on the playground or behind nearby barriers that protected them from the sniper's sight. Children looking out through windows on the sniper side of the school saw severe, bloody injuries through the window or were frightened by bullets breaking through windows. Children in classrooms on the other side of the school saw their teachers tape paper over windows and/or were ordered to hide in closets or under desks. They feared gang members were attacking the school and would enter to kill them.

One month after the sniper attack, 77% of children present on the playground under direct attack and 67% of children in the school had moderate to severe PTSD. In contrast, 74% of children who had already gone home at the time of the attack and 83% of children on a 3-week vacation from this year-round school had mild to no PTSD. Within each exposure level, children who knew the deceased classmate had significantly more symptoms of PTSD (Pynoos et al., 1987). Fourteen months later, children with greater exposure to the shooting continued to have significantly more symptoms and significantly greater severity of traumatic reactions. Children with lesser exposure had higher trauma scores if they knew the child who was killed or if they reported experiencing guilt feelings. Grief scores were associated with greater acquaintance with the deceased classmate, independent of exposure to the sniper attack. A child's previous trauma did not significantly affect trauma scores (Nader, Pynoos, Fairbanks, & Frederick, 1990).

Methods

In order to examine the effects of a parent's previous trauma on children exposed to traumatic events, the acute-phase clinical diagnoses and Childhood PTSD Parent Inventory (CPTSD-PI; Nader, 1984) of 92 children were reexamined. Twelve children were omitted from this review because 10 were missing clinician's diagnoses and 2 were missing data regarding theirs and their parents' previous traumas (8 exposed, 4 not exposed). Of the remaining 80 children, 48 were exposed (on the playground or in the school) and 32 were not exposed (on the way home, at home, out of the area) to the shooting.

All of the children on the playground during the sniper attack (estimated between 60 and 90) were invited to receive a clinical diagnostic interview with one of six members of the UCLA Trauma Team. A distinction was made between symptoms related to the sniper attack and those related to a previous experience. The unexposed group included 11 children randomly selected from the children unexposed to the shooting who had been interviewed in their classrooms using the Childhood Posttraumatic Stress Reaction Index (Frederick, Pynoos, & Nader, 1992) (12 were invited; one refused), 5 at-risk unexposed children (4 previous conduct disturbances and 1 depression), and 16 unexposed siblings of children in the exposed group. Because of sampling method and size, this particular review must be considered a clinical, descriptive examination of children.

Results

Subjects. The sniper attack was an event that traumatically affected children primarily as a result of exposure to a threat to life and the witnessing of injury or death (Nader *et al.,* 1990; Pynoos *et al.,* 1987). Fifty percent (24) of the children in this sample who were exposed to the attack had parents with previous traumas and 50% (24) had parents with no previous trauma. Of the 32 unexposed children, 19 (59%) had a parent with prior trauma(s) and 13 (41%) had parents with no prior traumas. For the total group, 43 (54%) of the children's parents had experienced a previous trauma and 37 (46%) children's parents had no previous trauma (Table 1).

Parent's Previous traumas and the Effects of the Sniper Attack. Although exposure to the attack was highly correlated with traumatic response—regardless of specific other factors such as grief or the child's previous trauma (Pynoos *et al.,* 1987)—all of the unexposed children with PTSD had parents with previous traumas. None of the unexposed children in this sample whose parents were free of previous trauma had PTSD. The five children in this sample who, although exposed, had no PTSD (including those with selected trauma symptoms or aggression), were in the school building rather than on the playground; they reported no prior traumas, and their parents reported no prior traumas.

Having a parent with a previous trauma was associated with the presence of symptoms, following the sniper attack, related to this or another stressful experience. All 8 (100%) of the unexposed children with no PTSD, no selected symptoms of PTSD, and no aggression in response to this sniper attack, whose parents had a previous trauma, were reexperiencing the

Table 1. Parent's Previous Trauma, Sniper Attack

		Parent trauma N = 24	No parent trauma N = 13
PTSD	Exposed	0	19
	Not exposed	3	0
No PTSD	Exposed	0	2
	Not exposed	8	10
Selected symptoms	Exposed	0	2
	Not exposed	3	1
Aggression	Exposed	0	1
	Not exposed	5	2
Total		43	37

symptoms of bereavement related to a previous loss or were reexperiencing specific traumatic symptoms related to a previous trauma (4 loss, 4 trauma). Of the 10 unexposed children with no PTSD, whose parents were previously untraumatized, only 1 of the 4 (25%) children with their own previous traumas was reexperiencing symptoms (Table 2).

The children of previously traumatized parents often reported a great deal of anxiety following the sniper attack. Children became fearful of a repetition of the parent's previous trauma or of harm to the parent. For example, a child who drew a heart with her mother's name in it tearfully described how, when her mother was 12, her stepgrandmother shot and killed her grandmother. After the sniper attack, the little girl, age 10, became very fearful that her mother would be killed. She had become anxious, hypervigilant, and unable to concentrate. Her sleep was disturbed and, in the night, she saw monsters, goblins, and her grandmother.

Previous studies have examined the caretaking child as a product of a parent's previous trauma (Armsworth, 1993). Although there was no direct inquiry about caretaking children in this study, a few children were so obviously parenting their parents that a note was made in the chart. At the beginning of the clinical diagnostic interview, children were asked to draw a picture of anything they wanted to and tell a story about it. A child who drew a picture of a deep, dark lake was one of the parenting children. She stated that she was drawing a park where she liked to play. She spent a great deal of time inking and reinking the lake. When the clinician commented that there must be things deep in that lake that no one could see, the child burst into tears. Since the sniper attack, the girl had been extremely worried that something would happen to her mother. Her mother had been traumatized by the traumatic death of her own mother.

Parent's Previous Traumas and Children's Previous Traumas. The sniper attack was an incident that affected a school of more than 1,100 children. The child's location in relationship to the sniper was more important to his or her reaction than prior experience, family circumstances, or other factors. Children's previous traumas did not significantly affect trauma scores (Nader *et al.,* 1990; Pynoos *et al.,* 1987). Half of the children in this sample had experienced previous traumatic events themselves. These previous traumas included accidental injury to children or relatives, witnessing family violence, or having a relative violently killed or injured. Seventy-four percent of children (32) in the parents with trauma group had been traumatized before the sniper attack, compared to only 22% of the children (8) in the parents without pervious trauma group (Table 3).

Inasmuch as some of the children of abused parents have been observed to repeat their parent's specific traumatic experience, repetition of specific parental trauma was examined. Previously traumatized parents of the children in this sample had been exposed to violent deaths or injuries of relatives, witnessed severe bloody injury, or experienced armed robbery, war, disasters, their child's sudden/accidental death or injury, their own injury, rape, or domestic violence. One had a nervous breakdown after personal illness and the multiple deaths of

Table 2. Unexposed Children, Sniper Attack

	% Parent with trauma	% Parent, no trauma
Traumatized	16	0
Reexperiencing	42	8
Selected symptoms	16	8
Aggression	26	15
Nonsymptomatic	0	69

Table 3. Child's Previous Trauma, Sniper Attack

		Parent trauma	No parent trauma
PTSD	Exposed	19	2
	Not exposed	1	0
No PTSD	Exposed	0	0
	Not exposed	8	4
Selected symptoms	Exposed	0	0
	Not exposed	1	0
Aggression	Exposed	0	0
	Not exposed	3	2

loved ones. The child's previous trauma most often did not replicate the parent's previous trauma. For example, a father with a severe accidental leg injury had four children whose close cousin (mother's side) was shot in the head. One of the children was also badly burned in an explosion. A grandmother had two grandchildren in her care severely burned. Her child was bitten by a dog and witnessed a robbery in which she was threatened by the robber. A parent was attacked sexually, and in the same year, her brother was shot, losing an eye and a lung. Her child was hit by a car at age 5, resulting in a persistent leg injury.

In two cases, the child's trauma somewhat resembled a parent's traumas. In the first, a mother (1) was raped and attempted suicide, and (2) on a later occasion, watched while a friend was hit by a car and the friend's leg was cut off. Her son, who was exposed to the sniper attack, was traumatized by the injury of his sister in an automobile accident. In the second instance, in a family with ongoing spousal abuse, the mother was once stabbed by the father. Her daughter witnessed a man being stabbed by another man.

Behaviors of Special Concern.   Following the attack, several specific characteristics eliciting concern were found in previously traumatized parents and other "red flag" behaviors were found in children. Awareness of the child's sniper-attack experience appeared frequently to reawaken symptoms in the parent from a previous trauma or loss, or it resulted in intense avoidance. As a result, the parent was either emotionally unable or unavailable to assist the child, or was intolerant of the child's posttrauma reaction. Additionally, some of the traumatized or previously traumatized parents became overprotective of their children following the traumatic event.

Following the sniper attack, 18 of the 54 exposed children in this sample exhibited behaviors of significant concern. These behaviors included fire setting, suicide attempts (e.g., 3 siblings took large doses of their father's medication), increased acts of aggression, dangerous climbing behaviors (e.g., a child climbing on car and rooftop), injuries, night terrors with sleepwalking (e.g., a child who awakens screaming and tries to run out of the front door in the night), severe depression with vomiting, incessant crying, freezing in front of oncoming automobiles, and risk of suicide. These behaviors were associated with parental psychopathology, parent's and/or child's previous trauma, unresolved traumatic grief, and child's psychopathology.

Hostage Taking and Suicide

A woman whose father had 10 years earlier committed suicide, and who had 3 years earlier divorced, was undergoing financial and emotional difficulties related to an on-the-job injury. In March 1987, she entered an elementary schoolyard through a side entrance, went into a fifth-grade classroom, and held the class and teacher at gunpoint. She dictated, to the teacher, a letter for the news media about her doctors, claiming inappropriate care. She waved two guns at the children, became agitated when other children appeared at the door to join the class, and accidently fired the gun, barely missing one child. Some of the children feared for their lives and the lives of their teacher and classmates. The teacher attempted to talk the woman out of killing herself. She asked the children if they wanted the woman to live, and they all yelled "Yes." When this was ineffective, she asked the children to put their heads down and pray that the woman did not shoot herself. The woman shot herself in the temple in front of the children. The woman slumped to the floor in the corner of the room. Blood poured from the side of her head and then from every opening in her face.

School staff escorted the children out of the room, called for help, and attempted to assist the woman. The fire alarm was sounded and all of the children in the school were ushered out onto the grounds and advised of the event. The hostage taking culminated in the assailant's death just before lunchtime. Psychologists and parents were called into the library area to comfort the exposed children. Other children had lunch inside their classrooms. A process of cleanup lasted into the night to prepare the school so that children could return to the classroom the next day.

Methods. All of the children from the fifth-grade classroom that was held hostage and the sixth-grade classroom next door were interviewed in semistructured clinical interviews, and their parents were interviewed separately. The clinical diagnoses and CPTSD-PI (Nader, 1984) of these children were reviewed for the purposes of examining the issue of transgenerational trauma.

Results: Parent's Previous Trauma and Children's Reactions.

Exposed Children. In this sample, 50% of the exposed children had a parent with a previous trauma and 50% had parents without previous trauma. Traumatic reaction to the hostage taking and suicide was highly correlated with exposure to the event. Of the 24 children who were present (one was home ill) in the classroom held hostage and exposed to the suicide, 18 (75%) were symptomatic whether or not they or their parents had a previous trauma. Of the 6 children who were present but not symptomatic (25%), 4 had no previous trauma and no parent with a previous trauma, 1 had a parent who had been in an airplane crash and had undergone successful therapeutic intervention, and 1 had a previous trauma during which both parent and child took successful action toward their own survival. Sixty-nine percent (11) of the children whose parent(s) had a previous trauma also had a previous trauma (2 were intrafamilial violence). Only 22% (2) of the children whose parents had no previous trauma had a previous trauma. The 3 exposed children who showed both an increase in mature and in regressive behaviors had a parent with a previous trauma. For example, 1 young girl, who insisted upon being talked to by her mother as though they were peers, also began playing with toys appropriate for a younger child. Three of the exposed children complained of persistent fatigue following the event; in all three cases, both parent and child had had a previous trauma.

Unexposed Children. Twenty children in the classroom next door to the classroom held hostage were also interviewed. These children were aware of the shooting only after it had occurred. They did not witness the event. The bullet that nearly missed one child in the classroom held hostage went through the wall of their classroom and lodged in a file cabinet. They were unaware of this when it occurred. Six of these children were referred for treatment. Three were reexperiencing the symptoms of a previous trauma, 1 was reexperiencing grief for a grandparent, 1 was evasive upon questioning, and 1 exhibited increased aggression and defiance. Of the 6 children, 5 (83%) had parents with a previous trauma, and the sixth had a mother who was prone to panic attacks.

Fourteen other children in the school, who were not directly exposed to the hostage taking and shooting, were symptomatic after the event. Eleven of these children (79%) had parents with previous traumas (2 with a family trauma). Among the other 3 children, 2 had parents whose own parents had died when they were young (ages 5 and 14) and 1 lived two houses down from the assailant. Of these 14 children, 4 had a previous trauma and 1 had a mother who had seizures.

DISCUSSION

The clinical examination of two groups of children exposed to catastrophic events suggests the transgenerational transmission of vulnerability. Traumatic events occurring in a group setting affected children with or without a parental history of trauma. Previous individual traumatic exposure, however, was more common among children with parents who had had a previous trauma. The parent's specific trauma was generally not repeated. Instead, children appeared more vulnerable to traumatic exposure of some kind and/or to increased symptoms.

More children in both groups whose parents had had a previous trauma had experienced a trauma of their own prior to the school event. These two samples were comprised of demographically very different groups of children. Although one group of children lived in a high-crime, low-socioeconomic region of Los Angeles in which children might be expected to have ample opportunity for traumatic exposure, the other group lived in an upper-middle-class area of Orange County, California, with a very low crime rate. The differences between children within each of these groups, in relationship to parents' previous trauma, lend strong evidence to an association between a parent's prior experience and a child's subsequent traumatic experience.

As has been found in studies of children of Holocaust survivors (Barocas & Barocas, 1980; Danieli, 1985; Klein & Kogan, 1986; Solomon et al., 1988) and of Vietnam veterans (Dan, 1995), the two studies described in this chapter suggest that children whose parents have been previously traumatized may have a subset of traumatic symptoms, specific psychological and behavioral disturbances, and increased vulnerabilities to or during traumatic exposure. Recognizing the legal significance of these findings, it is important to iterate that the children in this study who had PTSD were traumatized by the occurrence of an actual traumatic event. They did not have PTSD as a result of the parents' trauma but in relationship to the sniper attack or the hostage taking and witnessing of suicide. A parent's trauma does not guarantee that a child will be subsequently traumatized. Not all parents who have been traumatized have children who are subsequently traumatized (see Dan, 1995).

This study has, nevertheless, dynamically demonstrated the possibility of increased symptoms, following a traumatic event, for children whose parents have been previously traumatized. The increase in symptoms may be related to the parent's emotional unavailability or overprotectiveness as a result of their own experience. Caretaker unavailability, intolerance, and overprotection have all been associated with increased traumatic reactions in children (Bloch, Silber, & Perry, 1956; McFarlane, 1987; Nader & Pynoos, 1993; Silber, Perry, & Block, 1958). In addition, the child's traumatic exposure may result in the parent's reexperiencing aspects or symptoms of his or her own traumatic experience. Adults' traumatic reexperiencing, increased avoidance, and increased arousal have been found to create difficulties in the recovery of children following traumatic exposure (Nader, 1994). Whether these or other

factors are the primary contributors, the increased vulnerability of children during or following traumatic events suggests the need to include a parent's previous trauma among the list of
risk factors for increased symptomatology following traumatic events.

In examining the vulnerability of Holocaust-survivor offspring to increased traumatization from a traumatic event, Solomon *et al.* (1988) have elaborated possible contributing factors: (1) heightened vulnerability to stress among children of Holocaust survivors (see Danieli,
1980); (2) learned responses from parents; (3) the possible undermining of recovery by overprotective survivor parents; (4) a phenomenon similar to the increased intensity of a second
combat trauma (i.e., the parent's previous trauma serves as the previous event); and (5) a sense
of themselves as protectors of their surviving parents and as needing to undo the damage,
which may add stress and issues of failure during the potentially traumatic experience (here,
combat; see also Danieli, 1985). This study lends credibility to the relevance of these factors
for children of traumatized parents in general. Like Holocaust survivors, other traumatized individuals who are or become parents often exhibit overprotectiveness, emotional unavailability, reduced stress tolerance, and avoidance of traumatic issues, among other characteristics
that affect parenting behaviors and their results.

The findings described in this chapter have also indicated some of the protective factors
relevant to previous parental trauma. As has been suggested elsewhere, there is some evidence
that the parent's resolution of his or her traumatic experience or successful action taken during a traumatic experience may serve to minimize traumatic response (see Nader & Pynoos,
1993; Pynoos & Nader, 1988). Moreover, children whose parents have not been traumatized
have sometimes appeared to be less vulnerable than other children.

Conclusions

These two clinical studies have provided the opportunity for a preliminary examination
of the effects of parents' traumatic experience upon children. The results of these two studies
strongly suggest that children whose parent(s) are traumatized by violence or disaster may, in
fact, be more likely to be subsequently traumatized and are at risk of experiencing increased
symptoms following a traumatic event. Additional study is needed to confirm these results
and to examine their meaning. Danieli (1993) proposed that Holocaust-survivor parents who
teach their children, out of love, to be prepared for the traumas that they themselves have endured may inadvertently be teaching them that these traumas are to be expected in their lives
and may thus contribute to their vulnerability to a repetition of trauma. From transgenerational transmission described in the oral and written traditions of several cultures, it appears
that experiences that occur with intensity—positive or negative—are imprinted on the parent
or family in such a way that they emerge in subsequent generations. The separate studies of
Suomi, Calhoun, and Ward described earlier suggest that this imprint occurs and is transmitted genetically or biochemically. It is likely that loving and other verbal prescriptions, learned
behaviors, learned ideas, genetic or biochemical factors, and parenting styles contribute to
this phenomenon. The increased vulnerability to traumatization found in the two studies reported in this chapter suggests the advisability of intervention following traumatic exposure
to address symptoms and special issues with children whose parents have been previously
traumatized.

ACKNOWLEDGEMENTS: The author would like to thank the former UCLA Trauma, Violence, and
Sudden Bereavement Program for the opportunity to work with these children and parents, and
to thank Drs. Robert Pynoos, Margaret Stuber, Spencer Eth, Bill Arroyo, and Arturo Torres for

their collaboration. In addition, genuine appreciation is extended to Mary Avery of the San Diego District Attorney's office, to Mary Armsworth, and to Yael Danieli for the inspiration and opportunity to examine this issue.

REFERENCES

Armsworth, M. N. (1993, October 25). *Examining the intergenerational effects of trauma from multiple perspectives.* Paper presented at a symposium of the Annual meeting of the International Society for Traumatic Stress Studies, San Antonio, Texas.

Barocas, H., & Barocas, C. (1980). Wounds of the fathers: The next generation of Holocaust victims. *International Review of Psychoanalysis, 5,* 331–341.

Bloch, D., Silber, E., & Perry, S. (1956). Some factors in the emotional reaction of children to disaster. *American Journal of Psychiatry, 113,* 416–422.

Bowlby, J. (1969/1982). *Attachment.* New York: Basic Books.

Bowlby, J. (1973). *Separation.* New York: Basic Books.

Bowlby, J. (1980). *Loss.* New York: Basic Books.

Campbell, J. (1968). *The hero with a thousand faces* (2nd ed.). Princeton, NJ: Princeton University Press.

Curtis, G. C. (1963). Violence breeds violence—perhaps. *American Journal of Psychiatry, 120,* 386–387.

Dan, E. (1995). *Secondary traumatization in the offspring of Vietnam veterans with posttraumatic stress disorder.* Doctoral dissertation submitted to Fielding Institute, Santa Barbara, California.

Danieli, Y. (1980). Families of survivors of the Nazi Holocaust: Some long- and shot-term effects. In N. Milgram (Ed.), *Psychological stress and adjustment in time of war and peace* (pp. 000–000). Washington, DC: Hemisphere.

Danieli, Y. (1981, March 15–16). Exploring the factors in Jewish identity formation (in children of survivors). In *Consultation on the Psychodynamics of Jewish Identity: Summary of Proceedings* (pp. 22–25). American Jewish Committee and the Central Conference of the American Rabbis.

Danieli, Y. (1985). The treatment and prevention of long-term effects and intergenerational transmission of victimization: A lesson from Holocaust survivors and their children. In C. R. Figley (Ed.), *Trauma and its wake* (pp. 295–313). New York: Brunner/Mazel.

Danieli, Y. (1993, October 25). *Holocaust survivors and their children.* A discussion group on Transgenerational Trauma at the Annual Meeting of the International Society for Traumatic Stress Studies, San Antonio, Texas.

Feinstein, D., & Krippner, S. (1988). *Personal mythology.* New York: St. Martin's Press.

Frederick, C., Pynoos, R., and Nader, K. (1992). *Childhood Post-Traumatic Stress Reaction Index* (CPTS-RI), a copyrighted semistructured interview for children with traumatic exposure (available from one of the authors).

Freyberg, J. T. (1980). Difficulties in separation–individuation as experienced by offspring of Nazi Holocaust survivors. *Orthopsychiatry, 50*(1), 87–95.

Grisgam, C. (1988). *The healing emotion.* New York: Simon & Schuster.

Johnson, A. M., & Szurek, S. A. (1952). The genesis of anti-social acting out in children and adults. *Psychoanalytic Quarterly, 21,* 323–343.

Klein, H., & Kogan, I. (1986). Identification processes and denial in the shadow of Nazism. *International Journal of Psycho-Analysis, 67*(1), 45–52.

Ledgerwood, G. (1979). *Lecture on enlightenment.* Costa Mesa, CA: Yoga Center of California.

McFarlane, A. C. (1987). Posttraumatic phenomena in a longitudinal study of children following a natural disaster. *Journal of the American Academy of Child and Adolescent Psychiatry, 26*(5), 764–769.

Motoyama, H. (1992). *Karma and reincarnation.* New York: Avon Books.

Nader, K. (1997). Treating traumatic grief in systems. In C. R. Figley, B. E. Bride, and N. Mazza (eds.), *Death and trauma: The traumatology of grieving* (pp. 159–192). London: Taylor and Francis.

Nader, K. (1984). *Childhood post-traumatic stress disorder (PTSD), parent inventory.* A semi-structured interview about children, for parents of children with traumatic exposure, copyright, 1984, 1992.

Nader, K., & Pynoos, R. (1993). School disaster: Planning and initial interventions. *Journal of Social Behavior and Personality, 8*(5), 299–320.

Nader, K., Pynoos, R., Fairbanks, L., & Frederick, C. (1990). Children's PTSD reactions one year after a sniper attack at their school. *American Journal of Psychiatry, 147,* 1526–1530.

Nahwegahbow, B. (1995). Healer, Nishnawbe Health, Toronto, Canada. Personal communication, May.

Pynoos, R., Frederick, C., Nader, K., Arroyo, W., Eth, S., Nunez, W., Steinberg, A., & Fairbanks, L. (1987). Life threat and posttraumatic stress in school age children, *Archives of General Psychiatry, 44,* 1057–1063.

Pynoos, R. and ... violence: ...

Silber, E., Perry ... ster. *Psychiatry,* 21, 159–168.

Singer, M. (197... cept. *Arch...* ation of the superego lacunae con-

Solkoff, N. (19... of Orthops... of the literature. *American Journal*

Solomon, Z., M... eration Ho... tress disorder among second-gen- *sychiatry,* 145(7), 865–868.

Suomi, S. (199... sentation a... tions to stress in primates. A pre- ference, Alexandria, Virginia, Feb-

ruary 17.

Szurek, S. A. (1... *y,* 5, 1–6.

Ward, L. E. (19... *iiropractor,* 12(9), 4–13.

Ward, L. E. (19... national R... 's muscular dystrophy. *ICA Inter-*

Ward, L. E., W:... practic, 22... ing new frontiers. *Today's Chiro-*

Wasserman, S. ... '9.

Zeanah, C. H., ... ory and re... ent: Insights from attachment the-

or children exposed to community

IX

Infectious and Life-Threatening Diseases

34

AIDS and Its Traumatic Effects on Families

BARBARA H. DRAIMIN, CAROL LEVINE, and LOCKHART McKELVY

Hardly over, perhaps barely begun, the epic of acquired immunodeficiency syndrome (AIDS) involves multigenerational losses and redefinitions of individual, family, and community roles and responsibilities. An AIDS diagnosis dramatically alters the emotional climate of the family system. It creates a profound sense of dislocation in the timing and order of major life events. Years of parenting are compressed into a few, and roles are reversed. A 12-year-old girl changes her mother's diapers. A 65-year-old grandmother takes over the care of the seven children of her three dead daughters. A 17-year-old promises her dying mother that she will take care of her younger brothers and sisters, and not let them be separated.

The personal odyssey of a Brooklyn, New York, grandmother named Ada Setal resembles the stories being played out again and again in the United States and around the world today. Eddie, Ada's son, and Armida, the woman with whom he lived, were both infected with the human immunodeficiency virus (HIV). Their three children were also HIV-infected. When Eddie told his mother this devastating news and asked her to take the children because Armida was too ill to care for them, Ada wavered.

> I came home and thought about how I'd be treated by the church and the community. I thought, "If I take these children, I am going to be isolated, abandoned, left alone. I'm not going to be able to walk out of my house with my head up because there is going to be so much shame around me." I was only 51, but I saw myself as a woman with no future. (Setal, 1993)

Somehow fortified by her religious faith, she nonetheless took the children and struggled through a succession of deaths, becoming a community activist for children and families with AIDS in the process.

AIDS affected three generations in Ada Setal's family—her son and his girlfriend, their children, and herself. Yet her story is unusual only in that all three of her grandchildren were HIV-infected. Typically, most of the children born to an HIV-infected mother are not themselves

BARBARA H. DRAIMIN and LOCKHART McKELVY • The Family Center, 66 Reade Street, New York, New York 10007.   CAROL LEVINE • Families and Health Care Project, United Hospital Fund, 350 Fifth Avenue, New York, New York 10018.

International Handbook of Multigenerational Legacies of Trauma, edited by Yael Danieli. Plenum Press, New York, 1998.

infected. In the United States, the transmission rate of HIV from infected mother to fetus has been about 20–25%.

The generation most at risk for contracting HIV is young adults. As they grow ill and die, they leave the older and the younger generations to cope alone. Coping takes many forms. Once-independent young adults go home to die in their parent's care. Grandparents and extended families take in orphaned children. The oldest child becomes the parental figure and primary caregiver. Children enter foster care or are placed for adoption. Siblings are separated to make it more likely that relatives will be able to house them. Older children live on their own, often in precarious situations without adult supervision. Whatever the individual solutions, they reflect a world out of balance, a profound upheaval in the natural order that takes as a given that grandparents ought not to have to assume parenting responsibilities for two consecutive generations, and that parents should not have to bury their children.

This chapter describes the American experience, since that is the one the authors know intimately. Moreover, it focuses on families in which parents of children or adolescents have AIDS, and not on multigenerational traumas in families with gay men (see Lipmann, James, & Frierson, 1993; Macklin, 1989; Walker, 1991). Some excellent studies of the impact on families in other countries have been published (Brown & Sittitrai, 1995; Imrie & Coombes, 1995; Hunter, 1994). Most of these studies so far focus mainly on the service needs of affected communities, families, and children, and on the economic and structural dislocation of family life. There is little analysis yet on the impact of multigenerational legacies of AIDS-related trauma in other societies.

THE DEMOGRAPHICS OF AIDS

The World Health Organization (WHO) estimates that since the beginning of the pandemic, 18 million adults and 1.5 million children have been infected with HIV, and that over 4.5 million have developed AIDS. By the end of the century, WHO estimates that between 30 and 40 million people will have been infected with HIV. Although sub-Saharan Africa has been the hardest hit area, HIV is spreading rapidly in Asia. The toll in countries such as India and Thailand is particularly severe. The gender ratio has been equal in Africa, but in Asia, trends indicate more new infections among women than men. Everywhere in the world, the generation hardest hit has been young adults (World Health Organization, 1995).

AIDS is not a single epidemic, but a series of epidemics that began in different places around the world at different times and with different trajectories. Even within a single country, the path of HIV has varied. In the United States, for example, the epidemic in the West Coast city of San Francisco, California, has affected primarily gay men, while on the East Coast in Newark, New Jersey, male and female drug users and their sexual partners have predominated. A city as complex as New York has several epidemics, each with a distinctive profile.

How did this medical and social disaster happen so rapidly? The epidemic began slowly, almost imperceptibly. In the United States, the signal event was the report of the Centers for Disease Control and Prevention (CDC) in June 1981, that in Los Angeles, extremely rare cases of *Pneumocystis carinii* pneumonia (PCP) had been diagnosed in five previously healthy homosexual men (CDC, 1981a). This was not, of course, the actual beginning. One month later, the CDC reported that since January 1979, 26 homosexual men in New York City and California had been diagnosed with Kaposi's sarcoma, a rare cancer. Many had also been diagnosed with PCP and other viral diseases; eight had died (CDC, 1981b). In August 1981, the

CDC reported that five heterosexuals, including one woman, had been diagnosed with similar symptoms of severe immune deficiency now called AIDS (CDC, 1986).

In the nearly 15 years since AIDS was first identified, it has become endemic in the United States, particularly in poor communities of color. AIDS is now the leading cause of death for all Americans aged 25–44 and the leading cause of death among women aged 15–44 in New York and New Jersey (CDC, 1995a). In 1994, HIV infection became the fourth leading cause of years of potential life lost before age 65 (CDC, 1996). Among people in the United States infected with HIV between 1987 and 1991, one of four was under the age of 22 (Rosenberg, Biggar, & Goedert, 1994).

As of October 31, 1995, more than 500,000 AIDS cases had been reported to the CDC. More than half of these individuals have died (CDC, 1995b). The number of HIV-infected people who have not yet reached a diagnosis of AIDS in the United States is generally estimated at 750,000 to 1.5 million. In 1992, the CDC noted: "The recognition of a disease and its emergence as a leading cause of death within the same decade is without precedent" (CDC, 1992).

HIV infection is spreading most rapidly among women and adolescents. In 1994, women made up 18% of the total number of adult AIDS cases, nearly threefold more than the proportion of cases among women reported in 1985 (CDC, 1995a). These women—75% of them African American or Latina—are typically mothers and the primary caregivers for their children. An increasing percentage of young people are becoming infected through sexual activity. Between 1992 and 1993, the largest increases in AIDS case reporting occurred among persons aged 13–19 years and 20–24 years, heterosexual transmission accounted for 22% of the transmission in the younger group and 18% in the older group (CDC, 1994). Children born with HIV infection are now living into their teen years; many have become sexually active, and some have become pregnant. The National Institutes of Health study that showed a reduced rate of maternal–child HIV transmission in pregnant women taking zidovudine (AZT), for example, enrolled a 15-year-old girl as its youngest participant (Gelber & Kiselev, 1994).

Throughout the world, mothers are the primary caregivers of their children. Although fathers' deaths are certainly traumatic and may bring on family crises, it is mothers' deaths that most directly affect children's caregiving. In the United States, by the year 2000, an estimated 82,000–125,000 children and adolescents in the United States will have lost their mothers to AIDS (Michaels & Levine, 1992). The vast majority of these youngsters are not HIV-infected but are at serious risk for a range of emotional and behavioral problems. Their substitute caregivers are also under enormous emotional and financial stress. Michaels and Levine also estimate that the number of young adults (18 years and older) in the United States whose mother will die of HIV/AIDS–related causes will reach 35,100 by 1995 and 64,000 through the year 2000. The number of children worldwide who will have been orphaned by HIV/AIDS by the end of the decade has been estimated to be between 5 and 15.6 million (Chin, 1994; Mann & Tarantola, 1996; U.S. Agency for International Development, n.d.). The size of the range can be attributed to variations in the parameters and assumptions used in the models, as well as the different definitions used for orphan (children without mothers, or children who have lost either or both parents).

LITERATURE REVIEW

Before 1992, there were only a few references in the burgeoning AIDS literature to children surviving the death of a parent and their new caregivers. Most of the literature about AIDS and children focused on pediatric AIDS (Anderson, 1986, 1990; Pizzo & Wilfert, 1991).

Among the earliest references to affected, rather than infected, children are Walker's (1987) discussion of AIDS and family therapy, and Demb's (1989) clinical vignette about adolescent survivors of parents with AIDS. Macklin's (1989) was among the first collections to examine AIDS from a family perspective.

Several publications began to raise awareness of the problems of affected children and their new caregivers in 1992. Grosz and Hopkins (1992) described family circumstances affecting caregivers and siblings. Draimin, Hudis, and Segura (1992) outlined the mental health problems of well adolescents in families with AIDS. Michaels and Levine (1992) offered the first estimates of the numbers of children who would be left motherless in the United States because of AIDS.

These initial works were followed by Levine (1993), a collection of essays, including personal stories, that presented some innovative programs in New York City and analyzed some of the legal issues facing new caregivers. Levine and Stein (1994) focused on policy changes and services needed to assist orphaned children and their new caregivers. Dane and Levine (1994) explored the psychological and social aspects of bereavement in AIDS and described some programs for grieving children. Bauman and Wiener (1994) edited a series of papers on priorities in psychosocial research on pediatric HIV infection that includes several essays on uninfected children. Geballe, Gruendel, and Andiman (1995) is a collection of essays from medical, legal, psychosocial, and other perspectives. It also contains children's drawings. Boyd-Franklin, Steiner, and Boland (1995) deal with psychosocial and therapeutic issues, mostly focused on children with pediatric HIV infection.

Beyond these books, the number of articles on specific topics is growing. These include disclosure of a parent's or child's HIV status (Lipson, 1994), creating a legacy of memories through videotapes and other techniques (Taylor-Brown & Wiener, 1993), legal options (Herb, 1993; Pinott, 1993), bereavement (Boyd-Franklin, Drelich, & Schwolsky-Fitch, 1995; Mc-Kelvy, 1995), and psychotherapeutic techniques (McKelvy, 1995).

Recent publications in trauma theory as it relates to children have added to the understanding of the impact of an AIDS diagnosis. In particular, *Children in Danger* (Garbarino, Dubruow, Kostleny, & Pardo, 1992) describes children living in communities of poverty and violence, and examines the value of mental health treatment to help children resolve traumatic experiences. In writing about the psychological effects of specific traumas, Kerr (1991) identifies the long-term impact of unresolved feelings.

A book that examined parenting by women who lost their own mothers at young ages hints at the multigenerational impact of losing a parent to AIDS. Edelman (1995) describes mothers who are afraid they lack adequate parenting skills and, even more tragically, that they will not live past the age of their own mother's death. The author's sample consisted primarily of white, middle-class women who generally did not face the multitude of other stressors that saturate the lives of young people who have lost parents to AIDS. These factors almost surely complicate the losses she described.

Other literature has helped explain how emotions are transmitted in families. Most of this research has its roots in Freud's understanding of the unconscious and mental health as a result of early family relationships (Kerr, 1991). Bowen (1978) and many others have written about the now commonly held belief that families are emotional systems.

The literature to date reflects consensus that (1) services to meet the needs of all the involved generations should be improved and expanded; (2) research data, particularly long-term studies of children and new caregivers, is scarce; (3) the period before the parent's death should be emphasized in terms of making custody plans; and (4) relatively little attention is being paid to the problems faced by new caregivers.

WHO ARE THE FAMILIES WITH AIDS?

The children who struggle with AIDS in their families are typically living with their mothers in single-parent homes. Poverty, loss of community services, overcrowding in substandard housing, frequent displacement due to fire or criminal activity, and substance abuse are all characteristics of what Fullilove and Fullilove (1993) describe as the "seeding of the epidemic." The deterioration in communities erodes families' capacity to provide the emotional and financial support necessary for healthy functioning. Many children are raised in a perpetual shadow of scarcity. One Family Center client from New York City said, "I hate the end of every month, when we have no food." With poverty comes a reliance on subsidies and public housing, often in high-crime areas where random violence is common. Every family member faces the risk of stray bullets, robberies, and assault on a daily basis.

A more subtle erosion of a family's sense of self-esteem is caused by society's continued racial discrimination, especially within African American and Latino communities. Certain cultures, such as the Haitian immigrant population, are especially scapegoated because of their association with a high rate of HIV infection.

In New York City, 60% of the women with AIDS were exposed to HIV by sharing needles while using injection drugs (New York City Department of Health, 1995). Many of the absent fathers are also drug users, often with a history of incarceration. Because drug-using parents are preoccupied with their substance of choice, they have little time or patience for the demands of parenting. As a result, their children are at greater risk for exposure to child abuse and neglect (Zuckerman, 1994). Children who have been born to drug-using mothers are also at risk for low birth weight, being born addicted, developmental delays, and HIV, making them especially poorly equipped to confront the multiple stressors within the family. In addition, family members with a history of drug use or violence have generally learned how to avoid painful truths. The resulting habits of secrecy and isolation, coupled with poor communication skills, are greatly magnified by HIV.

Drug use, especially crack cocaine, has accelerated the phenomenon of "skip-generation parenting." Grandmothers have taken over when their own children have abdicated parenting responsibilities, or when they have chosen to remove their grandchildren from a dangerous environment. This phenomenon has particularly affected African American communities. As of 1990, 12% of black children in the United States were living with grandparents, compared to 5.7% of Hispanic children and 3.6% of white children (U.S. Bureau of the Census, 1991). The percentage of black children living with grandparents in some urban areas is significantly higher, with estimates ranging from 20% in a Head Start population in Oakland, California, to 30–70% in parts of Detroit, Michigan, and New York City (Minkler & Roe, 1993).

AIDS has created further pressures for alternative caregiving arrangements for children. Although data are scarce, it appears that when a mother dies of AIDS, children most often go to live—at least at first—with a grandmother or aunt. Sometimes the grandmother or aunt has already been taking care of the children. In a pilot study examining the outcome in 43 cases that were closed shortly after the mother's death, the New York City Division of AIDS Services found that 58% of the children went to live with grandmothers or aunts (Levine, Draimin, Stein, & Gamble, 1994).

Efforts to make permanent plans for children in families with AIDS are relatively recent. In Chicago, Illinois, 21 of 72 HIV-infected mothers who were interviewed indicated that they would like their mothers to take the children. Nine women designated their sisters, 20 were unable to identify anyone, and the remainder designated other relatives (LSC and Associates, 1993). It is unknown how many of these plans will actually work out, however, especially since only 14 mothers had made legal arrangements for their chosen caregiver. Nor do we fully understand the factors that influence placement choices. For example, one study looking at infants born to HIV-infected women in six regions of the United States concluded that maternal drug use may be the most important factor in determining whether a child lives with a biological parent. In all locations and for all racial and ethnic groups, newborns whose mothers used intravenous drugs were more likely to be placed with someone other than their mother (Caldwell *et al.,* 1992).

WHY AIDS IS UNIQUE

While any life-threatening illness has profound consequences to every generation that is affected, many aspects of AIDS distinguish it from other serious illnesses and make it even more difficult for the affected children, parents, and grandparents. In particular, the populations affected, the social stigma, the lack of a surviving parent, the transmissibility to children, and the number of losses experienced by affected families provide special challenges to every generation.

The populations that are most likely to have AIDS are homosexual men, drug users, and women and children of color. Discrimination against these populations in housing, health care, and insurance has been extensively documented. Moreover, there comes a time when the physical impact of HIV makes anonymity almost impossible. When the disease becomes physically apparent, so does a history of behaviors. Disclosing illness to family members may occur at the same time that drug-using behavior or sexual orientation is disclosed, adding layers of complexity to the trauma that is involved.

When other serious illnesses strike, there is usually a surviving parent who can take full responsibility for the care of the children. With AIDS, this is seldom the case. The other parent may be deceased, incarcerated, or simply absent; other surviving family members must step forward. At the same time that these relatives suffer the loss of a sibling or child, they must try to help surviving children deal with their own despair and loss.

The secrecy, stigma, and isolation that characterize AIDS are far greater than the stigma associated with other illnesses. Seldom is the same degree of moral responsibility attached to the lung cancer patient who smoked or the overweight executive who had a heart attack. In these instances, we extend caring and curing to all, recognizing that disease can, and often does, happen to anyone. By contrast, AIDS is more likely to be treated as a social and cultural curse, and a moral or religious punishment than as a medical condition.

Even within families, there can be an attempt to blame and ostracize an individual for "bringing this horrible disease into our home." Because of its association with unsafe drug use and sexual behavior, myths and misunderstandings abound. Truth is often hidden or denied. The moral judgments of family members may render any discussion of the illness and its origins completely taboo. Children of parents with AIDS may have fears of contagion that they are too embarrassed to share with anyone. The stigma is intensified by societal reaction. In a recent newscast, for example, a New York City television station publicized the plight of AIDS orphans while describing their parents as "junkies," reflecting the endemic failure to view drug addiction as a medical problem (WWOR, Channel 9 News, New York City, August 17, 1995). The self-esteem, pride, and self-image of the family are therefore affected by both the intrafamily and external oppression of those who are infected.

Another unique aspect of AIDS is that a mother can transmit the causative virus to her baby during pregnancy or delivery. Mothers who have infected their children speak openly about their fear of not living long enough to care for their children; others face the sadness of having to bury them. Their medical choices are complicated by recent research suggesting that identifying HIV-infected pregnant women and treating them with AZT may help reduce the rate of perinatal transmission (Connor et al., 1994). This raises complex and difficult questions about confidentiality, testing, and treatment. The need for intense counseling and education of pregnant mothers is clear. It is especially troubling that legislative efforts to mandate unconsented HIV testing for newborns or pregnant women portray mothers as more concerned about their privacy than about their babies' health. In this dichotomy, mothers are labeled "guilty" because of their HIV status, and their babies are characterized as "innocent."

A final, unique element of HIV is that many of the affected families have already suffered multiple losses. Rarely is a family dealing only with AIDS. In a study by Draimin et al. (1992), the average family with AIDS had experienced four major losses, defined as HIV diagnosis, death, incarceration, or divorce, within the last 2 years. These losses have devastated families and the communities in which they live.

HOW AIDS AFFECTS CHILDREN

Families with AIDS typically face a combination of challenges and traumatic stress whose "psychic scars" are passed on from one generation to the next. For the affected children, trauma comes early and with a vengeance.

In general, parents are largely responsible for the consistency, duration, and intensity of the feelings in the home. Their children absorb information on acceptable ways to express anger, love, and sorrow. Parental attitudes of self-esteem, hopelessness, and powerlessness, as well as the feelings of anxiety and fear associated with an AIDS diagnosis are also passed to the next generation (Halpern, 1990). Even if parents choose not to speak about their HIV status, children will sense danger in the home. Some of these emotional communications are passed between parent and infant nonverbally; later, language becomes another way to transmit emotions between generations.

In order to bond with an adult, infants require warmth, food, and language, either from their mothers or other consistent caregivers (Bowlby, 1973). The security provided by an attachment figure is vital to the child's ability to defend him- or herself against the anxiety caused by separation, discomfort, and unfamiliar surroundings. Unfortunately, mothers who spend the vast majority of their emotional resources simply struggling to survive may not able to provide what an infant needs to feel secure.

An AIDS diagnosis adds its own stressors and anxieties to an already overtaxed emotional family system. The effects of these multiple stressors "potentiate" each other (Rutter, 1979). In other words, the emotional impact of the combination of loss, poverty, drug-using parents, and AIDS in the family is far worse than these stressors experienced separately.

When children discover that a parent has been diagnosed with AIDS, they typically spend enormous amounts of energy defending themselves against the fears and fantasies that are associated with it. Children are afraid of contagion and how they will be viewed by their peers. Denial or desensitization is a common adaptive defense, learned from repeated exposure to guns, acts of violence, and the experience of other deaths in the family. Often children have known other people with HIV and many eventually become numb. When one teenager in a support group was asked if she was worried because her mother was in the hospital, she replied with a shrug, "I'm used to it."

Delinquent behavior is another common response to the disintegration of community structures. Some adolescent boys become particularly aggressive. One young man in psychotherapeutic treatment said, "I feel alive when I fight and I want to hurt people like I have been hurt." The challenges presented by an aggressive teenager are exacerbated by the mother's poor health. At a time when curfews and the obligation to attend school need to be reinforced, parents with AIDS may be too weak to assert their authority. Teenagers begin to identify with their aggressive environment and adapt to a world of violence by "gang banging," playing dangerous, thrill-seeking games, and relinquishing their ideas of a future. As one teen described in therapy, "I'm just grateful each New Year's Day to be alive." Young men and women who feel they lack a future may avoid long-term attachments, drop out of school, or refuse to plan ahead in any way. Their lives become governed by impulse, which often leads to sexual or drug-using behavior that puts them at high risk for contracting HIV. They are likely to pass on a "live fast, die hard" legacy to their own children.

Not every young person has the same reaction to living with a parent with AIDS. Some may respond by intensifying their attachment or becoming emotionally enmeshed to the point of sharing medical symptoms with ill parents. For example, some young girls who witness their mother's slow weight loss will lose their appetites. A teenage boy who lived alone with his mother was twice hospitalized at the same time that his mother was being treated for opportunistic infections. After many tests, the young man's "heart problems" proved inconclusive; however, his neurotic attachment to his mother was evident.

In a reversal of roles, young people may also manage their anxiety by caring for a parent. In one case, a teenage girl repressed her own fears and focused solely on the needs of her ailing mother, refusing all forms of outside help, including home and hospice care. Caretaking was a lifelong survival tool for this teenager, a common adaptation in drug-using families. Unfortunately, her caretaking did not flow from a fully realized sense of self, but instead from a "false self," which Winnicott (1990) describes as a seemingly responsible and responsive cover for an impoverished inner self. Sadly, the false self will not support the emotional demands of adulthood. As parents, "parentified" teens are at high risk for depression, experience intense feelings of longing and emptiness, and risk passing on to their offspring a tradition of excessive sacrifice.

In many cases, the fear, denial, and stigma associated with HIV may shroud the family in silence, preventing children from expressing their anxieties. One of the most traumatic experiences for both parents and children can be the feeling of total helplessness in the face of obvious physical or mental deterioration. Processing this type of trauma and anticipatory grief depends on communication, but many families overwhelmed with stress are not accustomed to analyzing and articulating emotions. Others view the expressions of feelings as futile or as a sign of weakness. Whatever the reason, the trauma of an impending parental death is intensified if the ideas and feelings that surround it remain family secrets.

Without therapeutic intervention, children may live with the unresolved effects of trauma for the duration of their lives. Kerr (1991, p. 293) notes, "Trauma does not ordinarily get better by itself. It burrows down further and further under the child's coping and defensive strategies." Bereaved young people who attempt to master their feelings either by acting out or by "parenting" their own parents ultimately pass along the experience of trauma to their children. Without a supportive extended family, social network, or a mental health professional, bereaved children who become parents will taint the emotional climate of their new families with a legacy of unresolved feelings about their own parent's death from AIDS.

HOW AIDS AFFECTS FAMILY CAREGIVERS

The role reversals that accompany the devastating course of illness are traumatic, but they are also adaptive. Faced with enormous barriers, many, perhaps most, families find some way to survive, at least in the short term. Until we have long-term research, however, we cannot say what may be the costs of coping on the family caregivers and on the children they try to raise.

The African American and Latino families that make up the vast majority of families affected by AIDS in the United States have much experience in finding their own solutions to caring for kin. "Informal adoption"—raising a child as one's own without any legal sanction—has long served as a traditional adaptation to a parent's economic or personal inability to nurture and support a child. Among the strengths of black families identified by Hill (1977) are "strong kinship bonds" and "adaptability of family roles." Similarly, Latino families practice informal adoption called *hijos de crianza;* typically children have *compadres* and *comadres* (godparents) who accept at birth responsibility for their care should the parents be unable to do so (Garcia-Preto, 1982).

However, AIDS—compounded with other contemporary social ills—is placing extraordinary pressures on these informal systems. Families must cope not only with the disease and death of one member, but of several. The stigmatized nature of the disease often isolates them from the few community resources that might be available. If drugs are involved, the older generation may also suffer the guilt of a perceived failure to raise their children properly and the pain of witnessing their own offspring mistreating the beloved next generation. At the same time, they may be overly involved with their adult children, enabling their dysfunctional behavior by giving them money and housing because they are unfamiliar with the various models of drug treatment—such as "tough love," narcotics anonymous, treatment communities, and so on—that may be more helpful (Walker, 1995).

In addition, family members today are often more isolated geographically from each other. The informal adoption of a Puerto Rican child whose parents are dead may mean that he or she is sent from the mainland to Puerto Rico, where he or she faces not only the aftereffects of loss but also of uprooting and adjusting to the differences between the mainland and the island culture.

Women have traditionally taken on the role of family caregiving. Many of the grandmothers and aunts who take over the care of children whose mothers died of AIDS have additional responsibilities caring for children, spouses, partners, elderly parents, and other relatives. Two general outcomes are predictable.

First, some of these women, no matter how willing and devoted, will be unable to continue to bear the escalating burdens of child rearing. Grandparents caring for their grandchildren sacrifice leisure time, health, and financial security. They may become angry, resentful, or emotionally exhausted as they confront the job of raising children who have lost developmental milestones, have poor eating habits, and are difficult to soothe (Minkler & Roe, 1993). Children with HIV have complex needs and require frequent medical appointments, psychotherapy, and special school programs. The final trauma for these grandparents is that they often survive the death of both their children and their grandchildren. In one study of black grandparents, health problems such as diabetes, hypertension, back problems, and low energy were often ignored because the health needs of the children took priority. Some of the grandparents viewed illness and death as their only escape from their burdens (Poe, 1992).

Second, there will be no new generation of grandmothers to take their place. The lost generation of daughters will become a lost generation of grandmothers. For children, this vacuum represents a serious break in family continuity, which is already fragile in many cases. For the child welfare system, the shortage of grandmothers will mean increased pressure on alternatives to family placements, such as foster or congregate care, possibly within a relatively short time, say 5–10 years.

Writing about African American families, Boyd Franklin, Aleman, Jean-Gilles, and Lewis (1995, p. 56) assert:

> The family myth that grandmothers and extended family caretakers are "towers of strength" is absolutely true, but it does not allow the caretakers to protest when their burdens become too great. As a result, help from extended family members, as well as from medical and social service systems, is usually not forthcoming. Too often, no one discovers the degree of burden until a caretaker has become completely overwhelmed and can no longer care for an HIV-infected child.

For parents with AIDS, the loss of their children either from AIDS or to their parents or other relatives is also traumatic. They suffer terrible guilt and the loss of autonomy that comes from the obligation to negotiate with relatives, or with child welfare agencies, for the right to visit their own children. These parents are no longer in charge of the lives of their children and are vulnerable to feeling rejected by their own children and disapproved of by their families. These feelings emerge especially at the beginning of each visit. Visitation is important, but it is difficult for everyone involved. Grandparents want to maintain ties between the parent and child, but after a visit, grandchildren may require days to settle down (Minkler & Roe, 1993).

"Skip-generation parenting" works in another direction as well. The younger generation may also be pressed to take on caregiving responsibilities out of the normal sequence of family life. While there are no data on the extent of the practice, and it is probably not typical, there are many anecdotal reports about teenagers and young adults (from ages 17 to 20) taking over the care of younger brothers and sisters while the parent is ill and after the parent's death. Sometimes these young people become the parent's primary caregiver during the illness, and it is the parent's wish that the oldest child or oldest girl take over the care of the family (Pinott, 1993). This "parentification" of teenagers will have long-term consequences for their own futures as well as for those of their younger siblings (Zayas & Romano, 1994). On the positive side, these adolescents may learn responsibility, effective coping mechanisms, and nurturing skills. However, they may also feel overwhelmed and resentful of having to assume such a caregiving role, especially when their peers are in school, at work, or simply having fun.

A possible service model for orphaned adolescents is shared foster family care. Traditionally, this option places both parent and child in a foster home; young mothers take full responsibility for their children but are offered support and guidance from the foster parents (Barth, 1994). Adolescents who become "parents" to their siblings could benefit from similar support.,

However, there are legal implications to arrangements in which an adolescent is the primary caregiver. For example, a medical provider may be reluctant to allow a teenager to consent to elective surgery for a younger sibling. If the arrangement comes to the attention of a lawyer, it may be possible for an older person to be named as coguardian. Assessing the stability and security of these new family configurations and finding ways to maintain viable households, while still allowing the young person in charge access to educational and career opportunities, is a formidable challenge.

The generational impact does not end with those already born. The continued spread of infection means teenagers or young adults will face the same excruciating dilemmas about custody of their babies faced by older cohorts of women, in some cases, their own relatives. The procedures, still new and exploratory, that now guide women toward permanency planning will have to be refined to address adolescent development and to deal with the reality of diminished family resources.

BREAKING THE LINK

How does one deal with loss after loss? How do the grandparent, parent, and child integrate these losses into their view of themselves and their world? How do they maintain hope and avoid despair? What happens to a family that has faced two or three generations of AIDS?

The cumulative effect of the generational losses, added to the losses from drugs and violence, devastates the social, cultural, and economic life of a community. Productive, or potentially productive, young adults cannot contribute to their families' and communities' income and welfare. More intangibly, the continuous psychic assault of deaths upon deaths in the repressive atmosphere of stigma and secrecy inhibits community mourning, healing, and growth.

Yet a reservoir of spiritual strength and resiliency still exists among individuals, families, and communities. Many grandparents have strong connections to the church, and their faith may bring some meaning to the random and seemingly endless tragedies that permeate their lives (Levine & Gamble, 1995). In some families, HIV has, ironically, been a source of positive change. Although no parent could wish HIV to be the catalyst for putting lives in order, many admit that it has forced them to become more responsible in their personal relationships, to remain drug free, and to devote quality time with their children. The Herculean efforts of these parents may help their children break out of the cycle of drug use, poverty, and AIDS.

In the face of enormously challenging conditions, some children in families with AIDS emerge relatively unscarred. Research has identified some of the characteristics that foster resilience. Rutter (1972) found that they had generally bonded with at least one parent or an extended family member. Typically, the most resilient children are girls who are intelligent and are able to respond to a challenging environment. These children have also been able to take advantage of available resources, such as schools, extended families, and religious institutions. Age is also an important factor: Children younger than 11 are three times more vulnerable to the long-term effects of trauma than older children (Davidson & Smith, 1990).

Garbarino et al. (1992) also note that self-esteem, confidence, and a good-natured disposition contribute to resilience, whereas Bowen (1978) sees the resilient child as the one who "differentiates" emotionally from the family system. Bowen has observed that resilient children are generally not the focus of the attacks or emotional brutality that occur within families with limited emotional resources. Combined with the brilliant adaptive responses of children in general, an arsenal to fight the traumatic effects of AIDS exists for some young people. The challenge is to find ways to enlarge it.

All members of a family affected by AIDS are likely to benefit from psychotherapeutic treatment. With proper support, families can learn communication skills that allow them to speak more openly and to grapple with the difficult topics of sex, drug use, disease, and death. Referrals to appropriate community resources may also provide families access to advocacy, entitlements, and legal and housing support.

A number of model programs have emerged to address the psychosocial needs of children and families infected, or affected, by AIDS. In New York City, Beth Israel Medical Center and the Special Needs Clinic at Columbia–Presbyterian Medical Center offer a full range of psychiatric services to all members of an affected family. At The Family Center, a freestanding service and research facility, a clinical social worker, an attorney, a nurse, a housing expert, and other family specialists work in the home to link families to health care systems and to create a custody plan for the children. Other innovative programs include the Children's Evaluation and Rehabilitation Center at the Rose Kennedy Center and the Community Consultation Center at Henry Street Settlement, which provide a full complement of counseling to families with AIDS, with a special focus on children.

Using a range of techniques—including multifamily groups that involve several generations, children's therapy groups, art therapy, reaction, and home-based care—each of these programs offer a helping hand that may be critical to survival. By tapping into the hidden strengths of most families and helping them to deal with the reality of illness and make viable plans for the future, their efforts may at least partially offset the multigenerational effects of the trauma of AIDS.

Model programs have also been developed in other parts of the world (WHO/UNICEF, 1994). The focus of many programs has been on strengthening the capacity of families and communities to provide for children and to support the caregivers who take over after the parent's death. Some of the services provided include medical care, housing, food, skills training, and education (payment of school fees is a particular problem in parts of Africa). Although the extended family as an institution has great resilience, it is being severely tested by extreme poverty, poor health of family members, and increased burdens of care. A review of the impact of AIDS on the urban Ugandan family, for example, found that AIDS disrupts family life in both material and intangible ways. Limits on a family's mobility—the freedom to take advantage of economic opportunities—because of caregiving burdens is one long-lasting effect (McGrath, Ankrah, Schumann, Nkrumba, & Lubeza, 1993). In Thailand, children, particularly daughters, are the traditional means of supporting parents in old age. AIDS is changing the roles.

> In accepting responsibility for their grandchildren from their deceased sons or daughters, grandparents will be facing increased family support costs at the same time they lose their traditional means of economic support. Given the advanced age of many elderly couples, the likely outcome is . . . that the pressures on young orphaned children to work will be immense. (Brown & Sittitrai, 1995, p. 145)

Despite the real differences in culture, resources, and experience with disease between the United States and other areas affected by the global epidemic, at the most basic human level, there are also strong similarities. Parents grieve the deaths of children; grandmothers take on the care of their grandchildren; children's lives are irrevocably altered by a parent's death. There is much to share, and much to learn from each other, even as we pursue different strategies to heal the wounds.

REFERENCES

Anderson, G..R. (1986). *Children and AIDS: The challenge for child welfare.* Washington, DC: Child Welfare League of America.

Anderson, G. R. (Ed.). (1990). *Courage to care: Responding to the crisis of children with AIDS.* Washington, DC: Child Welfare League of America.

Barth, R. (1994). Shared foster care. *The Source, 4*(11), 10–12.

Bauman, L., & Weiner, L. (Eds.). (1994). Priorities in psychosocial research in pediatric HIV infection. *Journal of Development and Behavioral Problems, 15*(3), S1–S78. Special supplement.

Bowen, M. (1978). *Family therapy in clinical practice.* New York: Aronson.

Bowlby, J. (1973). *Separation anxiety and anger.* Vol. 2 in J. Bowlby, series *Attachment and Loss.* New York: Basic Books.

Boyd-Franklin N., Drelich E., & Schwolsky-Fitch, E. (1995). Death and dying/bereavement and mourning. In N. Boyd-Franklin, G. L. Steiner, & M. G. Boland (Eds.), *Children, families, and HIV/AIDS: Psychosocial and therapeutic issues* (pp. 179–195). New York: Guilford.

Boyd-Franklin, N. Alemán, J., Jean-Gilles, M., & Lewis, S. (1995). Cultural sensitivity and competence. In N. Boyd-Franklin, G. L. Steiner, & M. G. Boland (Eds.) *Children, families, and HIV/AIDS: Psychosocial and therapeutic issues* (pp. 53–77). New York: Guilford.

Brown, T., & Sittitrai, W. (Eds.). (1995). *The impact of HIV on children in Thailand*. Bangkok: Thai Red Cross Program on AIDS.

Caldwell, M. B., *et al.* and the Pediatric Spectrum of Disease Clinical Consortium. (1992). Biologic, foster, and adoptive parents: Caregivers of children exposed perinatally to human immunodeficiency virus in the United States. *Pediatrics, 90,* 603–607.

Centers for Disease Control. (1981a). Pneumocystis pneumonia—Los Angeles. *Morbidity and Mortality Weekly Report, 30,* 250–252.

Centers for Disease Control. (1981b). Kaposi's sarcoma and Pneumocystis pneumonia among homosexual men—New York City and California. *Morbidity and Mortality Weekly Report, 30,* 305–307.

Centers for Disease Control and Prevention. (1986). *Reports on AIDS published in the* Morbidity and Mortality Weekly Report, *June 1981 through February 1986* (pp. 2–4). Springfield, VA: National Technical Information Service.

Centers for Disease Control and Prevention. (1992). Mortality patterns—United States, 1989. *Morbidity and Mortality Weekly Report, 41,* 121–125.

Centers for Disease Control and Prevention. (1994). Update: Impact of the expanded AIDS surveillance case definition for adolescents and adults on case reporting—United States, 1993. *Morbidity and Mortality Weekly Report, 43,* 160–161, 167–170.

Centers for Disease Control and Prevention. (1995a). Update: Acquired immunodeficiency syndrome—United States, 1994. *Morbidity and Mortality Weekly Report, 44,* 64–67.

Centers for Disease Control and Prevention. (1995b). First 500,000 AIDS cases—United States, 1995. *Morbidity and Mortality Weekly Report, 44,* 849–853.

Centers for Disease Control and Prevention. (1996). Update: Mortality attributable to HIV infection among persons aged 25–44 years—United States, 1994. *Morbidity and Mortality Weekly Report, 45,* 121–125.

Chin, J. (1994). The growing impact of the HIV/AIDS pandemic in children born to HIV-infected women. *Clinics in Perinatology, 21*(1), 1–114.

Connor, E. M., Sperling, R. S., Gelber, R., *et al.* (1994). Reduction of maternal–infant transmission of human immunodeficiency virus type 1 with zidovudine treatment. *New England Journal of Medicine, 331*(18), 1173–1180.

Dane, B. O., & Levine, C. (Eds.). (1994). *AIDS and the new orphans: Coping with death*. Westport, CT: Greenwood Publishing Group.

Demb, J. (1989). Clinical vignette: Adolescent "survivors" of parents with AIDS. *Family Systems Medicine, 7,* 339–343.

Davidson, J., & Smith, R. (1990). Traumatic experiences in psychiatric outpatients. In J. Garbarino, N. Dubruow, K. Kostleny, & C. Pardo (Eds.), *Children in danger: Coping with the consequences of community violence* (pp. 459–475). San Francisco: Jossey-Bass.

Draimin, B., Hudis, J., & Segura, J. (1992). The mental health needs of well adolescents in families with AIDS. *New York City Human Resources Administration Division of AIDS Services,* 31–35.

Edelman, H. (1995). *Motherless daughters: The legacy of loss*. Reading, MA: Addison-Wesley.

Fullilove, M. T., & Fullilove, R. E., III (1993). Understanding sexual behaviors and drug use among African-Americans: A case study of issues for survey research. In D. G. Ostrow & R. C. Kessler (Eds.). *Methodological issues in AIDS behavioral research* (pp. 117–131). New York: Plenum Press.

Garbarino, J., Dubruow, N., Kostleny, K., & Pardo, C. (Eds.). (1992). *Children in danger: Coping with the consequences of community violence*. San Francisco: Jossey-Bass.

Garcia-Preto, N. (1982). Puerto Rican families. In M. McGoldrick, J. K. Pearce, & J. Giordan. (Eds.), *Ethnicity and family therapy* (p. 172). New York: Guilford.

Geballe, S., Gruendel, J., & Andiman, W. (Eds.). (1995). *Forgotten children of the AIDS epidemic*. New Haven, CT: Yale University Press.

Gelber, R. D., & Kiselev, P. (1994). *Executive summary of ACTG 076*. Cambridge, MA: Cambridge Statistical and Data Analysis Center, Pediatric AIDS Clinical Trials Group, Harvard School of Public Health.

Grosz, J., & Hopkins, K. (1992). Family circumstances affecting caregivers and brothers and sisters. In A. C. Crocker, H. J. Cohen, & T. A. Kastner (Eds.), *HIV infection and developmental disabilities: A resource guide for service providers*. Baltimore: Paul H. Brookes.

Halpern, R. (1990). Poverty and early childhood parenting. Toward a framework for intervention. *American Journal of Orthopsychiatry, 60*(1), 6–18.

Herb, A. (1993). The New York State Standby Guardianship Law: A new option for terminally ill patients. In C. Levine (Ed.), *A death in the family: Orphans of the HIV epidemic* (pp. 87–93). New York: United Hospital Fund.

Hill, R. (1977). *Informal adoption among black families.* Washington, DC: National Urban League Research Department.

Hunter, S. (1994). *National assessment of children orphaned by AIDS.* Dar es Salaam Tanzania AIDS Project.

Kerr, M. (1991). Family systems theory and therapy. In A. Gurman & D. Kniskern (Eds.), *Handbook of family therapy* (Vol. 1, pp. 226–263). New York: Brunner/Mazel.

Imrie, J., & Coombes, Y. (1995). *No time to waste: The scale and dimension of the problem of children affected by HIV/AID in the United Kingdom.* Essex, UK: Barnardos.

Levine, C. (Ed.). (1993). *A death in the family: Orphans of the HIV epidemic.* New York: United Hospital Fund.

Levine, C., Draimin, B., Stein, G. L., & Gamble, I. (1994). *In whose care and custody? Placement and policies for children whose parents die of AIDS.* New York: The Orphan Project.

Levine, C., & Gamble, I. (1995). Enhancing children's spirituality: The role of new caregivers. *International Catholic Child Bureau News* special thematic edition on spirituality and AIDS.

Levive, C., & Stein, G. (1994). *Orphants of the HIV epideemic: Unmet needs in six U.S. cities.* New York: Orphan Project.

Lipmann, S. B., James, W. A., & Frierson, R. L. (1993). AIDS and the family: Implications for counseling. *AIDS Care, 5*(1), 71–78.

Lipson, M. (1994). Disclosure of diagnosis to children with human immunodeficiency virus or acquired immunodeficiency syndrome. *Journal of Developmental and Behavioral Pediatrics, 15*(3), 561–565.

LSC and Associates. (1993). *Report on the lives of Chicago women and children living with HIV infection.* Chicago: Author.

Macklin, E. D. (Ed.). (1989). *AIDS and families.* New York: Harrington Park Press.

Mann, J., & Tarantola, D. (Eds.). (1996). *AIDS in the world* (2nd ed.). New York: Oxford University Press.

McGrath, J. W., Ankrah, E. M., Schumann, D. A., Nkrumba, S., & Lubeza, M. (1993). AIDS and the urban family: Its impact in Kampala, Uganda. *AIDS Care 5*(1), 55–69.

McKelvy, L. (1995). Counseling children who have a parent with AIDS or who have lost a parent to AIDS. In W. Odets & M. Shernoff (Eds.), *The second decade of AIDS: A mental health practice handbook* (pp. 137–159). New York: Hatherleigh.

Michaels, D., & Levine, C. (1992). Estimates of the number of motherless youth orphaned by AIDS in the United States. *Journal of the American Medical Association, 268,* 3456–3461.

Minkler, M., & Roe, K. M. (1993). *Grandmothers as caregivers: Raising children of the crack cocaine epidemic.* Newbury Park, CA: Sage Publications.

New York City Department of Health. (1995, April–June). *New York City AIDS Surveillance Report.* New York: Author.

Pinott, M. (1993). Custody and placement: The legal issues. In C. Levine (Ed.), *A death in the family: Orphans of the HIV epidemic* (pp. 75–84). New York: United Hospital Fund.

Pizzo, P., & Wilfert, C. M. (Eds.). (1994). *Pediatric AIDS: The challenge of HIV infection in infants, children, and adolescents* (2nd ed.). Baltimore: Williams & Wilkins.

Poe, L. M. (1992). *Black grandparents as parents.* Berkeley, CA: Lenora Madison Poe.

Rosenberg, P., Biggar, R., & Goedert, J. (1994). Declining age at HIV infection in the United States. *New England Journal of Medicine, 330*(11), 789–790.

Rutter, M. (1972). *Maternal deprivation reassessed.* Middlesex, UK: Penguin.

Rutter, M. (1979). Protective factors in children's response to stress. In. M. Kent & J. Rolf (Eds.), *Primary prevention of psychopathology: Social competence in children* (pp. 49–74). Hanover, NH: University Press of New England.

Setal, A. (1993). A grandmother's view. In C. Levine (Ed.), *A death in the family: Orphans of the HIV epidemic* (pp. 40–46). New York: United Hospital Fund.

Taylor-Brown, S., & Weiner, L. (1993). Making videotapes of HIV-infected women for their children. *Journal of Contemporary Human Services, 74,* 468–480.

Terr, L. (1990). *Too scared to cry: How trauma affects children . . . and ultimately us all.* New York: Basic Books.

U.S. Agency for International Development (n.d. [1997]). *Children on the brink: Strategies to support children isolated by HIV/AIDS.* Washington, DC.

U.S. Bureau of the Census. (1991). *Current population reports: Marital status and living arrangements: March 1990,* series P-20, no. 450. Washington, DC: Government Printing Office.

Walker, G. (1987). AIDS and family therapy. *Family Therapy Today, 2*(2,6), pp. 2 and 6.

Walker, G. (1991). *In the midst of winter.* New York: Norton.

Walker, G., (1995). Family therapy interventions with inner-city families affected by AIDS. In W. Odets & M. Sher-
    noff (Eds.), *The second decade of AIDS: A mental health practice handbook* (pp. 85–114). New York: Hatherleigh.
Winnicott, D. W. (1990). The concept of a health individual. *Home is where we start from.* New York: Basic Books.
World Health Organization (1995). Provisional working estimate of adult HIV seroprevalences. *Weekly Epidemiolog-
    ical Record,* No. 50, December 15: 355–357.
Zayas, L., & Romano, K. (1994). Adolescents and parental death from AIDS. In B. O. Dane & C. Levine (Eds.), *AIDS
    and the new orphans: Coping with death.* Westport, CT: Greenwood Publishing Group.
Zuckerman, B. (1994). Effects on parents and children. In D. Besharov (Ed.), *When drug addicts have children*
    (pp. 49–63). Washington, DC: Child Welfare League of America

35

Daughters of Breast Cancer Patients
Genetic Legacies and Traumas

DAVID K. WELLISCH and ALISA HOFFMAN

INTRODUCTION

One could fairly ask, does a chapter on daughters of breast cancer have a rightful place in a book on multigenerational legacies of trauma—especially given that most of the chapters of this volume deal with the psychosocial sequelae of war, repressive governments, and urban violence? After some soul searching, we decided that the chapter deservedly belongs in the book. The protagonists of this chapter, daughters who are often also sisters, nieces, and granddaughters (or all of the above) of breast cancer patients, bear a genetic legacy of trauma, past visions of suffering, and fears from the past carried forth into the future. Their traumas, fears, and psychic scars do not come from a political regime, but rather from the possible mutation of a gene. This gene, now identified as BRCA-1 and BRCA-2 (for Breast Cancer 1, or Breast Cancer 2) has been localized on the short arm (small part) of chromosome 17 (Futureal *et al.*, 1994). Given this now-identified reality, these women must learn to live with several conflicts. On the one hand, the "perpetrator(s)" of their suffering (who has passed the increased risk and vulnerability for breast cancer on to them) is the same person (or often persons) with whom they empathize, or for whom they mourn and grieve. On the other hand, they have a vulnerability for which there is no definitive medical treatment at present. Thus, they must learn to cope with and adapt to a threat that has been termed the "Damocles Syndrome" (Koocher & O'Malley, 1981). The nature of these daughter's trauma differs from that of victims of political oppression in two distinct ways that greatly complicate their adjustment. First, their aggressor is internal, invisible, and, until fairly recently, mysterious and unknowable. This contrasts with victims of political repression in which the persecutor is external and distinct. Second, although for the victims/survivors of political persecution the trauma reverberates psychologically, the distinct physical threat generally ends. The Holocaust ended, as did World War II and Stalinist Russia. For the survivors of their mother's breast cancer, the physical threat will never end, the potential aggressor will never go away, die, be overthrown, or even be reduced in power or potential risk. In fact, the risk increases with age.

DAVID K. WELLISCH and ALISA HOFFMAN • Department of Psychiatry and Biobehavioral Sciences, Neuropsychiatric Institute, UCLA School of Medicine, Los Angeles, California 90024.

International Handbook of Multigenerational Legacies of Trauma, edited by Yael Danieli. Plenum Press, New York, 1998.

This chapter describes (1) the "real" physical and biological risk for this population and provides an overview of the literature about the psychological risk factors for this population; (2) the UCLA High Risk Clinic, and includes some outcome data on a subset of the population reflecting the impact of the management/intervention program; (3) a spectrum of coping/adjustment difficulties, with six associated case vignettes illustrating some of these difficulties; and (4) emerging perspectives on psychotherapies for these daughters of breast cancer patients to deal with their traumatic legacies and future coping/adaptational challenges.

PHYSICAL/BIOLOGICAL AND PSYCHOLOGIC RISKS

Physical/Biological Risks

The risk of breast cancer can be defined in at least three ways. These include (1) *absolute risk*—which relates to rate of mortality of or from cancer in a general population. Given 1,000 women, absolute risk is how many out of that 1,000 will get breast cancer in their lifetime; (2) *attributable risk*—which relates to how much risk could be prevented by altering factors of public health or mass behavior. Examples would be the public lowering of dietary fat consumption, or women lowering the average age by which they give birth; and (3) *relative risk*—which compares the incidence of breast cancer in a group with a particular risk factor to a population without that risk factor (Love, 1995). For the purposes of this section, particular emphasis will be placed on *relative risk,* the risk factor involved in having at least one first-degree relation (either a mother, daughter, or a sister) who has had breast cancer. Having at least one first-degree relation is a basic requirement for participation in the UCLA High Risk Clinic.

The greatest risk factor in *absolute risk* is age. As age increases, absolute risk also increases substantially. For example, the average risk of a Caucasian American developing breast cancer at age 30 is about 1 in 5,900. By the time the same woman is age 50, the average risk factor is about 1 in 590. By the time the same woman is age 80, the average risk is about 1 in 290 (Stomper, Gelman, Meyer, & Gross, 1990). Similarly, the risks of both developing and dying from breast cancer by decades (of age) increase over the life span. For the average Caucasian American woman, the risk over her entire life span (birth to age 110) is about 3.75%. This, however, is not evenly distributed over the decades. For example, a woman between 35 and 45 years of age has a probability of 0.88% of developing breast cancer and of 0.14% of dying from breast cancer. However, a woman between 65 and 75 years of age has a probability of 3.17% of developing breast cancer and of 0.43% of dying of breast cancer (Seidman, 1985). Ethnic differences in *absolute risk* do exist. A Caucasian woman, by age 75, has about a 8.2% probability of developing breast cancer; a black woman has about 7% probability, and a Japanese American woman has about a 5.4% probability (Berg, 1984). Reasons for these racial differences may refer back to the concept of attributable risk, with such issues as percentage of dietary fat consumed by ethnic groups being possibly causal (Hirohita, Nomura, Hankin, Kolorel, & Lee (1987).

As stated before, the term *relative risk* compares the incidence of breast cancer in a group with a specific factor and a comparable group without the same factor. When *relative risk* is described, the comparison group's risk is set at 1, with the risk group's calculated risk set at a figure above 1. Dupont and Page (1987) studied reproductive factors and risk of breast cancer. Regarding menstrual history, if age at menstruation is prior to 12 years, relative risk is calculated at 1.3. If menopause is after age 55, with greater than 40 menstruating years, relative risk is calculated at 2.0. Regarding pregnancy history, if a first child is born prior to age 20, relative risk is calculated at 0.8 (below 1, a preventive factor for breast cancer). This escalates to a relative risk of 1.4 if a first child is born after age 30. Nulliparity confers a relative risk of 1.6. Sattin *et al.* (1985) calculated relative risks of having a family history of breast cancer. Having any first-degree relative (mother, sister, daughter) confers a *relative risk* of 2.3. However, when the breast cancer was diagnosed in the relative, it confers a differential degree of *relative risk:* If the cancer was premenopausal in the first-degree relative, *relative risk* is calculated at 2.7, whereas if the cancer was postmenopausal, *relative risk* is calculated at 2.5. If a woman has both a mother and sister with breast cancer, *relative risk* is calculated at 13.6. Breast cancer in a second-degree relative (aunt, grandmother) confers a *relative risk* calculated at 1.5. However, these calculations are not straightforward, but form an interactional matrix. For example, there is an interaction for any given woman between her family history of breast cancer and her own history of onset of menses and time of pregnancy and first childbirth. In addition, age at which relative(s) was diagnosed with breast cancer is increasingly seen as important in risk calculation for a woman (see Claus, Risch, & Thompson, 1994).

Psychological Risk/Coping

Limited data exist at present to shed light on how high-risk women function and cope psychologically. In a study comparing high-risk women with a closely matched comparison group, no differences were found on psychological symptoms (Wellisch, Gritz, Schain, Wang, & Sian, 1991a). Kash, Holland, Halper, and Miller (1992) found 27% of high-risk women elevated on reported psychological symptoms to a level justifying psychological intervention. Kash, Holland, Osborn, and Miller (1995) later compared these high-risk women to normals, Hodgkin's survivors, and leukemia survivors, and did not find differences on a global measure of psychological symptoms. The high-risk women were, however, highest of the four groups on reports of depression and especially on feelings of alienation from others. A study of women at high risk for ovarian cancer (a close extension to women at high risk for breast cancer) used a path model to predict psychological distress. Overall, the sample showed moderately high levels of distress. High scores on monitoring were associated with high perceived risk, and elevated levels of intrusive thoughts and psychological distress (Schwartz, Lerman, Miller, Daly, & Masny, 1995).

Another way to assess the psychological status of high-risk women is through use of coping styles. In one study of women undergoing diagnosis of breast masses, (self)-identifiers used significantly less denial than did non(self)-identifiers. Self-identifiers were significantly more likely to have a family history of breast cancer (Styra, Sakinofsky, Mahoney, Colapinto, & Currig, 1993). Wellisch *et al.* (1991a) compared high-risk women to a comparison group on coping styles and found no differences between the two groups. The majority of both groups used high rates of problem-focused and seeking-of-support modes of coping. Neither group was prone to use avoidance or ruminative modes of coping. Josten, Evans, and Love (1985) identified a list of five key emotional states of high-risk relatives. These are applicable to women at high risk for breast cancer. They include (1) fear, (2) denial, (3) guilt, (4) anger, and (5) grief. This is by no means a complete list of key emotional conflicts or problems of this group, but it contains some of the key emotional conflicts presented by this population. Each of these will be personified in the case vignettes to be presented in the coping/adjustment difficulties section.

THE STRUCTURE OF THE UCLA HIGH RISK CLINIC

The UCLA High Risk Clinic was created in July 1993, and has been in existence for 26 months at the time of the writing of this chapter. In that time period, the clinic has enrolled and is following 275 women at high risk for breast cancer. To be enrolled, a woman must have at least one first-degree relative (either a mother or a sister) who has had breast cancer. At present, the clinic meets one-half day per week and sees 4–6 new patients and 2–4 follow-up patients during that clinic day. Demography on 160 of the clinic patients is presented in Table 1. As can be seen by the demographic data, the majority of patients are over age 40, but a significant minority (39%) are below age 40. A significant majority have had a mother with breast cancer, although a sizable minority (21%) have had either a sister, or a sister and a mother with breast cancer. Little, if anything, is known about the traumatic impact on having sister versus a mother with breast cancer. The demographics show an exact 50/50 split between patients who have and have not experienced a familial breast cancer death. Patients are generally seen for follow-up visits 6 months after the baseline visit, with ultrahigh-risk or ultra-anxious patients generally seen at 3-month intervals, four times annually. Most patients are seen twice annually.

Treatment in the High Risk Clinic is performed within a multidisciplinary team structure. The services offered and their providers are listed in Table 2. Patients come to the clinic and are seen by all the care providers in one place. This is an alternative to trying to find and assemble individual care providers such as mammographers, risk counselors, or psychologists in

Table 1. High Risk Clinic Patient Demographics ($N = 160$)

Age of high-risk patients		
20 to 40	39%	$N = 62$
41 to 60	54%	$N = 87$
Above 60	7%	$N = 11$
Ethnicity of high-risk patients		
Caucasian	94%	$N = 151$
Latina	2%	$N = 3$
Asian	4%	$N = 6$
Relationship to relative with breast cancer		
Daughter	78%	$N = 125$
Sister	13%	$N = 21$
Both	9%	$N = 14$
Relative's survival status		
Relative is feeling well	40%	$N = 64$
Relative's cancer is active; she is ill	10%	$N = 16$
Relative has passed away	50%	$N = 80$
Patient sought therapy to deal with breast cancer in relative		
Yes	25%	$N = 40$
No	75%	$N = 120$
Patient's self-rated grief (related to familial breast cancer)		
Minimal to low	44%	$N = 0$
Moderate to high	56%	$N = 90$
Patient's self-rated depression (related to familial breast cancer)		
Minimal to low	82%	$N = 131$
Moderate to high	18%	$N = 29$

Table 2. UCLA High Risk Clinic for First-Degree Relatives
of Breast Cancer Patients

Services offered	Provider
Risk counseling	Medical oncologist
Nutritional counseling	Physician specialist in nutritional medicine
Psychological counseling	Psychologists—2 Ph.D.'s, 1 M.A.
Breast evaluation—Exams, breast self-exam teaching	Nurse practitioner
Mammography	Radiologist—specialist in breast imaging
Exercise instruction	Kinesiologist

several different places. The team is then able to meet as a group and create a coordinated care plan to meet the needs of each patient. This creates elements of the "holding environment" (Winnicott, 1965) to be further discussed in the section on psychotherapy for trauma resolution. The roles of the team are seen as interfacing and facilitating the patient in learning the facts about genetics, risk, nutrition, and exercise, practicing interventions such as breast self-exams, and following treatment guidelines such as annual mammograms. Studies have demonstrated that high levels of breast-focused anxiety in this population can make breast self-examination impossible for high-risk women to perform (Kash *et al.*, 1992). This is a good example of a skill that requires the combined efforts of psychological stress/anxiety reduction (by the psychologist), skills training (by the nurse practitioner), and knowledge implementation (by the medical oncologist).

The initial baseline visit is usually the longest, the most involved, and the most emotionally intense for the new patient. This initial visit includes obtaining a basic medical history (including family medical history) by the nurse practitioner and a basic psychological history/database by the psychologist; initial risk counseling by the medical oncologist, and initial nutritional assessment and counseling by the nutritional physician; and initial exercise assessment and counseling by the exercise specialist. If needed, a mammography can be performed during the initial visit as well. In the first visit, the nurse practitioner begins assessment of and teaching breast self-exam (BSE) skills, first with a breast model and then with the patient on herself. The nurse practitioner also does a careful breast exam on the patient. The psychological testing that is performed in the first visit includes (1) the Center for Epidemiolgic Studies—Depression Scale (CES-D), (2) the Spielberger State–Trait Anxiety Inventory (STAI), and (3) a personal risk estimate of the patient's perceived risk of breast cancer in her lifetime on a scale from 0% to 100%.

The team meets as a group and creates a care plan for each patient based upon all of these contacts and databases.

The psychological structured interview for the first visit generally requires 40–90 minutes to administer. In this interview, the patient's experiences with her most significant relative with breast cancer are fully explored. In addition, her own psychological history, coping and adaptation modes, health management and compliance issues, and current personal stresses are also fully explored and discussed. This is often cathartic for the patient and of great importance to the staff in formulating a care plan.

Follow-up visits are generally less intensive and less involved than the initial visit. Every follow-up visit includes a breast exam by the nurse practitioner, further BSE teaching, a psychological follow-up interview by the psychologist, and the same protocol of psychological testing as at baseline. More risk counseling, nutrition counseling, exercise counseling, and

Table 3. Changes on Psychological Testing from Baseline to First Follow-Up Visit
($N = 77$ Patients)

Variable	Mean score at baseline visit	Mean score at 6-month follow-up visit	P
State anxiety symptoms (STAI-State)[a]	41.00% (SD 25.40)	36.32% (SD 13.01)	.13, ns
Trait anxiety symptoms (STAI-Trait)[b]	36.80% (SD 11.73)	35.55% (SD 11.57)	.20, ns
Depression symptoms (CES-D)[c]	10.51% (SD 11.81)	9.58% (SD 10.48)	.39, ns
Personal risk rating (0–100% estimate of lifelong risk)	54.37% (SD 22.60)	45.30% (SD 23.18)	.001

[a]40th percentile indicates significant symptoms of clinical anxiety state.
[b]40th percentile indicates significant core (chronic) anxiety.
[c]16 is cutting score for significant likelihood of diagnosis of depression.

possibly specialized medical evaluations (if lumps are detected) are often performed. A special, structured follow-up psychological interview probes stresses, impediments to change, successful changes, and unmet needs by the clinic. It also provides an opportunity for further elaboration and processing of important psychological issues noted in the initial interview. A group intervention program has been developed and will be implemented. It is described in the emerging perspectives on psychotherapy section of this chapter.

Data about changes on psychological tests from baseline to follow-up for a subset ($N = 77$) of the High Risk Clinic are shown in Table 3. As Table 3 reflects, state (current) anxiety is reduced between the baseline and follow-up visit. The reduction is to a level below clinically significant anxiety. As expected, trait (characterlogical) anxiety is not reduced between these two visits. The reduction of state anxiety perhaps reflects the relief the patient feels about being contained within the clinic structure that binds her anxiety. In contrast, depression symptoms, which we view as grief states rather than clinical depression, are scarcely reduced between these two visits. Exploring past traumas and losses may not allow the reduction of these symptoms compared with state anxiety. The reduction in personal risk rating of 9% is a major accomplishment for both staff and patients. It reflects the efforts by all of the staff, especially the oncologist risk counselor, to facilitate increased knowledge in addition to lowering anxiety. Perceived risk estimates can be viewed as highly correlated with the reduction of state anxiety. However, as encouraging as the data on personal risk rating reduction are, two cautions are necessary. First, an average risk rating of 45.30% is, in all likelihood, still far above what the "real" risk actually is for these patients (see Gail *et al.*, 1989). Thus, more work is clearly required in this area. Second, many follow-up visits have shown that these perceived risk ratings do not remain constant but fluctuate with the patient's level of anxiety and life stress.

COPING/ADJUSTMENT DIFFICULTIES RELATED TO FAMILY LEGACIES OF BREAST CANCER

At present, most factors specifically related to coping/adjustment difficulties of daughters of breast cancer patients are not sufficiently known. A study of 60 daughters of breast cancer patients suggests two variables: (1) the developmental stage of the daughter at the time of her mother's illness (adolescence being more stressful than preadolescence or adulthood), and (2) the survival status of the mother (death from breast cancer). Both variables predict less positive adaptation (Wellisch, Gritz, Schain, Wang, & Sian, 1991b). Compas *et al.* (1994) also showed adolescent girls whose mothers had breast cancer to display more symptoms of anxiety and depression than either preadolescents or young adults, a finding that appears to further validate the developmental variable. Studying children of breast cancer patients, Lichtman, Taylor, and Wood (1985) concluded that problems were more likely to occur in daughters than in sons. They suggest three factors that predict greater risk to and strain upon the mother–child relationship: (1) poorer prognosis (in the patient), (2) poor adjustment to the cancer (by the patient), and (3) more severe surgery (mastectomy vs. lumpectomy).

A constellation of three factors appears clinically particularly to bear upon the traumatic memories and coping/adaptation of our patient population. Depicted in Table 4, these include (1) the timing of mother's breast cancer (pre- or postmenopausal), which reliably divides daughters into those who were preadolescents or adolescents versus adults when their mothers were diagnosed: It also provides a quick but accurate estimate of the degree of biological risk of the daughter, since premenopausal breast cancer in the mother confers higher lifetime risk in the daughter (see Claus, Risch, & Thompson, 1990); (2) the mother's survival status: The daughters whose mothers and/or other female relatives died of their disease almost always presents more traumatic memories clinically; and (3) the quality of the mother–daughter relationship after the diagnosis: Does the daughter present the relationship as intact and well functioning, or as strained or broken in the wake of the illness, treatment, and (possibly) dying experience?

Table 4 presents a spectrum of coping/adjustment based on these factors, ranging from *Best* (Category 1) to *Worst* (Category 8). These factors are neither exhaustive nor inclusive. These merely serve as a clinical starting point. Other variables that deserve consideration may include how the family as a whole copes with the illness, the responsibilities presented to the child during the mother's illness, the parents' coping styles and capacities, the chronicity of the illness and the entire realm of the family's emotional atmosphere prior to the illness (functionality vs. pathology).

Clinical Vignettes

The following are six patient clinical vignettes derived from the High Risk Clinic patients at UCLA that represent varying levels of trauma and adjustment (see Table 1).

Vignette Number 1. Ms. M. represents coping/adjustment Level 1, the lowest level of trauma and the best level of adjustment. She is a 47-year-old, married executive whose mother was diagnosed with breast cancer 3 years ago at age 66. Her mother's illness was cured by a lumpectomy plus radiation to the local breast area. She reports that their relationship, which was quite good and harmonious prior to her mother's breast cancer, became closer and more (positively) bonded after the diagnosis. Her psychological needs are met by visiting the clinic twice a year, and she does not wish, nor clinically appear to require, additional psychological help outside the clinic. She reports her mother's breast cancer to have been a "wake-up call" to reassess and change her health habits. Her participation in the program led her to decrease her dietary fat consumption, exercise more regularly, take vitamins, and lose 5 pounds. Her psychological test scores in depressive and anxiety symptoms are all very low and in the normal range.

Table 4. Spectrum of Daughter's Coping/Adjustment Difficulties Based on Legacy of Trauma Associated with Mother's Breast Cancer

Daughter's coping/adjustment level	1 ("Best")	2	3	4	5	6	7	8 ("Worst")
Timing of mother's breast cancer	Postmenopausal	Postmenopausal	Postmenopausal	Premenopausal	Postmenopausal	Premenopausal	Premenopausal	Premenopausal
Mother's survival status	Survived	Died	Survived	Survived	Died	Died	Survived	Died
Status of relationship (postcancer)	Intact	Intact	Strained	Intact	Strained	Intact	Strained	Strained

Vignette Number 2.   Ms. J. represents coping/adjustment Level 3. She is a 41-year-old, married clerical worker whose mother was diagnosed 4 years earlier at the age of 61. Although her mother's illness was put in remission by mastectomy plus chemotherapy, she could not be told that she was cured. Reportedly always a nervous woman, the mother became obsessionally agitated and ruminative about this sense of threat. She became clinically depressed in the wake of her illness and treatment, and was placed on antidepressant medication in an attempt to reduce her ruminations about the possibility of recurrence. Having struggled to maintain boundaries with her mother, Ms. J. lost her ability to remain separate and found herself in a role reversal with a "needy, insatiable baby." Ms. J. indicated that all this had a strong impact on her own marriage, her ability to concentrate at work, and on her decision to not have children. Ms. J. reported that her relationship with her mother severely deteriorated. Her ability to be patient with and supportive of her mother seemed to erode. When Ms. J. first came to the clinic, she was well into the clinical range on tests of symptoms of both depression and anxiety. She was referred to, and accepted, individual therapy and was placed on antidepressant medication. She requested frequent visits to the High Risk Clinic and has been seen every 3 months for the last 2 years. Over that time, her symptoms have reduced but remain in the clinically significant range. On each visit to the clinic, every patient is asked to rate her estimation of her risk of breast cancer in her lifetime. This estimate can range from 0% to 100% (lifetime) risk. Ms. J.'s ratings have fluctuated from estimates of 100% perceived risk to 50% perceived risk. All her risk ratings are higher than her actual (real) lifetime risk. Along with all others in the High Risk Clinic, she has been repeatedly and intensively educated about the concept of lifetime (inherited) risk, real versus perceived risk, and given our estimates of her own risk based upon her family history, both orally and in the form of a chart to take home.

Two points seem especially important to consider in therapy for Ms. J. First, she cannot *get* support for her fears from her mother but must rather *give* support to her mother. Therapy reduces this traumatic absence of support. Second is the need to help Ms. J. set limits with her mother *without abandoning her.* This necessitates Ms. J. widening the base of support for her mother while setting limits with her in regard to her own time and availability. This may involve the clinic helping to find appropriate resources for Ms. J., such as a support group for her mother.

Vignette Number 3.   Ms. B. represents coping/adjustment Level 4. She is a 39-year-old housewife with one child. Her mother died 1 year ago, having been ill for about 3 years and experiencing monumental difficulties in coping with her breast cancer from diagnosis to death. Ms. B.'s father had died from complications of diabetes when she was an adolescent. Since then, her mother had raised her and her brother with a loving but highly anxious style. Although she was able to cope with normal everyday events, the mother's fragile emotional resources were easily overwhelmed by problems. Ms. B. and her brother became, in her own words, "crisis managers" and experienced role reversal with their mother. Breast cancer for Ms. B.'s mother was "the straw that broke the camel's back." She became chronically anxious, and as her disease progressed, she became utterly impaired with anxiety. Ms. B. related a closed loop phenomenon about her mother's inability to cope. As her mother experienced physical symptoms (pain, gastric distress, headaches, nausea), her anxiety level escalated. As her anxiety level increased, her mother focused more upon her somatic symptoms that, in turn, seemed to worsen with such an obsessive focus. Ms. B. and her brother arranged psychiatric help for their mother, who was minimally compliant with her therapy sessions, but essentially noncompliant with antianxiety medications. She repeatedly stated, "I just want this to be over. I just want to die already." As her illness progressed, Ms. B. felt uncomfortable leaving her mother alone at home. This led to another set of closed-loop dilemmas: Her mother also did not want to be alone, but felt guilty when she stayed with Ms. B. at her house, thinking that she was robbing her grandchild of her mother's attention. Yet feeling intruded upon, she would not accept a companion–aide in her own home. One day, Ms. B., sensing that her mother was saying good-bye, having not heard from her for several hours, went to her mother's home and found her unconscious. Her mother, indeed, had taken a massive overdose of pain medication. Not knowing what to do, whether she should attempt to save her mother or let her die as the mother so obviously wanted to, Ms. B. called for help. Her mother survived the overdose but refused to eat in the hospital after being revived. After extensive consultations between the staff and family, no intravenous feedings were attempted, and her mother died in the hospital about 10 days after her admission. This was the backdrop for Ms. B.'s early participation in the High Risk Clinic.

Ms. B.'s initial visit occurred before her mothers' suicide attempt. She was referred to, and accepted, individual, psychodynamically oriented psychotherapy. Prior to her mother's death, she reported extreme pressure and anxiety. Her test scores reflected high situational (state) anxiety with a core (trait) score of anxiety *not* in the clinical range. Thus, her core self was resolute and functional. However, as would be expected, her response to her present situation was highly pressured. After her mother's death, she reported a sense of peace regarding her mother. "She could not cope, she needed to die." For herself, she now experienced near panic. She asked, "Have I inherited her inability to cope if and when I get breast cancer?" She related substantially more fear about a potential inability to cope than about the possibility of getting breast cancer itself. She felt overburdened and overwhelmed with this traumatic legacy, which is based on identification with a mother who could not cope. Ms. B. was left with the internalized image of a mother drowning in anxiety about her own mortality.

This case calls for two therapeutic considerations. The first is dealing with Ms. B.'s ambivalent mourning and grief. Reconsideration of Freud's classic paper, "Mourning and Melancholia" (1915) is helpful here in Ms. B.'s vulnerability to identifying with her mother's style in the context of her own ambivalence (which includes anger and hatred) toward her mother. Helping her accept both her sadness over her mother's death and her own anger and frustration, culminating in the relief that her mother is gone, may possibly reduce the trauma. The second might be to refer her to group therapy with other daughters to be able to learn other styles of coping, thus opening up her (perceived) limited options of "only being like my mother."

Vignette Number 4.   Ms. W. represents coping/adjustment Level 5. She is a 35-year-old businesswoman who came to the clinic appearing profoundly sad, tense, and guarded. Her mother had died of breast cancer 2 years earlier. Although normally patients require from 40 minutes to up to 90 minutes to complete the baseline structured interview, Ms. W. took 2 hours. Both the story of her family of origin and that of her mother's breast cancer revealed the same basic theme, that is, her mother's inability to face up to and deal with harsh and ugly realities that demanded confrontation and action. In the family, the mother functioned as a "Stepford Wife." She lived in a state of fear and obsequiousness to her alcoholic, abusive husband, who terrorized the family. His emotional and physical abuse of Ms. W. evolved to sexual molestation when she became an adolescent. She bore all of it in silence until, when planning to leave home, she realized that her younger sister would be the next victim. She broke her silence and told her mother, feeling this would be an intolerable betrayal of her sister if she allowed it to happen. But her mother was unable to take action, and her sister, indeed, became the next victim.

Breast cancer became an extension of this process in which a malignant perpetrator was loose but could not be confronted. Her mother did not tell anyone she had a lump until the pain was beyond endurance, and the disease metastatic and incurable. Ms. W. returned home to nurse her mother through the terminal phase of her illness. She related, "Mother almost seemed relieved to die. It was a legitimate way to escape my father." In spite of this appalling history, Ms. W. had been able to marry and have a functional relationship but chose not to have children. She also became assertively self-reliant and successful in her business. We suggested psychotherapy; she cautiously assented. "It did not work," she complained, about the arrangements around the referral. Another referral was suggested, and again she felt it would not be possible due to "circumstances." She experienced the possibility of, in psychotherapy, facing her own mother's helpless dependency, her own sense of betrayal, and her rage, guilt, and fears as overwhelming. However, not unlike many women in our population, Ms. W. could not examine her own breasts without paralyzing anxiety and therefore had to return to the clinic frequently, allowing us to talk with her on this limited basis three to four times per year about her world of traumatic memories. She remains able to face these issues more than her mother but less than she would have if she used conventional psychotherapy. Our goal is to create a working alliance and facilitate trust with Ms. W. that will someday allow for conventional psychotherapy to heal the trauma of her past.

This case presents two major challenges for therapy: (1) of tolerating her resistances prior to even entering formal therapy; (2) of developing trust where little or none had been built in her family. Her transference reaction with the High Risk Clinic "family" is one of "Why should I trust your recommendations? I'll got it alone." Resolution will take a long period of interaction with the clinic prior to years of (formal) therapy.

Vignette Number 5. Ms. C. represents coping/adjustment Level 7. She is a 19-year-old, unemployed high school dropout. The staff of the High Risk Clinic was unclear as to how she actually supports herself. Her mother was diagnosed with a breast problem when Ms. C. was 14 years old. Upon reviewing the material Ms. C. brought with her about her mother, it was apparent that her mother had lobular carcinoma *in situ* (LCIS). By strict definition, this was really not cancer, but rather a precancerous condition from which about 17% of patients go on to develop actual cancer. LCIS puts a woman at 7.2 times the normal risk to develop cancer (Rosen, Lieberman, & Braun, 1987). The options available for LCIS are (1) bilateral mastectomy or (2) no treatment but close follow-up (Love, 1995). Unable to tolerate observation alone, her mother, then 38 years old, chose bilateral mastectomy. Because the procedure was performed at the height of the controversies surrounding silicone breast implants, the mother felt that she could neither have implants nor could she tolerate the more extensive tissue transfer techniques for breast reconstruction (Gabriel *et al.,* 1994; Shaw, 1995). Thus, she was left with no breasts, a radically altered body image, and a severely shaken sense of her femininity at age 38. Moreover, this coincided with Ms. C. becoming a very lithe, curvaceous, sexual young woman. She described her mother as first depressed by the loss of her breasts, but then turning angry. She tearfully related to us that her mother told her, "Everyone knows stress causes cancer. You have given me cancer. This is all your fault." Ms. C.'s response was to "get stoned," to spend her adolescence abusing alcohol, marijuana, and cocaine. She dropped out of high school and ended up in Los Angeles, about 300 miles from her parents' home. In her baseline visit to the High Risk Clinic, she was educated that (1) her mother almost certainly did not have actual cancer; (2) her mother's LCIS was not caused by stress from Ms. C.'s behavior during her early adolescence; and (3) based on her mother's experience, her risk of breast cancer was very modestly above a woman whose mother did not have LCIS. We do not know what this meant to her, as she never returned to the clinic.

Planning for therapy in this case reflects the age-related types of problems presented by Ms. C. to the Clinic. Her case makes it difficult to distinguish adolescent adjustment problems from her reactions to the trauma of her mother's breast situation. The first step with this 19-year-old is obviously to form a relationship that will allow for asking whether there is a reality beyond the mother's reality. The process that needs exploring with Ms. C. involved Mother's rage over her breast problem (leading to) displacement of blame onto Ms. C., (leading to) Ms. C. "numbing out" to cope, (leading to) Ms. C. fleeing from the entire family situation. As with Vignette Number 4, accepting slow progress and small gains is crucial.

Vignette Number 6.   Ms. A. represents coping/adjustment Level 8. She is a 49-year-old divorced woman with no children and has a very successful business to which she devotes the majority of her time and energy. Her mother was diagnosed with breast cancer when she was 12 and died 5 years later, when she was 17 years old, having received the standard treatment of that era, which included Halsted radical mastectomy, radiation therapy, and some chemotherapy. Her mother felt "deformed and mutilated" by her very extensive surgery and was further traumatized by the radiation that burned and scarred her skin. Control over side effects of chemotherapy was perfunctory and not well developed. Ms. A., then in the early phase of her own pubertal development, vividly remembers her mother as "on her hands and knees by her bedside vomiting on newspapers like a dog." She described her mother as "a brittle, proud, and narcissistic woman, totally involved with her looks and image." Her mother was clearly shattered, horrified, and ultimately enraged by this series of events. She forced her husband out of their bedroom and never again shared it with him until she died. She insisted that her daughter (Ms. A.) care for her and no one else. Eventually, she insisted that her daughter move in to her bedroom. Ms. A. described herself as "becoming her mother's slave" during that period. She tried hard to please and calm her but perpetually felt inadequate and unable to fulfill her mother's wishes. As was also typical of that era, a tense and fearful silence descended on the family about the illness. The word *cancer* was virtually never mentioned, not between Ms. A. and her mother, or between Ms. A. and her father, or between the family and the treating doctors. In the last few months of her mother's life, Ms. A. was a high school senior. She remained at home caring for her mother and did not attend school. She was taught how to inject her mother with morphine shots. When the dosages of morphine the doctors had authorized were not containing the mother's pain, they suggested to Ms. A. that "perhaps we should try a placebo. Her pain should be controlled by what we are giving her." Balking at this notion, this was the first time she remembers getting angry at adults who responded to her anger by changing their behavior. During the terminal phase of his wife's illness, her father would greet her mother only once a day, in the mornings, and then not return to her room at all. Ms. A. persisted in this almost indescribably difficult situation, not having a perspective that it could or should be different. She returned to finish school the following year, but felt out of sync with her classmates. She spent the next few years at home "being her father's housekeeper." Although she wished to go away to college, feeling too obligated to her father, she attended college while living at home. The experience left her feeling a "black anger." She is not sure whether she is angrier at her mother for "enslaving" her or at her father for not taking a stand and allowing her to be used in this fashion. Since that time her life has been dominated by (1) a strong sense of frustration and anger at people, no matter whether casual acquaintances or intimate relationships. In her own words, she has "a short fuse, or no fuse at all," and (2) a need to be in charge of others, to control others, to never again "be under anyone's thumb." These themes have been enacted on her life in three divorces and a very successful career in which she employs over 100 people in a garment manufacturing business. She describes her business as "a dog-eat-dog world where she is a top dog."

In the clinic, Ms. A. singularly stands out among the other 275 patients in having an uncanny ability to split and pit staff members against each other. In two separate situations during a recent visit, she caused staff members to feel humiliated, ashamed, and like failures; she provoked a senior staff member to angrily upbraid a junior staff member for perceived management errors with her. The staff have come to realize that she creates in them the same feelings she felt as a teenage girl trying to care for her enraged, dying mother. She creates a sense of failure, guilt, fear, and paralyzing inadequacy in the staff, much as she described having felt at that time. She had several bouts with psychotherapy, with highly regarded therapists in the community and scorned recommendations for therapy. We continue to see her twice per year in our clinic.

This case presents major challenges to the staff to contain and manage the stresses and provocations presented by this most difficult patient. Ms. A. is less able to "tell" than to "show" the staff what she experienced with her family/mother by means of projective identification (Adler, 1985). The rage she feels upon psychologically revisiting the illness experience with her mother has repeatedly driven her out of therapy. Thus, its management and containment by the staff is pivotal to treating her (Adler, 1985). Ms. A. shares many elements of psychological trauma of her daughters of breast cancer patients. These include role reversal, changes in short- and long-term life plans because of mother's illness, isolation combined with overwhelming responsibility for the mother's care, the father's regression and dependency, and familial silence that markedly intensifies all these problems (Wellisch *et al.*, 1991b). These need to be identified and worked through in therapy.

EMERGING PERSPECTIVES ON PSYCHOTHERAPY FOR TRAUMATIC LEGACIES

The words *emerging perspectives* in the title of this section are used pointedly and deliberately to signify that, to date, very limited data exist on psychotherapy with high-risk women (Kash *et al.*, 1995). Our clinic has been awarded a grant and has begun a nonrandomized clinical pilot trial of a model of group intervention for this population that will be described below. Thus, the following perspectives are based largely on clinical work rather than on databased outcome studies.

Psychological Aspects of the Clinic Structure and Milieu

The structure of a special, high-risk clinic such as the one at the UCLA Breast Center or at the Strang Cancer Prevention Center/Memorial Sloan–Kettering Cancer Center itself can be fundamental as a psychological intervention. Such clinics become special, safe "holding environments" (see Winnicott, 1965) for this unique population. The safety comes from the sense that the staff is highly knowledgeable about their risks both genetically, biologically, and psychologically. The continuity of the staff as they make follow-up visits to the clinic program adds to the sense of a safe and predictable environment. Physically, they feel confident in the nurse practitioner's skill to find anything suspicious in their breasts. Psychologically, these women know that there will be safety and empathic understanding in revealing their past experiences and traumas around familial breast cancer.

It is important to note that not all the patients in the program experience trauma-based symtomatology. In fact, the opposite is true. At least, by dint of baseline psychological testing, the majority are not symptomatic. For example, of the first 161 patients in the UCLA High Risk Clinic, 36 (22%) were at or above the cutting score of 16 on the CES-D. Of this same 161 patients, 72 (45%) were at or above the 40th percentile on the STAI, indicating significant symptoms of clinical (present state) anxiety. While the minority of these patients appear to need referral or triage to formal psychotherapy for trauma-based problems, all of these patients benefit from the therapeutic milieu created by the High Risk Clinic team structure.

Individual Therapy

To effectively deal with the core issues of this population, individual therapy needs to be dynamically oriented. This is especially true when the focus is the resolution of traumatically based symptomatology. To do relaxation therapy or cognitive therapy alone is to ignore or not reach the psychological strata where such trauma exists in these women. Several possible key foci of individual therapy were described elsewhere (see Wellisch, Hoffman, & Gritz, 1996). They include the following:

1. The fundamental act of asking the woman to talk about her familial cancer experience(s). As Vignette Number 6 illustrates, no one may have ever previously asked or given permission to the daughter to talk about these experiences. This may be especially true for daughters whose mothers had breast cancer in the 1950s and early 1960s, when silence about cancer was the operative behavioral/familial rule.

2. Exploring the relatively common theme of "I have decided not to have children." Of the six women in the vignettes, three had decided not to have children. Such decisions can be based on traumatic memories and/or fears of perpetuating such legacies in future generations. It can, at times, be based on false or misguided notions of risk. For example, Ms. C. in Vignette Number 5, had an inaccurate risk assessment to herself and future offspring based on her painful and traumatizing guilt toward her mother. Psychological exploration, support, and education may alter her sense of doom. However, education alone is rarely helpful to resolve such misperceptions (see Black, Nease, & Tosteson, 1995).

3. Exploring the presence of sexual conflicts in the daughter. Daughters may be coming into sexuality just as their mothers are (traumatically) losing theirs. This may result for the daughter in a trauma-based legacy of guilt around sexual expression. In addition, daughters may experience fear around sexual pleasure associated with breasts. In clinic interviews, some have stated, "That area (breasts) is off limits. I do not want to get used to pleasure from something I stand to lose." Vignette Numbers 4, 5, and 6 reflect elements of both of these issues. Ms. C. could not have sex without being "stoned," given that her mother was intensely threatened by and jealous of her daughter's intact body image and sexuality. For Ms. W. (Vignette Number 5), sexuality was always a dangerous, volatile area. Her inability to examine her own breasts is symptomatic of both fear and trauma. Ms. A. (Vignette Number 6) not only remained intact while her mother did not, but she also survived to become her father's substitute wife, further complicating her own psychosexual development. A key question in therapy for daughters seem to be, "Is it a betrayal of mother to have sexual pleasure, *including* breast-focused pleasure?"

4. Exploring fathers' roles in the resolution of trauma in their daughters. Was the father able to functionally cope with his wife's illness and then recover? Or did the father's own pathology further complicate the daughter's own recovery (see Wellisch, 1979)? Fathers have been reported to distance themselves from their daughters after their wife's death, or become dependent on and/or seductive with their daughters (as in Vignette Number 6, Ms. A.).

5. Exploring mother's own adaptation/coping style to her illness as a source of identification for daughter (see Stern, 1989). For example, was the mother an anxious denier (as in Vignette Numbers 2 and 3), or isolated and angry (as in Vignette Numbers 5 and 6)? In therapy, daughters can be encouraged to make different choices than their mothers if they themselves develop breast cancer. At the very least, therapy can help such daughters feel that they do not have to "go it alone" as their mothers often did emotionally.

6. Exploring for unresolved (now internalized) anger in the daughters about their forced participation in the experience of their mothers' illness. The key question is whether it has become a facet of a chronic dysphoria or low-level, persistent depression? Vignette Numbers 2 and especially 6 reflect this dynamic, both with a living and a deceased mother. How much this is an extension of the precancer relationship remains to be determined in psychotherapy. The adjunctive use of medication, especially antidepressants, can be important with this population. Hirschfeld and Goodwin (1988) state that the "use of psychopharmacological and psychotherapeutic approaches should not be considered an either/or proposition. The best clinical management often includes a combination of the two in a way that best meets the patient's individual treatment needs" (p. 434). This seems an apt treatment philosophy with such high-risk women.

Group Therapy

Group treatment is a very important intervention modality for this population. To our knowledge, only one small outcome study has been performed with high-risk women in a group psychoeducational mode (Kash et al., 1995). In this study, a 6-week program of education about risk, breast self-examination, and importance of adherence to screening guidelines was combined with psychological efforts to reduce the sense of isolation, encourage sharing of feelings and thoughts, and create a group milieu. As compared with a control group, the experimental group fared better with regard to decrease in perceived risk, lowering of perceived barriers to screening, and increase in knowledge about breast cancer. These changes persisted over time, up to 1-year follow-up. Our center is beginning a similar psychoeducational 6-week group intervention, with a strong psychological focus on the identification and resolution of grief states. Whether or not a death occurred in the family, significant losses are often present in our clinic population that has not been identified and mourned. What is not yet known about group interventions for this population to deal with trauma is whether they are better than individual intervention, whether they supplement individual intervention, or what the best group mix might contain. In our study, groups will be subdivided in regard to age (< 42 years vs. > 42 years), and in regard to loss status (mother died vs. mother survived), to see if one mix produces better outcomes. The study will incorporate elements of both cognitive therapy and relaxation therapy. These will be taught as well as practiced in a group context. This was an important element in a group outcome study with melanoma patients (Fawzy et al., 1990).

Family Therapy

Family therapy has not been reported in the literature for this population. It contains important possibilities for trauma resolution. We have experiences with several daughters spontaneously bringing their (breast cancer survivor) mothers with them to their appointments. The daughters' agendas in doing so have appeared to be, as in the words of one such daughter, "Let's finally face your breast cancer experience together fully by actually talking about it together." What we have witnessed in these powerful experiences is the breaking down of silence and of barriers between mothers and daughters that often lasted decades. Such mothers have related, "I tried to protect her from pain," with the realization that at least some of that pain was/is their own. The guilt of these mothers over the possibility of transmitting breast cancer to their daughter is enormous. This is a very potent modality to consider in trauma resolution for high-risk women. It is, after all, the context of the family of origin where such traumas originated.

CONCLUSION

This chapter must be viewed as a work in progress. Understanding both the traumas and especially interventions for these traumas in women at high risk for breast cancer are far from fully known. What is clear, however, is that this is a *heterogeneous* group of women, with a variety of predispositions, family circumstances, family experiences with illness, and risk factors. They cannot and must not be viewed as a homogenous group with one trauma and one characteristic response. Similarly, there is no "formula" or "model" for trauma resolution for this diverse group of women. We expect and hope that several pathways and models will be developed and evaluated in the future to remedy the traumas and enhance the coping and adaptation of these high-risk women.

REFERENCES

Adler, G. (1985). *Borderline psychopathology and its treatment.* New York: Jason Aronson.

Berg, J. W. (1984). Clinical implications of risk factors for breast cancer. *Cancer, 53,* 589–591.

Black, W. C., Nease, R. F., & Tosteson, A. N. A. (1995). Perceptions of breast cancer and screening effectiveness in women younger than 50 years of age. *Journal of the National Cancer Institute, 87*(10), 720–731.

Claus, B. E., Risch, N., & Thompson, W. D. (1990). Age at onset as an indicator of familial risk of breast cancer. *American Journal of Epidemiology, 131,* 961–972.

Claus, B. E., Risch, N., & Thompson, W. D. (1994). Autosomal dominant inheritance of early onset breast cancer. *Cancer, 73,* 643–651.

Compas, B. E., Worsham, N. L., Epping-Jordan, J. E., Grant, K. E., Mireault, G., Howell, D., & Molcarne, V. L. (1994). When Mom or Dad has cancer: Markers of psychological distress in cancer patients, spouses, and children. *Health Psychology, 13,* 507–515.

Dupont, W. D., & Page, D. L. (1987). Breast cancer risk associated with proliferative disease, age at first birth and a family history of breast cancer. *American Journal of Epidemiology, 125,* 769–777.

Fawzy, F. I., Cousins, N., Fawzy, N. W., Kemeny, M. E., Elashoff, R., & Morton, D. (1990). A structured psychiatric intervention for cancer patients. *Archives of General Psychiatry, 47,* 720–725.

Freud, S. (1915). Mourning and melancholia. In S. Freud (Ed.), *Standardized Works of Sigmund Freud, Vol. XIV.* London: Hogarth Press.

Futureal, A., Liu, Q., Shattuck-Eidens, D., Cochran, C., Harshman, K., & Tanigian, S. (1994). BRCA1 mutations in primary breast and ovarian carcinomas. *Science, 266,* 120–122.

Gabriel, S. E., O'Fallon, M., Kurland, L. T., Beard, C. M., Woods, M. D., & Melton, L. J. (1994). Risk of connective-tissue diseases and other disorders after breast implantation. *New England Journal of Medicine, 330*(24), 1697–1699.

Gail, M. H., Brinton, L. A., Byar, D. P., Corle, D. K., Green, S. B., & Schairer, C. (1989). Projecting individualized probabilities of developing breast cancer for white females who are being examined annually. *Journal of the National Cancer Institute, 81,* 1879–1886.

Hirohita, T. Nomura, A., Hankin, J. H., Kolorel, L. N., & Lee, J. (1987). An epidemiologic study on the association between diet and breast cancer. *Journal of the National Cancer Institute, 78,* 595–600.

Hirschfeld, R. M. A., & Goodwin, F. K. (1988). Mood disorders. In J. A. Talbott, R. E. Holes, & S. C. Yudofsky (Eds.), *Textbook of psychiatry* (p. 437). Washington, DC: American Psychiatric Press.

Josten, D. M., Evans, A. M., & Love, R. R. (1985). The cancer prevention clinic: A service program for cancer prone families. *Journal of Psychosocial Oncology, 3*(3), 5–20.

Kash, K. M., Holland, J. C., Halper, M. S., & Miller, D. G. (1992). Psychological distress and surveillance behaviors of women with a family history of breast cancer. *Journal of the National Cancer Institute, 84,* 24–30.

Kash, K. M., Holland, J. C., Osborne, M. P., & Miller, D. G. (1995). Psychological counseling strategies for women at risk for breast cancer. *Journal of the National Cancer Institute Monographs, 17,* 73–79.

Koocher, G. P., & O'Malley, J. F. (1981). *The Damocles syndrome: Psychological consequences of surviving childhood cancer.* New York: McGraw-Hill.

Lichtman, R. R., Taylor, S. E., & Wood, J. V., *et al.* (1985). Relations with children after breast cancer: The mother–daughter relationship at risk. *Journal of Psychological Oncology, 2,* 1–19.

Love, S. M. (1995). Dr. Susan Love's breast book (2nd ed.). New York: Addison-Wesley.

Rosen, P. P., Lieberman, P. H., & Braun, D. W. (1987). Lobular carcinoma of the breast. *American Journal of Surgical Pathology, 2,* 225–228.

Sattin, R. W., Rubin, G. L., Webster, L. A., Huezo, C. M., Wingo, P. A., Ory, H. W., & Layde, P. H. (1985). Family history and the risk of breast cancer. *Journal of the American Medical Association, 253,* 1908–1912.

Schwartz, M. D., Lerman, C., Miller, S. M., Daly, M., & Masny, A. (1995). Coping disposition, perceived risk, and psychological distress among women at increased risk for ovarian cancer. *Health Psychology, 14*(3), 232–235.

Seidman, H., Mushinski, M. H., Gelb, S. K., & Silverberg, E. (1985). Probabilities of eventually developing cancer—United States, 1985. *CA: A Cancer Journal for Clinicians, 35,* 36–56.

Shaw, W. W. (1995). Surgical reconstruction. In C. M. Haskell (Ed.), *Cancer treatment* (pp. 343–347). Philadelphia: Saunders.

Stern, D. N. (1989). The representation of relational patterns. In A. J. Sameroff & R. N. Emde (Eds.), *Relationships and relationship disorders* (pp. 52–69). New York: Basic Books.

Stomper, P. C., Gelman, R. S., Meyer, J. G., & Gross, G. S. (1990). New England Mammographic Survey, 1988: Public misconceptions of breast cancer incidence. *Breast Disease 3,* 1–7.

Styra, R., Sakinofsky, I., Mahoney, L., *et al.* (1993). Coping styles in identifiers and non-identifiers of a breast lump or a problem. *Psychosomatics, 34*(1), 53–60.

Wellisch, D. K. (1979). Adolescent acting out as a response to parental cancer. *International Journal of Family Therapy, 3,* 230–240.

Wellisch, D. K., Gritz, E. R., Schain, W., Wang, H., & Siau, J. (1991a). Psychological functioning of daughters of breast cancer patients: Part I. Daughters and comparison subjects. *Psychosomatics, 32,* 324–336.

Wellisch, D. K., Gritz, E. R., Schain, W., Wang, H., & Siau, J. (1991b). Psychological functioning of daughters of breast cancer patients: Part II. Characterizing the distressed daughter of the breast cancer patient. *Psychosomatics, 33*(2), 171–179.

Wellisch, D. K., Hoffman, A., & Gritz, E. R. (1996). Psychological concerns and care of daughters of breast cancer patients. In L. Baider & C. Cooper (Eds.), *Cancer and the family* (pp. 289–304). Sussex, UK: Wiley.

Winnicott, D. W. (1965). *The maturational processes and the facilitating environment.* New York: International Universities Press.

X

The Emerging Biology of Intergenerational Trauma

36

Psychobiology of Intergenerational Effects of Trauma
Evidence from Animal Studies

STEPHEN J. SUOMI and SEYMOUR LEVINE

INTRODUCTION: RATIONALE FOR ANIMAL STUDIES

Systematic scientific study of the effects of trauma on humans has always faced formidable methodological challenges and both ethical and practical obstacles. The most scientifically rigorous study designs—prospective longitudinal experiments, preferably double-blind in nature—are virtually nonexistent, appropriately precluded by the ethical standards of every civilized society. Instead, some reliance on retrospective data inevitably occurs, at least for part of the period under study (e.g., the time prior to the beginning of the trauma). Practical considerations also hinder prospective studies of the long-term consequences of trauma, especially those that involve life-span or multigenerational perspectives. It simply takes too long for humans to grow up (and old) for such prospective longitudinal studies to be feasible in most cases. As a result, retrospective reports provide the basis for much of our current knowledge base regarding long-term consequences of trauma.

This is not to say that retrospective data are without legitimacy or value in scientific inquiry. To the contrary, such data have clearly informed major areas of knowledge in traumatology and many other fields. Sophisticated epidemiological designs and analyses are currently at least on a par with most prospective approaches; there is nothing inherently nonscientific about such retrospective methodology. However, retrospective data of any and all forms are not sufficient in and of themselves to provide unambiguous scientific proof of causality, and that represents an absolute limitation.

In many areas of inquiry in traumatology, retrospective data are often rich in detail, objective in nature, and certifiably accurate (e.g., medical or archival records). Such retrospective data can be of great utility in understanding specific trauma-related phenomena. In

STEPHEN J. SUOMI • Laboratory of Comparative Biology, National Institute of Child Health and Human Development, Bethesda, Maryland 20892.   SEYMOUR LEVINE • Department of Psychology, University of Delaware, Newark, Delaware 19716.

International Handbook of Multigenerational Legacies of Trauma, edited by Yael Danieli. Plenum Press, New York, 1998.

contrast, for investigations focusing on the psychobiological correlates and consequences of trauma, reliance on retrospective approaches poses real problems. The biggest problem is that relevant retrospective psychobiological data rarely exist. The very kinds of measures typically used to document the psychobiological effects of stress and/or trauma (e.g., stress hormone levels, central neurotransmitter metabolite concentrations, or various measures of immunological functioning) are unlikely to be found in typical medical records, let alone in any sort of community or state archives.

Quantitative indices of these psychobiological measures are even less likely to be found in the memories of the vast majority of individuals who have experienced traumatic events or episodes. The human memory system is arguably one of the wonders of nature, and the capacity to recall specifics of circumstances, impressions, and emotions associated with trauma has provided the raw data for an expanding area of legitimate, indeed exciting, scientific inquiry and clinical application. However, experiences must be encoded as well as accessed for memory to be operative, and humans rarely, if ever, routinely monitor most of their psychobiological functioning in an objectively quantifiable fashion, let alone encode such information into memory. Of course, virtually all of us are aware of at least some of our visceral psychobiological experiences, especially during and following periods of stress (e.g., the experience of a "pounding" heart or the flushing of the face), and such memories are often intense and exceedingly long-lasting. However, it is difficult, if not impossible, to quantify such psychobiological memories in a scientifically useful fashion, especially when the memories go back many years and/or across generations.

Given the problems inherent in carrying out prospective longitudinal studies of long-term psychobiological consequences of trauma and the relative absence of relevant and scientifically useful retrospective data in humans, it should not be surprising that much of what we currently know in this area comes from research with animals. Prospective longitudinal experiments are the rule rather than the exception in animal studies of the psychobiology of stress. Current legal guidelines and ethical standards permit experimental designs with animals that involved preplanned exposure to stressful circumstances of systematically varied type, intensity, and duration, as well as the opportunity for rigorous and long-term follow-up. In these designs, variables deemed extraneous can be explicitly controlled for, in marked contrast to the "experiments of nature" that characterize much of human trauma research. Animal researchers are usually able to collect a much wider range of psychobiological measures in a more rigorous and direct fashion over more extended periods (including periods prior to exposure to trauma) than is typically feasible in human studies. Finally, and perhaps most relevant for this volume, the vast majority of animal species grow up much more rapidly and have considerably shorter life spans and generational turnovers than do humans. Thus, prospective experiments investigating long-term and intergenerational psychobiological consequences of stress in animals are clearly feasible and often practical, whereas comparable human research remains largely hypothetical.

Of course, findings from animal studies can be useful in furthering our understanding of the effects of trauma on humans only to the extent that there is generalizability between the human and animal phenomena under study (Harlow, Suomi, & Gluck, 1972). Such generalizations are not always possible. For example, given that humans have unique linguistic abilities in both the communicative and the mental imagery realms, it seems exceedingly unlikely that any animal model could be developed that would faithfully represent much of either realm. On the other hand, there are many aspects of psychobiological functioning in humans that are shared essentially in toto with many other animal species, homologous even down to the molecular level of gene functioning (Suomi & Immelmann, 1983). It is in these specific areas that animal models of psychobiological response to trauma are most likely to provide useful insights regarding possible cross-generational effects of trauma in humans.

BASIC PATTERNS OF PSYCHOBIOLOGICAL RESPONSE TO STRESS IN ANIMALS

Research on the effect of early experiences and, in particular, the influences of exposure to "trauma" early in ontogeny has been ongoing for at least four decades. Clearly, we have accumulated a greater understanding of the consequences of these experiences and some of the mechanisms underlying the variety of persistent changes that have been observed. For many reasons, the laboratory rodent has been the animal most extensively investigated. The laboratory rodent has a relatively short life span; thus, the long-term effects of neonatal trauma can easily be studied. The laboratory rodent breeds well in captivity; therefore, experimental subjects are readily available. Finally, it is possible to examine the neural correlates of the now well-documented changes in both behavior and physiological function that are altered by exposure to trauma neonatally. Examining changes in brain mechanisms that follow early experiences is difficult in primates and almost impossible in humans. What has become progressively clearer is that the effects of early experience with traumatic events depend upon a number of critical variables. Among these are (1) the age of onset of the experience, (2) the type of traumatic event, and (3) the intensity and duration of the experience. There are undoubtedly other variables that can modify outcomes. For example, there is increasing evidence that the genetic background of the organism can modify the outcome of exposure to early trauma.

Given the fact that this problem has been studied for many years, we do not attempt a comprehensive review of all the outcome measures that have been investigated. Rather, we focus on aspects of behavior associated with emotionality and on one of the major physiological systems associated with the response to stress, namely, the hypothalamic–pituitary–adrenal (HPA) axis. One of the major endocrine responses following exposure to stress is the increased secretion of specific hormones from the adrenal (glucocorticoids). In the rodent, the primary glucocorticoid is corticosterone (CORT), whereas in the primate and human, cortisol is synthesized and secreted by the adrenal. Release of the adrenal hormones is a result of a "neuroendocrine cascade" that involves specific release of a hormone, corticotropin-releasing hormone (CRH), from the brain, which, in turn, regulates the output of adrenocorticotropic hormone (ACTH) from the pituitary that is required to activate the adrenal to increase the secretion of glucocorticoids. Although much of the research on the effects of early experience on the endocrine response to stress has measured either CORT or cortisol as the dependent variable, it is always assumed that an increase in the levels of adrenal hormones reflects the response of the brain to stress.

In the original studies (Levine, Chevalier, & Korchin, 1956), infant rats were subjected to a brief daily exposure to a painful stimulus and were compared to another group of rats that were removed daily from their mothers for the same period of time but not subjected to the painful experience. An additional group received no experience and remained with the mother without any disturbance. As adults, these animals were tested in a learning paradigm that involved learning to avoid a noxious stimulus (conditioned avoidance learning). Surprisingly, the rats that either experienced the painful event or were removed from the mothers neonatally showed the appropriate adaptive response and learned to avoid the noxious stimuli very rapidly. In contrast, those animals who presumably had the best of all possible worlds failed to learn to avoid and showed excessive emotional reactivity when exposed to aversive stimuli as adults. Subsequent research (Levine, 1960), using a variety of behavioral probes designed to examine emotionality, demonstrated that these early experiences, traditionally called early handling (EH), resulted in an adult that was significantly less emotionally aroused. It is somewhat unfortunate that these procedures have been termed *early handling,* since this implies some form of positive physical contact, which is not at all descriptive of the actual experimental treatments and implies that these procedures involved stroking and gentling. The critical manipulation in these studies actually turned out to be the removal of the infant from the mother for brief periods of time. The additional exposure to painful stimuli did not seem to override the importance of the brief disruption of mother–infant interactions.

An extensive series of studies conducted for more than three decades (cf. Meany *et al.* [1993] for the most recent review) have examined the response of the HPA axis in EH rats. The results revealed changes in the endocrine responses to stress that were consistent with the reduction in emotional behavior. Thus, CORT secretion in response to a number of different stressors was reduced in EH animals when compared to their nontreated counterparts. Furthermore, following the initial increase in CORT, the EH rats showed a more rapid return to basal levels, indicating a more efficient negative feedback. Of particular importance is that these changes in the HPA axis of EH animals have been found to be a function of permanent structural and functional alterations of the brain mechanisms that are part of the regulation of the HPA axis (Meany *et al.,* 1993). The crucial message is that there is a great deal of plasticity in developing nervous systems, which can be affected by early experiences and appear to permanently alter later neuroendocrine activity. To what extent other brain structures are also affected remains to be determined.

We have discussed the EH model at length since it has received a great deal of attention. This, however, is only one of several experimental manipulations that have been observed to have long-term effects. Other neonatal experiences result in outcomes that are paradoxical to those seen with EH. Recently, two different methods of maternal separation in rats have been shown to result in an hyperactive HPA axis, as well as increased emotionality. Whereas the EH paradigm involved removing the rat pup from the mother for periods of time between 5 and 15 minutes per day, the critical period for these treatments is between 3 and 14 days of age. If the length of separation is increased to 3 hours daily during this period, the adult rat now exhibits a significantly greater CORT response than the pups that were separated for 15 minutes daily (Meaney *et al.,* 1993). Further prolonged daily separated animals show a greater increase in corticotropin releasing factor (CRF mRNA) when compared to nonhandled (NH) and handled subjects (Plotsky & Meaney, 1993). These results are very recent; thus, behavioral changes have not been explored extensively. However, the evidence does suggest that there are changes in the central nervous system (CNS) that are consistent with the hyperactivity of the HPA axis in these animals.

Recently, a different type of maternal separation has been shown to also produce persistent changes in HPA function. In these studies, pups are separated from the mother for 24 hours at different ages. If pups are separated early in development (days 3–4) and then reunited with the mother, they exhibit a pattern of HPA hyperactivity when tested as juveniles. In contrast, if the separation occurs between days 11–12, these animals hyposecrete ACTH and CORT (Van Oers & Levine, 1998, unpublished observations). There is also evidence that deprivation between days 3–4 results in long-term functional and structural changes in the brains of the early deprived rats (Levine, 1994). Thus far, there have been no behavioral studies conducted using this model of maternal deprivation. Thus, it appears that all forms of early experiences that we presume to be traumatic result in permanent alterations in the CNS regulation of the neuroendocrine responses to stress in these rodents. There is no evidence that these changes are reversible.

There is also evidence for intergenerational effects of EH. In an extensive series of studies, Denenberg and colleagues (Denenberg, 1970; Deneberg & Whimby, 1963) examined the influence of the mothers' postnatal experience on their offspring. The primary measures used were body weight and open field behavior (a presumed measure of emotionality). Although there was clear evidence of intergenerational effects, they were complex and depended not only on the maternal postnatal experience but also interacted with the rearing conditions (cf. Denenberg, 1970).

Most of the research on intergenerational effects has studied behavior as the outcome variable. Levine (1967) reported that weanling rats of EH mothers showed a reduced CORT response to novelty when compared to weanlings of nonhandled mothers. Handling the pups of previously handled mothers did not affect the CORT response, whereas EH of offspring of NH mothers once reduced the CORT response to the same level that was seen in the pups of EH mothers.

PRIMATE STUDIES OF PSYCHOBIOLOGICAL RESPONSIVENESS TO STRESS

The knowledge base regarding the psychobiological consequences of stress in primates is considerably less extensive than it is in rodents, both in terms of breadth and depth. However, those findings that have emerged from stress research with primates have been remarkably congruent with what is known for rodents, at least where straightforward comparisons have been feasible. In this respect, there have been relatively few surprises to date.

On the other hand, the rich behavioral and emotional repertoires and cognitive capabilities of monkeys and apes provide opportunities for modeling aspects of human stress response patterns that are simply not feasible with rodents. Significantly, it is possible with primates to investigate patterns of covariance between specific behavioral and emotional responses and concomitant psychobiological reactions during and following stressful periods. Many of these behavioral and emotional response patterns seem remarkably congruent with those seen in humans. The correspondence between human and nonhuman primates is perhaps even greater for most physiological systems, which is not surprising in light of the extensive genetic overlap among monkeys, apes, and humans (e.g., humans share approximately 94% of their genes with rhesus monkeys and over 98% with chimpanzees; cf. Lovejoy, 1981). These behavioral and emotional patterns provide a face validity for primate models that simply cannot be matched by those with rodents.

A case in point can be seen in studies of psychobiological response to social separation in primates. Short-term separation from family and/or friends is essentially as obsequious a phenomenon for most wild-living monkeys and apes as it has been for humans throughout recorded history. Such separations can be stressful or routine (or both), depending on the circumstances and the individuals involved. For example, virtually every rhesus monkey infant born into a wild troop experiences repeated short-term separations from its mother when she consorts with different adult males during the troop's annual breeding season (Berman, Rasmussen, & Suomi, 1994). The universal reactions of these infants to such involuntary maternal separation is one of significant behavioral disruption and physiological arousal, much as Bowlby has described for human infants experiencing involuntary maternal separation (Bowlby, 1960, 1973). Although most of these rhesus monkeys youngsters soon get over their initial period of protest and subsequently seek out the company of other troop members during their mothers' absence, about 20% instead become lethargic and withdraw from all social contact (Suomi, 1991), reminiscent of Bowlby's description of separation-induced "despair" in some human infants and children.

Experimental studies of social separation in captive nonhuman primates have been carried out under a variety of laboratory conditions for over 30 years. These studies of mother–infant separation have consistently found that, as in the wild, captive-living infant monkeys and apes initially respond to separation with behavioral agitation, characterized by dramatic increases in locomotor activity and "coo" vocalizations, and a cessation of exploratory and play behaviors. Maternal separation also typically activates the HPA axis, as indexed by sharp increases in levels of plasma cortisol and ACTH, and increased turnover of the noradrenergic system, as indexed by decreased cerebral spinal fluid levels of norepinephrine (NE) and increased levels of the NE metabolite 3-methoxy-4-hydroxyphenylglycol (MHPG), as well as elevated heart rate, indicating sympathetic arousal.

Although most infant monkeys in these laboratory studies begin to return to preseparation levels of behavioral and physiological functioning within a few hours, some individuals continue to display profound behavioral and physiological reactions for several days, if not longer, as is the case for some individuals in the wild. Virtually all of these young separated monkeys essentially show spontaneous recovery when reunited with their mothers, although physical contact with mother remains elevated, and social play reduced, relative to preseparation levels, for days or even weeks following reunion (e.g., Seay, Hansen, & Harlow, 1962).

Many investigators have noted the parallels between these reactions to separation and Bowlby's characterization of prototypical separation reactions in human infants and young children. Parametric studies have demonstrated that numerous factors can influence various features of reaction to maternal separation in nonhuman primates, including species, age at separation, nature of the attachment relationship with mother prior to separation, duration of separation, nature of the separation (and reunion) environment, and availability of substitute caretakers during the time away from the mother (e.g., Mineka & Suomi, 1978). What is clear, however, is that forced separation from the mother is almost always a traumatic experience for primate infants, at least initially, and it almost always results in profound behavioral and emotional disruption, along with dramatic activation of several physiological systems. It is also clear that there are marked individual differences within primate species in the relative severity and duration of separation-induced distress.

An increasing body of data has documented long-term consequences for at least some individuals who have experienced traumatic maternal separation early in life. These individuals tend to react to subsequent stressful situations with exaggerated behavioral and physiological reactions (e.g., greater and more prolonged elevation of cortisol levels) relative to individuals who did not experience the early trauma or those who did but whose reactions at the time were mild. Other forms of early trauma or stress (e.g., exposure to extreme fear-provoking stimuli) appear to have generally parallel psychobiological consequences (cf. Suomi, 1995).

In some cases, the long-term effects of early stress or trauma are expressed in domains seemingly far removed from the initial experience. For example, squirrel monkey males who experienced brief maternal separations in their first few months of life undergo puberty many months earlier on average than nonseparated cagemates (Levine, Weiner, & Coe, 1993). Rhesus monkey adolescents who experienced maternal deprivation during their first 6 months of life tend to consume significantly more alcohol in a "happy hour"–like situation than monkeys reared by their mothers during that initial 6 months (Higley, Hasert, Suomi, & Linnoila, 1991). Rhesus monkey females who were neglected or abused by their own mothers during infancy have a much higher incidence of neglecting and/or abusing their own firstborn offspring than primiparous females who received normal caregiving from their own mothers during infancy (Ruppenthal, Arling, Harlow, Sackett, & Suomi, 1976; Seay, Alexander, & Harlow, 1964). Adolescent male rhesus monkeys who likewise experienced inadequate parenting as infants are much more likely to exhibit explosive bouts of impulsive aggression and have lower rates of central serotonin turnover than their normally reared agemates (Higley, Linnoila, & Suomi, 1994). These diverse examples clearly demonstrate that early experience with trauma can have significant long-term (and sometimes lifelong) consequences for both behavioral and psychobiological functioning.

What about the possibility of cross-generational transmission of some effects of early trauma in primates? Are there ways in which trauma experienced in one generation of primates can be "transmitted"—in the form of behavioral and/or psychobiological dysfunction—to the next generation? With humans, the answer seems to be relatively clear, as evidenced by numerous chapters in this volume. Humans, of course, can use oral and written language to recall and retell past experiences, including pleasant as well as terrifying ones, to members of subsequent generations. Nonhuman primates have neither oral nor written language (as we know it). Are there other ways by which traumatic experiences of one generation of monkeys or apes could have specific and significant behavioral and psychobiological consequences for subsequent generations? The data to date suggest at least three modes for such cross-generational transmission in primates. The first mode is via observational learning; the second encompasses maternal treatment of offspring, and the third involves prenatal mechanisms. Each is considered in turn.

Cross-Generational Transmission via Observational Learning

One potential way for the effects of trauma experienced by members of one generation to be passed on to the next generation is via observational learning. Among humans, observational learning provides a highly efficient means of transmitting certain types of information between individuals or groups. Observational learning and related forms of knowledge acquisition (e.g., social facilitation, imitation, and direct modeling) do not require language to be effective as "teaching devices" (although appropriate use of language usually facilitates the process) and hence can be used with individuals who are not fluent in the language of the "teacher" or "model," such as preverbal infants and toddlers or members of a different culture.

The degree to which animals are capable of learning via observation has been the subject of considerable research and even more debate over the years. At issue have been arguments regarding the operational definition of observational learning, sufficient and necessary conditions for its demonstration, the nature and scope of information that can be effectively transmitted, and differences between and within species in its efficacy. Although a discussion of these issues is well beyond the scope of this chapter, it is worth noting that (1) simian primates (i.e., monkeys, apes, and humans) are usually considered to have the most advanced observational learning capabilities among all animals (e.g., Seyfarth & Cheney, 1990), and (2) some types of information are much more readily and effectively transmitted via observational means than are others. For example, capuchin monkeys (Cebus apella), a species of primates with unusual tool-using capabilities, are quite capable of using observational learning techniques to discover the location of preferred food types but are surprisingly unable to learn how to use a particular tool to access such food by watching the performance of a skilled model; instead, they must learn individually on a trial-and-error basis (Visalberghi & Fragaszy, 1990).

In contrast, chimpanzee juveniles apparently acquire considerable tool-using proficiency simply by watching their mothers in action.

The potential for observational learning to provide a mechanism for cross-generational transmission of the effects of trauma is nicely illustrated through some elegant experiments by Susan Mineka and her colleagues regarding the acquisition of snake "phobias" by rhesus monkeys born and raised in captivity (Mineka, Davidson, Cooke, & Keir, 1984). The original impetus for these studies came from the long-standing observation by researchers working with captive primates that whereas virtually every wild-caught subject brought into laboratory settings spontaneously exhibited an intense fear of snakes, few if any laboratory-born subjects ever displayed any evidence of fearful or avoidant behavior, or any indications of emotional arousal, when exposed to live or artificial snakes. Such observations obviously challenged previous assumptions that primates have an "innate" fear of snake-like stimuli and additionally raised the question as to how wild-born monkeys and apes actually acquired their "universal" snake phobia.

Mineka hypothesized that observational learning might provide the vehicle by which fear of snakes could be acquired by primates growing up in habitats that contained snakes—that youngsters might learn such fears by observing the reactions of their mothers and others in their social group to the presence of snakes and other potential predators. In an exquisitely controlled series of studies, she was able to demonstrate clearly and convincingly that juvenile monkeys previously indifferent to live snakes quickly acquired an intense fear of snake stimuli when they observed another monkey (especially their mother) exhibit a fearful reaction to their presence. The juveniles' acquired fearful responses included visceral as well as behavioral components. Most importantly, the emergence of such psychobiological reactions in the presence of a fearful model was immediate (always within a single exposure) and essentially permanent (virtually impossible to extinguish) (Mineka *et al.*, 1984).

It is easy to see how such a mechanism for acquiring fear of potentially lethal stimuli would be adaptive in the wild. This very specific form of observational learning is quickly and permanently acquired. Furthermore, it occurs without requiring the juvenile to have any actual physical contact with snakes (e.g., a bite or constriction) in order to develop an intense aversion to them or to similar stimuli. Indeed, one can envision how generation after generation of rhesus monkeys could readily sustain such an intense aversion without any individual actually getting killed or injured by snakes throughout this process.

This example serves as an illustration of how the consequences of traumatic experience for certain individuals might be passed on to progeny via observational learning mechanisms. To the extent that such individuals continued to exhibit emotionally intense reactions in the face of stimuli associated with the original trauma, the likelihood that their offspring would acquire a parallel behavioral and psychobiological response set to the same or similar stimuli would clearly be enhanced if such observational learning mechanisms were indeed operative. Unfortunately, to date, there have been precious few studies directly examining whether observational learning of specific fears associated with previous trauma actually occurs among wild-living primates, although the data that do exist appear promising. For example, Seyfarth, Cheney, and Marler (1980) demonstrated that young vervet monkeys rapidly learn to respond to different alarm calls by older group members with predator-specific escape behaviors (e.g., seeking cover in response to a "raptor" call vs. climbing a tree in response to a "snake" call). Such learning undoubtedly occurs via observation of the specific escape behaviors (and associated emotional arousal) shown by adults, especially kin, and apparently does not require observation of actual predation to be effective.

Thus, there exist at least some data from both laboratory and field studies suggesting that monkeys can indeed pass specific fears on to the next generation. To be sure, a great deal remains to be learned about this phenomenon, including sufficient and necessary conditions for its occurence, the magnitude and duration of physiological concomitants, and its specificity and generalizability to other stimuli and situations. Nevertheless, the evidence to date clearly establishes that observational learning can provide one pathway for intergenerational transmission of the consequences of trauma, a pathway that does not require either spoken or written language to be effective.

If monkeys are indeed capable of developing aversive psychobiological response patterns to stimuli toward which they observe their parents responding with fear and avoidance, it would seem likely that humans have at least as powerful observational learning capabilities. Such capabilities need not require language for effective cross-generational transmission; indeed, they might occur in spite of language. Perhaps the most striking aspect of the observational learning of specific fears in monkeys is its permanence: Mineka and her colleagues expressed some surprise as to how difficult it was to extinguish such emotional response patterns once acquired. Other investigators (e.g., LeDoux and his colleagues) have demonstrated a limbic system–based emotional memory system that operates essentially independent of any cortical input (such as linguistic information; cf. LeDoux, 1986). It may well be that emotional responses acquired via observational learning in humans are similarly highly resistant to extinction. If such responses are not dependent on language for either their acquisition or their long-term maintenance, then it may also be the case that language-based interventions or therapies might be relatively ineffective in extinguishing such acquired fears.

Cross-Generational Transmission via Effects on Maternal Behavior

A second way in which the consequences of traumatic stress can be transmitted to the next generation is through effects on maternal behavior. This can occur in primates when trauma and its sequelae compromise an individual's capabilities as a parent. Inadequate parenting, in turn, can affect an offspring's well-being and adaptive capabilities, both in the short and long term. Such effects include physiological functioning as well as behavioral competence.

Unlike the case for observational learning of trauma consequences, the database in primates documenting long-term effects of inadequate parenting on progeny is quite impressive. Over 30 years ago, Harlow and his colleagues demonstrated convincingly that rhesus monkey "motherless mothers," that is, females who were raised in isolation, with surrogates or with peers—but not with their own mothers—were at exceedingly high risk for showing major deficits in their care of firstborn offspring, including high rates of neglect and abuse (Seay *et al.*, 1964). Subsequent research in Harlow's laboratory demonstrated that (1) the nature and duration of the early deprivation was predictive of subsequent deficits in maternal behavior; (2) there were several ways in which the risk for "motherless mothers" exhibiting inadequate maternal behavior could be significantly reduced; these "interventions" were most effective when they were introduced during these females' juvenile and adolescent years; and (3) even in the absence of such intervention (and especially in its presence), the risk for inadequate maternal behavior by motherless mothers toward their second-born and subsequent offspring was greatly reduced (Ruppenthal *et al.*, 1976). These findings suggested that even the most severe early deprivations need not inevitably result in aberrant maternal behavior; instead, effective preventive interventions could be developed in most cases.

Other primate researchers have examined the effects on maternal behavior of less severe and long-lasting environmental stressors than total maternal deprivation initiated at birth. For example, Rosenblum and his colleagues demonstrated that changes in food accessibility and availability for mothers had clear-cut "carryover" effects to their treatment of offspring, over and above any effects on their interactions with others in their social group (Andrews & Rosenblum, 1994). Other researchers have found predictable relationships between changes in a mother's position in her group's dominance hierarchy and disruption of her behavior with her offspring. These effects, seen in both laboratory and field studies, are most pronounced when mothers exhibit dramatic drops in status, but they also can occur in the face of general instability of dominance relationships (e.g., that result from changes in overall group composition).

What is the nature and extent of cross-generational psychobiological consequences of stress or trauma experienced by a mother? One general consequence that seems to transcend the specific types of trauma experienced by the mother involves the compromising of a secure attachment relationship with her infant. Offspring of stressed-out monkey mothers are much less likely to develop and maintain secure attachment relationships than those whose mothers live in stable, benign social settings. In turn, infants with insecure attachments are less likely to use their mothers as a secure base to explore their physical and social environment throughout their first year of life (Suomi, 1995). One long-term consequence emerges in play patterns with peers. Monkey juveniles with insecure maternal attachments typically play less often and are less sophisticated in their interactions with securely attached peers. When they reach adolescence, monkeys who grew up with insecure early attachments are at risk to develop impulsive, socially incompetent, and often inappropriately aggressive patterns of response to seemingly neutral social stimuli. They usually end up at or near the bottom of their peer group's dominance hierarchy (Higley & Suomi, 1996).

Perhaps the most dramatic long-term consequence for offspring of mothers exposed to stress is their own subsequent psychobiological responses to novel and/or stressful stimuli or circumstances. In a word, offspring of stressed-out mothers tend to overreact both behaviorally and physiologically to their own encounters with stress. For example, infants and juvenile monkeys with anxious attachments react to brief separation not only with more extreme and more prolonged behavioral disruption, but also with higher and longer lasting elevations of plasma cortisol, greater central NE turnover, and a greater degree of immune system suppression than their securely attached agemates (Suomi, 1995). Other risks associated with disrupted early maternal experiences may be more subtle, sometimes masked for years. For example, Rosenblum and his colleagues found that monkeys whose mothers experienced variable food availability when they were infants were in turn much more behaviorally and physiologically reactive (e.g., greater HPA activation and monoamine turnover) when exposed to a pharmacological challenge as adolescents (Rosenblum et al., 1994).

One of the most intriguing long-term consequences of disruption of an infant's early attachment relationship with its caregiver is the effect on its own capabilities as a parent when it becomes an adult. An increasing body of data collected in both laboratory and field environments has documented remarkable specificity of cross-generational consequences of deficits in parenting behavior: Female monkey infants who experienced certain abnormalities in the care they received from their own mothers (or substitute caregivers) tend to exhibit virtually identical or highly similar abnormalities toward their own offspring when they become parents themselves. Such cross-generational specificity is especially clear-cut in terms of patterns of ventral–ventral contact (cradling) between monkey mothers and infants.

Numerous studies have shown that ventral–ventral contact is crucial for developing and sustaining normal attachment relationships in Old World monkeys and apes. Typically, infants in these species spend virtually all of their initial days and weeks of life in ventral–ventral contact with their mother, and they gradually reduce the frequency and duration of such contact in the ensuing weeks and months. Indeed, some investigators have viewed ventral–ventral contact as a rough index of, or proxy for, maternal "warmth." At any rate, several studies have reported a highly predictive relationship between the precise amount and developmental pattern of ventral–ventral contact a female receives from her mother as an infant and the amount and patterning of contact she directs toward offspring when she becomes a mother herself. For example, females who experienced greater than normal amounts of ventral–ventral contact as infants tend to contact their own infants excessively, whereas females who were relatively contact-deprived as infants tend to be contact-shy with their own offspring (Fairbanks, 1989). These predictive relationships are especially strong when the early contact experience is most aberrant, as in the case of peer- or surrogate-reared females (Champoux, Byrne, Delizio, & Suomi, 1992).

Recent theoretical and empirical work on long-term consequences of differential early attachment relationships in humans has also focused on possible cross-generational continuities in attachment style, including specific parenting behaviors. The results to date have generally been highly congruent with the primate data described earlier. For example, mothers who experienced secure attachments as infants and young children tend to develop secure attachments with their own infants, whereas those who experienced avoidant, ambivalent, or disorganized attachment with their mothers tend to promote avoidant, ambivalent, and disorganized-like attachments, respectively, as mothers themselves. Current attachment theorizing attributes these infancy-to-parenthood continuities in attachment type to internalized "working models" initially based on early memories and periodically transformed by more recent experiences (e.g., those accrued during adolescence). Such "working models" are generally thought to involve complex cognitive imagery and mental representational capabilities not usually ascribed to monkeys or even to apes. However, the primate data clearly suggest that such "advanced" human cognitive capabilities need not be prerequisites for cross-generational transmission of specific patterns of parental behavior. Indeed, they raise the distinct possibility that more "primitive" emotional memory processes might also be involved in the parallel human phenomenon (cf. Suomi, 1995).

Cross-Generational Transmission via Prenatal Mechanisms

A third way in which the psychobiological consequences of trauma might be transmitted across generations of primates involves prenatal mechanisms. According to this view, normal developmental processes transpiring during gestation might be comprised as a result of stress experienced by the mother-to-be during her pregnancy. Such effects could occur either by relatively direct means, for example, via transmission of maternal cortisol across the placental barrier resulting in fetal exposure to high and/or chronic glucocorticoid elevation, or through more indirect mechanisms, for example, changes in fetal nutrition resulting from stress-induced changes in maternal eating behavior, or fetal reactions to stress-induced physical and/or physiological changes in the intrauterine environment.

Recent research by Schneider and her colleagues strongly suggests that such prenatal mechanisms are more than merely hypothetical in nature (Schneider, 1992). These researchers subjected pregnant rhesus monkeys to brief (10 minutes) periods of exposure to a mild stressor 5 days per week for 8 weeks during pregnancy (normal gestation for rhesus monkeys is 21–22 weeks). The daily stressor involved removing each pregnant female from her home cage, placing her in a smaller cage in a darkened room, and randomly administering three 10-second noise bursts from a 1300 Hz horn at 115 db over a 10-minute period, then returning the pregnant female to her home cage. This procedure routinely produced short-term behavioral agitation and brief cortisol elevation in the pregnant females but no obvious effects on their home-cage behavior or food consumption. The offspring of these females were then compared with offspring of females who had not been exposed to the noise stressor, but whose living arrangements and diets were otherwise identical during pregnancy. Both prenatally stressed and control infants were nursery-reared from birth and socialized with peers in order to eliminate potential variance resulting from differential postnatal treatment by their mothers, and their subsequent behavioral, cognitive, and physiological development was systematically monitored as they grew up in comparable physical and social environments.

Schneider and her colleagues found significant differences between prenatally stressed and control infants on numerous measures, both behavioral and physiological, throughout development. In general, the prenatal exposure to stress had the effect of making these monkeys more reactive to mildly stressful events and situations throughout development. For example, when these monkeys were placed in a novel playroom filled with toys and unfamiliar peers, they were less likely to explore the playroom, manipulate the toys, or initiate interactions with peers than were the offspring of control mothers who had not experienced the stress during pregnancy. Prenatally stressed monkeys also exhibited greater and more prolonged elevation of plasma cortisol and ACTH during their playroom sessions than did their agemates who were not prenatally stressed. Similar behavioral and physiological differences emerged when these monkeys were briefly separated from their respective social groups as juveniles and adolescents. Thus, 10-minute daily exposure to unpredictable noise over an 8-week period during pregnancy was sufficient to produce long-term behavioral and physiological effects in the offspring under subsequent conditions of environmental novelty and challenge (Clarke & Schneider, in press).

Schneider and her colleagues also studied another group of rhesus monkey infants whose mothers had experienced a physiological stressor on a daily basis over the same part of pregnancy as described earlier. In this case, the stressor involved exogenous adminstration of ACTH, which had the effect of briefly raising these females' plasma cortisol levels even though they remained in their home cases during this procedure. The postnatal effects on their offspring were remarkably similar to those resulting from prenatal exposure to the unpredictable noise. These youngsters likewise exhibited increased stress reactivity, as indexed by behavioral disruption and elevated plasma cortisol and ACTH, when faced with novel or challenging situations throughout development (Schneider, 1992).

These findings suggest that different types of prenatal stress that result in maternal glucocorticoid elevation have common consequences, most notably the tendency to "overreact" both behaviorally and physiologically to postnatal environmental challenges. In this respect, prenatally stressed monkeys clearly resemble individuals who experienced trauma in their early postnatal life, either directly or indirectly, as a result of their mothers' previous experience with trauma. The common feature is increased reactivity to subsequent environmental stressors. Such increased reactivity clearly does not require human linguistic or other advanced cognitive capabilities to become a prominent part of an individual's psychobiological response repertoire.

INTERACTIONS AND IMPLICATIONS

The research described in the preceding sections provides clear-cut evidence, obtained from prospective longitudinal experiments, demonstrating that nonhuman primates are indeed capable of transmitting long-term psychobiological effects of trauma across generations via at least three different mechanisms. In each case, the long-term effects include physiological as well as behavioral features or propensities, and in two of the three cases, the mechanisms of transmission have been documented in natural social groups of primates living in the wild as well as those studied in laboratory settings. None of the three mechanisms—observational, maternal, and prenatal—require language capabilities on the part of either the initiating or receiving generation for the transmission to take place.

These three mechanisms differ considerably with respect to the potential specificity and timing of the cross-generational transmission. Observational learning, in theory, is quite specific with respect to the type of stimulus that generates the cross-generational psychobiological effects; on the other hand, it can transpire at any time and to anyone in an individual's social sphere. Psychobiological effects of trauma transmitted via maternal behavior patterns involve a much wider range of stimuli and situations that potentially can affect how a mother acts, but such effects are typically limited to offspring and, then, largely to their period of maternal dependence. Effects of trauma that are transmitted via prenatal mechanisms can theoretically come from anything that raises a pregnant female's cortisol levels, but those effects are obviously limited to the period of pregnancy and affect only the fetus. Despite these differences, it can be argued that each mechanism can produce remarkably similar consequences for those in the next generation—increased behavioral and physiological reactivity in the face of environmental novelty and/or challenge.

Although these three pathways for cross-generational transmission can be distinguished from one another on a number of dimensions, they clearly need not be mutually exclusive. Rather, it is easy to envision how they might interact within a given individual and/or have cumulative effects for that individual. Consider, for example, what might transpire if a rhesus monkey female in the middle of her second pregnancy lived through a series of violent thunderstorms that uprooted many trees and bushes, killing some members of her social group, including relatives, in the process. One immediate consequence would be acute and dramatic elevation of the female's cortisol levels during the storms, producing effects on the fetus that would be reflected postnatally in increased psychobiological reactivity to subsequent stressful situations.

In addition, the habitat destruction and social disruption created by the series of storms might well have long-term consequences for the young mother after her infant was born. Specifically, her food supply might be more variable and less predictable, the habitat destruction might make her and the rest of her social group more vulnerable to predation, and her position in the group's dominance hierarchy might plummet as a result of loss of social support her now-deceased relatives might have provided. Each of these factors could compromise the care of her new infant, increasing its psychobiological reactivity in the face of subsequent stressors over and above any bias resulting from its prenatal stress experiences. In contrast, the consequences of the same factors for the female's firstborn offspring would likely be considerably less than those for its younger sibling, because it had not received comparable prenatal stress and, being older, would not have been as dependent on the mother during the time her maternal capabilities were being influenced by long-term sequelae of the storms.

Finally, the infant who experienced the storm prenatally might additionally be especially sensitive to the effects of subsequent violent storms, particularly if it witnessed storm-related fear responses by its mother to flashes of lightning or claps of thunder. To be sure, its older sibling (and others in the social group) might also witness the mother's reactions and indeed might have some of their own. However, it seems likely that the infant's psychobiological reaction would be even more extreme because (1) the mother would have greater salience as a model, and (2) the infant's threshold for responding would be lower and the magnitude and duration of response greater as a long-term consequence of the previous prenatal and maternal experiences. Such exaggerated responses to tropical storms might well be expected to continue throughout the infant's lifetime—and possibly be transmitted to any offspring she herself might have in the future.

This admittedly hypothetical example illustrates one way in which different modes of cross-generational transmission of psychobiological effects of trauma can interact and/or have cumulative long-term consequences for certain individuals. While carefully controlled prospective laboratory experiments can clearly identify, differentiate, and even isolate specific modes, nature is usually much messier in its "natural experiments." This is doubtlessly as true for humans as it is for rhesus monkeys and other primates.

What implications do these studies of the cross-generational psychobiological consequences of trauma in nonhuman primates have for consideration of the human case? To be sure, monkeys are not furry little humans with tails but rather members of other species, albeit with considerable genetic overlap and some commonality in evolutionary history. Furthermore, as previously mentioned, monkeys and apes lack the linguistic capabilities that make our history, our cultures, and our experiences—both good and bad—uniquely human. Nevertheless, it seems hard to believe that the same mechanisms that permit cross-generational transmission of psychobiological effects of trauma in nonhuman primate species would not be operative in humans as well. Such mechanisms require no special cultural traditions, special instructions, or advanced cognitive or linguistic capabilities to transpire—and they have undoubtedly transpired generation after generation for millions of years in our closest primate relatives. On the other hand, our unique human capabilities do enable us to study these phenomena, to try to comprehend how and why they occur, and to consider how they might contribute to cross-generational effects of trauma on ourselves and our progeny. We will fail to engage such capabilities at our own peril.

REFERENCES

Andrews, M. W., & Rosenblum, L. A. (1994). The development of affiliative and agonistic social patterns in differentially reared monkeys. *Child Development, 65,* 1398–1404.

Berman, C. M., Rasmussen, K. L. R., & Suomi, S. J. (1994). Responses of free-ranging rhesus monkeys to a natural form of social separation: I. Parallels with mother–infant separation in captivity. *Child Development, 65,* 1028–1041.

Bowlby, J. (1960). Grief and mourning in infancy and early childhood. *Psychoanalytic Study of the Child, 15,* 9–52.

Bowlby, J. (1973). *Separation.* New York: Basic Books.

Champoux, M., Byrne, E., Delizio, R., & Suomi, S. J. (1992). Motherless mothers revisited: Rhesus maternal behavior and rearing history. *Primates, 33,* 251–255.

Clarke, A. S., & Schneider, M. L. (in press). Prenatal stress alters social and adaptive behavior in adolescent rhesus monkeys. *Annals of the New York Academy of Science.*

Denenberg, V. H. (1970). Experimental programming of life histories and the creation of individual differences: A review. In M. R. Jones (Ed.), *Miami Symposium on Prediction of Behavior,* pp. 62–98. Coral Gables, FL: University of Miami Press.

Deneberg, V. H., & Whimby, A. E. (1963). Behavior of adult rats is modified by the experiences their mothers had as infants. *Science, 142,* 1192–1193.

Fairbanks, L. A. (1989). Early experience and cross-generational continuity of mother–infant contact in vervet monkeys. *Developmental Psychobiology, 22,* 669–681.

Harlow, H. F., Suomi, S. J., & Gluck, J. P. (1972). Generalization of behavioral data between nonhuman and human animals. *American Psychologist, 27,* 709–716.

Higley, J. D., Hasert, M. L., Suomi, S. J., & Linnoila, M. (1991). A new nonhuman primate model of alcohol abuse: Effects of early experience, personality, and stress on alcohol consumption. *Proceedings of the National Academy of Science, 41,* 308–314.

Higley, J. D., Linnoila, M., & Suomi, S. J. (1994). Ethological contributions. In R. T. Amerman (Ed.), *Handbook of aggressive behavior* (pp. 17–32). New York: Raven Press.

Higley, S. J., & Suomi, S. J. (1996). Reactivity and social competence affect individual differences in reaction to severe stress in children: Investigations using nonhuman primates. In C. R. Pfeffer (Ed.), *Intense stress and mental disturbances in children* (pp. 3–58). New York: American Psychiatric Press.

LeDoux, J. E. (1986). Sensory systems and emotion: A model of affective processing. *Integrative Psychiatry, 4,* 237–248.

Levine, S. (1960). Stimulation in infancy. *Scientific American, 202,* 80–86.

Levine, S. (1967). Maternal and environmental influences on the adrenocortical response to stress in weanling rats. *Science, 156,* 258–260.

Levine, S. (1994). The ontogeny of the hypothalamic pituitary adrenal axis: The influence of maternal factors. In E. R. de Kloet, E. C. Azmitia, & P. W. Lamgfield (Eds.), *Annals of the New York Academy of Sciences, 746,* 275–293.

Levine, S., Chevalier, J. A., & Korchin, S. J. (1956). The effects of early shock and handling on later avoidance learning. *Journal of Personality, 24,* 475–493.

Levine, S., Weiner, S. G., & Coe, C. L. (1993). Temporal and social factors influencing behavioral and hormonal responses to separation in mother and infant squirrel monkeys. *Psychoneuroendocrinology, 18,* 297–306.

Lovejoy, C. O. (1981). The origins of man. *Science, 211,* 341–350.

Meaney, M. J., Aitken, D. H., Sharma S., Viau, V., Sarrieau, A. (1989). Postnatal handling increases hippocampal glucocorticoid receptors and enhances adrenocortical negative-feedback efficacy. *Neuroendocrinology, 55,* 204–213.

Meany, M. J., Bhatnagar, S., Larocque, S., McCormick, C., Shanks, N., Sharma, S., Smythe, J., Viau, V., & Plotsky, P. M. (1993). Individual differences in the hypothalmic–pituitary–adrenal stress response and the hypothalmic CRF system. In C. Rivier & Y. Tachet (Eds.), *Annals of the New York Academy of Sciences, 697,* 70–85.

Mineka, S., & Suomi, S. J. (1978). Social separation in monkeys. *Psychological Bulletin, 85,* 1376–1400.

Mineka, S., Davidson, M., Cooke, M., & Keir, R. (1984). Observational conditioning of snake fear in rhesus monkeys. *Journal of Abnormal Psychology, 93,* 355–372.

Plotsky, P. M., & Meaney, M. J. (1993). Early postnatal experience alters hypothalamic releasing factor (CRF) mRNA, median eminence CRF content and stress induced release in adult rats. *Molecular Brain Research, 18,* 195–200.

Rosenblum, L. A., Coplan, J. D., Friedman, S., Bassoff, T., Gorman, J. M., & Andrews, M. W. (1994). Adverse early experiences affect noradrenergic and serotonergic functioning in adult primates. *Biological Psychiatry, 35,* 221–227.

Ruppenthal, G. C., Arling, G. L., Harlow, H. F., Sackett, G. P., & Suomi, S. J. (1976). A 10-year perspective on motherless mother monkey behavior. *Journal of Abnormal Psychology, 85,* 341–349.

Schneider, M. L. (1992). Delayed object permanence in prenatally stressed rhesus monkey infants. *Occupational Therapy Journal of Research, 12,* 96–110.

Seay, B. M., Alexander, B. K., & Harlow, H. F. (1964). Maternal behavior of socially deprived rhesus monkeys. *Journal of Abnormal and Social Psychology, 69,* 345–354.

Seay, B. M., Hansen, E. W., & Harlow, H. F. (1962). Mother–infant separation in monkeys. *Journal of Child Psychology and Psychiatry, 3,* 123–132.

Seyfarth, R. M., & Cheney, D. L. (1990). *How monkeys view the world.* Chicago: University of Chicago Press.

Seyfarth, R. M., Cheney, D. L., & Marler, P. (1980). Monkey responses to three different alarm calls: Evidence for predator classification and semantic communication. *Science, 210,* 801–803.

Suomi, S. J. (1991). Primate separation models of affective disorders. In J. Madden (Ed.), *Neurobiology of learning, emotion, and affect* (pp. 195–214). New York: Raven Press.

Suomi, S. J. (1995). Influence of Bowlby's attachment theory on research on nonhuman primate biobehavioral development. In S. Goldberg, R. Muir, & J. Kerr (Eds.), *Attachment theory: Social, developmental, and clinical perspectives* (pp. 185–201). Hillsdale, NJ: Analytic Press.

Suomi, S. J., & Immelman, K. (1983). On the product and process of cross-species generalization. In D. W. Rajecki (Ed.), *Studying man studying animals* (pp. 203–223). New York: Plenum Press.

Visalberghi, E., & Fragaszy, D. M. (1990). Do monkeys ape? In S. Parker & K. Gibson (Eds.), *Language and intelligence in monkeys and apes* (pp. 247–273). Cambridge, UK: Cambridge University Press.

37

Phenomenology and Psychobiology of the Intergenerational Response to Trauma

RACHEL YEHUDA, JIM SCHMEIDLER, ABBIE ELKIN,
SKYE WILSON, LARRY SIEVER, KAREN BINDER-BRYNES,
MILTON WAINBERG, and DAN AFERIOT

INTRODUCTION

The literature describing the effects of the Holocaust on offspring of survivors has developed in a parallel fashion to the literature describing the effects of the Holocaust on its survivors. Early descriptions of the "Survivor Syndrome" arose as clinicians began to realize that classical psychoanalytic views of depression, mourning, and responses to trauma did not provide an adequate framework for understanding and treating Holocaust survivors. The classic observations describing severe symptomatology, maladjustment, and impairment of functioning were made on treatment-seeking individuals, many of whom were being evaluated for compensation or reparations, who did not benefit from psychoanalytic therapy (e.g., Chodoff, 1963; Eitinger, 1961; Krystal, 1968; Neiderland, 1969).

The literature on the effects of offspring also began with clinical anecdotal observations that children of Holocaust survivors appeared to display an increased incidence of psychological problems (Rakoff, 1966; Rakoff, Sigal, & Epstein, 1976; Trossman, 1968) that were also not resolved by classic psychoanalytic therapy (Barocas & Barocas, 1983; Danieli, 1981). These observations appeared soon after the descriptions of concentration camp syndrome. The early observations comparing children of survivors, then mostly children and adolescents, to those of nonsurvivor children and adolescents are noteworthy. Rakoff *et al.* (1976) and Sigal and Weinfeld (1985) indicated a greater incidence of depression, anxiety, and maladaptive behavior such as conduct disorder, personality problems, inadequate maturity, excessive dependence, and poor coping problems in them. Offspring of Holocaust survivors were also

RACHEL YEHUDA, JIM SCHMEIDLER, ABBIE ELKIN, SKYE WILSON, LARRY SIEVER, KAREN BINDER-BRYNES, MILTON WAINBERG, and DAN AFERIOT • Mount Sinai Traumatic Stress Studies Program, Mount Sinai School of Medicine and Bronx Veterans Affairs Hospital, Bronx, New York 10468.

International Handbook of Multigenerational Legacies of Trauma, edited by Yael Danieli. Plenum Press, New York, 1998.

reported to have more physical ailments (Waldfogel, 1991) and were described as having a general vulnerability to stress (Barocas & Barocas, 1983; Danieli, 1981). In one of the more provocative findings, Solomon, Kotler, and Mikulincer (1988) reported that offspring of Holocaust survivors were more likely than other soldiers to develop posttraumatic stress disorder (PTSD) following deployment in the Lebanon War. This finding further served to underscore the idea of offspring of survivors as more fragile and vulnerable. Barocas and Barocas (1983) commented not only on the alarming number of children of survivors seeking and requiring help, but also on the nature of their symptoms. They stated that offspring of Holocaust survivors "present symptomatology and psychiatric features that bear a striking resemblance to the concentration camp survivor syndrome described in the international literature," and that these children "show symptoms that would be expected if they actually lived through the Holocaust" (p. 332). The observation that children of trauma survivors display PTSD symptoms, but to a lesser extent, was also observed by Rosenheck and Nathan (1985) in their study of children of Vietnam combat veterans. Rosenheck and Nathan termed this phenomenon *secondary traumatization.*

Interestingly, there was an apparent backlash to observations of symptomatology in Holocaust survivors and observations of pathology in their offspring. In contrast to the findings of impairment in Holocaust survivors, for example, a literature arose describing exceptional coping skills among survivors that focused on predictors of subsequent well-being, particularly in nonclinical populations (Dimsdale, 1974; Harel, Kahana, & Kahana, 1988; Kahana, Harel, & Kahana, 1988; Leon, Butcher, Kleinman, Goldberg, & Almagor, 1981). These studies focused on the remarkable adaptive and reintegrative capacities of Holocaust survivors, who demonstrated good social and family functioning, high socioeconomic achievement, good coping skills, and other personal achievements. Interestingly, the describers of coping and resilience chose to call into question the earlier observations of impairment in Holocaust survivors (Harel *et al.,* 1988) on methodological and other grounds, rather than resolve the diversity of opinions and data by acknowledging the broad spectrum of responsivity to trauma, as, for example, Danieli (1981, 1982) was astutely able to do.

There were similar negative responses in the literature on offspring of Holocaust survivors. Many investigations reported a failure to observe differences in psychopathological features characterizing children of survivors (Aleksandrowicz, 1973): Studies of coping and adjustment again found no significant differences between offspring of Holocaust survivors and matched controls on measures of well-being (Zlotogorski, 1983), MMPI-derived (Minnesota Multiphasic Personality Inventory) measures of global mental health (Last & Klein, 1981), or anxiety, depression or adjustment (Rose & Garske, 1987). Again, the best defense mounted against the studies depicting severe psychopathology was a methodological attack. Solkoff's critical review (1992) concluded that almost no study of children of Holocaust survivors fulfilled the necessary methodological criteria of subject selection and other experimental biases. This indictment attempted to render all conclusions in the literature about pathology in offspring practically useless. It is noteworthy that others also reacted quite sharply to methodological biases in studies of offspring that demonstrate weaknesses in these individuals as a group (e.g., Silverman, 1987). Nonetheless, the clinical literature, seemingly oblivious to the implications of these studies, continued to provide case reports and other anecdotal observations of pathology in offspring (Danieli, 1981), and continued to explore treatment strategies for this group (e.g., Kestenberg, 1980; Kinsler, 1981). Thus, with few exceptions, the literature on offspring of Holocaust survivors is divided into two "camps": those who described the adverse effects of the Holocaust, and those failing to note these detrimental effects.

The polarized spectrum of opinions regarding the long-term effects of the Holocaust and the failure to deal systematically or scientifically with this wide diversity is unusual and also informative. Also interesting is the relative failure of the Holocaust literature to become integrated with the larger emerging literature focusing on the effects of other types of trauma exposure. Of particular note in this regard is the conspicuous absence of the concept of PTSD from the Holocaust literature, especially in articles that have been published after 1980, which marked the formal entrance of PTSD into the psychiatric nosology. The heterogeneity reflected in the Holocaust literature is certainly compatible with (and may have contributed to the development of) the now well-established idea that the long-lasting effects of trauma, as reflected by the presence of PTSD, appear in some but not all severely traumatized individuals. Yet only very few studies to date have applied the formal diagnostic criteria for PTSD to Holocaust survivors (Kaminer & Lavie, 1991; Kuch & Cox, 1992; Yehuda, Kahana, Southwick, & Giller, 1994; Yehuda *et al.*, 1995b; Yehuda *et al.*, 1995c), and even fewer have invoked this idea in considering intergenerational syndrome (for exception, see Solomon *et al.*, 1988). It is clear that if Holocaust survivors and their children had been considered from the vantage point of either having or not having posttraumatic stress syndrome, this might have helped clarify prior observations of other aspects of posttraumatic adaptation such as affect dysregulation, character changes, psychiatric comorbidity, and resilience, and might have provided a more cohesive literature. Similarly, exploring the effects of the Holocaust on offspring based on whether they may have been raised by more or less symptomatic parents might yield similar clarity with regard to intergenerational syndromes.

The opposing views of survivors and offspring speaks to the ambivalence of mental health professionals who are searching for the most appropriate way to describe and view victims of trauma (Danieli, 1982; Yehuda & Giller, 1994). To describe severe symptoms as a consequence of trauma exposure, on the one hand, serves to validate the experience of the victim by acknowledging that the traumatic events, rather than some personal flaw, were the cause of resulting symptoms. On the other hand, an acknowledgment of the profound effects of trauma may also serve further to victimize and stigmatize the survivor by implicitly suggesting a permanent damage, which may be quite contradictory to the survivors' perception that they have overcome adversity. Such a view may also promote hopelessness and pessimism in survivors, who may already be prone to these experiences. This issue is further compounded by the catastrophic magnitude of the Holocaust itself. Because the Holocaust was not only a personal trauma for the survivor, but also a conspiracy to eradicate the entire Jewish race, the Holocaust literature becomes much more than a vehicle for describing an individual's struggle with the effects of trauma, but also becomes a historical record of the persecution of the Jews and their ability to overcome this oppression.

Thus, the dilemma that is invariably created is how one goes about documenting the horrors and the permanent scars created by the racial prejudice as a result of the Holocaust while at the same time demonstrating the dignity of the Jewish people and their capacity to survive. To describe Holocaust survivors and their children as vulnerable, particularly if this has biological dimensions, is to document traits similar to the ones that were actually used to justify the extermination of the Jews. On the other hand, to mitigate the scars of the Holocaust is equally problematic and serves as an obstacle to providing the needed resources to help survivors overcome their mental health symptoms. The scientist investigating the effects of the Holocaust must acknowledge the social, political, and humanistic forces that may serve to shape mental health descriptions of the Holocaust in no less serious a manner than the clinician who must explore these very same issues in the context of their implications for countertransference.

When our research group began investigating the phenomenology and neurobiology of posttraumatic adaptations in Holocaust survivors, our aim was to try to view the Holocaust survivor with a lens similar to that which we had been using to study combat veterans. For example, we attempted to utilize the diagnosis of PTSD to subgroup Holocaust survivors. Furthermore, we were interested in examining Holocaust survivors on the same psychological and biological measures that had served to differentiate combat veterans from normal controls. Although we recognized that there were substantial differences between combat veterans (especially Vietnam veterans) and Holocaust survivors (e.g., in length of time since the focal trauma, nature and severity of the trauma, occupational functioning of survivors, incidence of substance abuse, etc.), we believed that it was essential to study Holocaust survivors with the same paradigm, so that both similarities and differences between these groups could be explored. We hypothesized that to the extent that there were commonalities in behavioral and neuroendocrine parameters between Holocaust survivors and other groups of trauma survivors, the variables being examined would explain core features of the response to trauma. To the extent that there would be differences between groups of trauma survivors based on the nature of the trauma, the findings would be less applicable to features of the general response to trauma. This approach allowed an operational scientific perspective with relatively unbiased observation and was hypothesis driven. Indeed, to date, we have been able to demonstrate both similarities (Yehuda *et al.*, 1994, 1995b) and differences (Yehuda *et al.*, 1996) between Holocaust survivors and other trauma survivors using this approach.

In our studies of adult offspring of Holocaust survivors, we attempted to utilize a similar approach to the one used in the study of Holocaust survivors. We believed that by using the same descriptive and biological measures that have been used to study Holocaust survivors, it would be possible to determine similarities and differences between these two groups in a more precise way, and to specifically test the hypothesis that adult children of Holocaust survivors are similar to Holocaust survivors. To the extent that there are commonalities in behavioral and neuroendocrine parameters between Holocaust survivors and other groups of trauma survivors, we hypothesized that these variables might explain core features of the intergenerational syndrome. However, since one of the main features of our work with Holocaust survivors has been the recognition of heterogeneity in this group, a critical variable in our studies of offspring has been to try to determine the parameters that describe individual differences.

Indeed, the problem of how to select appropriate offspring for study and conceptualize their clinical or psychological status has been challenging. In this context, one of the major methodological criticisms that has arisen in studies of Holocaust survivors and offspring of survivors concerns potential biases in the selection of subjects. It is clearly recognized that individuals who agree to participate in this kind of research are a self-selected group and may be quite different from individuals that choose not to participate. Although this kind of bias is inherent in all clinical research studies, it is important to keep this caveat in mind. Obviously, one can only speculate about what could be learned from individuals who decide not to participate in research.

This chapter illustrates the approaches used by our group to arrive at different types of comparisons. Three such approaches and studies are described. The first approach has been to try and examine the relationships between offspring and their own parents. A second approach has been to compare first- and second-generation Holocaust survivors without consideration of familial relationship (i.e., comparing a group of Holocaust survivors to a group of similarly selected but not related offspring of Holocaust survivors) on variables of interest. A third approach has been to explore different subgroups of second-generation offspring and compare these subgroups to demographically matched controls (i.e., Jewish adults with non-European-born parents). The following represents preliminary findings from work in progress.

STUDY 1: EXAMINING THE RELATIONSHIP BETWEEN PTSD SYMPTOMS IN PARENTS AND THEIR OFFSPRING

Rationale

Barocas and Barocas (1983) and Rosenheck and Nathan (1985) suggested that offspring of Holocaust survivors have similar symptoms to those of their parents. The implicit suggestion in these studies was that children "acquire" symptoms that they see their parents experience. Indeed, Solomon *et al.* (1988) suggested that the increased incidence of PTSD following the Lebanon War in the offspring of Holocaust survivors may have been a direct result of the PTSD in the parents:

> The PTSD in the second generation may involve an unmasking of Holocaust-related disturbances or reflect responses that the children "learned" from their survivor parents. For example, the second generation PTSD casualty may have more war-related nightmares than his control group peers because he had seen and heard his parents venting their emotion (p. 868).

No study that we knew of systematically assessed psychiatric diagnoses in parents and their offspring. We were specifically interested in determining whether there would be significant correlations between the PTSD symptoms of the parents and the offspring.

Subject Recruitment

In our initial recruitment, we began by asking the Holocaust survivors we had studied whether they would be interested in telling their children about the research project. The Holocaust survivors in these studies had all been interned in Nazi concentration camps. They were randomly selected from publicly available lists of Holocaust survivors provided by the local historical society and local synagogue membership rosters. They were invited through a mailing to participate in studies exploring the biological basis of survival and adaptation. Subjects who agreed to participate provided written, informed consent and received medical clearance by one of the study physicians. None of the subjects were treatment seekers. Almost all of the Holocaust survivors with children that we studied were amenable to telling their children about the study. Parents were told that children interested in participating in the project should contact the local study coordinator for further information. From this effort, 19 children called us and agreed to participate in the research. Note that although the sample size is relatively small, the subjects were recruited through a relatively nonbiased procedure.

Methods

The 19 second-generation offspring were interviewed using the same structured instruments and ratings as their parents. They were asked whether they felt the Holocaust had been traumatic. They were further queried about PTSD symptoms. The Clinician-Administered PTSD Scale (CAPS; Blake *et al.*, 1990) was used to quantify the frequency and intensity of current and lifetime PTSD in response to the trauma of the Holocaust in these offspring. Subjects also filled out the Dissociative Experiences Scale (DES; Bernstein & Putnam, 1986). Additional information included presence of current and lifetime psychiatric diagnoses as determined by the Structured Clinical Interview for the DSM-III (SCID; Spitzer, Williams, & Gibbon, 1987). A comprehensive trauma history was obtained using the Antonovsky Scale (Antonovsky, 1979), and the Recent Life Events Scale (Kahana & Kahana, 1982).

The responses of the 19 parents and offspring on each individual item of the CAPS and the DES were correlated. Nine of the parents were men, and 10 were women. Eleven of the 19 pairs were of the same sex. Given the small number of subjects and the large number of correlations, the results should not be considered definitive. These are pilot data that are being presented to illustrate the approach we have been trying to develop in our studies.

Results and Conclusions

Nine of the 19 parents met diagnostic criteria for current PTSD according to the CAPS, and 11 of the 19 met diagnostic criteria for past PTSD. Table 1 shows the correlations between the individual PTSD symptoms in the parents and children. Most of the symptoms were not correlated; however, positive correlations were present for flashbacks, avoidance of situations that are reminders of the Holocaust, emotional detachment, and physiological reactivity. Additionally, there was a significant association between dissociative experiences as reflected by DES scores in parents and children.

There are several reasons to be cautious in interpreting these findings. First, the number of subjects is small, and the number of correlations is relatively large. Second, it is unclear from this study whether these current symptoms in either the parent or the children reflected long-term symptoms. However, according to the diagnostic interview, all but 2 of the parents that did not meet current criteria for PTSD also did not meet past criteria for PTSD. Similarly, the parents who did meet criteria for PTSD reported suffering from PTSD symptoms on a chronic basis, but generally tended to indicate that symptoms currently were less severe than they had been in the past.

The results indicate that the level of severity of some PTSD symptoms in parents and their own children are correlated, which supports the suggestions of Barocas and Barocas

Table 1. Correlations between PTSD Symptoms Severity in Holocaust Survivors and their Biological Offspring (*n* = 38)

Symptom	*r*	*p**
B1 intrusive thoughts	.06	
B2 distress at reminders	.00	
B3 flashbacks	.46	.025
B4 nightmares	.33	.085
C1 avoidance of thoughts	.09	
C2 avoidance of situations	.43	.03
C3 psychogenic amnesia	.24	
C4 diminished interest	**	
C5 emotional detachment	.52	.01
C6 restricted range of affect	.26	
C7 sense of foreshortened future	.28	
D1 difficulties with sleep	.10	
D2 irritability	.08	
D3 impaired concentration	.12	
D4 hypervigilence	.09	
D5 increased startle	.10	
D6 physiological reactivity	.63	.002
DES scores	.55	.01

*one-tailed
**two-tailed

(1983), Rosenheck and Nathan (1985), and Solomon *et al.* (1988). There appears to be no specific pattern regarding which of the 17 core symptoms of PTSD are more likely to be correlated between parent and child. In fact, at least one symptom from each of the three symptoms clusters were correlated. Thus, to the extent that the symptoms of PTSD are correlated between parent and child, there does not appear to be a systematic preference for a particular symptom cluster. These results provide at least preliminary support that offspring may be influenced by the symptoms of their parents.

STUDY 2: COMPARING FIRST- AND SECOND-GENERATION SURVIVORS ON BIOLOGICAL VARIABLES: A PILOT STUDY

Rationale

Given that parents and offspring may share symptoms in common, it was reasonable to explore the extent to which first- and second-generation survivors are similar in regard to a biological alteration. Our objective was to compare the urinary cortisol excretion of Holocaust survivors with and without PTSD to those of offspring.

We chose to measure cortisol because levels of this hormone have been found to be altered in individuals with PTSD. Cortisol is a hormone that is released by the adrenal gland. In response to stress, several biological systems are activated in order to allow the body to become mobilized for the "fight-or-flight" reaction (Munck, Guyre, & Holbrook, 1984). During stress, the brain also signals the pituitary gland to stimulate the release of cortisol from the adrenal gland. The function of cortisol in response to stress is to shut down the other biological reactions that have been turned on in order to cope with the short-term demands of a stressor (Munck *et al.,* 1984). If cortisol did not shut off these other reactions, they would do long-term damage to the body. Therefore, it is possible to conceptualize cortisol as an "anti-stress" hormone, because if an organism were unable to produce cortisol in sufficient amounts in response to stress, this would have deleterious consequences.

In conditions of acute and chronic stress, and in certain types of psychiatric disorders that are associated with stress, such as major depression, cortisol levels are high (Mason, Giller, Kosten, Ostroff, & Podd, 1986; Sachar, Hellman, & Roffwarg, 1973), but this sometimes reflects the fact that the hypothalamic–pituitary–adrenal (HPA) axis has grown resistant to the effects of cortisol (Yehuda, Southwick, Krystal, Charney, & Mason, 1993b). The dexamethasone suppression test (DST) has been used as a probe of the HPA axis (Carroll, 1982). Dexamethasone is a synthetic glucocorticoid that mimics the effects of cortisol and allows testing of the effectiveness of the HPA axis in shutting off a stress response. Under normal conditions, the administration of dexamethasone results in a suppression of the body's own cortisol. This indicates that the negative feedback of cortisol is intact and the body is capable of responding to stress or glucocorticoids. However, under conditions of hypercortisolism, such as is observed in major depression, dexamethasone often fails to shut down cortisol levels, resulting in a response called a "nonsuppression." Such a response suggests a defect in the sensitivity of cortisol receptors.

Studies in combat veterans' PTSD have shown that cortisol levels are lower in trauma survivors with PTSD compared to normals and other psychiatric groups (Yehuda *et al.,* 1990, 1993b). Furthermore, individuals with PTSD respond to the administration of dexamethasone by suppressing their own cortisol levels to a greater extent than normals do (Yehuda, Boisoneau, Lowy, & Giller, 1995a; Yehuda *et al.,* 1993b). The hypersuppression of cortisol in response to dexamethasone suggests that the cortisol (or glucocorticoid) receptors in PTSD are very sensitive (Yehuda, Giller, Southwick, Lowy, & Mason, 1991; Yehuda *et al.,* 1995a). Importantly, the hypersuppression is the opposite of the nonsuppression response to dexamethasone observed in depression (Yehuda *et al.,* 1991, 1996). These and other (Yehuda *et al.,* 1996) results suggest that unlike depressed patients who seem relatively unresponsive to the environment, trauma survivors with PTSD may be exquisitely sensitive to external events. The more sensitive cortisol system may account for why trauma survivors show exaggerated responses even to nondangerous environmental stimuli (Yehuda *et al.,* 1996).

Recently, we observed that Holocaust survivors with PTSD also showed significantly lower mean 24-hour cortisol excretion compared to both Holocaust survivors without PTSD and comparison subjects not exposed to the Holocaust (Yehuda *et al.,* 1995b). In this study, 24-hour urine samples were collected, and the following day, subjects were evaluated for the presence and severity of past and current PTSD and other psychiatric conditions. The results demonstrated a significant relationship between cortisol levels and avoidance symptoms. We concluded from these findings that low cortisol levels are associated with PTSD symptoms of a clinically significant nature, rather than occurring as a result of exposure to trauma per se.

Recruitment

For the present study, rather than asking the children of survivors of parents we had already identified to participate as we had done in Study 1, we placed ads in local newspapers around the New York metropolitan area. Many offspring also called us in response to hearing about our research through local television and newspaper articles, and seeing advertisements for our group therapy program.

Methods

Twenty-four offspring participated in the study. For this first preliminary study, the only inclusion criterion was that the subjects have at least one parent who was a Holocaust survivor. Typically, however, most were the offspring of two Holocaust survivors, and almost all had at least one parent who survived concentration camps. None of the offspring were taking any psychotropic medications or drugs that could interfere with cortisol levels. This group was compared to a sample of Holocaust survivors, who were further subgrouped according to the presence ($n = 31$) or absence ($n = 34$) of a PTSD diagnoses (as determined using the CAPS). Data from 46/65 of these patients have recently been reported in Yehuda *et al.* (1995b). However, for that study, subjects with comorbid Axis I diagnoses and those taking psychotropic medications were excluded from the analysis. Since the completion of the study, the sample of survivors has been expanded. Furthermore, because presence of Axis I disorder was not an exclusion criterion in the offspring, we included Holocaust survivors who also had Axis I conditions ($n = 10$): Of the 24 offspring studied, 4 were men and 20 were women. Of the Holocaust survivors studied, 23 were men and 42 were women.

Urine was collected, beginning at 9:00 A.M., in exact 24-hour portions in 2-liter polyethylene bottles kept in freezers in the subjects' residences in order to ensure stability of cortisol. Collections were scheduled to occur on days when subjects planned to be home for the 24-hour period. Clinical assessments took place following the completion of the 24-hour collection, usually within the same week. Urinary-free cortisol levels were determined by using an extraction procedure and radio immunoassay kit from Clinical Assays, Inc.

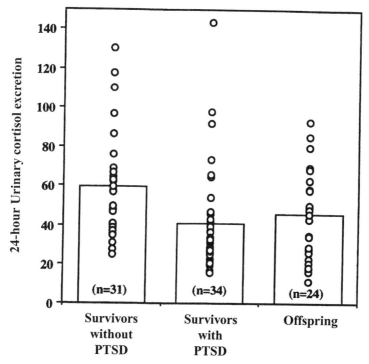

Figure 1. 24-hour urinary cortisol excretion in Holocaust survivors and offspring. (Circles represent raw data for individual cases.)

Results and Conclusions

Overall analysis of variance (ANOVA) demonstrated a main effect of group ($F = 4.04$; $df = 2.86$; $p = .02$). The mean urinary cortisol excretion of Holocaust survivors with and without PTSD was significantly different. The mean cortisol levels were comparable to what we reported previously; however, the PTSD group contains a larger range of values due to the inclusion of some subjects with comorbid major depressive disorder. Post hoc testing using the Scheffe test showed that the offspring group was not significantly different from either survivor group. The results are graphically portrayed in Figure 1. As can be seen by examining the individual scatter points, many of the offspring had cortisol levels that could be considered extremely low (i.e., under 25 ug/day).

STUDY 3: EXPLORING SUBGROUPS OF OFFSPRING AND COMPARING URINARY CORTISOL EXCRETION IN OFFSPRING TO THAT OF DEMOGRAPHICALLY MATCHED NORMALS

Rationale

As more offspring began calling in response to advertisements to participate in the research, we searched for ways to subgroup these individuals based on traumatic experiences or clinical symptomatology. Just as considering Holocaust survivors as a group without consideration of

PTSD diagnoses would have obscured important findings, we felt equally that the offspring of Holocaust survivors should be subgrouped according to similar parameters.

Method

We considered two possible ways to subgroup the offspring of Holocaust survivors. The first was on the basis of whether these individuals met or did not meet the diagnostic criteria for an Axis I psychiatric disorder, as assessed by the SCID. In reviewing the diagnostic history of the 23 offspring described in Table 2 (one SCID could not be completed), we learned that only 10 of these subjects had no current or past psychiatric disorder. Seven of the 23 met criteria for past major depression, and 3 met diagnostic criteria for anxiety disorder (i.e., 2 with past panic disorder, and 1 with past generalized anxiety disorder). Five had current psychiatric disorder (1 met criteria for major depression, 1 for generalized anxiety disorder, 1 for both major depression and generalized anxiety disorder, 1 for attention deficit disorder with depression, and 1 for bulimia with dysthymia and secondary depression).

A major focus of the assessment of offspring was their own history of traumatic events. We were interested in determining whether offspring of Holocaust survivors would be more vulnerable to developing PTSD in response to stressful events. We used several scales to help offspring identify their traumatic events including the Traumatic History Questionnaire (Green *et al.,* unpublished) and the Antonovsky Scale (Antonovsky, 1979). We then queried subjects about PTSD using the CAPS (Blake *et al.,* 1990). This interview was done by asking the subject which traumatic event or events they experienced as the worst, and perhaps might be the focus of PTSD symptomatology. In response to this question, 12/23 of the offspring spontaneously indicated that hearing about their parents' experiences in the Holocaust constituted their trauma (even though almost all of them had undergone extremely stressful events such as being mugged or assaulted, being in motor vehicle accidents, etc.). As being "confronted" with information about trauma exposure in others qualifies in the DSM-IV conception of Criterion A, we felt that we could consider the possibility that offspring may indeed develop PTSD symptoms in response to hearing about their parents' experiences during the Holocaust, particularly if they subjectively stated that such information elicited fear, helplessness, or horror. The other 11 either indicated no traumatic event or stressful events that would not meet the criteria for PTSD under the current DSM-IV stressor criterion (such as losing a sibling or father, having an illness, etc.). The subgroups were similar to each other in total scores on the Traumatic History questionnaire (i.e., the groups were comparable in the extent of "trauma" exposure exclusive of the Holocaust trauma). Subjects also filled out the Civilian Mississippi PTSD Scale (Keane, Caddell, & Taylor, 1991), and the Impact of Events Scale (Horowitz, Wilner, &

Table 2. Mean + *SD* for Mississippi and Impact of Event Scores in Offspring Subgrouped on the Basis of Meeting or Not Meeting Diagnostic Criteria for an Axis I Disorder and Comparison Subjects

Scale	Offspring: Axis I	Offspring: No Axis I	Comparison group
Mississippi PTSD Scale	75.0 + 20.8*	77.65 + 20.4*	59.9 + 7.0
IES total	10.6 + 8.4*	13.9 + 9.3*	1.1 + 2.6
IES Intrusive	6.6 + 5.3*	7.1 + 5.4*	0.9 + 2.5
IES Avoidance	4.0 + 4.0*	0.2 + 0.6*	0.2 + 0.6

*Significantly different than comparison group.

Alvarez, 1979). In filling out the latter scale, subjects were instructed to use the "Holocaust" as the "event."

Using both these methods to subgroup patients, cortisol levels and PTSD symptoms were assessed and compared with a nonoffspring comparison group.

Results and Conclusions

Figure 2 shows the scatterplot of 24-hour urinary cortisol excretion in the offspring group when they are divided based on meeting and not meeting criteria for other Axis I disorders. As can clearly be seen when the offspring group was subdivided in this manner, significantly lower cortisol values were observed in the group without Axis I disorder. An overall ANOVA demonstrated a significant main effect of group $F = 4.98$; $df = 2.30$; $p = .01$. Post hoc testing revealed that the offspring group without Axis I disorder had significantly lower cortisol levels compared to the other two groups. The mean $\pm SD$ urinary cortisol excretion for the offspring group without Axis I disorder was 37.9 ± 20.8. In contrast, the mean cortisol level in the offspring group with Axis I disorder was 60.0 ± 24.0. The mean for comparison subjects was 66.5 ± 30. When scores on the Civilian Mississippi PTSD Scale and the Impact of Events Scale were tabulated, overall ANOVA revealed significant group differences on the Mississippi Scale ($F = 3.36$; $df = 2.29$; $p = .05$), the Impact of Event Total Score ($F = 8.65$; $df = 2.27$; $p = .001$), and Intrusive ($F = 5.76$; $df = 2.27$; $p = .008$) and Avoidance ($F = 8.99$; $df = 2.27$; $p = .001$) subscale scores. In all cases, however, the F tests reflected the fact that both offspring groups were significantly higher on these measures than the comparison group. Post hoc testing showed that the two offspring groups were comparable on these self-reports, as indicated in Table 2.

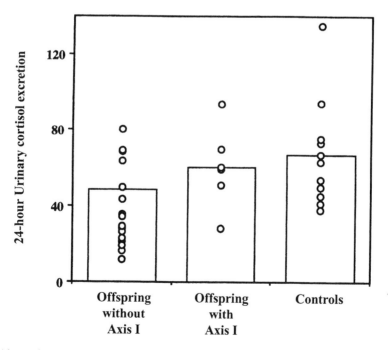

Figure 2. 24-hour urinary cortisol excretion in offspring with or without Axis I disorder and controls. (Circles represent raw data for individual cases.)

Figure 3 shows the scatterplot of 24-hour urinary cortisol excretion in the offspring group when they were divided on the basis of reporting the Holocaust as their major traumatic event during the clinician-rated PTSD interview. As can be clearly seen, when the offspring group was subdivided in this manner, significantly lower cortisol values were observed in the group reporting distress in response to Holocaust-related material. An overall ANOVA demonstrated a significant main effect of group $F = 5.93$; $df = 2.30$; $p = .007$. The mean $\pm$ *SD* urinary cortisol excretion for the offspring group without Holocaust trauma was 54.1 ± 25.7. In contrast, the mean cortisol level in the offspring group with Holocaust trauma was 32.4 ± 14.2. The mean for comparison subjects was 66.53 ± 30. These distinctions do not consider current diagnostic status of the subjects.

When scores on the Civilian Mississippi PTSD Scale and the Impact of Events Scale were tabulated, overall ANOVA revealed significant group differences on the Mississippi Scale ($F = 6.66$; $df = 2.29$; $p = .004$). However, in this case, the offspring groups with and without Holocaust trauma were significantly different. The mean Mississippi PTSD Scale score for offspring with Holocaust trauma was 68.3 ± 14.5, and the mean score for offspring with Holocaust trauma was 84.3 ± 21.6. Note that the mean Mississippi PTSD Scales score for offspring without Holocaust trauma did not differ from the mean Mississippi PTSD Scale score for the comparison subjects (i.e., 59.9 ± 7.0).

Figure 4 graphs the mean Impact of Events Scores in the three groups. ANOVA showed a significant main effect for total Impact of Events scores ($F = 10.9$; $df = 2.27$; $p = .009$), Intrusive subscale scores ($F = 8.46$; $df = 2.27$; $p = .001$), and Avoidance subscale scores ($F =$

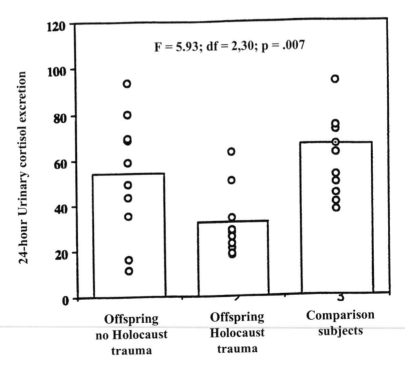

Figure 3. Urinary cortisol excretion in offspring of Holocaust survivors and controls. (Circles represent raw data for individual cases.)

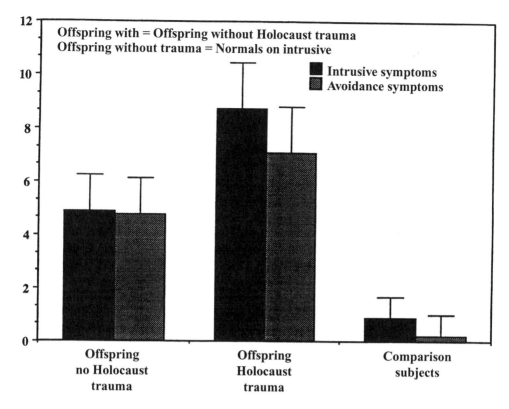

Figure 4. Intrusive and avoidance symptoms in offspring of Holocaust survivors and controls. (Data represent ± standard deviation for intrusive and avoidance symptoms as scored on the Impact of Event Scale.)

8.90; $df = 2.27$; $p = .001$). Figure 5 shows that offspring with Holocaust trauma were significantly more symptomatic on almost each symptoms as assessed by the CAPS. Thus, offspring who report that the Holocaust was the significant traumatic event in their lives also appear to suffer from PTSD symptoms in response to the Holocaust. As Figure 5 indicates, the most common symptoms endorsed were distress at reminders of the Holocaust, emotional detachment, intrusive and distressing thoughts about the Holocaust, sense of foreshortened future, restricted affect, and sleep difficulties. By comparison, offspring without Holocaust trauma reported negligible levels of these symptoms.

In summary, the results indicate that low cortisol levels in offspring of Holocaust survivors were associated with the tendency of these individuals to indicate distress about the trauma of the Holocaust and to have PTSD symptoms in response to Holocaust-related events that they heard about.

The etiology of the PTSD symptoms and low cortisol levels in the offspring studied is currently unknown. There are many potential models that could explain these findings, but more information must be acquired before any of these models can be confidently applied to these observations. The absence of objective and definitive knowledge about the diagnostic status or severity of the trauma of the parent(s) is a critical omission to the biological data obtained in this study. However, such knowledge is not typically available in studies of offspring of trauma survivors. In fact, except for the preliminary observations in Study 1, no investigation of which

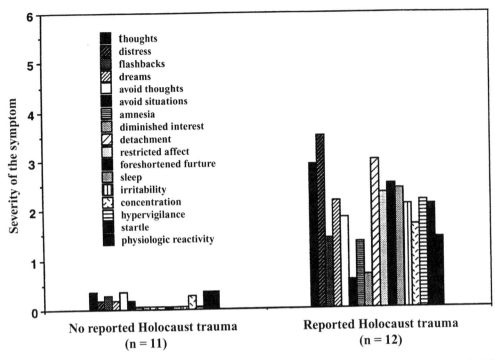

Figure 5. PTSD symptoms in offspring with and without "Holocaust trauma." Data represent mean scores for 17 PTSD symptoms as scored on the Clinician Administered PTSD Scale (CAPS).

we are aware has actually compared the level of PTSD or other psychiatric symptoms in parents and offspring. By omitting these data, studies of offspring assume a homogenous syndrome in the parents. However, our studies of Holocaust survivors have clearly indicated that not all survivors have suffered chronic PTSD symptoms, regardless of the magnitude in all survivors. Therefore, information about parental symptoms and trauma exposure must be considered in formulating a hypothesis of the etiology of PTSD symptoms and biological alterations in offspring. To the extent that such knowledge could be obtained, then it might be possible to determine whether the same biological or psychological risk factors that contribute to the chronic nature of symptoms in the Holocaust survivor parent are relevant to the biological and clinical picture of offspring, or whether symptoms in offspring are due to the impact of psychological or biological impairments in their parents. Although the present studies have not addressed the larger question of the etiology of the intergenerational syndrome, they do provide the first biological validation that the symptoms described by offspring as being related to the Holocaust appear, indeed, to reflect a type of posttraumatic response. The best conclusion from these studies to date is that the offspring of Holocaust survivors may be more psychologically and "biologically" vulnerable to stress and trauma for a host of reasons yet to be elucidated.

ACKNOWLEDGMENTS: The authors wish to acknowledge the following individuals who have contributed to the studies of Holocaust survivors that provided the basis for these investigations: Drs. Earl L. Giller, Jr., M.D., Ph.D.; Boaz Kahana, Ph.D.,; Steven Southwick, M.D.; John W. Mason, M.D. This work was supported by NIMH grant MH-49536.

REFERENCES

Aleksandrowicz, D. R. (1973). Children of concentration camp survivors. In E. J. Anthony & C. Koupernik (Eds.), *The child in his family: Vol. 2: The impact of disease and death* (pp. 385–392). New York: Wiley.

Antonovsky, A. (1979). *Health, stress and coping.* San Francisco: Jossey-Bass.

Antonovsky , A., Maoz, B., Dowty, N., & Wijsenbeek, B. (1971). Twenty-five years later: A limited study of the sequelae of the concentration camp experience. *Social Psychiatry, 6,* 186–193.

Barocas, H., & Barocas, C. (1983). Wounds of the fathers: The next generation of Holocaust victims. *International Review of Psychoanalysis, 5,* 331–341.

Bernstein, E. M., & Putnam, F. W. (1986). Development, reliability, and validity of a dissociation scale. *Journal of Nervous Mental Disease, 174,* 727–735.

Blake, D., Weathers, F., Nagy, D., Kaloupek, G., Klauminzer, D., Charney, D., & Keane, T. (1990). A clinician rating scale for current and lifetime PTSD. *Behavior Therapist, 13,* 187–188.

Carroll, B. J. (1982). The dexamethasone suppression test for melancholia. *British Journal of Psychiatry, 140,* 292–304.

Chodoff, P. (1963). Late effects of the concentration camp syndrome. *Archives of General Psychiatry, 8,* 323–333.

Danieli, Y. (1981). Differing adaptational styles in families of survivors of the Nazi Holocaust: Some implications for treatment. *Children Today, 10,* 6–10.

Danieli, Y. (1982). Families of survivors of the Nazi Holocaust: Some short and long-term effects. In C. D. Spielberger, I. G. Sarason, & N. A. Milgram (Eds.), *Stress and anxiety* (Vol. 8, pp. 405–421). New York: McGraw-Hill/Hemisphere.

Dimsdale, J. G. (1974). The coping behavior of Nazi concentration camp survivors. *American Journal of Psychiatry, 131,* 792–797.

Eaton, W. W., Sigal, J. J., & Weinfeld, M. (1982). Impairment in Holocaust survivors after 33 years: Data from an unbiased community sample. *American Journal of Psychiatry, 139,* 773–777.

Eitinger, L. (1961). Pathology of the concentration camp syndrome. *Archives of General Psychiatry, 5,* 371–380.

Green, B. Trauma history questionnaire. Available from the author.

Harel, Z., Kahana, B., & Kahana, E. (1988). Psychological well-being among Holocaust survivors and immigrants in Israel. *Journal of Traumatic Stress, 1,* 413–429.

Horowitz, M., Wilner, N., & Alvarez, W. (1979). Impact of event scale: A measure of subjective distress. *Psychosomatic Medicine, 41,* 209–218.

Kahana, B., Harel, Z., & Kahana, E. (1988). Predictors of psychological well-being among survivors of the Holocaust. In J. Wilson, Z. Harel, & B. Kahana (Eds.), *Human adaptation to extreme stress* (pp. 171–192). New York: Plenum Press.

Kahana, E., & Kahana B. (1982). The elderly care research center life events scale: Adaptation. In D. J. Mangen & W. A. Peterson (Eds.), *Clinical and social psychology* (vol. 1, pp. 145–193). Minneapolis: University of Minnesota Press.

Kaminer, H., & Lavie, P. (1991). Sleep and dreaming in Holocaust survivors: Dramatic decrease in dream recall in well-adjusted survivors. *Journal of Nervous and Mental Disease, 179,* 664–670.

Keane, T. M., Caddell, J. M., & Taylor, K. L. (1991). The Civilian Mississippi PTSD Scale. Boston: National Center for Posttraumatic Stress Disorder.

Kestenberg, J. L. (1972). Psychoanalytic contributions to the problems of children of survivors from Nazi persecution. *Israel Annals of Psychiatry and Related Disciplines, 10,* 311–325.

Kestenberg, J. S. (1980). Psychoanalyses of children of survivors from the Holocaust: Case presentation and assessment. *Journal of the American Psychoanalytic Association, 28,* 775–804.

Kinsler, F. (1981). Second generation effects of the Holocaust: The effectiveness of group therapy in the resolution of the transmission of parental trauma. *Journal of Psychology and Judaism, 6,* 53–66.

Klein, H., Zellermayer, J., & Shana, J. (1963). Former concentration camp inmates on a psychiatric ward. *Archives of General Psychiatry, 8,* 334–342.

Krystal, H. (Ed.). (1968). *Massive psychic trauma.* New York: International Universities Press.

Kuch, K., & Cox, B. J. (1992). Symptoms of PTSD in 124 survivors of the Holocaust. *American Journal of Psychiatry, 149,* 337–340.

Last, U. (1989). The transgeneration impact of Holocaust trauma: Current state of the evidence. *Institutional Journal of Mental Health, 17,* 72–89.

Last, U., & Klein, H. (1981). Impact de l'holocauste: Transmission aux enfants de vecu des parents [Impact of the Holocaust: Transmission of the parents' experiences to their children]. *L'Evolution Psychiatrique, 41,* 375–388.

Leon, G., Butcher, J. N., Kleinman, M., Goldberg, A., & Almagor, M. (1981). Survivors of the Holocaust and their children. *Journal of Personality and Social Psychology, 41*, 503–516.

Mason, J. W., Giller, E. L., Kosten, T. R., Ostroff, R. B., & Podd, L. (1986). Urinary free-cortisol levels in post-traumatic stress disorder patients. *Journal of Nervous Mental Disease, 174*, 145–159.

Munck, A., Guyre, P. M., & Holbrook, N. J. (1984). Physiological functions of glucocorticoids in stress and their relation to pharmacological actions. *Endocrinological Review, 93*, 9779–9783.

Nadler, A., & Ben-Shushan, D. (1989). Forty years later: Long-term consequences of massive-traumatization as manifested by Holocaust survivors from the city and the kibbutz. *Journal of Consulting and Clinical Psychology, 57*, 287–293.

Niederland, W. G. (1969). The problem of the survivor. In H. Krystal (Ed.), *Massive Trauma.* New York: International Universities Press.

Novac, A. (1993, May). Clinical heterogeneity in children of Holocaust survivors. *Psychiatry Newsletter of the World Psychiatric Association*, pp. 24–26.

Rakoff, V. (1966). A long-term effect on the concentration camp experience. *Viewpoints, 1*, 17–20.

Rakoff, V., Sigal, J. J., & Epstein, N. (1976). Children and families of concentration camp survivors. *Canada's Mental Health, 14*, 24–26.

Rose, S., & Garske, J. (1987). Family environment, adjustment, and coping among children of Holocaust survivors: A comparative investigation. *American Journal of Orthopsychiatry, 57*, 332–344.

Rosenheck, R., & Nathan, P. (1985). Secondary traumatization in the children of Vietnam veterans with posttraumatic stress disorder. *Hospital and Community Psychiatry, 36*, 538–539.

Rubinstein, I., Cutter, F., & Templer, D. I. (1989–1990). Multigenerational occurrence of survivor syndrome symptoms in families of Holocaust survivors. *Omega, 20*, 239–244.

Sachar, E. J., Hellman, L., & Roffwarg, H. P. (1973). Disrupted 24-hour patterns of cortisol secretion in psychotic depression. *Archives of General Psychiatry, 28*, 19–24.

Sigal, J. J. (1976). The effects of parental exposure to prolonged stress on the mental health of the spouse and children. *Canadian Psychiatric Association Journal, 21*, 169–172.

Sigal, J. J., & Weinfeld, G. (1985). Control of aggression in adult children of survivors of the Nazi persecution. *Journal of Abnormal Psychology, 94*, 556–564.

Silverman, W. K. (1987). Methodological issues in the study of transgenerational effect of the Holocaust: Comment on Nadler, Kav-Venaki, and Gleitman. *Journal of Consulting and Clinical Psychology, 55*, 125–126.

Solkoff, N. (1992). Children of survivors of the Nazi Holocaust: A critical review of the literature. *American Journal of Orthopsychiatry, 62*, 342–358.

Solomon, Z., Kotler, M., & Mikulincer, M. (1988). Combat-related posttraumatic stress disorder among second-generation Holocaust survivors: Preliminary findings. *American Journal of Psychiatry, 145*, 865–868.

Spitzer, R. L., Williams, J. B. W., & Gibbon, M. (1987). Structural Clinical Interview for DSM-III-R (SCID). New York: New York State Psychiatric Institute, Biometrics Research.

Stokes, P. E., Stoll, P. M., Koslow, S. H., Maas, J. W., Davis, J. M., Swann, A. C., & Robins, E. (1984). Pretreatment DST and hypothalamic–pituitary–adrenocortical function in depressed patients and comparison groups. *Archives of General Psychiatry, 41*, 257–267.

Trossman, B. (1968). Adolescent children of concentration camp survivors. *Canadian Psychiatric Association Journal, 13*, 121–123.

Waldfogel, S. (1991). Physical illness in children of Holocaust survivors. *General Hospital Psychiatry, 14*, 267–269.

Wilson, A., & Fromm, E. (1982). Aftermath of the concentration camp: The second generation. *Journal of the American Academy of Psychoanalysis, 10*, 289–313.

Yehuda, R., Boisoneau, D., Lowy, M. T., & Giller, E. L., Jr. (1995a). Dose-response changes in plasma cortisol and lymphocyte glucocorticoid receptors following dexamethasone administration in combat veterans with and without posttraumatic stress disorder. *Archives of General Psychiatry, 52*, 583–593.

Yehuda, R., Elkin, A., Binder-Brynes, K., Kahana, B., Southwick, S. M., Schmeidler, J., Giller, E. L., Jr. (1996a). Dissociation in aging Holocaust survivors. *American Journal of Psychiatry, 153*, 935–940.

Yehuda, R., & Giller, E. L. (1994). Comments on the lack of integration between the Holocaust and PTSD literatures. *PTSD Research Quarterly, 5*, 5–7.

Yehuda, R., Giller, E. L., Southwick, S. M., Lowy, M. T., & Mason, J. W. (1991). Hypothalamic–pituitary–adrenal dysfunction in post-traumatic stress disorder. *Biological Psychiatry, 30*, 1031–1048.

Yehuda, R., Kahana, B., Binder-Brynes, K., Southwick, S., Zemelman, S., Mason, J. W., & Giller, E. L., Jr. (1995b). Low urinary cortisol excretion in Holocaust survivors with posttraumatic stress disorder. *American Journal of Psychiatry, 152*, 982–986.

Yehuda, R., Kahana, B., Schmeidler, J., Southwick, S. M., Wilson, S., & Giller, E. L., Jr. (1995c). Impact of cumulative lifetime trauma and recent stress on current posttraumatic stress disorder symptoms in Holocaust survivors. *American Journal of Psychiatry, 152,* 1815–1818.

Yehuda, R., Kahana, B., Southwick, S. M., Giller, E. L., Jr. (1994). Depressive features in Holocaust survivors with post-traumatic stress disorder. *Journal of Traumatic Stress, 7,* 699–704.

Yehuda, R., Resnick, H., Kahana, B., & Giller, E. L., Jr. (1993a). Persistent hormonal alterations following extreme stress in humans: Adaptive or maladaptive? *Psychosomatic Medicine, 55,* 287–297.

Yehuda, R., Southwick, S. M., Krystal, J. M., Charney, D. S., & Mason, J. W. (1993b). Enhanced suppression of cortisol following dexamethasone administration in combat veterans with posttraumatic stress disorder and major depressive disorder. *American Journal of Psychiatry, 150,* 83–86.

Yehuda, R., Southwick, S. M., Nussbaum, G., Wahby, V., Giller, E. L., Jr., & Mason, J. W. (1990). Low urinary cortisol excretion in patients with posttraumatic stress disorder. *Journal of Nervous and Mental Disease, 178,* 366–369.

Yehuda, R., Teicher, M. H., Levengood, R., Trestman, R., & Siever, L. J. (1996). Circadian rhythm of cortisol regulation in PTSD. *Biological Psychiatry, 40,* 79–88.

Zlotogorski, Z. (1983). Offspring of concentration camp survivors: The relationship of perceptions of family cohesion and adaptability of levels of ego functioning. *Comprehensive Psychiatry, 24,* 345–354.

38

Initial Clinical Evidence of Genetic Contributions to Posttraumatic Stress Disorder

JOHN H. KRYSTAL, LINDA M. NAGY, ANN RASMUSSON,
ANDREW MORGAN, CHERYL COTTROL,
STEVEN M. SOUTHWICK, and DENNIS S. CHARNEY

There are few topics in the field of traumatic stress studies that clinicians approach more ambivalently than considerations of genetic factors associated with vulnerability or resistance to traumatization. Historically, individuals suffering from combat-related posttraumatic stress disorder (PTSD) received diagnoses including "soldier's heart" or "neurocirculatory asthenia," and were frequently viewed as possessing characteristics that cast them in a disparaging light, such as "constitutional inferiority" and "lack of virility" (Campbell, 1918; see Krystal *et al.,* 1989). Early studies implicated race as an important factor influencing the vulnerability to psychological stress (cf. Dunn, 1942). However, these studies attempted to use flawed clinical data to support widely held societal prejudices against minority groups, similar to early misguided efforts to characterize the inheritance of intelligence (Gould, 1981). Similarly, German authorities abused genetic arguments to justify denying the claims of Jewish survivors of the Nazi concentration camps for reparation for long-term psychiatric sequelae of their traumatization (Eisler, 1963/1964, 1967; Kestenberg, 1980). The relatively greater progress made in characterizing the environmental factors that influence subsequent stress response, such as the importance of early childhood trauma (Herman, 1992; Krystal, 1988) and the impact of parental traumatization on parent–child relationships (Danieli, 1980; Oliver, 1993; Rosenheck, 1986), further compounds concerns about overestimating genetic factors associated with PTSD.

Yet the pull to study genetic aspects of PTSD is compelling. It grows out of efforts to explain different vulnerabilities to traumatization and distinct patterns of stress response. First, there is increasing evidence that parental PTSD increases the vulnerability to PTSD in their

JOHN H. KRYSTAL, LINDA M. NAGY, ANN RASMUSSON, ANDREW MORGAN, CHERYL COTTROL, STEPHEN M. SOUTHWICK, and DENNIS S. CHARNEY • Clinical Neurosciences Division, National Center for PTSD, VA Connecticut Healthcare System, West Haven Campus, West Haven, CT 06516.

International Handbook of Multigenerational Legacies of Trauma, edited by Yael Danieli. Plenum Press, New York, 1998.

children, without a validated explanatory model for this effect (Solomon, Kotter, & Mikulincer, 1988). Second, the debate over the establishment of PTSD in DSM-III (American Psychiatric Association, 1980) focused attention on the need to establish exposure to traumatic stress as the predominating etiological factor for PTSD. However, a series of excellent epidemiological studies succeeded in demonstrating the critical pathogenic role of extreme stress for PTSD (Centers for Disease Control Vietnam Experience Study, 1988; Egendorf, Kadushin, Laufer, Rothbart, & Sloan, 1981; Gleser, Green, & Winget, 1981; Kilpatrick *et al.*, 1989; Kulka *et al.*, 1990). As a result, the research focus has been shifting to other issues, including genetically transmitted risk factors for traumatization and resilience. Third, a careful exploration of genetic traits that predispose to traumatization may reveal characteristics that might be advantageous outside of the extraordinary singularity of traumatic stress, such as bravery, cautiousness, moral rigor, and artistic capacities (Campbell, 1918; Dunn, 1942). Fourth, recent research on PTSD has begun to characterize the neurobiology of this disorder, implicating neurobiological systems whose genetic regulation has been increasingly well delineated (Hyman & Nestler, 1993). Finally, human genetic studies of PTSD trail preclinical research on distinct genotypic patterns of uncontrollable stress response by almost two decades (Krystal, 1990).

Genetic epidemiological models for PTSD begin by acknowledging the multifactorial nature of this disorder (Kendler & Eaves, 1986; True *et al.*, 1993). Generally speaking, the variance in predicting who will develop PTSD (V_{PTSD}) may be explained by the sum of the variance contributed by genetic contributions to PTSD vulnerability (V_G), the variance contributed by common or shared family environmental factors (V_C), and the variance arising from unique factors associated with an individual subject (V_E). Thus the total vulnerability to PTSD may be characterized using the following equation:

$$V_{PTSD} = V_G + V_C + V_E$$

For the purposes of genetic epidemiological studies, it is important to remember that the particular traumatic stress for each individual studied potentially influences this model in two ways: as common environmental influences, and as unique factors. Thus the total environmental influence on a trait would be the sum of V_C and V_E. Family study methods examine *familial* contributions to PTSD vulnerability but do not permit determining the relative genetic and common environmental contributions, represented as the sum of V_G and V_C. However, twin studies comparing monozygotic and dizygotic twins do permit examination of the relative contributions of genetics and family environment.

Application of a genetic epidemiological approach to the study of PTSD requires consideration of the role of the exposure to the traumatic event. The requirement of a particular environmental exposure to reveal an underlying vulnerability to pathology in PTSD may be analogous to phenylketonuria, where a metabolic defect is not evident unless vulnerable individuals are exposed to a poorly tolerated amino acid. Furthermore, the multifactorial nature of PTSD has long suggested to clinicians that heritable and environmental contributions to PTSD were reciprocally related, that is, the stronger the heritable contribution to PTSD, the lower the intensity of the stress needed to cause PTSD (reviewed in Davidson, Swartz, Storck, Krishnan, & Hammett, 1985). However, because the expression of vulnerability to PTSD may not be expressed unless individuals are exposed to extreme stressors, it may be manifest in family members in other forms that could include biological, cognitive, and personality traits, as well as other psychiatric diagnoses.

This chapter reviews the growing number of clinical studies evaluating the contribution of heritable factors to vulnerability to PTSD. In doing so, it provides an initial framework for interpreting genetic contributions to this disorder. There is a growing diversity of approaches to the study of genetic contributions to psychiatric disorders, character traits, or biological characteristics. To date, there have been no published direct-interview family studies or molecular genetic studies of PTSD patients. Thus, this chapter reviews studies employing two methodologies: family history studies and twin studies.

FAMILY HISTORY STUDIES

Family history studies evaluate the association of psychiatric diagnoses in the family members affected with PTSD in comparison with the family members of another group of patients or healthy subjects. In contrast to the family study method, where family members are interviewed directly in order to determine their lifetime diagnoses, family history studies indirectly assess the diagnoses of family members. In other words, the subject is interviewed about the psychiatric histories of his or her relatives. A validated, structured psychiatric interview for family history assessment has been developed to standardize the collection of information (Andreason, Endicott, Spitzer, & Winokur, 1977). However, family history studies may have limited sensitivity, resulting in underestimation of the occurrence of the disorder within a family and vulnerability to recall biases on the part of the interviewed subjects (Chapman, Mannuzza, Klein, & Fyer, 1994; Kendler *et al.*, 1991; Orvaschel, Thompson, Belanger, Prusoff, & Kidd, 1982).

Although scanty, the preponderance of evidence collected from family history studies suggests that there is an increased risk for PTSD in individuals with a family history of psychiatric illness. For example, one study of firefighters exposed to a brushfire disaster found that 6 of 9 (67%) firefighters who developed chronic PTSD had family histories of psychiatric illness compared to 7 of 34 (20%) firefighters who did not develop PTSD (McFarlane, 1988). In a study of World War II prisoners of war, there was a trend for veterans with a family history of alcoholism, but not other mental illnesses, to have increased likelihood of developing PTSD (Speed, Engdahl, Schwartz, & Eberly, 1989). Similarly, a study conducted in young adults suggested that a family history of anxiety was associated with a threefold increased risk for PTSD after controlling for other risk factors (Breslau, Davis, Andreski, & Peterson, 1991).

Two family history studies conducted in populations with combat-related PTSD suggest that chronic PTSD is associated with a higher rate of familial psychopathology, particularly alcoholism, depression, and anxiety disorders (Davidson *et al.*, 1985; Davidson, Smith, & Kudler, 1989). The earlier of these studies suggested that first-degree relatives of Vietnam veterans with chronic PTSD had higher rates of alcoholism or drug abuse (60%) compared to the first-degree relatives of patients with depression (26%) or generalized anxiety disorder (38%). The first-degree relatives of patients with PTSD also had higher rates of generalized anxiety (22%) compared to the relatives of depressed patients (4%), but not the relatives of generalized anxiety disorder patients (14%). The siblings of Vietnam veterans with chronic PTSD had a higher uncorrected morbidity risk for alcoholism (12%) than did patients with either depression (1.7%) or generalized anxiety disorder (0%), where there was no increased morbidity risk in the parents of these patients. In their second study, Davidson and colleagues were unable to replicate the finding that siblings and parents of patients with PTSD had more elevated rates of anxiety disorders than patients with major depression and alcoholism, or healthy control subjects. However, the parents and siblings of patients with PTSD had higher rates of anxiety disorders, particularly generalized anxiety, than did combat veterans who did not develop PTSD. Also, the children of PTSD and generalized anxiety disorder patients had higher rates of generalized anxiety than did the children of depressed patients. These studies raise the possibility that familial anxiety disorders might contribute to the vulnerability to developing combat-related PTSD.

One factor influencing the findings of family history studies of PTSD are cohort effects, that is, generations who differ with respect to the prevalence of characteristics, such as substance abuse. Given the elevated prevalence of substance abuse among soldiers in the Vietnam war (Kulka *et al.,* 1990), one might be concerned that cohort effects might influence the relative prevalence of substance-abuse disorders in the siblings of Vietnam combat veterans with PTSD. Perhaps reflecting these cohort effects, Davidson and colleagues (1989) found that alcoholism and drug-abuse rates were elevated in the parents and siblings of Vietnam veterans relative to the parents and siblings of World War II veterans. Also, the children of Vietnam veterans with PTSD had a greater risk of developing a chronic psychiatric illness. Again, these effects must be viewed as familial; that is, the study was unable to differentiate the impact of serving in the Vietnam war on parenting from the genetic traits of the veterans studied.

Nagy *et al.* (in review) recently conducted a family history study evaluating the extent to which comorbid panic disorder or vulnerability to yohimbine-induced panic attacks in PTSD patients may be explained by a familial vulnerability for panic attacks. The overlap of panic disorder and PTSD has been of interest in light of evidence that panic disorder rates are elevated in PTSD populations (Kulka *et al.,* 1988; Breslau *et al.,* 1991). This overlap is also suggested by the phenomenological similarity between naturally occurring (Mellman & Davis, 1985) and lactate-induced (Rainey *et al.,* 1987) flashbacks and panic attacks in PTSD patients. Further, yohimbine, a drug that stimulates central noradrenergic activation, provoked panic attacks and flaskbacks in a subgroup of PTSD patients (Southwick *et al.,* 1993) and panic disorder patients (Charney, Woods, Krystal, Nagy, & Heninger, 1992) even though it failed to have this effect in many other diagnostic groups, including alcoholics, schizophrenics, depressed patients, generalized anxiety disorder patients, obsessive–compulsive disorder patients, and healthy subjects. Thus, clinical and neurobiological data warranted the investigation of familial predictors of naturally occurring and yohimbine-stimulated panic in PTSD patients.

Despite the convergence of phenomenological and biological findings, the study by Nagy *et al.* (in review) did not find familial evidence of overlap between panic disorder and PTSD. This study found lower rates of panic disorder in family members of patients with PTSD and comorbid panic disorder (3.1%) or PTSD alone (2.7%) relative to the family members of patients with panic disorder (15.9%). The rates of panic disorder in relatives of patients with PTSD and healthy controls (0%) did not significantly differ. However, the rates of PTSD were elevated in the family members of PTSD patients with (7.2%) and without (12.2%) comorbid panic disorder relative to the absence of PTSD in the relatives of both panic disorder patients and healthy controls. The presence or absence of a yohimbine-induced panic attack did not differentiate the pattern of psychiatric illness in the first-degree relatives of PTSD patients.

TWIN STUDIES

There have been two reports from twin studies related to PTSD. Twin studies are a particularly powerful approach for studying the genetic and environmental contributions to the likelihood of exhibiting a particular trait. Twin studies take advantage of the fact that twins are generally raised in the same environment. Therefore, if monozygotic (identical) twins share a trait more frequently than dizygotic (fraternal twins), it is assumed that the trait is transmitted genetically rather than environmentally. There are limitations to these models. For example, monozygotic twins may not be truly identical in many cases. For example, they may develop as mirror images of each other with opposing laterality, a process that may be influenced by the timing of the separation of the identical twins during embryonic development (Faber, 1981). Although not yet applied to PTSD, two strategies have been applied elsewhere that provide additional insight into genetic and environmental contributions to a particular trait, including studies of twins reared apart and cross-fostering studies (Faber, 1981; Kety, 1987).

A twin study of 4,029 twin pairs who served during the Vietnam War era suggested that genetic factors contributed to many features of their military experience that influenced the degree of likelihood that they would be involved in combat-related trauma (Lyons *et al.*, 1993). Monozygotic (MZ) twins were approximately twice as similar as dizygotic (DZ) twins in their likelihood of their volunteering for service in Southeast Asia (MZ =-.4, DZ = .22; heritability = .36), serving in Southeast Asia (MZ = .41, DZ = .24; heritability = .47), being exposed to a similar degree of combat (MZ = .53, DZ = .30; heritability = .47), and receiving combat decorations (MZ = .52, DZ = .23; heritability = .54). There were no significant effects in this study associated with the shared environment (i.e. $V_C = 0$). This study suggested that genetic factors associated with the likelihood of experiencing situations that might generate PTSD might have influenced the rates of the subsequent development of PTSD in these individuals. These findings are consistent with an increasing number of studies (Burnam *et al.*, 1988; Helzer, Robbins, & McEvoy, 1987) indicating that premorbid factors, such as personality disorder, influenced exposure to potentially traumatic stressors.

Twins from the same twin sample also provided evidence that the development of PTSD symptoms was influenced by both unique environmental (V_E) and genetic factors (V_G) (True *et al.*, 1993). In this study, combat exposure correlated strongly with the reexperiencing cluster of symptoms, the avoidance cluster of symptoms, and guilt, but not arousal symptoms, consistent with studies in Israeli combat veterans (Solomon & Canino, 1990). Among the total sample of twins, including those who had and had not served in Vietnam, both genetic and environmental factors contributed to the development of PTSD symptoms (Table 1).

Symptoms from each cluster showed greater within-pair correlations for MZ relative to DZ twins, with an identified contribution from unique environmental factors controlling for combat exposure. In contrast to familial models, the shared environment did not contribute highly to any symptom within the PTSD symptom cluster, with the exception of avoidance of activities (adjusted $d^2 = .34$). These data indicate that genetic factors contribute to PTSD vulnerability. They also strongly suggest that the elevated rates of PTSD in the relatives of combat veterans with PTSD reflect genetic influences rather than shared family environment. Consistent with these findings, a much smaller twin study found that PTSD was more prevalent in the twins diagnosed with anxiety disorders than in twins diagnosed with other diagnoses (Skre, Onstad, Torgersen, Lygren, & Kringlen, 1993). This study also found higher rates of PTSD in the small number of MZ twins with PTSD relative to DZ twins with PTSD (Skre *et al.*, 1993).

Although not explicitly related to PTSD, a recent twin study informs considerations of the interactive effects of a major stressful life event and depression (Kendler *et al.*, 1995). This study of 1,082 female twin pairs found that stressful life events, such as assault, serious marital problems, job loss, and serious illness increased risk of developing depression within 1 month of the event. Also, having an identical twin with depression was associated with a greater risk of developing depression than was having a fraternal twin with depression, while having a healthy identical twin was more protective against developing depression than was having a healthy fraternal twin. Furthermore, there were multiplicative interactive effects of having a genetic predisposition for depression in the face of a recent major life stress. The interactive effects of environmental and genetic factors from this study are illustrated in Figure 1.

Although this study did not report the prevalence of PTSD in its sample, these data support the interactive effects of stress and psychopathology.

Table 1. PTSD Symptoms in Monozygotic and Dizygotic Twins Adjusting for Combat Exposure

Symptom	Monozygotic correlations (s_1, s_2)	Dizygotic correlations (s_1, s_2)	Environment adjusted e^2	Additive genetic adjusted h^2
Reexperiencing				
Painful memories	.35	.24	.44	.13
Dreams/nightmares	.38	.19	.44	.30
Event happening again	.37	.18	.49	.28
Avoidance				
Avoided activities	.41	.11	.42	.00
Loss of interest	.32	.15	.67	.30
Felt distant	.38	.18	.59	.35
Life is not meaningful	.38	.16	.61	.34
Arousal				
Sleep disturbance	.33	.11	.67	.10
Irritable, short-tempered	.34	.16	.64	.30
Angry, aggressive	.37	.15	.62	.31
Trouble concentrating	.31	.15	.67	.28
Easily startled	.38	.20	.56	.32
Only DSM-III				
Felt guilt	.28	.15	.50	.26
Memory problems	.32	.16	.67	.30

Modified from True *et al.* (1993).
e^2 = variance from environmental influences, including the trauma.
h^2 = variance from genetic influences.

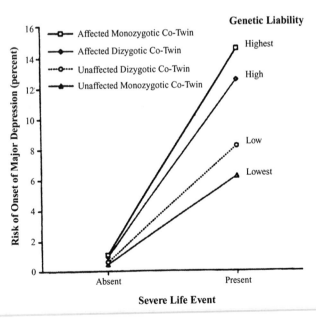

Figure 1. Risk of onset of major depression per person-month as a function of genetic liability and the presence or absence of a severe stressful life event in that month among 2,060 female twins. Genetic liability is reflected by both the zygoisty of the twin and the lifetime history of major depression in the co-twin. The results presented above are those predicted by the best-fitting logistic regression equation that contains control variables and the main effects of the life event and genetic risk factors. A severe life event is defined as assault, serious marital problems, divorce/break-up, or death of a close relative (from Kendler *et al.*, 1995, p. 837).

COMMENT AND FUTURE DIRECTIONS

A growing body of data suggests that genetic factors contribute to PTSD. PTSD appears to be associated with other anxiety disorders in a still undetermined fashion. No single diagnosis is of sufficient prevalence in the family members of patients diagnosed with PTSD to question the validity of PTSD as a distinct diagnosis. The increased risk for PTSD among individuals with anxiety disorders and the increased prevalence of anxiety disorders in the offspring of PTSD patients supports this connection but does not yet explain the nature of the relationship. Familial factors undoubtedly contribute to the rates of psychiatric problems in the offspring of combat veterans with PTSD. Consensus may emerge after the family history studies conducted in veterans with PTSD are integrated with the findings of studies that must eventually be conducted in probands with non-combat-related PTSD.

Future studies will introduce new complications. For example, it is not yet clear whether the genetic predisposing factors associated with one type of traumatic stress are similar to that associated with vulnerability to a different type of stressor. Also, we do not yet know whether the genetic factors predisposing to PTSD in males are similar to genetic factors associated with PTSD in females, and concerns about this issue have been raised for other disorders (Kosten, Rounsaville, Kosten, & Merikangas, 1991). Furthermore, it is not clear whether the genetic factors associated with vulnerability to later symptomatic presentations associated with infantile or childhood traumatization are similar to those associated with adult traumatizations. With such large and important gaps in our understanding of the genetics of PTSD, it is clearly a time for caution in the interpretation of any particular study. Perhaps it is also a time for generativity as the gaps in our knowledge base serve to stimulate future research.

Several important steps will undoubtedly be taken by the field of traumatic stress studies. One necessary step in the characterization of genetic contributions to PTSD is the completion of studies incorporating a growing number of rigorous genetic designs, such as family interview studies, that may more accurately characterize the prevalence of psychiatric disorders in the family members of PTSD patients relative to other disorders. The existing family history studies provide an important initial step but are not definitive. The family interview studies also provide a foundation for initiating molecular genetic linkage studies, incorporating a spectrum of powerful techniques that may help to identify the contributions of particular genes to traumatic stress response.

An important second step will be to characterize genetic factors associated with resilience following exposure to extreme stress. Although the prevalence of the PTSD diagnosis in 15.2% of Vietnam theater veterans speaks to the chronicity of this disorder, approximately half of the veterans with a lifetime history of this diagnosis no longer met diagnostic criteria at follow-up (Kulka *et al.,* 1990). Several factors appear to be associated with coping and recovery following traumatic stress exposure. For example, one study of American prisoners of war in Vietnam following 1969, found that successful coping was associated with introversion, whereas veterans who coped less well tended to be outgoing and extroverted (Ursano, Wheatley, Sledge, Rahe, & Carlson, 1986). Studies have found genetic contributions to introversion and extroversion (cf. Cloninger, 1991), suggesting at least one potential bridge between genetic and clinical descriptive studies. The comorbid conditions of antisocial personality, alcoholism, and substance abuse have been cited as commonly associated with chronic PTSD in combat veterans (Sierles, Chen, McFarland, & Taylor, 1983) and in the family members of combat veterans (Davidson *et al.,* 1985, 1989). These comorbid conditions with increasingly well-characterized genetic transmission (Cloninger, 1987) may predict a lack of resiliency among traumatized veterans (Cowen & Work, 1988; Garmezy, Masten, & Tellegen, 1984) or behavior patterns, such as repetitive exposure to violence in drug-using subcultures, that may exacerbate the course of PTSD (Lyons, 1991). Because resiliency factors influence the course of PTSD, subgroups of traumatized patients may recover and, as a result, fail to be included in genetic studies of this disorder. Thus, resiliency factors may contribute significantly to the findings of studies drawn from clinical samples of PTSD patients.

A third step that may be useful in characterizing genetic contributions to traumatic stress response would be to shift the emphasis from diagnoses to specific traits. For example, it has been difficult to find a single gene that explains alcohol dependence in all affected individuals; however, a gene involved in serotonin synthesis has already been implicated in violent behavior exhibited by impulsive alcoholics (Nielsen et al., 1994). Alternatively, one might focus on particular traits that might predispose individuals to a spectrum of diagnoses, the display of which depends on environmental factors during development. One trait that has received significant attention due to its association with anxiety disorders is behavioral inhibition in children (Kagan, Reznick, & Snidman, 1988). Behavioral inhibition is a laboratory-based measure of the tendency to restrict behavior in the presence of an unfamiliar environment. Behavioral inhibition was initially found to be more prevalent in the offspring of patients with panic disorder and agoraphobia (Rosenbaum et al., 1988) and subsequently was found to be associated with other parental anxiety disorders as well (Rosenbaum et al., 1991). These traits may have parallels in the provocative studies conducted in rhesus monkeys. These studies suggest that inherited factors producing increased reactivity to relatively mild stressors predict the pattern of response to a major stressor, maternal deprivation (see Suomi & Levine, Chapter 36, this volume). The evaluation of the patterns of inheritance of this and other well-defined and well-quantified traits could be informative in the families of patients with PTSD.

There also is an increasing need to link pathophysiological and etiological models for PTSD in the pursuit of enhancing the efficacy of pharmacotherapies for this disorder. The only current study attempting to bridge this gap to date (Nagy et al., in review) did not find that responsivity to yohimbine differentiated the pattern of psychiatric disorder in family members of patients with PTSD. Yet the growing literature on the neurobiological foundations of PTSD (Charney, Deutsch, Krystal, Southwick, & Davis, 1993; Krystal et al., 1989) provides new research directions that grow out of preclinical research findings. For example, a recently completed study suggested that patients with combat-related PTSD tended to respond to either yohimbine or the serotonin partial agonist, m-chlorophenyl-piperazine (mCPP), but not to both agents with a panic attack (Southwick et al., 1997) It is not yet known whether yohimbine and mCPP differentiate stable subtypes of PTSD with differential involvement of noradrenergic and serotonergic systems, or whether the differential responses to these drugs reflect state-related factors.

Preclinical research suggests that different inbred mice strains respond to inescapable stress with consistent and differential involvement of monoamine neurotransmitter systems, resulting in mice strains with preferential dopaminergic, noradrenergic, and serotonergic responses to stress (Anisman, Grimmer, Irwin, Remington, & Sklar, 1979; Shanks & Anisman, 1989; Zacharko, Lalonde, Kasian, & Anisman, 1987). These mice strains respond to inescapable stress with a characteristic behavioral disruption syndrome, sometimes referred to as "learned helplessness." The rodent strains with prominent noradrenergic activation tended to be better protected from the disruptive effects of inescapable stress by prestress administration of a noradrenergic reuptake blocker than by a serotonin reuptake blocker, whereas rodent strains with more prominent serotonergic responses exhibited superior protective effects when pretreated with a serotonin reuptake blocker (Shanks & Anisman, 1989).

Information regarding genetically determined patterns of stress response could lead to a rational matching of subgroups of PTSD patients to optimally effective treatments. Currently, there is no established strategy for determining the optimal match of particular PTSD patients with particular treatment modalities. However, if human serotenergic and noradrenergic patterns of stress response (Southwick *et al.,* 1997) parallel those reported in animals (Shanks & Anisman, 1989), then one would predict that pharmacological challenge studies and ultimately patterns of allelic expression would predict patterns of pharmacotherapy response. As a corollary, the failure to match an appropriate population of PTSD patients to an appropriate pharmacotherapy may have contributed to the lack of efficacy observed in a study evaluating desipramine treatment for PTSD (Reist *et al.,* 1989). While not yet applied to PTSD, the strategy of treatment matching based on clinically evident traits has been applied with success in other areas of psychiatry, particularly the field of alcoholism research (Kadden, Cooney, Getter, & Litt, 1989).

In closing, genetic studies of PTSD are challenged by the complexity of studying an environmentally triggered disorder and burdened by the heightened responsibility to ensure that genetic traits predisposing individuals to developing this disorder do not acquire pejorative implications. The promise of genetic studies is the better understanding of vulnerability, course, and pathophysiology of PTSD. In acquiring better predictors of vulnerability and resistance to traumatization, ultimately, clinicians and society might develop the capacity to intervene to reduce the incidence of PTSD. Understanding genetically determined patterns of stress response would illuminate all aspects of pathophysiological study of this disorder and potentially lead to more effective treatment, and treatments that are better geared to fit the needs of particular patterns of stress response. Currently, the lofty goals of genetic studies of PTSD seem quite distant within the context of a relatively small number of studies published in this area. Yet the field of traumatic stress studies awaits the development of this exciting and promising area of study.

ACKNOWLEDGMENTS: The authors acknowledge the helpful contributions of Bonnie Becker and Yael Danieli to this chapter. This work was supported by funds from the Department of Veterans Affairs to the National Center for PTSD, the VA–Yale Alcoholism Research Center (JK), and a Merit Review Grant (LN).

REFERENCES

American Psychiatric Association. (1980). *Diagnostic and statistical manual of mental disorders* (3rd ed). Washington, DC: Author.

Andreason, N. C., Endicott, J., Spitzer, R. L. & Winokur, G. (1977). The family history method using diagnostic criteria, reliability and validity. *Archives of General Psychiatry, 34,* 1229–1235.

Anisman, H., Grimmer, L., Irwin, J., Remington, G., & Sklar, L. S. (1979). Escape performance after inescapable shock in selectively bred lines of mice: Response maintenance and catecholamine activity. *Journal of Comparative Physiology and Psychology, 93,* 229–241.

Breslau, N., Davis, G. C., Andreski, P., & Peterson, E. (1991). Traumatic events and posttraumatic stress disorder in an urban population of young adults. *Archives of General Psychiatry, 48,* 216–222.

Burnam, M. A., Stein, J. A., Golding, J. M., Siegel, J. M., Sorenson, S. B., Forsythe, A. B., & Telles, C. A. (1988). Sexual assault and mental disorders in a community population. *Journal of Consulting Clinical Psychology, 56,* 843–850.

Cadoret, R. J., O'Gorman, T. W., Troughton, E., & Hayweood, E. (1985). Alcoholism and antisocial personality: Interrelationships, genetic and environmental factors. *Archives of General Psychiatry, 42,* 161–167.

Campbell, C. M. (1918). The role of instinct, emotion and personality in disorders of the heart: with suggestions for a clinical record. *Journal of the American Medical Association, 71,* 1621–1626.

Centers for Disease Control Vietnam Experience Study. (1988). Health status of Vietnam veterans: I. Psychosocial characteristics. *Journal of the American Medical Association, 259,* 2701–2707.

Chapman, T. F., Mannuzza, S., Klein, D. F., & Fyer, A. J. (1994). Effects of informant mental disorder on psychiatric family history data. *American Journal of Psychiatry, 151,* 574–579.

Charney, D. S., Deutch, A., Krystal, J. H., Southwick, S. M., & Davis, M. (1993). Psychobiological mechanisms of posttraumatic stress disorder. *Archives of General Psychiatry, 50,* 294–305.

Charney, D. S., Woods, S. W., Krystal, J. .H., Nagy, L. M., & Heninger, G. R. (1992). Noradrenergic neuronal dysregulation in panic disorder: The effects of intravenous yohimbine and clonidine in panic disorder patients. *Acta Psychiatrica Scandinavia, 86,* 273–282.

Cloninger, C. R. (1991). Neurogenetic adaptive mechanisms in alcoholism. *Science, 236,* 410–416.

Cowen, E. L., & Work, W. C. (1988). Resilient children, psychological wellness, and primary prevention. *American Journal of Community Psychology, 16,* 591–607.

Crowe, R. R. (1974). An adoption study of antisocial personality. *Archives of General Psychiatry, 31,* 785–791.

Danieli, Y. (1980). Families of survivors of the Nazi Holocaust, some long and some short term effects. In N. Milgram (Ed.), *Psychological Stress and Adjustment in Time of War and Peace,* Washington, DC: Hemisphere.

Davidson, J., Smith, R., & Kudler, H. (1989). Familial psychiatric illness in chronic posttraumatic stress disorder. *Comprehensive Psychiatry, 30,* 345–399.

Davidson, J., Swartz, Z., Storck, M., Krishnan, R., & Hammett, E. (1985). A diagnostic and familial study of posttraumatic stress disorder. *American Journal of Psychiatry, 142,* 90–93.

Dunn, W. H. (1942). Emotional factors in neurocirculatory asthenia. *Psychosomatic Medicine, 4,* 333–354.

Egendorf, A., Kadushin, C., Laufer, R. S., Rothbart, G., & Sloan, L. (1981). *Legacies of Vietnam: Comparative adjustment of veterans and their peers.* New York: Center for Research Policy.

Eisler, K. R. (1963/1964). Die ermordung von wieveilen seiner KINDER muss ein Mensch symptomfrei ertragen können, um eine normale Konstitution zu haben? [The murder of how many of one's children must a person be able to bear, without symptoms, in order to be considered to have a normal constitution?] *Psyche, 5*(17), 241–291.

Eisler, K. R. (1967). Perverted psychiatry? *American Journal of Psychiatry, 123,* 1352–1358.

Farber, S. L. (1981). *Identical twins reared apart: A reanalysis.* New York: Basic Books.

Garmezy, N., Masten, A. S., Tellegen, A. (1984). The study of stress and competence in children: A building block for developmental psychopathology. *Child Development, 55,* 97–111.

Gleser, G. C., Green, B. L., & Winget, C. (1981). *Prolonged psychosocial effects of disaster: A study of Buffalo Creek.* New York: Academic Press.

Gould, S. J. (1981). *The mismeasure of man.* New York: Norton.

Helzer, J. E., Robbins, L. N., & McEvoy, L. (1987). Post-traumatic stress disorder in the general population: Findings of the Epidemiologic Catchment Area Survey. *New England Journal of Medicine, 317,* 1630–1634.

Herman, J. L. (1992). *Trauma and recovery.* New York: Basic Books.

Hyman, S. E., & Nestler, E. J., (1993). *The molecular foundations of psychiatry.* Washington, DC: American Psychiatric Association Press.

Kadden, R. M., Cooney, N. L., Getter, H., & Litt, M. D. (1989). Matching alcoholics to coping skills or interactional therapies: Posttreatment results. *Journal of Consulting and Clinical Psychology,* 698–704.

Kagan, J., Reznick, J. S., & Snidman, N. (1988). Biological basis of childhood shyness. *Science, 240,* 167–171.

Kendler, K. S., & Eaves, L. J. (1986). Models for the joint effect of genotype and environment on liability to psychiatric illness. *American Journal of Psychiatry, 143,* 279–289.

Kendler, K. S., Kessler, R. C., Walters, E. E., MacLean, C., Neale, M. C., Heath, A. C., & Eaves, L. J. (1995). Stressful life events, genetic liability, and onset of an episode of major depression in women. *American Journal of Psychiatry, 152,* 833–842.

Kendler, K. S., Silberg, J. L., Neale, M. C., Kessler, R. C., Heath, A. C., & Eaves, L. J. (1991). The family history method: Whose psychiatric history is measured? *American Journal of Psychiatry, 148,* 1501–1504.

Kestenberg, M. (1980, August). *Discriminatory aspects of the German restitution: Law and practice.* Paper presented to the First World Congress of Victimology, Washington, DC.

Kety, S. S. (1987). The significance of genetic factors in the etiology of schizophrenia: Results from the National Study of Adoptees in Denmark. *Journal of Psychiatric Research, 21,* 423–429.

Kilpatrick, D. G., Saunders, B. E., Amick-McMullan, A., Best, C. L., Veronen, L. J., & Resnick, H. S. (1989). Victim and crime factors associated with the development of crime-related post-traumatic stress disorder. *Behavior Therapy, 20,* 199–214.

Kosten, T. R., Rounsaville, B. J., Kosten, T. A., & Merikangas, K. (1991). Gender differences in the specificity of alcoholism transmission among the relatives of opioid addicts. *Journal of Nervous and Mental Diseases, 179,* 392–400.

Krystal, H. (1988). *Integration and self-healing: Affect, trauma, alexithymia.* Hillsdale, NJ: Analytic Press.

Krystal, J. H. (1990). Animal models for post-traumatic stress disorder. In E. Giller (Ed.), *The Biological Assessment and Treatment of PTSD* (pp. 3–26). Washington, DC: American Psychiatric Association Press.

Krystal, J. H., Kosten, T. R., Perry, B. D., Southwick, S., Mason, J. W., Giller, E. L., Jr. (1989). Neurobiological aspects of PTSD: Review of clinical and preclinical studies. *Behavioral Therapy, 20,* 177–198.

Kulka, R. A., Schlenger, W. E., Fairbank, J. A., Hough, R. L., Jordan, B. K., Marmar, C. R., & Weiss, D. S. (1990). *Trauma and the Vietnam war generation: Report of findings from the National Vietnam Veterans Readjustment Study.* New York: Brunner/Mazel.

Lyons, J. A. (1991). Strategies for assessing the potential for positive adjustment following trauma. *Journal of Traumatic Stress, 4,* 93–111.

Lyons, M. J., Goldberg, J., Eisen, S. A., True, W., Tsuang, M. T., Meyer, J. M., & Henderson, W. G. (1993). Do genes influence exposure to trauma? A twin study of combat. *American Journal of Medicinal Genetics (Neuropsychiatric Genetics), 48,* 22–27.

McFarlane, A. C. (1988). The etiology of post-traumatic stress disorders following a natural disaster. *British Journal of Psychiatry, 152,* 116–121.

Mellman, T. A., & Davis, G. C. (1985). Combat-related flashbacks in posttraumatic stress disorder: Phenomenology and similarity to panic attacks. *Journal of Clinical Psychiatry, 46,* 379–382.

Nagy, L. M., Morgan, C. A., III, Miller, H. L., Southwick, S. M., Merikangas, K. R., Krystal, J. H., & Charney, D. S. (in review). Genetic epidemiology of panic attacks and noradrenregic response in post-traumatic stress disorder: A family history study.

Oliver, J. E. (1993). Intergenerational transmission of child abuse: Rates, research, and clinical implications. *American Journal of Psychiatry, 150,* 1315–1324.

Orvaschel, J., Thompson, W. D., Belanger, A., Prusoff, B. A., & Kidd, K. K. (1982). Comparison of the family history method to direct interview: Factors affecting the diagnosis of depression. *Journal of Affective Disorders, 4,* 49–59.

Rainey, J. M., Aleem, A., Ortiz, A., Yeragani, V., Pohl, R., & Berchou, R. (1987). A laboratory procedure for the induction of flashbacks. *American Journal of Psychiatry, 144,* 1317–1319.

Reist, C., Kauffmann, C. D., Haier, R., Sangdahl, C., DeMet, E. M., Chicz-DeMet, A., & Nelson, J. N. (1989). A controlled trial of desipramine in 18 men with posttraumatic stress disorder. *American Journal of Psychiatry, 146,* 513–516.

Rosenbaum, J. F., Biederman, J., Gersten, M., Hirschfeld, D. R., Meminger, S. R., Herman, J. B., Kagan, J., Reznick, J. S., & Snidman, N. (1988). Behavioral inhibition in children of parents with panic disorder and agoraphobia: A control study. *Archives of General Psychiatry, 45,* 463–470.

Rosenbaum, J. F., Biederman, J., Hirschfeld, D. R., Bolduc, E. A., Faraone, S. V., Kagan, J., Snidman, N., Reznick, J. S. (1991). Further evidence of an association between behavioral inhibition and anxiety disorders: Results from a family study of children from a nonclinical sample. *Journal of Psychiatric Research, 25,* 49–65.

Rosenheck, R. (1986). Impact of post-traumatic stress disorder of World War II on the next generation. *Journal of Nervous and Mental Disease, 174,* 319–327.

Shanks, N., & Anisman, H. (1989). Strain-specific effects of antidepressants on escape deficits induced by inescapable shock. *Psychopharmacology, 99,* 122–128.

Sierles, F. S., Chen, J. J., McFarland, R. E., & Taylor, M. A. (1983). Posttraumatic stress disorder and concurrent psychiatric illness: A preliminary report. *American Journal of Psychiatry, 140,* 1177–1179.

Skre, I., Onstad, S., Torgersen, S., Lygren, S., & Kringlen, E. (1993). A twin study of DSM-III-R anxiety disorders. *Acta Psychiatrica Scandinavia, 88,* 85–92.

Solomon, S. D., & Canino, G. J. (1990). Appropriateness of DSM-III-R criteria for posttraumatic stress disorder. *Comprehensive Psychiatry, 31,* 227–237.

Solomon, Z., Kotler, M., & Mikulincer, M. (1988). Combat-related posttraumatic stress disorder among second-generation Holocaust survivors: Preliminary findings. *American Journal of Psychiatry, 145,* 865–868.

Southwick, S. M., Krystal, J. H., Bremner, J. D., Morgan, C. A., III, Nicolaou, A., Navy, L. M., Johnson, D. R., Heninger, G. R., Charney, D. S. (1997). Noradrenergic and serotonergic function in post-traumatic stress disorder. *Archives of General Psychiatry, 54,* 246–254.

Southwick, S. M., Krystal, J. H., Morgan, C. A., Johnson, D. R., Nagy, L. M., Nicolau, A., Heninger, G. R., Charney, D. S. (1993). Abnormal noradrenergic function in post traumatic stress disorder. *Archives of General Psychiatry, 50,* 266–274.

Speed, N., Engdahl, B., Schwartz, J., & Eberly, R. (1989). Posttraumatic stress disorder as a consequence of the POW experience. *Journal of Nervous and Mental Diseases, 177,* 147–153.

True, W. R., Rice, J., Eisen, S. A., Heath, A. C., Goldberg, J., Lyons, M. J., & Nowak, J. (1993). A twin study of genetic and environmental contributions to liability for posttraumatic stress symptoms. *Archives of General Psychiatry, 50,* 257–264.

Ursano, R. J., Wheatley, R., Sledge, W., Rahe, A., & Carlson, E. (1986). Coping and recovery styles in the Vietnam era prisoner of war. *Journal of Nervous and Mental Disease, 174,* 707–714.

Zacharko, R. M., Lalonde, G. T., Kasian, M., & Anisman, H. (1987). Strain-specific effects of inescapable shock on intracranial self-stimulation from nucleus accumbens. *Brain Research, 426,* 164–168.

Conclusions and Future Directions

YAEL DANIELI

The preceding thirty-eight chapters represent a pioneering effort to portray a comprehensive picture of the "state of the art" in the study of multigenerational transmission of trauma. The goal of this book is to map the international landscape of this emerging field by bringing together the work of different scholars/researchers from around the world. This volume reveals how they view, understand, and conceptualize the multigenerational legacies of trauma of multiple populations and places their findings within the multidimensional, multidisciplinary, integrative (TCMI) framework (see the Introduction). For some of these populations, this is the first time such issues have appeared in print.

FINDINGS: THE UNIVERSALITY OF MULTIGENERATIONAL TRANSMISSION OF TRAUMA

The evidence presented in the various chapters leads to the conclusion that the intergenerational transmission of trauma indeed exists. It occurs across populations within groups exposed to trauma. The book provides a solid clinical, theoretical, and empirical basis for understanding the multigenerational legacy of trauma and strongly suggests that it is a universal phenomenon.

In view of this overwhelming evidence, it is surprising that this topic is totally absent from, or only implicit in, "current" work such as Van der Kolk, McFarlane, and Weisaeth (1996) and Marsella, Friedman, Gerrity, and Scurfield (1996), respectively. It is also surprising that the concept of multigenerational legacies of trauma is deemed "rather inappropriate" by Figley and Kleber (1995), who (incorrectly) conclude that "[The] disturbances of the offspring of war survivors are not so much an issue of transmission of trauma as an issue of a specific socialization" (p. 87). Such views render the "socializations" devoid of both their trauma-related content and meaning. To the contrary, as Auerhahn and Laub (Chapter 1, this volume) ironically comment, the posttraumatic stress disorder (PTSD) literature accepts that therapists suffer from vicarious traumatization when working with trauma victims, yet disputes

YAEL DANIELI • Director, Group Project for Holocaust Survivors and Their Children; Private Practice, 345 East 80th Street, New York, New York 10021.

International Handbook of Multigenerational Legacies of Trauma, edited by Yael Danieli. Plenum Press, New York, 1998.

whether children of survivors are seriously affected by identification with their traumatized parents (see also *event countertransference;* e.g., Danieli, 1984). Moreover, Yehuda *et al.* (Chapter 37, this volume) find that low cortisol levels in offspring of Holocaust survivors are associated with their tendency to indicate distress about the trauma of the Holocaust and to have PTSD symptoms in response to Holocaust-related events that they hear about.

Although multigenerational consequences (Albeck, 1994) of trauma clearly exist, their phenomenology, etiology, and the precipitating conditions for their emergence are highly complex. Among children of survivors who suffer pathological consequences, for example, a heuristic explanation from an *intrafamilial* perspective alone consists of at least three components: (1) the parents' trauma, its parameters, and the offspring's own relationship to it; (2) the nature and extent of the conspiracy of silence surrounding the trauma and its aftermath; and (3) their parents' posttrauma adaptational styles (Danieli, 1985).

In agreement with numerous clinicians working with children and grandchildren of survivors of the Nazi Holocaust, Auerhahn and Laub (Chapter 1, this volume) state that these offspring are "burdened by memories which are not their own," and that the Holocaust is a core existential and relational experience for both generations. Consistent with most of the authors in this volume who approach their subjects from a clinical perspective, they conclude that massive trauma shapes the internal representation of reality of several generations, becoming an unconscious organizing principle passed on by parents and internalized by their children, and constituting the matrix within which normal developmental conflict takes place. Holocaust studies such as these, and their empirical counterparts, inspired much of the succeeding research on multigenerational legacies of other traumata.

In her review of empirical studies of the *nature* and *prevalence* of multigenerational effects of the Nazi Holocaust among North American nonclinical samples of children of survivors, Felsen (Chapter 2, this volume) concludes that while they do not, as a group, demonstrate psychopathology, they do share a psychological profile. Solomon (Chapter 3, this volume) reaches similar conclusions in her review of published empirical studies (of comparable variables) carried out in Israel. She adds that those who fail to cope suffer deeper and more intense distress than those who are not children of survivors (see also in this volume Rosenheck and Fontana, Chapter 14, on Vietnam veterans in the United States, and Nader, Chapter 33, on children exposed to a violent event).

Yehuda *et al.* (Chapter 37, this volume) demonstrate empirically that offspring of Holocaust survivors appear to have a similar neuroendocrine status to that of Holocaust survivors with PTSD, and that they may be more *psychologically* and *biologically* vulnerable to stress and trauma than controls. They also conclude that the "intergenerational syndrome" may have a phenomenology and *neurobiology* similar to that of PTSD.

Numerous authors in this volume, like Felsen (Chapter 2), find from empirical studies of family communication patterns that when *intrafamilial* communication about the parents' traumatic experiences is hindered, children suffer adverse effects, including problems of identity.[1] Felsen's review, however, reports differences between Israeli and North American samples in this regard, reflecting distinctions across *historical, sociocultural,* and *political* dimensions, among others.

These and other identity dimensions (e.g., *ethnic, religious*) are included in Erős, Vajda, and Kovacs (Chapter 19), and in the comparative study by Rosenthal and Völter (Chapter 18) of families of victims, perpetrators, and bystanders conducted in Israel, West Germany, and the

[1] See Nagata, Chapter 7; Op den Velde, Chapter 9; Lindt, Chapter 10; Aarts, Chapter 11; Rosenheck and Fontana, Chapter 14; Hunter-King, Chapter 15; Ancharoff *et al.*, Chapter 16; Rosenthal and Völter, Chapter 18; Baker and Gippenreitner, Chapter 25; Becker and Diaz, Chapter 26; Draimin *et al.*, Chapter 34; Wellisch and Hoffman, Chapter 35.

former East Germany. (A comparison of these families can also be found in Auerhahn and Laub, Chapter 1.)

Many of the variables investigated in the studies of offspring of the Nazi Holocaust reported here were also studied either clinically or empirically by contributors to this book exploring other populations. Their findings are mostly similar, yet interesting differences also emerge. Numerous authors note the *heterogeneity* of findings.[2] Several authors offer explanations for their findings and for the discrepancies between clinical and empirical reports; they grapple with numerous methodological issues and make recommendations for further work.

Focusing on indigenous peoples, a number of authors illustrate the interplay among multiple dimensions. They chronicle the attempts by European colonialism to destroy the peoples, their culture, and their indigenous governing structures (especially Odejide, Chapter 23, and Gagné, Chapter 22), thereby creating a system of *economic* dependency (Gagné, Chapter 22).

In Australia (Raphael, Swan, & Martinek, Chapter 20) and North America (Duran *et al.*, Chapter 21; Gagné, Chapter 22), for example, family structures and *cultural* identities were systematically assaulted by the forced removal of children into residential schools that were degrading and abusive. These practices led to significantly greater rates of alcoholism, drug abuse, domestic violence, crime, and suicide among the Aboriginal and Native communities than in the populations at large. These destructive behaviors have, in turn, had traumatogenic intergenerational effects on indigenous peoples. Everything that created security and order in their lives was ruptured. Their "soul wound" (Duran *et al.*, Chapter 21) was inflicted by ongoing, multidimensional trauma.

In his chapter on Hibakusha Nisei (children of atomic-bomb survivors), Tatara (Chapter 8) also demonstrates that a full understanding of the intergenerational consequences of massive traumatization is possible only through a multidimensional (e.g., physiological, cultural, sociopolitical, and economic) perspective. The same holds true for Buchanan's (Chapter 31) examination of the current world literature on international child maltreatment.

UTILITY OF THE MULTIDIMENSIONAL INTEGRATIVE (TCMI) FRAMEWORK

Given their findings, it is apparent that the study of multigenerational trauma requires a multidisciplinary, multidimensional integrative framework and, indeed, most of the contributors to this volume, working from the perspective of their own disciplines, acknowledge the need for such an approach. The Introduction to this volume offers an integrative framework that underscores the complex interplay of multiple dimensions both in describing traumata and the multigenerational responses to them.

The TCMI framework is versatile. In addition to the benefits listed in the Introduction, it can be used to focus in depth on a single dimension of an issue, or population, or to examine a wider field. Even when one maintains a "narrow" focus, the model provides a comprehensive contextual matrix to be kept in mind to illuminate possible omissions and interactions. For example, note the conspicuous absence of possible intergenerational consequences in the literature on rape trauma and rape treatment, as if the victim lives at least partially in a familial vacuum (Pynoos & Eth, 1985; Remer & Elliott, 1988a, 1988b; see also Danieli, 1994a). The framework is meant to help decipher, disentangle, and clarify complex

[2]Systematically introduced earlier (Danieli, 1985; Introduction, this volume; e.g., see Nagata, Chapter 7; Op den Velde, Chapter 9; Hunter-King, Chapter 15; Edelman *et al.,* Chapter 27; Yehuda *et al.,* Chapter 37; see also Major, 1996).

issues and guard against unidimensional reductionistic impulses and interdimensional displacements and substitutions that so often occur in the literature. See the analysis in Becker and Diaz (Chapter 26) for an example of the relationship between the "social process" and intrafamily dynamics, of "antifacism as a substitute mourning" in Rosenthal and Völter (Chapter 18), and, the description in Odejide *et al.* (Chapter 23) of ethnic conflicts that filled the power vacuum created by the end of colonialism and were transformed, at their worst, into fierce political and economic warfare.

Buchanan's (Chapter 31) framework is similar to the one proposed herein. She examines the current, multidisciplinary world literature on intergenerational child maltreatment, or what has become known as the "cycle of abuse." Her central thesis is that there are four cycles, rather than one, that operate both within and outside the family: sociopolitical and cultural (extrafamilial); psychological and biological (intrafamilial). She concludes that if patterns of intergenerational child maltreatment are to be broken, interventions need to be focused on the separate mechanisms that operate within each cycle. Comparative/interactional studies such as Simons and Johnson's (Chapter 32) and Rousseau and Drapeau's (Chapter 28) are informed by a multidimensional orientation. Findings by Rousseau and Drapeau (Chapter 28) suggest that culture influences the way in which the impact of trauma is mediated both through family variables and through implicit and explicit familial discourse around trauma. The developmental stage of the child also appears to interact with the different modes of familial transmission of trauma.

Aspects of the Time Dimension

Rousseau and Drapeau (Chapter 28) are among the few investigators who give prominence to the crucial dimension of time in understanding the complex process of intergenerational trauma. While it is sometimes implied in the trauma literature, it has generally been underemphasized. Focusing on the time dimension may shed light on the impact of trauma on both the perspective and time orientation of survivors and the generations before and after them.

The time orientation is an individual's temporal organization of experience, usually conceived in terms of past, present, and future, and often endowed with different weights, degrees of attentiveness, and cognitive or emotional investments. Trauma affects one's relationship to the totality of one's lifeline: to birth and death, developmental stages, transitions, and changes.

The importance of time is also acknowledged by the inclusion of symptom C.(7) in the DSM-IV diagnosis of PTSD: "sense of a foreshortened future (e.g., does not expect to have a career, marriage, children, or a normal life span" (p. 428). (See Terr, 1985, pp. 61–63, for a discussion of time distortion in traumatized children.)

Many of the chapters in this book corroborate the conceptualization of trauma as *rupture* resulting in *fixity,* reflected in the victim/survivor's experience of being *frozen in time* (e.g., Hardtmann, Chapter 4; Bar-On, Ostrovsky, & Fromer, Chapter 5; Hunter-King, Chapter 15). Lomranz, Shmotkin, Zechovoy, and Rosenberg (1985) confirm empirically that the time orientation of survivors "reflects their Holocaust experience," and conclude that "time orientation is a concomitant to catastrophic and extremely stressful events" (p. 234). From a multigenerational perspective, Klain (Chapter 17) states: "If we can say that this [patriarchal] society has not changed, or has changed very little . . . since the Roman and Turkish times, then we must conclude that, in fact, *it has no history."* He also describes mechanisms of transmission that ensure the maintenance and perpetuation of this static living in the traumatic rupture.

Some of the authors also concur with the conception of *bidirectional transmission* of trauma (Elder, Caspi, & Downey, 1986). Perhaps the most striking examples of this are found in Draimin, Levine, and McKelvy's (Chapter 34) analysis of the HIV/AIDS global epidemic, which illustrates the distortions of the normal cycle of all generations and ages. "The generation of young adults has been hardest hit, adding extra burdens to the older generation and foreclosing options for the young" (see also Wellisch & Hoffman, Chapter 35). Raphael *et al.* (Chapter 20) write of the "stressed grannies" who must assume their children's parenting role.

Conversely, in the bidirectionality of the concept of time used, herein lies a central element for healing: the hope and promise enshrined in future generations. Ornstein (1981) views grandparenting and the creation of postwar "adoptive" extended families as highly adaptive and healing, especially for aging survivors (see also Bar-On, 1994).

Several authors[3] write about children born, or already alive, during the trauma period. In these cases, the trauma impacts the whole family during the same time span. This is a different situation from the parents' or grandparents' trauma affecting generations born *after* the trauma. McFarlane, Blumbergs, Policansky, and Irwin (1985) have shown in disaster studies that ongoing parental PTSD is one of the most significant variables leading to disaster-related morbidity in the child (see also Green, Karol, & Grace, 1994; with regard to crime, see Nader, Chapter 33).

Another important issue is the moment in history that the victim/survivor designates as the beginning of his or her identity and heritage. (Does it reach back to biblical times? After the Holocaust? Does he or she claim the totality of his or her history, or only a portion of it?) The variety of dimensions the individual involves in the recovery process is related to his or her healing and the availability of resources for growth and strength (Danieli, 1981b, 1994a). Hardtmann (Chapter 4) observes that when children of Nazis grew up with faceless and "history-less" parents, they had problems developing their own identities. Several parts of the book, particularly those focusing on indigenous peoples, repressive regimes, and infectious diseases, elaborate on the complexity of *ongoing,* as distinct from *discrete,* trauma. For example, Raphael *et al.* (Chapter 20) observe that it is difficult to distinguish particular intergenerational transmission when considerable vulnerability must be related to the extensive and pervasive ongoing effects of dislocation, depression, deprivation, and discrimination (see also Buchanan, Chapter 31; Simons & Johnson, Chapter 32).

Unresolved trauma results in an absence of closure in the lives of victim/survivors and their children. Hunter-King (Chapter 15) observes that, in the case of those missing in action in Vietnam, the grief is timeless; the lack of resolution ensures the passage of trauma to the next generation. In Argentina and Chile, the relatively more democratic successors to repressive regimes have still failed to account fully for those who "disappeared."

Changes are also possible along the time dimension. Most children of survivors remember their family's and war history "only in bits and pieces," and experience the *healing of the narrative* as most integrative and therapeutic (Danieli, 1993). The activity of rebridging is often experienced as healing the family wound, which may free one to go on with life more fully. Keller (1988) reported that the older the offspring, the more likely they were to describe their families as less adaptive, and their parents as engaging in indirect communication about the Holocaust. However, there seem to be reparative processes later in the lives of these offspring. They perceive themselves as less depressed and less anxious than they were when younger (Schwartz, Dohrenwend, & Levar, 1994). Parts V, VI, and VII of this volume discuss the effects of sociopolitical changes, or lack thereof, on legacies of trauma.

The time dimension is integral to Keilson's (1992) theory of sequential traumatization, and to Duran *et al.*'s (Chapter 21) definition of trauma: "Historical trauma response" consists

---

[3]See Becker and Diaz, Chapter 26; Edelman *et al.,* Chapter 27; Rousseau and Drapeau, Chapter 28; Simpson, Chapter 29; Ghadirian, Chapter 30.

of a constellation of features in reaction to the multigenerational, collective, historical, and cumulative psychic wounding over time, both in their victims' life span and across generations.

Resilience

The utility of the TCMI framework is further illustrated by its applicability to the seeming debate in the literature over vulnerability versus resilience. As mentioned in the Introduction, the TCMI framework enables discussion of "vulnerability *or* resilience" as "vulnerability *and* resilience." This is preferable to the unidimensional perspective, which is simplistic at best, and meaningless and wrong at worst.

Solomon (Chapter 3) suggests that more attention should be paid to positive effects that arise from trauma. Felsen (Chapter 2) concludes that along with vulnerabilities, there is evidence of significant ego strengths, as illustrated by both high achievement motivation and increased empathic capacities. Increased empathic capacities are mentioned by many other authors.[4] Draimin *et al.* (Chapter 34) also mentions "a reservoir of spiritual strength" in families with HIV/AIDS. O'Shane, quoted in Raphael *et al.* (Chapter 20), reflects: "I recognized the thing that happened to the thousands of other Aboriginal families like our family and I marvelled that we weren't all stark, raving mad." Krystal *et al.* (Chapter 38) further suggest that resilience, like vulnerability to traumatization, is modulated genetically. In addition, the genetic effect on resilience may be mediated by effects on affiliative behaviors.

Baker and Gippenreitner (Chapter 25) conclude that whether the grandparents actually physically survived Stalin's Purge of the mid-1930s was less important than the strength and values passed on to their grandchildren through the knowledge of what had happened to them. "Disconnected" grandchildren were less clear about who they were or where they were going, as they attempted to function in the Russia of the 1990s. "Connected" grandchildren had a sense of identity firmly rooted in family experience. The grandchildren's *social functioning* correlates positively with *active protest* (see also Kupelian, Kalayjian, & Kassabian, Chapter 12), efforts to research a family member's experience of the Purge, and the perception that the Purge had a positive influence on their lives (for additional examples of positive outcomes, see also Nagata, Chapter 7; Hunter-King, Chapter 15; Danieli, 1985).

Satir (1972), too, writes of the "nurturing" strength of family roots and the importance of connections across generations, concepts reflecting the protective functions of the family. (See also Winnicott's "holding environment," cited by Becker & Diaz, Chapter 26, and Rutter's concept of *permitting circumstances* that parents need in order to parent, cited by Buchanan, Chapter 31.)

In this context, resilience is related to continuity, transmission without cutoff, and preserving the connections with the past, without letting them become so rigid as to become *perversions of freedom* (Danieli, 1991; see also Klain, Chapter 17). However, once the threatening period is over and survival strategies and defenses have outlived their usefulness, they may nevertheless persist and become adaptational styles of the family and the culture (Danieli, 1985; see also Spicer, 1971).

Felsen (Chapter 2) offers the example of the *culturally* valued emphasis on the family demonstrated by Eastern European Jewry. This provided the survivors with the defenses and coping mechanisms that allowed them to make the leap of hope necessary to establish new

---

[4]On empathic capacities, see, e.g., Nagata, Chapter 7; Op den Velde, Chapter 9; Lindt, Chapter 10; Ancharoff *et al.,* Chapter 16; Baker and Gippenreitner, Chapter 25; Becker and Diaz, Chapter 26.

families after the Holocaust. But this adaptation also took its toll on survivors' offspring, who exhibited increased difficulties around separation–individuation. Such negative consequences must be taken into account with the potentially highly adaptive role of the family in the context of severe traumatization and loss.

The findings in this volume clearly show the importance of cultural roots and practices in creating stability, and the deleterious and even tragic effects on future generations when the culture is weakened or destroyed.

Cross (Chapter 24), too, chronicles the positive effects of culture and family strength in creating coping strategies. Referring to the adaptive and protective value of the *multidimensional mind-set* (Webber, 1978), Cross explains that by resisting negative elements of the culture that enslaved them, but incorporating protective, positive, and functional ones, most notably the Christian religion, former slaves were able "to exit slavery with far more psychological strengths and resources than psychological defects and dysfunctionalities." Ghadirian (Chapter 30) emphasizes the contribution of spiritual, religious, and sociocultural beliefs to resilience. Trials and suffering may actually serve a positive function in overcoming adversity and lead to personal growth in victim/survivors and their offspring. Illuminating as they are, all these studies demonstrate the need for future research on the relationship between culture and traumatization on succeeding generations.

Theoretical Frameworks

Different writers use different concepts and related methodologies stemming from existing, generally complementary, although sometimes seemingly contradictory theoretical frameworks. While part of what distinguishes this book is its diversity, many of the authors choose similar ways of looking at the issues, leading to some overlap and yet maintaining coherence among their viewpoints.

Suomi and Levine (Chapter 36), Krystal *et al.* (Chapter 38), and Yehuda *et al.* (Chapter 37), for example, use animal models, and genetic and biological frameworks, respectively. Hardtmann (Chapter 4), Op den Velde (Chapter 9), and Aarts (Chapter 11) utilize primarily the intrapsychic/psychodynamic approaches, such as psychoanalytic object relations theories, while Klain (Chapter 17) applies psychoanalytic and group analytic concepts. Ancharoff, Munroe, and Fisher (Chapter 16) apply "assumptive world" and constructivist self-development theories.

Quite a few of the chapters borrow various family system theory and family theory concepts (Nagata, Chapter 7; Baker & Gippenreitner, Chapter 25). Nagata (Chapter 7) also uses life-span developmental theory.

Several authors combine and integrate concepts from different theoretical frameworks (e.g., Buchanan, Chapter 31; Becker & Diaz, Chapter 26; Simpson, Chapter 29; Nagata, Chapter 7). Gagné (Chapter 22) integrates sociological and psychological concepts with Third World development dependency theory to explore the prevalence of PTSD in First Nations.

Many of these concepts derive from theories aimed at analyzing and interpreting everyday life. Some of the writers also utilize or propose concepts that seem to have originated more directly from, and are thus inherent to, the universe of trauma and are particularly relevant to multigenerational trauma theory. Notably, Felsen (Chapter 2) includes a dimension of *being* (vs. doing) as part of a general conceptual framework to organize and unify the diverse clinical and empirical observations about offspring of survivors of the Nazi Holocaust. Becker and Diaz (Chapter 26) include the concept of "the third traumatic sequence" (Keilson, 1992[5]; see also Op den Velde, Chapter 9), as well as trauma-related formulations by Winnicott (1973, 1974, 1976) and Kinston and Cohen (1986). In a similar vein, Duran *et al.* (Chapter 21) define *historical trauma response* or "intergenerational posttraumatic stress disorder" as a constellation of features in reaction to the multigenerational, collective, historical, and cumulative psychic wounding over time: the "soul wound."

MECHANISMS OF THE TRANSMISSION OF TRAUMA

The mechanisms of transmission emerging from this book range from the molecular genetic on the one end, to the political on the other; that is, they range from the basic biological to the complex psychological—psychodynamic constructs at the individual level, and from the intrafamilial to the extrafamilial—the socioethnocultural, to the political. Logically, the authors' descriptions and explanations of the transmission processes and their contents are often determined by the dimension(s) they choose to focus on, and their theoretical orientations and disciplines. Yet considering the richness and variety of the materials covered in this book, the mechanisms depicted are surprisingly consistent and few in number. Moreover, various modes of trauma transmission are not likely to be mutually exclusive; rather, for most individuals, they reflect some overlap and a cumulative effect. While it sometimes seems artificial to place divisions among interrelated mechanisms, researchers must isolate them in order to target appropriate interventions.

Krystal *et al.* (Chapter 38) review the evidence supporting a genetic contribution to the vulnerability to developing PTSD. They suggest that the overall adaptiveness or maladaptiveness of particular genetic traits may depend on the environment in which individuals bearing these traits exist.

Suomi and Levine (Chapter 36) provide clear-cut evidence obtained from prospective longitudinal experiments that demonstrates that nonhuman primates are indeed capable of transmitting long-term psychobiological effects of trauma across generations via at least three different mechanisms: observational, maternal, and prenatal. In each case, the long-term effects include physiological as well as behavioral features or propensities, and in two of the three cases, the mechanisms of transmission have been documented in natural social groups of primates living in the wild, as well as in those studies conducted in laboratory settings. None of the three mechanisms requires language capabilities on the part of either the initiating or receiving generation for the transmission to take place.

Hardtmann (Chapter 4), Aarts (Chapter 11), and Becker and Diaz (Chapter 26), among others, draw on psychoanalytic object relations theories to provide detailed, poignant descriptions of the processes and mechanisms of transmission that deepen the insight into the pathogenesis in the second generation. They cite *denial, splitting, identification, projection,* and *projective identifi-*

---

[5]In his theory of sequential traumatization, Keilson (1992) coined the phrase *third traumatic sequence* to refer to the postwar period that followed both the occupation, with its terror (first sequence), and the direct persecution, including deportations (second sequence). Having followed up 2,000 child survivors in The Netherlands, he concluded that "approximately twenty-five years later, children who experienced a favorable second but adverse third traumatic sequence will display development features which are less favorable than those of children presenting an adverse second but favorable third traumatic sequence" (p. 440). Similar to Danieli (see section on the *conspiracy of silence* in the Introduction), a poor postwar environment could intensify the preceding traumatic events and, conversely, a good environment could mitigate some of the traumatic effects. Op den Velde (Chapter 9) adds that when understanding and support are adequate, the postwar period does not have to be, by definition, a traumatic sequence.

cation. One such example is the interaction between parent and child that can become a repetition of an aggressor–victim dyad from the traumatic past, after first becoming an intrapsychic conflict and, subsequently, through projective identification, seeking an outlet in object relations.

These mechanisms are both very similar to the process of the original victimization and maintain the victimization process. On every level, we psychologically or literally expel troubling matters: as individuals, families, communities, societies, nations, and the international community (Hardtmann, Chapter 4; Baker & Gippenreiner, Chapter 25; Simpson, Chapter 29; see elaboration by Klain, Chapter 17). Society as a whole can behave as if it had PTSD. The same mechanisms of defense have both personal and societal dimensions.

From *this* point of view, the most malignant component of the transmission is the raw, unintegrated affect that has never been processed in the parents' generation and, consequently, becomes internalized in the children in another place and time.

For Ancharoff *et al.* (Chapter 16), intergenerational transmission refers to *thoughts, feelings, behaviors,* and *disrupted schemata or traumatic beliefs* of the traumatized parents that are generated from the survivors' experiences. The survivors transmit them to their children through *silence* and *underdisclosure,* (age-inappropriate) *overdisclosure, identification*— observation, modeling, and emulating (e.g., survivor's propensity for hypervigilance), and isomorphic *reenactment.* In the latter mechanism, the survivor's trauma experience is created in the offspring, perhaps unconsciously, but forcefully, transmitting the parent's worldview.

Participants in this process are secondarily traumatized (Figley, 1983). Their affective experience is of projective identification that may generate certain countertransference reactions in psychotherapists (Danieli, 1984, 1994c). Kestenberg (1989) coins the term *transposition* to describe the tendency of Holocaust survivors' offspring to transpose the present into the past and to live in their fantasy during the Holocaust. Pynoos (1996) elaborates on the "traumatic expectations" parents transmit to their children.

Nagata (Chapter 7) views family relationships as accountable to the standards of loyalty and justice upheld by previous generations, and, as such, families transmit rules, dispense "credits" for fulfilling obligations, and "debits" for unfulfilled obligations. They also transmit ethnic values, family myths, loyalties, secrets, and expectations. The uncompleted actions of past generations may impinge on relationships within the new generation.

Kupelian *et al.* (Chapter 12) state that the Armenians perpetuated a distinct ethnic identity by adapting their family structure to centuries of persecution. Functionally, presence of the *persecutory oppositional pressure* (Spicer, 1971) became integral to multigenerational family structure and identity. *Informal* structures of transmission include *family* and *community* (e.g., food, stories, songs, friends, and language). *Formal* means include reestablishing institutional structures. The church has been central to the preservation of cultural identity, particularly against forced assimilation.

Duran *et al.* (Chapter 21) explore the mechanisms that render *historical trauma* an *ongoing* process. These include pressures brought on by *acculturation stress* and the aftereffects of *racism, oppression,* and *genocide.* They also point to "a less murderous form of genocide in the Native community, sometimes labeled cultural genocide" which refers to "actions that are threatening to the integrity and continuing viability of peoples and social groups" (Legters, 1988, p. 769). These actions include the prohibition of religious freedom.

Current classifications of mechanisms of transmission include the heritability (Kendler, 1988, also in Krystal *et al.,* Chapter 38; Schwartz *et al.,* 1994) and the biopsychosocial (Engel, 1977, 1996) models. Novac (1994; Novac & Hubert-Schneider, 1998) proposes that the transmission of trauma includes three major biopsychosocial components: transmission of information, transmission of acquired traits, and intrafamilial traumatization (biological dysregulation), which are concomitant and potentially constant new sources of traumatization.

Examining the influence of remote historical events on recent interethnic conflicts in the former Yugoslavia, Klain (Chapter 17) describes the multigenerational transmission of "inherited" emotions from psychoanalytic and group analytic points of view. Processes and mechanisms of transmission, such as *paranoid projections fed by stereotypes, group superego,* and *group memory,* lead to transgenerational remembrance of injury, murder, and destruction that are laid at the door of the "enemy people" or nation as a whole. He differentiates between vehicles of transmission, which he terms mediators of "inherited" emotions, and *what* they transmit.

The mediators of "inherited" emotions, which he lists and illustrates extensively, are the *patriarchal family,* the *superego, folklore, church/religion,* and *myths.* These powerful mechanisms transmit *deep hate and rage, revenge, guilt, shame,* and *authority.* They also operate on larger groups that may encompass the neighborhood, the town, or the state, which is conceived as a widened family of a patriarchal type, in which all authority lies in the hands of its leader. This endangers democracy for the present and future generation.

Korbin (in Buchanan, Chapter 31) suggests that in coming to internationally accepted definitions of child abuse, there is a need for both an emic approach, where the local community makes the definitions, and an etic approach, where there is an international consensus on types of behavior toward children that are deemed abusive (see the same classification in Rousseau & Drapeau, Chapter 28).

Simons and Johnson (Chapter 32) examine competing explanations for the intergenerational transmission of domestic violence in three generations: role modeling, family relationships, and antisocial orientation perspectives. In contrast to past research findings that children who witness violence between their parents or who are subjected to severe physical discipline often grow up to be violent toward their spouses and offspring, their analyses show that the relationship between childhood exposure to domestic violence and the perpetration of such behavior as an adult is mediated by the extent to which the person displays an antisocial orientation acquired in childhood as a result of ineffective parenting. These findings are consistent with criminological theories.

CONSPIRACY OF SILENCE

An overwhelming finding throughout the chapters in this volume is the "conspiracy of silence" that far too often follows the trauma(ta) (see discussion in the Introduction). According to most contributors, the conspiracy of silence is the most prevalent and effective mechanism for the transmission of trauma on all dimensions. Both intrapsychically and interpersonally protective, silence is profoundly destructive, for it attests to the person's, family's, society's, community's, and nation's inability to integrate the trauma. They can find no words to narrate the trauma story and create a meaningful dialogue around it. This prevalence of a conspiracy of silence stands in sharp contrast to the widespread research findings that social support is the most important factor in coping with traumatic stress.

Nagata (Chapter 7) reports that more than twice as many Sansei whose fathers were in camps died before the age of 60, compared to Sansei whose fathers were not interned (see also Eitinger, 1980, about survivors of the Nazi Holocaust, and Edelman, Kordon, & Lagos, 1992, about fathers of the disappeared in Argentina). Nagata speculates that there may be a link between the early deaths of the Nisei fathers and their general reluctance to discuss the internment. Pennebaker, Barger, and Tiebout's (1989) research suggests that avoidance of discussing one's traumatic experience may negatively affect physical health, and Sansei in the present study reported that their Nisei fathers were much less likely to bring up the topic of internment than were their mothers.

The conspiracy of silence is also used *as a defense* for trying to prevent total collapse and breakout of intrusive traumatic memories and emotions. Like paper, it is a very thin and flimsy protection that rips easily. Auerhahn and Laub's (Chapter 1) focus on children's conflicting attempts both to know and to defend against such knowledge emerges as a central theme in many of the chapters.

Aarts (Chapter 11) concludes that the conspiracy of silence, encouraged by societal, cultural, and political silence, is generally understood to be at the core of the dynamics that may lead to more or less serious symptomatology in the second generation. Op den Velde (Chapter 9) demonstrates that when offspring of war sailors and participants in the resistance observed the "family secret," separation and identification problem arose. Lindt (Chapter 10) states that children of collaborators, who had to hide who they are, have great difficulty in sharing in the experience of liberation: "to be allowed to be there with one's story."

To this day, only meager attention has been paid to the offspring of veterans of World War II. Bernstein (Chapter 6) chronicles the isolation and emotional distance and emptiness created when World War II prisoners of war avoided close emotional relationships with their spouses and children.[6] Except in the literature on Vietnam veterans, "good" wars are not supposed to have "bad" consequences. This holds true for veterans of Israel's War of Independence as well (Bar-On *et al.,* Chapter 5).

In studies of Israel, West Germany, and the former German Democratic Republic, Rosenthal and Völter (Chapter 18) find that the phenomenon of collective silence had endured despite the emergence in recent years of a more open social dialogue about the Holocaust. Their case analyses clearly show that silence and family secrets and myths constitute some of the most effective mechanisms that ensure the traumata's continued impact on the family's second or third generation.

These findings raise the important question of whether silence is part, or an extension of, the trauma (e.g., Kupelian *et al.,* Chapter 12), or whether it is a qualitatively different "trauma *after* the trauma" (Rappaport, 1968, p. 730; emphasis added). Does the posttrauma environment pose a *new* set of events that the victim needs to complete or resolve in addition to the initial victimization?

The process of confronting multigenerational trauma has taken over five decades to unfold, stage by stage. First, as Aarts notes in Chapter 11, the barriers of silence needed to be removed in order for society in general, and politicians in particular, to address the individual and collective needs of victims of World War II. Indeed, it took a social movement in order to arouse interest not only of policymakers but also of most mental health professionals (Herman, 1992).

Though descriptions of what is now understood as posttraumatic stress have appeared throughout recorded history, the development of the field of traumatic stress, or traumatology, has been episodic, marked by interest and denial, and plagued with serious errors in diagnostic and treatment practices (Herman, 1992; Mangelsdorf, 1985; Solomon, 1995). Indeed, one of the most prevalent and consistent themes during this century has been the denial of psychic trauma and its consequences (Lifton, 1979), particularly in the myriad deadly conflicts that find their multigenerational origins in history, the nonresolution of which ensures their perpetuation.

---

[6]See also Op den Velde, Chapter 9; for comparison, see Crocq, Macher, Barros-Beck, Rosenberg, and Duval, 1993; Harel, Kahana, and Wilson, 1993; Tennant, Goulston, and Dent, 1993.

Politically dictated or officially sanctioned silence is part of the system of terror of any tyrannical regime, and extreme versions of this are found in Kupelian *et al.* (Chapter 12) and Ghadirian (Chapter 30). One can only marvel at the international dimensions of the conspiracy of silence, as shown by the slowness of the world community to acknowledge and act on the terrible events in the former Yugoslavia (Klain, Chapter 17), as well as in Rwanda and Burundi.

THE IMPORTANCE OF CULTURE AS TRANSMITTER, BUFFER, AND HEALER

Most authors see culture as integral to understanding the predicament of the survivors' families, particularly where their cultural identity played a role in their victimization. The very notion of intergenerational transmission is implied in the concept of culture (Marsella *et al.*, 1996), and "bears directly upon the puzzle of how society is possible" (Elder *et al.*, 1986, p. 295). From a multidimensional approach, in some cases, healing requires restoring the *cultural context* and culturally appropriate therapies.

Kupelian *et al.* (Chapter 12) review the crucial role of culture—family, community, language, church—in maintaining Armenian identity during the diaspora. Kinzie, Boehnlein, and Sack's study of the effects of massive trauma on Cambodian parents and children (Chapter 13) and Rousseau and Drapeau's (Chapter 28) examination of the impact of culture on the transmission of trauma among Southeast Asian and Latin American children point to the traumatic effects of the destruction of culture.

Culture influences the way the impact of trauma is mediated, and cultural continuity can play a protective role while facilitating the grieving process. In Nagata's study of Japanese American internees (Chapter 7), a major after-effect of internment was the accelerated loss of the Japanese language and culture, along with continued uncertainty about their status. This phenomenon of trauma-related *accelerated deacculturation* is also emphasize in Kinzie *et al.* (Chapter 13).

The intentional, brutal, and largely effective efforts to destroy indigenous cultures as part of colonization are the central element in Part VI of this volume. It is particularly noteworthy that this trauma is, in the words of Raphael *et al.* (Chapter 20), "enduring and unquantifiable," and it is perpetuated by the continuing destruction of their culture and disruption of any effort to pass it along to future generations (Duran *et al.*, Chapter 21; Gagné, Chapter 22). This *historical trauma* is a cumulative, unresolved trauma, and the final irony is that to survive, people must assimilate into the very culture that has destroyed their own (Duran *et al.*, Chapter 21; see also Kleber, 1995; Robin, Chester, & Goldman, 1996).

Odejide *et al.*'s (Chapter 23) analysis of the Nigerian civil war points to ethnic clashes based on differences in cultures as one of the major reasons for war. As in the chapters on succeeding generations of Cambodians and Japanese, a major consequence of intergenerational transmission in shown to be the breakdown of social values. His recounting of fiction to tell this story is unique to the book and is a technique rich for anecdotal information and comparisons.

Hunter-King (Chapter 15) finds that "typical" military wives who have firmly adopted the "military culture" are more likely to rear children who can adjust to their father's missing-in-action (MIA) status.

Given the strong role of the destruction of cultural foundations in intergenerational transmission of trauma, it is not surprising that several authors stress the importance of incorporating elements of traditional culture into the *healing* process through the development and usage of culturally appropriate therapies.

Duran *et al.* (Chapter 21) insist on the necessity for cultural revitalization that would include "indigenous therapies" to replace the hegemonic approach of "postcolonial therapies" based on European concepts of healing. However, they also recognize the need to combine the modern (i.e., psychotherapy) with traditional ceremonies. Raphael *et al.* (Chapter 20) agree and list several approaches that build on Aboriginal holistic views of mental health.

Some authors mention the need for therapy that is less centered on the individual and family, as in the West, and more oriented to groups and society. Moreover, Simpson (Chapter 29) speaks of the need to heal the effects of unresolved conflicts on communities and nations.

Societies, cultures, and religions differ in their emphasis on the individual versus the social/collective. A child of survivors of the Nazi Holocaust exclaimed: "On Yom Kippur, Jews say, 'we have sinned, we have done. . . .' Nowhere does it say, 'I have done. . . .' It is all 'we.' It's never individual, it's always the community. It may say something about our reaction to the Shoah [Holocaust] that it is not a personal thing, but it is what has happened to *us,* and that goes transgenerationally."

The concept of culturally sensitive therapies leading to the restoration of traditional skills and values, when combined with a program of national reconciliation, offers hope to the remnants of indigenous people, as well as to former warring parties. Both Bar-On *et al.* (Chapter 5), in the context of generations of the Holocaust, and Klain (Chapter 17), in the case of the former Yugoslavia, emphasize that it is necessary to bring people together who were on opposite sides during civil wars. The emphasis must be on children and on utilizing group treatment modalities. A central challenge is to transform the destructive use of culture into a healing one.

RECOMMENDATIONS FOR THE FUTURE

In this groundbreaking volume of work on multigenerational trauma in a multidimensional framework, many contributors propose further areas of inquiry to advance this critically important field.

Methodological Considerations

As yet, empirical research in the field of intergenerational trauma is in its infancy, but its social and public health significance is ever growing. Given a lifetime PTSD rate of 7.8% in the U.S. general population (Kessler, Sonnega, Bromet, Hughes, & Nelson, 1995), even if only a minority is or will be involved in parenting, the number of children upon whom intergenerational effects will have an impact is enormous. In other groups and societies, where the rates of trauma exposure are much higher, an even greater proportion of the population is affected, with consequent intergenerational implications.

One leading recommendation is for improved research methodology representing all points of view, through better sampling and more valid tools. Some analyses of intergenerational patterns reveal significant between-group differences, while others do not, and it was found that the combination of survey and in-depth interviews was particularly useful in uncovering such a range.

Researchers should also attempt to replicate and expand on the exploratory work contained in this volume, not only to understand the legacies of unique experiences, but also to clarify the impact of differing cultural and situational factors on traumatic response.

Prospective investigations of the intergenerational psychobiological consequences of stress in human populations are also sorely needed, but as Suomi and Levine (Chapter 36) *psycho-somatic-*

acknowledge, such studies are more feasible and practical in animals than in humans (for an exception, see Elder *et al.,* 1986).

Further molecular genetic studies of PTSD should be conducted in order to identify genes that modulate the vulnerability as well as resilience to traumatization (Krystal *et al.,* Chapter 38).

There is a need for comparisons among similar populations, particularly where there is as yet only the most rudimentary information from which inferences may be drawn (Raphael *et al.,* Chapter 20), and multidimensional cross-cultural comparisons that include sources of resilience. In addition, some contributors recommend systematic comparative studies of individual and societal traumata, as well as families in which one or both parents have been traumatized. It is also worth exploring whether both parents have shared specific traumatic experience(s). In all these endeavors, researchers should strive for agreement on definitions, rather than use ad hoc terms that can undermine the discipline.

Keeping in mind their contextual parameters, future research should gauge the usefulness and applicability of numerous concepts that emerge from the book along different dimensions and in differing (cultural) settings.

In planning multicultural comparisons, investigators should consider the relative centrality of the family and differing emphases on the individual versus the collective/social in different cultures.

Clinical Considerations

As noted in the Introduction and described in this volume, many of the clinical features reported in the majority of the chapters fit the syndrome of PTSD. Many offspring of survivors of trauma, however, struggle with problems of a psychosomatic and/or characterological nature, yet these are not included in the construct of PTSD. The evidence presented herein calls for expanding the current diagnostic criteria for the disorder. Moreover, this volume suggests that a new framework—Trauma and the Continuity of Self: A Multidimensional Multidisciplinary Integrative (TCMI) Framework—is needed to understand and treat trauma along all dimensions and across cultures.

Similarly, to meet the complex needs of survivors and their families, any program must be comprehensive, integrative, and linked to formal and informal networks of all relevant services and resources in the local and global community.

Additional efforts must be made by clinicians working with indigenous people. They must develop competence in the local culture in order to correct the persisting cultural hegemony of Euro-American therapeutic models that follow a postcolonial paradigm. The earlier section on culture contains a discussion of mechanisms of healing that exist on a cultural level.

One of the key clinical recommendations suggested by many of the findings is the need to take a full intergenerational history of trauma and PTSD evidence as a routine part of history-taking and diagnostic evaluations. This is particularly true for "children" who meet criteria for PTSD, and those who often fail to present family background.

As the history is being taken, the guiding dynamic principle of integration should inform the choice of therapeutic modalities, techniques, or interventions. The central therapeutic goal is to integrate rupture, discontinuity, and disorientation. An extremely useful diagnostic and therapeutic method is to construct a multigenerational family tree. Although this may trigger an acute sense of pain and loss, it serves to recreate a sense of continuity and coherence damaged by the traumatic experiences. One invaluable yield of exploring the family tree is that it opens communication within families and between generations, and makes it possible to work-through toxic family secrets. Breaking the silence about traumatic experiences within the family is generally helpful in (family) therapy, but it is particularly crucial for aging survivors and their offspring (Danieli, 1981a, 1994b). Whether family therapy is feasible or not, and regardless of the therapeutic modality used, individuals and families should be viewed within the context of their multigenerational family tree, with its unique dynamics, history, and culture (Danieli, 1993).

As for the mix of therapeutic modalities urged by Danieli (1989, 1993), Felsen (Chapter 2) points to the potential usefulness of cognitive therapy in enhancing the individual's resilience and in emphasizing self-statements that empower the victim/survivor as opposed to blame or victimize him- or herself.

This book cautions policymakers that the trauma-related decisions they make, which they may assume have only short-term consequences (if any), may actually have lifelong and multigenerational effects. The findings of many contributors to this volume have far-reaching implications for the *prevention* of social and political upheaval. As for designing means of prevention, some of Klain's "mechanisms of inherited emotions," for example, may be used to transmit messages and emotions of peace and tolerance instead of hatred and revenge. Outside the realm of traditional mental health practices, a number of peace-related organizations have sprung up to avert further outbreaks of violence. Among these is the German-based Action Reconciliation Service for Peace (ARSP), whose motto is "Learning from History, Taking a Stand Today, Building a Positive Future." For almost 30 years, ARSP has had volunteers in the countries affected by World War II to work with the peoples who suffered during the Nazi regime. They believe there can be no true reconciliation without atonement, without acknowledging German responsibility for Nazi crimes (see other examples in Dubrow, Liwski, Palacios, and Gardinier, 1996).

The future is ever more problematic in settings where ongoing conflicts and difficult living conditions spawn multigenerational consequences of chronic trauma.

Issues and Populations Warranting Further Exploration

Despite the range of populations addressed in this volume, several traditional categories of "individual" and "group" victims have not been included in this multigenerational survey. One such category is that of rape victims, who have been studied widely, but very little is known about their children (Remer & Elliott, 1988a, b). Another category includes the offspring of Korean and other Asian women who were kept as "sex slaves" by the Japanese occupying forces during World War II, an atrocity that they admitted only recently.

Other topics worth exploring, which are given limited treatment herein, are the sexual abuse of children and the "false memory syndrome," both issues of great intergenerational importance, and the multigenerational effects of parental dissociative identity disorder.

Studies on the multigenerational legacies of natural disasters should be extended to focus on children born after the trauma. Similarly, studies addressing families with/of diethylstilbestrol (DES) daughters should expand the work of Draimin *et al.* (Chapter 34) and Wellisch and Hoffman (Chapter 35) on the intergenerational effects of AIDS and breast cancer, respectively. In addition, it behooves us to ensure the end of discrimination against women with AIDS (probably mothers) with regard to the availability of treatment.

The issues raised in this volume may also be applicable to other populations who have suffered massive psychic trauma that put people at risk for similar sequelae. These would include the Palestinians, Irish, Turks/Greeks/Cypriots, Kurds, Afghans, and Afghanis. Additionally, populations traumatized by recent catastrophic events in places such as Somalia, Rwanda, and Burundi have suffered, and will undoubtedly continue to suffer, intergenerational effects. They will require both immediate interventions and long-term preventive strategies.

The role of gender in the transmission of traumatic history should be further explored cross-culturally (Felsen, Chapter 2; Solomon, Chapter 3; Hunter-King, Chapter 15; Klain, Chapter 17). Baker and Gippenreitner (Chapter 25) also highlight the special role of women as *messengers* of family values, traditions, and memories.

A growing number of populations face the daunting circumstances of ongoing traumatic stress. It would be valuable to study the sources of their resilience and vitality as these become more important not only for them but also for the communities of which they are part, and internationally. It is, therefore, both a clinical and a social policy task to incorporate the TCMI framework in designing longitudinal intervention, postvention, and prevention programs. Many contributors to this volume urge that future research systematically explore the interaction between various dimensions included in the framework (Nagata, Chapter 7; Rousseau & Drapeau, Chapter 28; Buchanan, Chapter 31).

On Justice

In a recently published interview, Judge Richard Goldstone (1995), who at the time was Chief Prosecutor for the War Crimes Tribunals for the Former Yugoslavia and Rwanda, stated:

> I have no doubt that you cannot get peace without justice. . . . If there is not justice, there is no hope of reconciliation or forgiveness because these people do not know who to forgive [and they] end up taking the law into their own hands, and that is the beginning of the next cycle of violence. . . . I don't think that justice depends on peace, but I think peace depends on justice. (p. 376)

Many of the authors discuss various aspects of justice. The findings uniformly suggest that the process of redress and the attainment of justice are critical to the healing for individual victims, as well as their families, societies, and nations. Klain (Chapter 17) underscores its importance for succeeding generations "to break the chain of intergenerational transmission of hatred, rage, revenge, and guilt."

Justice is understood here both in terms of the administration of a formal and fair judicial process and the implementation of judgments of courts, and also in terms of the complete reparation to victims by governments and by society as a whole. This process must include the investigation of crime, identification and bringing to trial of those responsible, the trial itself, punishment of those convicted, and appropriate restitution.

As quoted in the Introduction to this volume in connection with a study done in 1992 for the United Nations Commission on Human Rights, examining the "Right to Restitution, Compensation and Rehabilitation for Victims of Gross Violations of Human Rights and Fundamental Freedoms" (Danieli, 1992; see also Stamatopoulou, 1996), I suggested a number of essential elements. These include reestablishing the victim's value, power, and dignity; rehabilitation, restoration, and compensation; and recognition and apology, followed by commemoration, memorials, and continuing education. Finally, the provision and maintenance of justice must be (re)incorporated into the legal structure, with mechanisms for monitoring, conflict resolution, and preventive intervention.

In cases where this could be done, the process contributed substantially to the sense of closure. The best-known international examples are the Nuremberg and Tokyo war crimes trials, and the trial of Adolph Eichmann. The developments following Japanese American internment during World War II further illustrate some of these elements. However, 37 years passed before the Commission on Wartime Relocation and Internment of Civilians concluded that "a grave injustice was done to American citizens and resident aliens of Japanese ancestry" (Commission on the Wartime Relocation and Internment of Civilians, 1982, p. 18).

Interviewees in the Sansei Project (Nagata, Chapter 7) made it clear that redress payments were one act, albeit inadequate, that recognized significant wrongdoing on the part of the government. The legislation was passed in 1988, with a largely symbolic, one-time payment of $20,000 to each surviving internee and an official government apology.

As Montville (1987) notes, a perpetrator's explicit expression of acknowledgment and remorse has enormous value in healing the victim (on atonement, see Bar-On *et al.,* Chapter 5). In contrast, Prime Minister Howard of Australia, for example, decided not to apologize for the treatment of the Aboriginal people on the grounds that the current generation of (white) Australians was not responsible for earlier misdeeds. In many instances discussed in this volume, the achievement of all the elements of justice proved elusive. All are key factors in the intergenerational transmission of trauma.

Victims and their offspring who have been wronged by a government or society, for example, find it considerably more difficult to begin the healing process if the responsible individuals cannot be identified and punished for their crimes (Raphael *et al.,* Chapter 20; Duran *et al.,* Chapter 21; Gagné, Chapter 22; Cross, Chapter 24).

The attempted genocide of the Armenians stands as one of the most grievous instances of injustice in this century, one in which none of the necessary steps for resolution of the trauma have been taken by the perpetrators, the Turks (Kupelian *et al.,* Chapter 12). Not only does the current generation of Turks refuse to acknowledge, apologize, and compensate for the genocide, its ongoing campaign of denial, delegitimization, and disinformation affects the Armenians as a psychological continuation of persecution.

In parts of Latin America, justice continues to be denied, defeating the full realization of democracy (Becker & Diaz, Chapter 26; Edelman *et al.,* Chapter 27). Impunity, by definition, is the opposite of justice (Roht-Arriaza, 1995). Why, then, would it be embraced? One reason—in parts of Latin America and South Africa—is that it was a requirement by military dictatorships or the racial minority government for relinquishing power or negotiating a peace settlement (Shriver, 1995).

A second reason behind the acceptance of impunity is the belief that "forgive and forget" is the route to follow in order to heal societies torn apart by conflict. However, the critical question remains: What does it do for a society if individual and groups claims to justice are set aside in the name of what is purported to be the greater good (see also Duffy, 1996)?

The creation of "truth commissions"[7] would seem to be an integral tool of justice. In many cases, however, such commissions have not identified those responsible and have been accompanied by amnesty laws or pardons that enshrine impunity. An example is the Guatemalan Commission on Clarification of the Past currently under way.

In South Africa's Truth and Reconciliation Commission, pardons are granted for any actions taken during the apartheid years if they were for political reasons and there is full disclosure. Simpson (Chapter 29) scathingly criticizes the commission, calling this "flight into reconciliation" an imposed conspiracy of silence that fails to deal with the multigenerational effects of trauma. As far as individual victims or groups are concerned, this process is a poor substitute for justice. Simpson refers to the case of the South African mother who, seeking

---

[7]Thirteen states have implemented or are currently implementing amnesties and pardons: South Africa, El Salvador, Guatemala, Honduras, Nicaragua, Haiti, Argentina, Uruguay, Chile, Brazil, Suriname, Peru, and the Philippines.

punishment for those who killed her son a year ago, was told not to rake up the past! For the victims, according to Edelman *et al.* (Chapter 27), impunity has become "a new traumatic factor" so detrimental that it renders closure impossible. For their societies, moreover, impunity may contribute to a loss of respect for law and government, and in a subsequent increase in crime.

One significant trend countering such amnesties and pardons is found in the creation by the United Nations Security Council of two ad hoc international criminal tribunals for the former Yugoslavia and Rwanda. Since the tribunals are subsidiary bodies of the Security Council, whose decisions are binding on all United Nations member states, these tribunals are vested with considerable authority. However, given their slow and tentative beginnings, and the degree of resistance to them, their long-term success is far from certain.

The decades-long effort to establish a permanent International Criminal Court is currently closer to becoming a reality through the action of the United Nations. This points toward a trend that would favor punishment, rather than amnesty and pardons, for those responsible for crimes (see, e.g., Bassiouni, 1997).

Emboldened by the world's indifference to the Armenian genocide, Hitler proceeded with the systematic attempt to annihilate the Jewish people. Much preventable pain is likely to occur in the future if atrocities are not stopped, and justice is not done in the present. The struggle for victims and the generations that follow them is to defy the dominance of evil and find a way to restore a sense of justice and compassion to the world. Victim/survivors of trauma feel a need to bear witness, to speak the truth, to urge the world, to ensure that such injustices never happen again. But some cannot say "Never again," because it has happened again—in Cambodia, Rwanda, and elsewhere.

This book is a record of humanity's unremitting shame. As the twentieth century draws to a close, the contributors trace some of the elemental threads of this century's tragic tapestry. Nevertheless, the reader may find hope in the courage and dignity chronicled in these chapters and in the genuine commitment of so many serious scholars to accumulate and apply knowledge to make the world a better place for our generation, and for generations to come.

REFERENCES

Albeck, J. H. (1994). Intergenerational consequences of trauma: Reframing traps in treatment theory—a second-generational perspective. In M. B. Williams & J. F. Sommer, Jr. (Eds.), *Handbook of post-traumatic therapy* (pp. 106–125). Westport, CT: Greenwood/Praeger.

Bar-On, D. (1994). *Fear and hope: Life-stories of five Israeli families of Holocaust survivors, three generations in a family.* Tel Aviv: Lochamei Hagetaot-Hakibbutz Hameuchad. (Hebrew)

Bassiouni, M. C. (1997, Spring). From Versailles to Rwanda in seventy-five years: The need to establish a permanent international criminal court. *Harvard Human Rights Journal, 10,* 11–62.

Bowen, M. (1978). *Family therapy in clinical practice.* New York: Aronson.

Commission on the Wartime Relocation and Internment of Civilians. (1982). *Personal justice denied.* Washington, DC: U.S. Government Printing Office.

Crocq, M.-A., Macher, J.-P., Barros-Beck, J., Rosenberg, S. J., & Duval, F. (1993). Posttraumatic stress disorder in World War II prisoners of war from Alsace-Lorraine who survived captivity in the USSR. In J. P. Wilson & B. Raphael (Eds.), *International handbook of traumatic stress syndromes* (pp. 253–261). New York: Plenum Press.

Danieli, Y. (1981a). On the achievement of integration in aging survivors of the Nazi Holocaust. *Journal of Geriatric Psychiatry, 14*(2), 191–210.

Danieli, Y. (1981b, March 15–16). Exploring the factors in Jewish identity formation (in children of survivors). In *Consultation on the psycho-dynamics of Jewish identity: Summary of proceedings* (pp. 22–25). American Jewish Committee and the Central Conference of American Rabbis. New York.

Danieli, Y. (1984). Psychotherapists' participation in the conspiracy of silence about the Holocaust. *Psychoanalytic Psychology, 1*(1), 23–42.

Danieli, Y. (1985). The treatment and prevention of long-term effects and intergenerational transmission of victimization: A lesson from Holocaust survivors and their children. In C. R. Figley (Ed.), *Trauma and its wake* (pp. 295–313). New York: Brunner/Mazel.

Danieli, Y. (1989). Mourning in survivors and children of survivors of the Nazi Holocaust: The role of group and community modalities. In D. R. Dietrich, & P. C. Shabad (Eds.), *The problem of loss and mourning: Psychoanalytic perspectives* (pp. 427–460). Madison, CT: International Universities Press.

Danieli, Y. (1991, January 6). *Reflections on perversions of freedom after the fall of the wall*. Presentation to the Intergenerational Community Meeting of the Group Project for Holocaust Survivors and their Children. New York.

Danieli, Y. (1992). Preliminary reflections from a psychological perspective. In T. C. van Boven, C. Flinterman, F. Grunfeld, & I. Westendorp (Eds.), The Right to Restitution, Compensation and Rehabilitation for Victims of Gross Violations of Human Rights and Fundamental Freedoms. *Netherlands Institute of Human Rights [Studie-en Informatiecentrum Mensenrechten], Special issue* No. 12 (pp. 196–213). Also published in N.J. Kritz (Ed.). (1995). *Transitional justice: How emerging democracies reckon with former regimes*. (Vol. 1, pp. 572–582). Washington, DC: United States Institute of Peace.

Danieli, Y. (1993). The diagnostic and therapeutic use of the multi-generational family tree in working with survivors and children of survivors of the Nazi Holocaust. In J. P. Wilson & B. Raphael (Eds.), *International handbook of traumatic stress syndromes* (pp. 889–898). New York: Plenum Press.

Danieli, Y. (1994a). Trauma to the family: Intergenerational sources of vulnerability and resilience. In J. T. Reese & E. Scrivner (Eds.), *The law enforcement families: Issues and answers* (pp. 163–175). Washington, DC: U.S. Department of Justice, Federal Bureau of Investigation.

Danieli, Y. (1994b). As survivors age—Part I. *National Center for Post Traumatic Stress Disorder Clinical Quarterly, 4*(1), 1–7.

Danieli, Y. (1994c). Countertransference, trauma and training. In J. P. Wilson & J. Lindy (Eds.), *Countertransference in the treatment of post-traumatic stress disorder* (pp. 368–388). New York: Guilford.

Danieli, Y. , Rodley, N. S., & Weisaeth, L. (1996). Introduction. In Y. Danieli, N. S. Rodley, & L. Weisaeth (Eds.), *International responses to traumatic stress: Humanitarian, human rights, justice, peace and development contributions, collaborative actions and future initiatives* (pp. 1–14). Published for and on behalf of the United Nations. Amityville, NY: Baywood.

Danieli, Y., Rodley, N. S., & Weisaeth, L. (Eds.). (1996). *International responses to traumatic stress: Humanitarian, human rights, justice, peace and development contributions, collaborative actions and future initiatives*. Published for and on behalf of the United Nations. Amityville, NY: Baywood.

Dubrow, N., Liwski, N. I., Palacios, C., & Gardinier, M. (1996). Traumatized children: Helping child victims of violence. In Y. Danieli, N. S. Rodley, & L. Weisaeth (Eds.), *International responses to traumatic stress: Humanitarian, human rights, justice, peace and development contributions, collaborative actions and future initiatives* (pp. 327–346). Published for and on behalf of the United Nations. Amityville, NY: Baywood.

Duffy, H. (1996). The truth behind reconciliation. In Fundacion Myrna Mack (compiladora) *Amnistia y Reconciliacion Nacional: Encontrando el Comino dela Justicia* [Amnesty and national reconciliation: Finding the way of justice]. Guatemala: F & G Editores. (Spanish)

Edelman, L., Kordon, D., & Lagos, D. (1992). Argentina: Physical disease and bereavement in a social context of human rights violations and impunity. In L. H. M. van Willigen (Chair), *The Limitations of current concepts of post traumatic stress disorders regarding the consequences of organized violence*. Session presented at the World conference of the International Society for Traumatic Stress Studies, Amsterdam, The Netherlands.

Eitinger, L. (1980). The concentration camp syndrome and its late sequelae. In J. E. Dimsdale (Ed.), *Survivors, victims, and perpetrators: Essays on the Nazi Holocaust* (pp. 127–162). New York: Hemisphere.

Elder, G. H., Jr., Caspi, A., & Downey, G. (1986). Problem behavior and family relationships: Life course and intergenerational themes. In A. Sorensen, F. Weinert, & L. Sherrod (Eds.), *Human development and the life course: Multidisciplinary perspectives* (pp. 293–340). Hillsdale, NJ: Erlbaum.

Engel, G. L. (1977). The need for a new medical model: A challenge for biomedicine. *Science, 196,* 129–136.

Engel, G. L. (1996). From biomedical to biopsychosocial: I. Being scientific in the human domain. *Families, Systems and Health: Journal of Collaborative Family Health Care, 14*(4), 425–433.

Figley, C. R. (1983). Catastrophes: An overview of family reactions. In C. R. Figley & H. I. McCubbin (Eds.), *Stress and the family: Coping with catastrophe* (Vol. 2, pp. 3–20). New York: Brunner/Mazel.

Figley, C. R., & Kleber, R. J. (1995). Beyond the "victim": Secondary traumatic stress. In R. J. Kleber, C. R. Figley, & B. P. R. Gersons (Eds.), *Beyond trauma: Cultural and societal dynamics* (pp. 75–98). New York: Plenum Press.

Goldstone, R. (1995). Interview with Judge Richard Goldstone. *Transnational Law and Contemporary Problems, 5,* 374–385.

Green, B. L., Karol, M., & Grace, M. C. (1994). Children and disaster: Age, gender and parental effects on PTSD symptoms. *Journal of the American Academy of Child and Adolescent Psychiatry, 30,* 945–951.

Harel, Z., Kahana, B., & Wilson, J. P. (1993). War and remembrance: The legacy of Pearl Harbor. In J. P. Wilson & B. Raphael (Eds.), *International handbook of traumatic stress syndromes* (pp. 263–274). New York: Plenum Press.

Herman, J. (1992). *Trauma and recovery.* New York: Basic Books.

Keller, R. (1988). Children of Jewish Holocaust survivors: Relationship of family communication to family cohesion, adaptability and satisfaction. *Family Therapy, 15,* 223–237.

Keilson, H. (1992). *Sequential traumatization in children.* Jerusalem: Hebrew University, Magnes Press.

Kendler, K. S. (1988). Indirect vertical cultural transmission: A model for nongenetic parental influences on the liability to psychiatric illness. *American Journal of Psychiatry, 145*(6), 657–665.

Kessler, R. C., Sonnega, A., Bromet, E., Hughes, M., & Nelson, C. B. (1995). Posttraumatic stress disorder in the National Comorbidity Survey. *Archives of General Psychiatry, 52,* 1048–1060.

Kestenberg, J. S. (1989). Transposition revisited: Clinical, therapeutic, and developmental considerations. In P. Marcus & A. Rosenberg (Eds.), *Healing their wounds: Psychotherapy with Holocaust survivors and their families* (pp. 67–82). New York: Praeger.

Kinston, W., & Cohen, J. (1986). Primal repression: Clinical and theoretical aspects. *International Journal of Psychoanalysis, 67,* 337–355.

Kleber, R. (1995). Epilogue. In R. J. Kleber, C. R. Figley, & B. P. R. Gersons (Eds.), *Beyond trauma: Cultural and societal dynamics* (pp. 299–305). New York: Plenum Press.

Legters, L. H. (1988). The American genocide. *Policy Studies Journal, 16*(4), 768–777.

Lifton, R. J. (1979). *The broken connection.* New York: Simon & Schuster.

Lomranz, J., Shmotkin, D., Zechovoy, A., & Rosenberg, E. (1985). Time orientation in Nazi concentration camp survivors: Forty years after. *American Journal of Orthopsychiatry, 55*(2), 230–236.

Major, E. F. (1996). The impact of the Holocaust on the second generation: Norwegian Jewish Holocaust survivors and their children. *Journal of Traumatic Stress, 9*(3), 441–454.

Mangelsdorf, A. D. (1985). Lessons learned and forgotten: The need for prevention and mental health interventions in disaster preparedness. *Journal of Community Psychology, 13,* 239–257.

Marsella, A. J., Friedman, M. J., Gerrity, E. T., & Scurfield, R. M. (Eds.). (1996). *Ethnocultural aspects of posttraumatic stress disorder: Issues, research, and clinical applications* Washington, DC: American Psychological Association.

McFarlane, A. C., Blumbergs, V., Policansky, S. K., & Irwin, C. (1985). *A longitudinal study of psychological morbidity in children due to a natural disaster.* Unpublished manuscript. Department of Psychiatry, Flinders University of South Australia, Bedford Park, South Australia.

Montville, J. V. (1987). Psychoanalytical enlightenment and the greening of diplomacy. *Journal of the American Psychoanalytic Association, 37,* 297–318.

Novac, A. (1994, May). Clinical heterogeneity in children of Holocaust survivors. *Newsletter of World Psychiatric Association,* pp. 24–26.

Novac, A., & Hubert-Schneider, S. (1998). Acquired vulnerability: Comorbidity in a patient population of adult offspring of Holocaust survivors. *American Journal of Forensic Psychiatry, 19*(2), 45–58.

Ornstein, A. (1981). The effects of the Holocaust on life-cycle experiences: The creation and recreation of families. *Journal of Geriatric Psychiatry, 145*(2), 135–163.

Pennebaker, J. W., Barger, S. D., & Tiebout, J. (1989). Disclosure of trauma and health among Holocaust survivors. *Psychosomatic Medicine, 51,* 577–589.

Pynoos, R. S. (1996, March). *The repercussion of traumatic expectations within and across the generations.* Presentation at the 6th IPA Conference on Psychoanalytic Research, London, England.

Pynoos, R. S., & Eth, S. (1985). Children traumatized by witnessing acts of personal violence: Homicide, rape or suicide behavior. In S. Eth & R. S. Pynoos (Eds.), *Post-traumatic stress disorder in children* (pp. 45–70). Washington, DC: American Psychiatric Press.

Rappaport, E. A. (1968). Beyond traumatic neurosis: A psychoanalytic study of late reactions to the concentration camp trauma. *International Journal of Psychoanalysis, 49,* 719–731.

Remer, R., & Elliott, J. (1988a). Characteristics of secondary victims of sexual assault. *International Journal of Family Psychiatry, 9,* 373–387.

Remer, R., & Elliott, J. (1988b). Management of secondary victims of sexual assault. *International Journal of Family Psychiatry, 9,* 389–401.

Robin, R. W., Chester, B., & Goldman, D. (1996). Cumulative trauma and PTSD in American Indian communities. In A. J. Marsella, M. J. Friedman, E. T. Gerrity, & R. M. Scurfield (Eds.), *Ethnocultural aspects of posttraumatic stress disorder: Issues, research, and clinical applications* (pp. 239–253). Washington, DC: American Psychological Association.

Roht-Arriaza, N. (Ed.). (1995). *Impunity and human rights in international law and practice.* New York: Oxford University Press.

Satir, V. (1972). *Peoplemaking.* Palo Alto, CA: Science and Behavior Books.

Schwartz, S., Dohrenwend, B. P., & Levav, I. (1994). Nongenetic familial transmission of psychiatric disorders? Evidence from children of Holocaust survivors. *Journal of Health and Social Behavior, 35,* 385–402.

Shriver, D. W., Jr. (1995). *An ethic for enemies: Forgiveness in politics.* New York: Oxford University Press.

Solomon, Z. (1995). Oscillating between denial and recognition of PTSD: Why are lessons learned and forgotten? *Journal of Traumatic Stress, 8*(2), 271–282.

Spicer, E. H. (1971). Persistent cultural systems: A comparative study of identity systems that can adapt to contrasting environments. *Science, 174,* 795–800.

Stamatopoulou, E. (1996). Violations of human rights: The contribution of the United Nations Centre for Human Rights and the High Commissioner for Human Rights. In Y. Danieli, N. S. Rodley, & L. Weisaeth (Eds.), *International responses to traumatic stress: Humanitarian, human rights, justice, peace and development contributions, collaborative actions and future initiatives* (pp. 101–129). Published for and on behalf of the United Nations. Amityville, NY: Baywood.

Symonds, M. (1980). The "second injury" to victims. *Evaluation and Change* [special issue], 36–38.

Tennant, C. C., Goulston, K., & Dent, O. (1993). Medical and psychiatric consequences of being a prisoner of war of the Japanese: An Australian follow-up study. In J. P. Wilson & B. Raphael (Eds.), *International handbook of traumatic stress syndromes* (pp. 231–239). New York: Plenum Press.

Terr, L. C. (1985). Children traumatized in small groups. In S. Eth & R. S. Pynoos (Eds.), *Post-traumatic stress disorder in children.* [The Progress in Psychiatry Series, David Spiegel, Series Ed.] (pp. 45–70). Washington, DC: American Psychiatric Press.

Van der Kolk, B. A., McFarlane, A. C., & Weisaeth, L. (Eds.). (1996). *Traumatic stress: The effects of overwhelming experience on mind, body and society.* New York: Guilford.

Webber, T. L. (1978). *Deep like the rivers.* New York: Norton.

Winnicott, D. W. (1965). *The maturational processes and the facilitating environment.* London: Hogarth Press.

Index